HANDBOOK OF AFFIRMATIVE PSYCHOTHERAPY WITH LESBIANS AND GAY MEN

Handbook of Affirmative Psychotherapy with Lesbians and Gay Men

Kathleen Y. Ritter
Anthony I. Terndrup

Foreword by Sari H. Dworkin

THE GUILFORD PRESS
New York   London

© 2002 The Guilford Press
A Division of Guilford Publications, Inc.
72 Spring Street, New York, NY 10012
www.guilford.com

Printed in the United States of America

This book is printed on acid-free paper.

Last digit is print number: 9 8 7 6 5 4 3 2 1

Library of Congress Cataloging-in-Publication Data

Ritter, Kathleen.
  Handbook of affirmative psychotherapy with lesbians and gay men /
Kathleen Y. Ritter, Anthony I. Terndrup.
     p. cm.
  Includes bibliographical references and index.
  ISBN 1-57230-714-5 (hardcover)
    1. Gays—Mental health. 2. Lesbians—Mental health. 3. Psychotherapy. 4. Gays—
Mental health services. I. Terndrup, Anthony I. II. Title.

RC451.4.G39 R55 2002
616.89′14′08664—dc21   2001040743

About the Authors

Kathleen Y. Ritter, PhD, is Professor of Counseling Psychology at California State University, Bakersfield, and maintains a private practice. She has extensive experience counseling, teaching, and presenting workshops focused on working with sexual minority clients. With Craig O'Neill, she wrote *Coming Out Within: Stages of Spiritual Awakening for Lesbians and Gay Men* and *Righteous Religion: Unmasking the Illusions of Fundamentalism and Authoritarian Catholicism.*

Anthony I. Terndrup, PhD, is a senior staff therapist at the Pastoral Counseling Center of the Mid-Willamette Valley in Corvallis, Oregon, and a member of the graduate faculty in Counselor Education at Oregon State University. He is Past President of the Association for Gay, Lesbian and Bisexual Issues in Counseling (a division of the American Counseling Association). For over 15 years, he has served sexual minority clients in a variety of clinical settings, including psychosocial rehabilitation, private practice, college counseling, and pastoral care.

Together, Drs. Ritter and Terndrup have presented over 30 continuing education workshops on sexual orientation for mental health professionals across North America.

Foreword

remember meeting Kathleen Ritter and Anthony Terndrup at a meeting of the Association for Gay, Lesbian and Bisexual Issues in Counseling (AGLBIC) many years ago (before AGLBIC was an official division of the American Counseling Association). They were already doing research together on lesbian and gay issues. I learned that Dr. Ritter was heterosexual and knew that this would come as a surprise to many lesbian and gay mental health professionals. At that time, the prevalent belief was that only lesbians and gays did research on sexual minority issues. The few presentations on lesbian and gay issues at the convention of the American Counseling Association were known, or at least assumed, to attract only lesbian and gay audiences to listen to lesbian and gay presenters.

I am glad to say that we have come a long way since then, although there is still a distance to go. How thrilling it is to see the number of articles, books, and dissertations that now focus on lesbian, gay, bisexual, and transgender (LGBT) issues. As a researcher and teacher about LGBT issues and a private practitioner working primarily with LGBT clients, I find it especially gratifying to see the number of students, LGBT and heterosexually identified, who are interested in working in this area.

Nevertheless, in spite of having made strides since homosexuality was removed from being classified as pathology, we still have a long way to go. On the one hand, there are now practice *Guidelines for Psychotherapy with Lesbian, Gay, and Bisexual Clients*, published by the American Psychological Association (2000). On the other hand, there are still therapists who believe in and practice reparative therapy and researchers who focus on whether or not homosexuals can change to heterosexuals. While the majority of the research studies with this population no longer focus on attempting to prove that LGB people are healthy, collaborative research conducted by the American Psychological Association and the American Counseling Association on healthy LGB students in public schools shows that counselors feel woefully uneducated about LGB issues. Training of mental health professionals is improving regarding education about LGB clients, but there are still many graduate programs and many textbooks that barely touch on these important issues.

The world operates from a heterosexual ideology, and this book reviews how this heterosexist framework impacts our work and the lives of LGB people. The authors include earlier theories about prejudice and what we can glean from these studies in our work. I am reminded of a candidate for a position at my university who, like Dr. Ritter, was heterosexually identified but did much work with LGB couples. She stated how when her daughter talked about falling in love with a man, she said to her daughter, "You know, you might fall in love with a woman." This is someone who has moved outside of the heterosexist framework. Unfortunately, few heterosexual parents take this stance with their children and few educators, researchers, and clinicians view the world through this LGB-affirmative stance.

I have been greatly impressed by the comprehensive nature of the information in this book. As the authors state, most therapeutic implications for work with LGB clients are based on anecdotal evidence from therapists rather than on empirical data. Yet the amount of research reviewed here and the implications drawn from that research are outstanding. The authors come through on their promise to "view minority sexual orientations through the lens of theory and science." No matter how knowledgeable readers believe themselves to be on LGB issues, and whether they are students, therapists, educators, or researchers, they will be pleased at how much they will learn from this book. As a researcher and writer on bisexual issues in therapy, I am painfully aware that the work on bisexuality is still in its infancy. Thus, it is important to note that while bisexual issues are not a main focus of this book, wherever there is some research and/or therapeutic information specific to bisexual persons, it is included in the text.

This book is well organized, moving from the framework of the ideology of heterosexuality to sexual identity models and developmental issues to specific client concerns. I was pleased to see that sections on minority concerns, language differences, career issues, healthcare, and sex therapy were included. Not only are LGB clients discussed throughout the book, but their families of origin and families of procreation are extensively considered as well. The authors take theories based on heterosexual people that most of us have been taught within our training programs and explore how these theories can be used to help us work with sexual minorities. Gay men and lesbians are treated separately in almost every chapter in recognition of their differing concerns. These are among the major strengths of this book.

Another particularly noteworthy strength is the attention given to areas rarely addressed in books on LGB issues. Recently, LGB-affirmative therapists have realized that the healthcare system presents unique challenges for LGB clients. While we are used to seeing chapters on HIV and AIDS, this book addresses how heterosexist beliefs can impede LGB people from seeking the care that they need. The authors address issues such as breast cancer and why lesbians face risks different from those of many heterosexual women. They also address how gay men's culture can impact how gay men interact with the healthcare system.

The chapter focusing on minority issues includes not only the groups usually represented in multicultural texts but also information about immigrants. Class issues are also addressed, a topic not often covered in multiculturally based texts. Drs. Ritter and Terndrup help the therapist to work with the many intersections of identity that may impact the minority LGB client. They also provide a framework for assessment that looks at the interactions of sexual minority identity with other important aspects of identity. These include but are not limited to racial/ethnic identity, gender identity, class identity, and/or disability identity. The mental health professional will find specific ways to approach therapeutic concerns in these areas and throughout the book as well.

Dr. Ritter is especially knowledgeable about the religious struggles that many LGB clients face. Her previous book *Coming Out Within: Stages of Spiritual Awakening for Lesbians and Gay Men* (coauthored with Craig O'Neill) has helped many LGB clients with their religious struggles, and Chapter 13 builds on that. Since it is struggles with religion that often bring LGB clients to therapy, therapists need guidance about how to address this issue. Anecdotally I can attest to the fact that the majority of my LGB clients either have begun therapy with this issue, or this issue arose at some point in the therapeutic process. I learned new ways to handle religious concerns from this chapter.

From this brief preview, I hope that I have created excitement about what is to be learned from this book. My association with Drs. Kathleen Ritter and Anthony Terndrup has been a fruitful relationship. They work hard to further what has become known as affirmative psychotherapy for LGB clients. Their work ultimately betters the lives of LGB people, and along the way their work furthers research, education, and practice.

SARI H. DWORKIN, PHD
Coordinator and Professor, Counselor Education Program,
Department of Counseling and Special Education,
California State University, Fresno, California;
President, Division 44, Society for the Psychological Study
of Lesbian, Gay, and Bisexual Issues of the
American Psychological Association

Acknowledgments

We are deeply indebted to Sharon Panulla, former Senior Editor at The Guilford Press, for inviting us to write this book. We commend her for persisting with us over the years when our writing was interrupted by full-time jobs, the birth of Kathleen's three grandchildren, Anthony's relocation, and the completion of his doctoral work. During early writing and revisions, her suggestions and those of two other editors, Susan Marples and Rochelle Serwator, were very helpful. After Sharon left Guilford, we were extremely fortunate to have been assigned Barbara Watkins as our editor. Like Sharon, Barbara was continually supportive and patient with us as our temporal constraints, again, limited the time we were able to spend on the manuscript. Her insights and advice contributed to making this book one of which we are very proud.

Together and separately we have presented numerous workshops on issues related to minority sexual orientations, and many of the ideas from these sessions, as well as helpful comments from participants, have provided the foundation for this book. Conversations with our students and clients also have enriched the material. We especially want to thank Sari H. Dworkin for writing the foreword to the book and Robert L. Barret, John C. Gonsiorek, and Christine M. Browning for reviewing the manuscript. John C. Gonsiorek, along with Maryka Biaggio, offered constructive suggestions during the early writing of Chapter 8.

The staff at Guilford was extremely efficient and helpful during the production phase. We are particularly indebted to Anna Nelson in the production department, and Marian Robinson, Katherine Lieber, Abby Peck, and Kim Miller in the marketing department. We also appreciated the creative work of Bessie Tsouplakis who designed the jacket of the book, the careful copy editing of Lori Jacobs, and the efforts of Guilford exhibits manager, Dorothy Avery. Our fondest and most profound thanks, however, go to our partners, John Ritter and Tom Eversole, upon whose unconditional love and support we relied to complete this book. We deeply appreciate them both.

Contents

HANDBOOK OF AFFIRMATIVE PSYCHOTHERAPY WITH LESBIANS AND GAY MEN

Introduction

This book is written for psychologists, family therapists, mental health counselors, social workers, and other clinicians who wish to enhance their psychotherapeutic treatment of gay, lesbian, and bisexual clients. Sexual minorities present in therapy with essentially the same kinds of problems as heterosexuals, including difficulties with relationships and work. In addition, Hancock (1995) identified six specific treatment issues of gay, lesbian, and bisexual clients: coming out, anti-gay and other prejudice, relationship issues, concerns of gay and lesbian youth, gay and lesbian parenting, and family-of-origin dynamics. Regardless of the treatment focus, however, anything less than an affirmative stance in which individuals are treated with positive regard can further undermine their self-esteem (Isay, 1996). Even the neutral therapeutic posture advocated by psychoanalytic theory may be problematic and insufficient for lesbian, gay, and bisexual clients who require an affirmative approach that communicates the belief that homosexuality is a natural developmental outcome for numerous individuals (Frommer, 1994; Liddle, 1999a). Accordingly, Falco (1996) believes that "the self" of most gay, lesbian, and bisexual clients is "constricted," due to numerous acts of nondisclosure, self-censoring, and vigilance (p. 401). If these individuals are denied positive and affirming psychotherapy, their self-esteem can deteriorate rather than improve.

AFFIRMATIVE PSYCHOTHERAPY

Clinicians of all sexual orientations can work successfully with sexual minorities as long as they are accepting of their clients' homosexuality and are (reasonably) free of heterosexist bias and homophobic prejudice (Baron, 1996; A. C. Bernstein, 2000; Cabaj, 1996b; Stein, 1996b, 1999). In fact, one study of 40 gay and 40 lesbian participants (M. R. Moran, 1992) found that the counselor's experience and expertise were more salient concerns for these clients than the therapist's sexual orientation. The "basic psychodynamic elements that make any psychotherapeutic interaction work are the trust and motivation of the patient and the integrity, warmth, knowledge, and genuineness of the therapist" (Marmor, 1996, p. 542). Moreover, it is crucial that clinicians understand the degree to which heterosexism in society shapes the context of lesbian, gay, and bisexual experience (Phillips & Fischer, 1998) as well as the "specific subcultural network systems" (Marmor, 1996, p. 543) of sexual minority groups. Further, therapists must examine their own dynamics in the areas of self-concept, sexual identity, and attitudes toward these client populations (Gelso, Fassinger, Gomez, & Latts, 1995; Reiss, 1987) and be aware of their own anti-homosexual and heterosexist biases that can appear as "unworked-through countertransferences" (L. S. Brown, 1996, p. 900).

Some sexual minorities prefer to see a gay, lesbian, or bisexual therapist because they believe these clinicians share similar backgrounds and values, are free of heterosexist bias, and understand their situations quicker and more easily than does a heterosexual therapist (Cabaj, 1996b; Hughes, Haas, Razzano, Cassidy, & Matthews, 2000; Isay, 1991; R. D. Schwartz, 1989). In this regard, some clients are annoyed with having to bring their therapists "up to speed" about the societal constraints in their lives (A. C. Bernstein, 2000, p. 446), and others feel that the need to educate their counselors interferes with rapport, trust, and progress in therapy (Dworkin, 1996). Sometimes, the problems of transference (e.g., elevating the therapist to a position of success in the gay and lesbian world) and countertransference (e.g., assuming commonality of experience with clients when none or little exists) are compounded when sexual minority counselors and clients interact. In these instances, roles and boundaries often lack definition, overlap, or both (e.g., therapists serving as mentors for clients who are coming out, or encountering them at various gay or lesbian events). Whereas mirroring and positive identification are crucial elements in affirmative psychotherapy with sexual minorities, homosexual clients and therapists may encounter reciprocal blind spots, mutual internalized homophobia, or eroticized transference and countertransference.

While lesbian, bisexual, and gay clinicians who work with sexual minority clients are examining ethical issues of this nature, (presumably) heterosexual therapists treating homosexual patients in previous eras rarely engaged in this degree of introspection. Accordingly, Krajeski (1986) commented on the "unwarranted certitude and dogmatism in the past" (p. 22), given that the pre-1980 psychoanalytic literature did not include even a single reference to possible countertransference issues with homosexual patients!

When compared with majority culture clients, numerous concerns relative to assessment, diagnosis, and intervention mandate that traditional approaches be modified when treating sexual minorities. Ethical concerns must be reformulated, and treatment considerations adapted relative to such issues as ethnicity, career choice and satisfaction, chemical dependency, health concerns, spirituality, sexuality, and family (nuclear and biological) dynamics. Further, due to the societal stigma that these clients inescapably internalize, a perspective that accounts for the developmental experiences of gay, lesbian, or bisexual individuals is important. It is for the purpose of providing this context that *Handbook of Affirmative Psychotherapy with Lesbians and Gay Men* was written.

PSYCHOTHERAPY LITERATURE

Until the 1970s, virtually all the writing about psychotherapy with sexual minorities assumed that homosexuality was pathological. Accordingly, treatment was aimed at curing patients or clients of this condition and orienting them to heterosexuality. During the

1980s and 1990s, the tone of the literature fortunately shifted and a focus affirming of gays and lesbians emerged in virtually all areas, except for traditional psychoanalysis (Stein & Cabaj, 1996). C. Silverstein (1991, 1996) discussed this body of literature and concluded that it could be divided into three areas. The first area concerned the effect of external stressors (all of which are discussed in various chapters of this book) on the lives of gay, lesbian, and bisexual individuals. The majority of published material was found in this domain, the central theme of which was coping with discrimination. The second area of focus related to the internalization of societal stigma and its consequences for the mental health of sexual minorities. Specifically, the internal psychological processes associated with emotional pain were examined, with the largest number of papers devoted to "the effects of low self-esteem and self-hate, or what has been called *internalized homophobia*" (C. Silverstein, 1996, p. 7). The third and smallest emphasis in the literature concerned psychotherapy techniques. Included were descriptions of group modalities, assertiveness training, and behavioral therapy to improve sexual functioning.

GUIDELINES FOR PSYCHOTHERAPY

Along similar lines, Division 44 of the American Psychological Association created a task force for the dual purpose of (1) determining the scope and focus of the psychotherapy literature related to lesbian, gay, and bisexual clients, and (2) developing professional practice guidelines for service delivery to these consumers. Three members of the team began their work by reviewing the literature on psychotherapy with lesbians and gay men between 1987 and 1993 (Acuff, Cerbone, & Shidlo, 1996). After locating and examining 272 articles, the working group found that the number of these writings declined from 1987 (< 50 published) to 1993 (< 10 published), and that only 35 (12.9%) were specifically related to treatment (i.e., group therapy, psychoanalysis [$n = 22$], and transference issues). The remainder of the articles (87.1%) concerned an array of issues that provided a context for psychotherapy (adolescence, HIV, substance abuse, couples and families, etc.). One of the more salient impressions of the task force was that much conceptualization of problem areas existed and few directions for interventions, given that the preponderance of the literature was theoretical in nature and virtually no empirical studies or explorations of specific treatment methods were located.

To provide practitioners with (1) a frame of reference for the treatment of lesbian, gay, and bisexual clients and (2) basic information and further references in the areas of assessment, intervention, identity, relationships, and the education and training of psychologists, the Council of Representatives of the American Psychological Association adopted *Guidelines for Psychotherapy with Lesbian, Gay, and Bisexual Clients* (American Psychological Association, 2000). The 16 guidelines are aspirational in intent and are built on the American Psychological Association's *Ethical Principles of Psychologists and Code of Conduct* (1992), and other policies of the Association, as well as those of additional mental health organizations. The literature reviewed by the task force discussed in the previous paragraph forms the foundation of the Guidelines, which differs from standards (which are considered mandatory) in that they are recommendations for specific professional behavior, endeavor, or conduct for psychologists. Given, however, that the Guidelines are built on an extensive body of theoretical and contextual literature related to the practice of psychotherapy with sexual minority clients, ideally they can have an impact on professional practice as well as inspire a body of research that can provide empirical validation. Following, under four major sections, is a list of the *Guidelines for Psychotherapy with Gay, Lesbian, and Bisexual Clients.**

Attitudes toward Homosexuality and Bisexuality

- *Guideline 1.* Psychologists understand that homosexuality and bisexuality are not indicative of mental illness.
- *Guideline 2.* Psychologists are encouraged to recognize how their attitudes and knowledge about lesbian, gay, and bisexual issues may be relevant to assessment and treatment and seek consultation or make appropriate referrals when indicated.
- *Guideline 3.* Psychologists strive to understand the ways in which social stigmatization (i.e., prejudice, discrimination, and violence) poses risks to the mental health and well-being of lesbian, gay, and bisexual clients.
- *Guideline 4.* Psychologists strive to understand how inaccurate or prejudicial views of homosexuality or bisexuality may affect the client's presentation in treatment and the therapeutic process.

Relationships and Families

- *Guideline 5.* Psychologists strive to be knowledgeable about and respect the importance of lesbian, gay, and bisexual relationships.
- *Guideline 6.* Psychologists strive to understand the particular circumstances and challenges facing lesbian, gay, and bisexual parents.
- *Guideline 7.* Psychologists recognize that the families of lesbian, gay, and bisexual people may include people who are not legally or biologically related.
- *Guideline 8.* Psychologists strive to understand how a person's homosexual or bisexual orientation may have an impact on his or her family of origin and the relationship to that family of origin.

Issues of Diversity

- *Guideline 9.* Psychologists are encouraged to recognize the particular life issues or challenges experienced by lesbian, gay, and bisexual members of racial and ethnic minorities that are related to multiple and often conflicting cultural norms, values, and beliefs.
- *Guideline 10.* Psychologists are encouraged to recognize the particular challenges experienced by bisexual individuals.
- *Guideline 11.* Psychologists strive to understand the special problems and risks that exist for lesbian, gay, and bisexual youth.
- *Guideline 12.* Psychologists consider generational differences within lesbian, gay, and bisexual populations and the particular challenges that may be experienced by lesbian, gay, and bisexual older adults.

• *Guideline 13.* Psychologists are encouraged to recognize the particular challenges experienced by lesbian, gay, and bisexual individuals with physical, sensory, and/or cognitive/emotional disabilities.

Education

• *Guideline 14.* Psychologists support the provision of professional education and training on lesbian, gay, and bisexual issues.
• *Guideline 15.* Psychologists are encouraged to increase their knowledge and understanding of homosexuality and bisexuality through continuing education, training, supervision, and consultation.
• *Guideline 16.* Psychologists make reasonable efforts to familiarize themselves with relevant mental health, educational, and community resources for lesbian, gay, and bisexual people.

FOCUS OF TREATMENT

In addition to the task force of the American Psychological Association (discussed previously), others (Bieschke, Eberz, Bard, & Croteau, 1998; Cabaj & Klinger, 1996; Falco, 1996) also have noted that the psychotherapy literature related to lesbian, gay, and bisexual (LGB) clients is based more on the clinical experience of therapists than on treatment research, and that no systematic approaches to psychotherapy unique to homosexual individuals have been formulated. Further, there are virtually no empirical process or outcome studies available that measure the effectiveness of various conceptual of strategic approaches to therapy or treatment methods; the handful that do exist are believed to have considerable methodological weaknesses (Dunkle, 1994; Fassinger, 2000). In fact, "almost nothing is known empirically about the effectiveness of theoretical approaches for LGB clients beyond the general literature on therapy process, outcome, and efficacy" (Fassinger, 2000, p. 124). If readers thus are expecting to find research-based, population-specific interventions to use with sexual minorities, they will find them neither in this book nor in the professional journals. In other words, "the fact that the evolution of the new models of psychotherapy is in its early stages is evident in the literature" (Krajeski, 1986, p. 22).

Many clinicians seem to agree with Falco (1996), who contends that "the therapist's preferred style of psychotherapy probably makes little difference: effective [gay or] lesbian-affirmative therapy can be based upon a dynamic, cognitive-behavioral, humanistic–existential, Jungian, Gestalt, systems theory, and perhaps any other approach" (p. 409). She and other clinicians stress, however, the importance of using modifications that incorporate the issues and stressors inherent in living as gay, lesbian, or bisexual in a heterosexually constructed world. In fact, such adaptations are critical given the societal stigma and marginalization that these clients experience, as well as the difference in their developmental trajectories when compared with normative heterosexual maturation.

Therapists working with homosexually oriented clients must have a considerable amount of information regarding the environment in which these individuals reside, the conditions of their reality, and the unique problems and dynamics arising from their minority sexual orientations (L. S. Brown, 2000; Browning, Reynolds, & Dworkin, 1991; Falco, 1996; Liddle, 1999a; J. C. Phillips & Fischer, 1998; Platzer, 1998; Roth & Murphy, 1986; Shannon & Woods, 1991; Stein, 1988, 1996b). In fact, treatment that is informed by the context of gay, lesbian, and bisexual experience is essential for affirmative psychotherapy because unique psychosocial stressors influence the presentation of their illnesses and symptoms and shape the types of concerns that these individuals bring to treatment (Cabaj & Klinger, 1996; Gonsiorek, 1991; J. C. Phillips & Fischer, 1998). This book pulls together existing research and discourse, as well as explores their implications for treatment.

OVERVIEW OF THE BOOK

The first part of the book lays a foundation for understanding the social, developmental, and political context of gay, lesbian, and bisexual experience. Chapter 1 establishes a fundamental premise that heterosexist assumptions and stereotypes have a negative impact on sexual minorities, just as sexism and racism oppress women and people of color. An awareness of this basic principle is crucial when working with bisexual, lesbian, and gay clients, many of whom seek psychotherapy to address the harmful effects of discrimination and prejudice. Chapter 2 summarizes past and current perspectives on minority sexual orientation, including its multidimensional complexity. With this knowledge of historical and contemporary constructions of homosexuality (both social and personal), clinicians are better able to offer the psychoeducation necessary to help clients see that many of their difficulties stem not from their own deficiencies but from society's perception of their sexuality and worth. Chapter 3 describes biological, familial, and psychosocial variables thought (by some) to be related to the development of minority sexual orientations and preconceptualizes and reformulates psychodynamic explanations of homosexuality. These perspectives can be especially helpful to clients and their families, many of whom seek therapy to understand the etiology of minority sexual orientation. Chapter 4 reviews legal issues that affect sexual minorities and often lead them to therapy.

Part II addresses identity formation and developmental considerations specific to lesbian, gay, and bisexual clients. Because effective psychotherapy is based on an accurate understanding of developmental principles, these chapters describe theoretical adaptations that account for the differing, but nonetheless normative, developmental trajectories of sexual minorities. Accordingly, Chapter 5 outlines theoretical models for understanding gay and lesbian identity formation, while Chapters 6 and 7 discuss developmental issues for sexual minority adolescents and adults.

Part III examines key areas of affirmative practice, starting with psychodiagnostic considerations. Chapter 8 thus describes how predictable behavioral patterns or emotional reactions during the "coming-out" process may be mistaken for psychiatric disorders. Based on the models summarized in Chapter 5, Chapter 9 illustrates therapeutic applications across five phases of identity development designed to facilitate the formation of positive identifications in sexual minority clients. Chapter 10 addresses culture-specific dynamics and considerations and applications to psychotherapy, as well as discussing the interactive processes of sexual minority and racial/cultural identity formation for lesbians, bisexuals, and gay men of color.

Also related to affirmative practice, the next three chapters specifically focus on work, health, and spirituality. Accordingly, Chapter 11 examines the effects of heterosexism in the workplace and on sexual minority career development, including trade-offs individuals often must make between job satisfaction and identity formation. Chapter 12 summarizes health concerns that affect sexual minority clients and often lead them to therapy. Part III concludes with a discussion in Chapter 13 relating to the influence of religion and spirituality on gay, lesbian, and bisexual persons. Given that many clients struggle with moral questions about homosexuality, religious concerns are treated in some detail. In this regard, Chapter 13 assesses the viability of traditional religion for sexual minorities, addresses religious-based conversion, and offers affirmative interventions for revitalizing religion and reformulating spirituality.

Part IV addresses family units with gay, lesbian, and bisexual members. Chapter 14 discusses various relationship patterns among sexual minorities and members of their families of origin, particularly their parents. As with the discussions of identity formation, parental reactions and associated counseling strategies are outlined for use at various stages in therapeutic work with these families. Chapter 15 considers same-sex couples in terms of heterosexism, gender role socialization, and stages of relationship development. Chapter 16 examines their sexual functioning, with special attention to the effects of internalized oppression and gender role conditioning on erotic interactions. Further, categories of sexual dysfunctions according to the fourth edition of the *Diagnostic and Statistical Manual of Mental Disorders* (DSM-IV; American Psychiatric Association, 1994) are reconceptualized for use in treatment with gay and lesbian individuals and couples. The final chapter (17) describes the origins and psychodynamics of families headed by sexual minority parents. The book concludes with an extensive Resources section to which clinicians can refer in providing affirmative psychotherapy to lesbians, bisexuals, and gay men.

Part I

SOCIAL, DEVELOPMENTAL, AND POLITICAL FOUNDATIONS

1

Heterosexism:
A Fundamental Reality

Heterosexist stereotypes impose heavy physiological and psychological burdens on sexual minorities of all ages and ethnic backgrounds. Accordingly, a far greater percentage of lesbian or gay individuals have received mental health services than have heterosexuals (Bradford, Ryan, & Rothblum, 1994; Cochran & Mays, 2000b; Dworkin, 2000a; Gonsiorek & Weinrich, 1991; Hughes et al., 2000; Razzano, Hamilton, & Hughes, 2000; Rudolph, 1988). Heterosexism is *oppressive*, a word that *Webster's* dictionary defines as "weighing heavily on the mind, spirits, or senses; causing physical or mental distress" (McKechnie, 1971, p. 1256). Morgan (1992, 1997) found that nearly three-quarters of lesbians, in particular, seek counseling, compared with less than one-third of heterosexual women (29%). Results of one study of lesbians of color (*n* = 568) revealed that 84% of Latina and Asian American subjects had used mental health services, compared with 75% of the Native American and 68% of the African American lesbians (Morris, 2000). In spite of the widespread use of psychotherapy and recent studies showing satisfaction with the services offered (M. A. Jones & Gabriel, 1999; Liddle, 1999b; Morris, 2000), up to 50% of sexual minority clients in other, and sometimes older, studies have reported dissatisfaction with their experiences (Liddle, 1999b; Platzer, 1998; Rudolph, 1988). Many said they felt misunderstood by well-meaning clinicians who often overlooked the impact of oppression on their clients' lives or were uninformed about minority sexual orientations. Further, numerous surveys of both practitioners and students consistently found that they lack information about lesbians, gay men, and bisexuals or hold negative attitudes toward them (Dworkin, 2000a; R. J. Green, 2000; Liddle, 1995, 1996, 1999a; J. C. Phillips & Fischer, 1998; Prairielands, 2000), and no area of the mental health profession appears to be immune from heterosexist bias (American Psychological Association, 2000; Committee on Lesbian and Gay Concerns, 1991; DeCrescenzo, 1983/1984; Garnets, Hancock, Cochran, Goodchilds, & Peplau, 1991; Rudolph, 1988; Tievsky, 1988; Wisniewski & Toomey, 1987).

This book is based on the phenomenon that people who are sexually and emotionally attracted to persons of the same sex (i.e., *lesbians* and *gay men*) and of both sexes (i.e., *bisexuals*) share common characteristics with other minority groups and are similarly oppressed socially, culturally, and politically. These common attributes and experiences include (Herek, 1991) the following:

- Being subordinate segments of a larger society.
- Exhibiting features that are devalued by the dominant segments of society.
- Being bound together as a community because of these characteristics.
- Receiving differential treatment because of these traits.

Although bisexuals, lesbians, and gay men meet these criteria for minority group status, their subordinate position on the social hierarchy often goes unrecognized or is discounted. Clinicians who work with sexual minority populations need to focus on the status of these clients as *minority* group members and the impact of this social position on their individual and collective lives. To reinforce this perspective, as well as to avoid repetition, then, the term *sexual minorities* is used interchangeably with *gay men, lesbians, and bisexuals* throughout this book. This chapter discusses the fundamental reality of heterosexist oppression and briefly describes the negative impact of heterosexist assumptions on the psychosocial, vocational, and spiritual development of gay, lesbian, and bisexual persons. In addition, this chapter addresses and considers correlates of heterosexism and its adverse effects on mental health.

The social, cultural, and political oppression of sexual minority groups is maintained by *homophobia* and *heterosexism*. *Homophobia* is described both as an irrational fear of homosexuality (Bhugra, 1987) and as an intolerance of any sexual differences from an established norm (Gramick, 1983a). According to Neisen (1990), however, the concept has become so expanded and extended over time that much of its meaning has been lost. For example, *homophobia* seldom refers to a phobic or fearful response, as the term itself implies. Often, though, it is used to indicate *anti-homosexual prejudice* (Haaga, 1991) and thus to characterize a wide range of negative emotions, attitudes, and behaviors toward lesbians and gay men. In addition to other experts (Morin, 1977; Morin & Garfinkle; 1978), Neisen (1990) discussed the need to redefine *homophobia* as *heterosexism* in order to incorporate the pervasive ramifications of the social environment which places a superior value on heterosexuality. Thus, although *heterosexism* is the more accurate terminology, this book uses these terms interchangeably in accordance with common usage in the literature; *heterosexism* is preferred over *homophobia,* but both of these designations are employed to accurately reflect the material being cited.

Accordingly, *heterosexism* has been defined as "a world-view, a value-system that prizes heterosexuality, assumes it as the only appropriate manifestation of love and sexuality, and devalues homosexuality and all that is not heterosexual" (Herek, 1986b, p. 925). Similarly, the concept has been described as the institutional promotion of heterosexual life and the concurrent subordination of gay, lesbian, and bisexual experience. Thus considered, the term promotes an understanding of the associations between and among various forms of oppression experienced by members of other minority groups. Like *racism* and *sexism*, for example, *heterosexism* is based on unfounded prejudices (Neisen, 1990). In addition, all three types of oppression separate the powerful and the powerless into mutually exclusive categories: White people over people of color, men over women, and heterosexual over nonheterosexual (W. L. Williams, 1987). Chapter 10 discusses the multiplicative effects of these *isms* converging to oppress sexual minorities of color.

HETEROSEXIST ASSUMPTIONS AND THEIR NEGATIVE IMPACT

Assumptions based on heterosexism pervade U.S. society and affect the intrapsychic dynamics of gay, lesbian, and bisexual individuals such that many, as noted previously, seek psychotherapy to deal with the psychological distress, depression, and loneliness that result (Shidlo, 1994a). Heterosexist expectations also have an impact on sexual minorities to some degree in nearly all other domains. Specifically, their influence on the psychosocial, career, and spiritual development of gay men, lesbians, and bisexuals is outlined in the following illustrations and further discussed in subsequent chapters.

Psychosocial

From the moment of childbirth, most parents assume that their newborn infants will grow and develop heterosexually, and thus they begin to socialize them into gender roles that complement those of the other sex. In due course, preschool children practice the complementary gender roles of husband and wife as well as "Mommy" and "Daddy" in the corner playhouse of the nursery school or kindergarten. Throughout early, middle, and late childhood, girls are teased good-naturedly about having boyfriends while boys are taunted humorously about having girlfriends. During adolescence, heterosexual dating is taken for granted as a teenage rite of passage eventually leading to courtship, engagement, and marriage. As unconscious or innocent as they seem, these heterosexist expectations marginalize sexual minority youth, not only during childhood and adolescence but into their adulthood and old age (see Chapters 6 and 7).

Vocational

From the classrooms of middle America to the boardrooms of corporate America, heterosexist assumptions confine the career choices and constrict the upward vocational mobility of gay, lesbian, and bisexual adults. For example, many local communities suspect that sexual minority teachers will either neglect or impede the presupposed heterosexual growth and development of their school-age children. As a result, self-affirming and self-disclosing sexual minorities frequently rule out careers in elementary and secondary education. Many corporations assume that heterosexual marriages will stabilize the lives of their executives and project positive images to the business world, and, hence, managers and administrators often are hired and promoted on the basis of their marital status. In both cases, the career development of bisexuals, gay men, and lesbians is restricted (see Chapter 11 for additional details).

Spiritual

From their initiation ceremonies to their burial rites, many religious traditions are permeated by beliefs and practices that assume the moral and spiritual superiority of heterosexuality. In this regard, many traditional religions consecrate heterosexual love and marriage while condemning gay and lesbian commitments and covenants. Numerous religious institutions further restrict their leadership to heterosexually married or celibate clergy and organize the lives of their faith communities around the experiences and expectations of "traditional families." Hence, even those sexual minorities who do not feel particularly abandoned or betrayed by their religious traditions frequently feel excluded and alienated from institutional religion (O'Neill & Ritter, 1992). Consequently, many bisexuals, lesbians, and gay men feel deprived of the comfort and consolation that faith communities offer to other oppressed minorities. (These concepts are discussed further in Chapter 13.)

POPULAR OPINION

Public opinion relative to rights and opportunities for gay, lesbian, and bisexual citizens is mixed but in most areas is considerably more favorable than in years past. The discussions that follow examine various data sets and compare the positive and negative aspects of each.

Favorable

Postelection survey data estimating the impact of sexual minority issues during the 1996 campaign (D. M. Smith, 1997) reflected that "the principle of protecting gay people from job discrimination has emerged as a moderate, mainstream issue" (p. 8) with a 70% support rate among respondents. Voters were more ambivalent toward same-sex marriage in general but supported extending some of its specific advantages to gay and lesbian partners, such as allowing them the same hospital visitation rights (82%), inheritance rights (62%), healthcare benefits (52%), and social security benefits (46%) as heterosexual spouses. Slightly more favorable findings were noted in a *Newsweek* poll conducted 4 years later (Leland, 2000) when 58% of the respondents favored the receipt of benefits from a partner's health insurance and 54% from the partner's social security earnings.

A 1996 Gallup poll (Saad, 1996) also found a substantial increase in Americans' tolerance of lesbians and gay men in everyday society. For example, when asked if homosexuals should or should not have equal rights in terms of job opportunities, 84% responded favorably, compared with 74% in 1992 and 59% in 1982. When asked further to distinguish between occupations, Americans seemed to have little problem accepting sexual minorities as salespersons (90% in 1996) yet more difficulty approving them as clergy or high school teachers (60%) and elementary educators (55%). According to a Gallup press release, these 1996 percentages reflect a "wholesale change in public attitudes" (p. 1) from 1977, when only 27% favored gays as elementary school teachers and 36% as religious leaders. Similarly, 1998 General Social Survey (GSS) data indicated that moral approval of gay and lesbian sexual relations increased over 150% during a 25-year period, with 28.2% of respondents indicating that same-sex behaviors were "not wrong at all" in 1998 compared with 11.2% in 1973 (National Opinion Research Center, 1998).

Unfavorable

At the same that an increasingly larger percentage of Americans refuse to condemn same-sex intimate relationships, the GSS data described previously (National Opinion Research

Center, 1998) revealed nonetheless that 58.6% of respondents thought these encounters were "always wrong." When these 1998 opinions are compared with data from the 1973 GSS, only a 13.9% decrease in negative response was noted during the 25-year period. In all other areas measured by the GSS or Gallup poll relative to homosexual citizens, negative opinion decreased substantially. A 2000 *Newsweek* poll (Leland, 2000), however, found the decline in negative opinion to be sharper; that is, "fewer (46 percent, down from 54 percent in 1998) say they believe homosexuality is a sin" (p. 49). When compared with the 58.6% of 1998 GSS respondents (if, indeed, the methodologies employed would allow comparison), this decline of over 20% could be seen as striking. In any case, these high percentages of unfavorable opinion, when contrasted with the support shown in areas such as the equal right to employment, would appear to indicate Americans make a distinction between the social and sexual activities of lesbians and gay men.

As indicated earlier, the Gallup poll (Saad, 1996) found that for the first time, a majority (60%) of Americans approved of gay men and lesbians as clergy or teachers. On the other hand, however, approximately 40% of Gallup respondents believed that homosexuals should not be allowed to enter these occupations, and 16% either responded "no" or had "no opinion" when asked whether homosexuals should have equal job opportunities. The 1996 postelection poll data (D. M. Smith, 1997) revealed considerable heterosexist bias and negative public opinion (18% to 54%) relative to extending various privileges to lesbian and gay relationships. Similarly, the 2000 *Newsweek* poll data revealed the 57% of respondents were opposed to gay marriage, 50% said that gays should not adopt, 35% opposed them serving openly in the military, and 36% said that gays should not be allowed to teach elementary school (Leland, 2000).

Due to the widespread nature of these unfavorable attitudes, virtually all lesbians, bisexuals, and gay men are aware that there still is a substantial segment of the population that is unwilling to support them or their civil rights (Leland, 2000). Most of these sexual minority individuals have been adversely affected, in some way or another, by this antagonistic climate. In addition to both ordinary and unique problems of living, then, they bring these internalized attitudes to therapy.

MEDIA

Popular opinion is shaped by film, as well as by electronic and printed media. When gay, lesbian, and bisexual characters appear in mainstream movies, for example, they usually are portrayed as scoundrels, or as figures who are suffering intensely; rarely, however, are they presented as humans living ordinary lives (Faderman, 1997). Likewise, on television, they ordinarily play supporting roles that reinforce the heterosexual order. Thus, negative, stereotypical, or narrow typecasting rarely allows viewers to see accurate portrayals of sexual minorities that counter explicit homophobia or implicit heterosexism. As these representations go unchallenged, the common decency of good taste that shields most other minority groups from ridicule by entertainers or misrepresentation by reporters does not extend to bisexuals, lesbians, and gay men (Gross, 1991).

The lack of media visibility, positive and otherwise, often has extended to collections in academic libraries. For example, Whitam (1991) reviewed three sociology journals from 1977 through 1988 and found only three articles related to gay and lesbian populations. He contended that sociology textbooks also slight the subject of homosexuality and ignore many of the historical events which have had a profound effect on the sociological development of the gay and lesbian community. Similarly, Clark and Serovich (1997) examined 13,217 articles in 17 marriage and family therapy journals published between 1975 and 1995. Only 77 articles (0.006%) focused on gay, lesbian, or bisexual issues; employed sexual minorities as a sample; or used sexual orientation as a variable. The literature reviewed for this book, similarly, revealed a large number of post-1988 journal references from diverse fields, including counseling, psychology, human sexuality, psychotherapy, social psychology, and social work, but only a handful in marriage and family therapy. A recent surge in the number of periodicals devoted specifically to gay, lesbian, and bisexual issues was detected, however. Though the depiction of homosexuality and bisexuality obviously is improving both quantitatively and qualitatively in the academic press, the historical neglect and misrepresentation of sexual minorities has without a doubt left a negative impression in the minds of scholars, researchers, and practitioners.

The increased circulation of periodicals affirming homosexuality has not reached many public libraries, because few subscribe to these journals or to publications directed toward regional lesbian and gay communities (Fejes, 1991). On the other hand, popular periodicals in libraries, such as *Newsweek*, *Time*, and *U.S. News & World Report*, are replete with articles discussing gay and lesbian people and their lives. Although this expanded media attention undoubtedly has contributed positively to the improvement in public opinion regarding civil rights protections for sexual minorities, the current situation is not entirely favorable. Unfortunately, magazine features specifically about bisexuals, lesbians, and gay men sometimes reinforces perceived differences rather than similarities between them and their heterosexual counterparts, thus further polarizing the sexual majority and sexual minorities.

STEREOTYPES

Differences between majority and minority groups become institutionalized when dominant groups assume the power of establishing norms from which subordinate groups are seen to deviate. These differences are perceived as deficits, or as failures of the minority to meet the standards of the majority. This institutionalization of differences creates stereotypes which reduce the full humanity of others to a handful of deviant traits, limiting them socially and disempowering them psychologically (de Monteflores, 1986). Accordingly, findings from two studies indicated that lesbians and gay men were perceived as needing counseling, occasionally using drugs, having no religious identification, opportunistic, impulsive, and insensitive (Jenks, 1988; Van de Ven, 1995). Though these stereotypes obviously represent judgmental attitudes, they most likely also reflect the stigmatizing effects of heterosexism.

Like negative stereotypes about other subordinate groups, heterosexist assumptions about gay men, lesbians, and bisexuals are shaped by cultural ideologies that legitimize the oppression of minorities (Herek, 1991). Many people still subscribe to Freud's inversion theory (Kite & Deaux, 1987; Lhomond, 1993) which suggests that gay men are similar to heterosexual women and that lesbians are similar to heterosexual men. Accordingly, gay men often are assumed to possess culturally defined feminine attributes and thus are described as "sissies" or seen as fitting the "gay-pretty-boy stereotype"; similarly, lesbians frequently are believed to exhibit socially determined masculine characteristics and therefore are thought of as "tomboyish" (Innala & Ernulf, 1994; McConaghy & Zamir, 1995). Consequently, "feminine" men repeatedly are presumed to be gay and "masculine" women presupposed to be lesbian (Blinde & Taub, 1992; Herek, 1984, 1991; Kite & Deaux, 1986, 1987).

Because gender nonconformity is devalued more in men than in women (Page & Yee, 1985), gay men repeatedly are depreciated on the basis of a hypothetical association between male homosexuality and femininity. Ironically, however, lesbians are not appreciated more because they are stereotyped as being masculine; that is, a lesbian's "masculinity" does not compensate sufficiently for her biological femininity. The quality of being female, whether biologically or psychologically, still ranks lowest on the social hierarchy and renders men as well as women subject to oppression. As a result, in the United States and in most Western societies, people who show any variance from popular conceptions of masculinity and femininity develop the sense that they are outsiders (Isay, 1989). This sense of isolation from family, friends, and the broader society leads many to psychotherapy to address their pain.

CORRELATES OF HETEROSEXISM

Like other forms of oppression, such as racism and sexism, heterosexism has been correlated with a number of variables that legitimize and reinforce negative attitudes and behaviors (Patel, Long, McCammon, & Wuensch, 1995; Simon, 1995). From his own work and the research of others, Herek (1984) identified seven characteristics of people with negative attitudes toward lesbians and gay men. Accordingly, these individuals are likely to:

- Hold traditional attitudes toward gender roles
- Not have engaged in homosexual behaviors or not have identified as lesbian or gay
- Have peers who manifest negative attitudes
- Have little contact with lesbians and gay men
- Be older and less educated
- Live in rural areas, the Midwest, or the South
- Be strongly and conservatively religious

Similarly, data from a national sample of 2,308 adults revealed that people are more likely to hold negative attitudes toward gay men and lesbians if they are politically conservative, male, married or widowed, older, less educated, southern, or religious (Seltzer, 1992). The following discussions examine these correlates more closely.

Conservative Attitudes

Although each oppressive system has its own ideological foundation and structure, heterosexism reflects the same general psychological constructs and processes as racism and sexism. In other words, many people who are heterosexist are also racially prejudiced and sexually conservative. Accordingly, Ficarrotto (1990) surveyed 48 female and 31 male Caucasian heterosexuals and found that social prejudice and sexual conservatism independently and equally predict the homophobic (i.e., heterosexist) personality. Other research has shown that people with hostile or negative attitudes toward lesbians and gay men tend to adhere to traditional ideologies of family and gender (Herek, 1988; Van de Ven, Bornholt, & Bailey, 1996), conservative thoughts about sex roles (Britton, 1990), and conventional beliefs about female sexuality, male dominance, and feminism (Lottes & Kuriloff, 1992).

Fear of Being Homosexual

Heterosexism, often also called homophobia, has been associated with the secret fear of being homosexual (Forstein, 1988). Some male perpetrators of homophobic violence, for example, are assumed to assault gay men rather than affirm unacceptable same-sex attractions within themselves. These aggressors are unable to accept their sexual interests in other men and, thus, are uncomfortable and insecure with their own sexual orientation. Because acknowledging these feelings would threaten their vulnerable sense of masculine heterosexuality, many of these assailants project their same-sex attractions onto their victims whom, in turn, they blame and punish for arousing homosexual interests in them (Groth & Burgess, 1980).

A more common strategy for managing the fear of being gay or lesbian is heterosexual marriage (Bridges & Croteau, 1994; Buxton, 1991; D. F. Smith & Allred, 1990; van der Geest, 1993; Whitney, 1990). In this regard, Ross (1983) documented the lives of over 500 heterosexually married homosexual men from five different countries. His data demonstrated the degree to which some gay men have internalized societal homophobia and heterosexism and, in their efforts to avoid and escape anti-gay prejudice, "have been duped into self-hatred and stifling themselves in nuptial closets" (p. x). He concluded that more homosexual men marry in societies that are less tolerant of homosexuality. Similarly, Coleman (1982) studied 31 men who worried about their same-sex feelings and behaviors and thus decided to marry women because of pressures from family and society. Some of these men believed that heterosexual marriage would help them overcome their homosexual attractions.

Male Attitudes

In samples of the general population, men consistently tend to express more hostility and negative affect than do women toward sexual minorities in general, and gay men in particular (Herek, 1988; Kite, 1992; Kurdek, 1988a; Whitley, 1988). One meta-analysis of 112 studies, published between 1965 and 1996, found that attitudes of heterosexual men are more negative than those of heterosexual women toward homosexual people and behavior (Kite & Whitley, 1996). The extent of this anti-gay prejudice was demonstrated by male subjects in one study who responded with significantly less help than did female subjects to a male stranger's request for help when he wore a T-shirt bearing a pro-gay slogan (P. A. Russell & Gray, 1992).

As mentioned previously, one set of explanations for homophobia in men claims that core male gender identity, male role, or heterosexual masculinity is somehow threatened by gender nonconformity in other men (Herek, 1986a; Kerns & Fine, 1994; Pleck, Sonenstein, & Ku, 1994; Reiter, 1991; Stein, 1996b). Herek (1986a) contends that men affirm their heterosexual masculinity by expressing who they are *not;* that is, they define themselves in opposition to gay males. This continuous externalization of the threat keeps the masculine ego safe (Moss, 1992) and thereby protects the privileged position of the heterosexual male in society. The "strong linkage of masculinity with heterosexuality in American culture . . . creates considerable pressures (both social and psychological) for males to affirm their masculinity through rejection of that which is not culturally defined as masculine (male homosexuality) and that which is perceived as negating the importance of males (lesbianism)" (Herek, 1991, p. 65).

Accordingly, Franklin (1998) examined the motivations and attitudes of presumably heterosexual males who had assaulted gay men and concluded that "antigay violence can be seen primarily as an extreme manifestation of pervasive cultural norms rather than as a manifestation of individual hatred" (p. 20). Her findings reflected a multiple determinism and an interplay of hierarchical gender norms, peer dynamics, youthful thrill seeking, and economic and social disempowerment as mutually reinforcing factors in leading men who typically did not see themselves and hate-filled extremists to commit acts of anti-gay violence. Franklin, in essence, found that her subjects were not motivated by "a simple and singular psychological element such as hatred or repressed homosexuality" (p. 19) but, rather, seemed to be demonstrating their masculinity, garnering social approval, and alleviating boredom.

Peer Attitudes and Personal Contact

People who perceive that their friends express similar negative attitudes toward sexual minorities generally feel supported in their antagonism toward lesbians and gay men (Herek, 1986b, 1988). Conversely, individuals report greater alienation from the wider society when they hold more positive attitudes toward sexual minorities (Wells & Daly, 1992). In some social circles, then, people are considered "in" if they are intolerant and "out" if they are tolerant of gay and lesbian people. Accordingly, tolerant and intolerant subjects react differently when they believe they are interacting with lesbians or gay men (Kite & Deaux, 1986).

In addition to peer attitudes, individual contact and social exchange with gay men and lesbians influence personal opinions about sexual minorities (Herek, 1986b, 1988; Lance, 1987). Studies reflect a reciprocal relationship between social contact and positive attitudes; in other words, the more association and disclosure, the more favorable the relationships and fewer the negative stereotypes (Herek & Capitanio, 1996; Pagtolun-An & Clair, 1986). Having gay or lesbian friends and liking those individuals, similarly, has been associated with feeling comfortable around sexual minorities and experiencing little bias or prejudice toward them (Gentry, 1987; Jussim, Nelson, Manis, & Soffin, 1995). On the other hand, limited contact with lesbians and gay men has been correlated with negative attitudes toward homosexuals (Herek, 1984). These unfavorable opinions are likely to persist as long as interaction is minimal between people of differing sexual orientations. In two instances, fewer heterosexual men reported knowing a gay man than women reported knowing a lesbian (Whitley, 1990), and three-fourths of sexual minorities in a national telephone survey described socializing only with nonheterosexuals ("Results of Poll," 1989). As long as these relationship patterns continue, negative attitudes are likely to persist and heterosexist assumptions to go unchallenged.

Demographics: Age, Education, and Region

As previously reported in this chapter, both Herek (1984) and Seltzer (1992) identified correlations between negative attitudes toward homosexuals and age, education, and region of residence. A close relationship between these three demographic variables and social tolerance also was detected when Dejowski (1992) analyzed more than 14,000 responses to sociodemographic surveys issued between 1973 and 1988. People who were older and less educated and from small towns, rural areas, and southern states were found to be less tolerant toward lesbians and gay men. A poll by *U.S. News & World Report* (Shapiro, Cook, & Krackow, 1993) similarly revealed that of those groups *least* likely to know a homosexual, 67% are retired, 63% have less than a high school education, 55% live in the southern–central states, and 54% live in small towns. Conversely, of those *most* likely to know a gay or lesbian person, 58% are between ages 35 and 64, 63% are college graduates, and 58% live in the suburbs. In a national telephone survey of 937 adults (Herek & Glunt, 1993), interpersonal contact was more likely to be reported by respondents who were young, female, highly educated, and politically liberal.

There are few studies of attitudes toward sexual minorities in nonurban and rural United States because since most research has been conducted among urban populations. Thus, most reports of the lives of rural lesbians and gay men are anecdotal or narrative. Nonetheless, social isolation, loneliness, invisibility, lack of role models, and severe anxiety over being discovered are commonly described (D. R. Atkinson & Hackett, 1995; D'Augelli, 1989b; McCarthy, 2000). Numerous social, political, financial, and religious constraints exist in rural communities where traditional morals, values, and behaviors prevail (H. B. McDonald & Steinhorn, 1993). Given the traditional expectations for marriage and family life, people who do not marry draw attention to themselves. D'Augelli (1989b), however, contends that life is somewhat easier for an unmarried lesbian than for a gay man because single men almost always are assumed to be homosexual. In addition, Sears (1991b) discusses regional pressures faced by southern lesbians and gay men, namely, the importance of family name and honor; race, gender, and class boundaries; and fundamentalist religion. According to H. B. McDonald and Steinhorn (1993), life in some parts of rural America is "like living in a goldfish bowl," where almost everyone knows everyone else's daily activities, associations, and "comings and goings" (p. 129). Consequently, lesbians and gay men feel the constant pressure to be discreet, to remain invisible, and to socialize with extreme selectivity. In this regard, one study of 34 rural lesbians (ages 19 to 53) found that many of their close friends and supporters also were lesbians (D'Augelli, Collins, & Hart, 1987).

On a more positive note, a recent issue of the national gay and lesbian magazine *The Advocate* (2000) published a special report on the growing number of sexual minorities in small-town and rural United States. Bull (2000b) noted that the decision of many to remain in their local areas "is a reversal of the great gay migration of the latter half of the 20th century" (p. 66) when many lesbians and gay men moved to cities where they believed they could live openly and free from discrimination. Now, often facilitated by the Internet, political organizations, and community centers, social groups can be found in less populated areas of the United States. Progress is much more complicated than in more transient large cities where people are far less involved in the lives of their neighbors. On the other hand, however, individuals who have earned the respect of friends and community members over the years often find that this personal support and inclusion continues after their sexual orientations are known publicly.

Religious Beliefs

Heterosexist attitudes have been correlated with extremely conservative or fundamentalist religious beliefs that reinforce rigid distinctions between masculine and feminine characteristics, along with defining the spiritual life in terms of good and evil acts and the afterlife in terms of eternal salvation and damnation. Further, pious extremism and doctrinaire religiosity regularly are used to motivate and morally justify prejudice and animosity toward gay men and lesbians (Britton, 1990; Crawford & Solliday, 1996; Fisher, Derison, Polley, & Cadman, 1994; Forstein, 1988; Herek, 1988; Hunsberger, 1996). Although most studies measure the beliefs of Christian fundamentalists, Hunsberger (1996) extended his investigation to include samples with Muslim, Hindu, and Jewish backgrounds. Interestingly, he found that fundamentalists within each of the four religious groups tended to be authoritarian and to have hostile attitudes toward homosexuals.

VanderStoep and Green (1988) tested a path model constructed from variables thought to predict negative attitudes toward same-sex relations. Responses from 201 college students supported their hypothesis that religiosity predicts ethical conservatism, which in turn predicts bias against gay and lesbian intimacy. Maret (1984) also found support for this finding when he studied 151 New Jersey fundamentalist and nonfundamentalist college students. Results indicated that fundamentalists were more conservative and significantly less accepting of same-sex relations than nonfundamentalists because they believed that the practices "are strictly forbidden within a literal and inerrant biblical interpretation" (p. 206).

Similarly, McFarland (1989) studied the discriminatory attitudes of 99 female and 74 male Caucasian religious Christian undergraduates and divided their responses into four categories: fundamentalism, extrinsic, intrinsic and "quest" (open-minded search for truth). Fundamentalism correlated positively with discriminatory attitudes toward women and homosexuals but negatively with anti-Black attitudes. The results of Herek's (1987) study of 126 White heterosexual students on eight university campuses may provide insight into this finding. He divided his sample into extrinsics (those whose religious orientation was a self-serving, instrumental approach conforming to social conventions) and intrinsics (those for whom religion provided a meaningful framework for a comprehensive understanding of life) and found that extrinsics were more prejudiced against racial minorities whereas intrinsics were more biased against gay men and lesbians. Herek (1987) suggested that an intrinsic orientation does not generally foster acceptance of others (as is commonly thought) but, rather, encourages tolerance of groups accepted by contemporary Judeo-Christian teachings. In other words, intrinsics (and possibly fundamentalists) who belong to denominations that condemn homosexuality are more likely to be critical than those who belong to denominations with a more accepting stance. An intrinsic orientation, then, "is associated with tolerance toward groups identified as deserving of tolerance by one's religious philosophy" (p. 40).

Dictatorial religious beliefs undoubtedly have motivated numerous fundamentalist clergy and fervent devotees to wage spiritual warfare on homosexuality in the name of God (Ritter & O'Neill, 1996). Similarly, religious conversion therapists, equally impassioned by religious zeal and conviction, wage their own form of warfare against human spirits as they persist in their efforts to convert lesbians and gay men to heterosexuality despite no empirical evidence that such treatments are effective (Haldeman, 1991, 1994, 1995; see Chapter 13 for additional discussion).

EFFECTS OF HETEROSEXISM ON MENTAL HEALTH

This chapter previously introduced the fundamental reality on which this book is based: that sexual minorities share common characteristics with other subordinate groups and, therefore, are oppressed social, culturally, and politically in the United States. Stigmatization negatively affects mental health and intrapsychic processes, often producing debilitating emotional stress and high levels of internalized homophobia (DiPlacido, 2000; Dupras, 1994; Fein & Neuhring, 1981; Herek, Cogan, & Gillis, 2000; McDougall, 1993; Rosario, Rotheram-Borus, & Reid, 1996; Ross, 1990; Rosser & Ross, 1989; Shidlo, 1994a). For example, 741 New York City gay men were sampled and found to suffer from numerous "minority stressors," namely, internalized homophobia, stigma, and experiences of discrimination and violence. Those with high levels were two to three times as likely to suffer from high levels of distress (Meyer, 1995). As a result of these environmental forces, then, lesbians and gay men experience higher rates of psychological distress than do heterosexuals and seek counseling or psychotherapy far more often.

Allport (1954) contended that "no one can be indifferent to the abuse and expectations of others" and that "ego defensiveness will frequently be found among members of groups that are set off for ridicule, disparagement, and discrimination" (p. 143). Accordingly, people who are stereotyped and stigmatized are likely to experience a broad range of intrapsychic and interpersonal consequences. Allport (1954) referred to these effects as "traits due to victimization" or "persecution-produced traits." These unfavorable outcomes include the following:

- Social withdrawal and passivity
- Obsessive anxiety, suspicion and insecurity
- Personal and social denial of minority group membership
- Self-hating dominant group identification

Many of these characteristics apply to gay men, lesbians, and bisexuals, as well as to other oppressed minorities. The following discussions briefly describe these attributes.

Social Withdrawal and Passivity

Therapists should keep in mind the extent to which fears of discrimination and rejection keep their gay, lesbian, and bisexual clients socially withdrawn, passive, and otherwise reluctant to disclose their sexual orientations. For example, a national telephone survey required 27,000 calls in order to locate 800 people who would admit being gay to a stranger. In Kansas alone, 1,650 calls and 55 hours were required to locate one self-identified gay person. Of those contacted, 70% had told their families and 50% had told coworkers of their sexual orientation (in both cases, considerably fewer women than men had disclosed). Varying by the region of the country, between 23% and 40% had *not* informed their families that they were gay or lesbian; between 37% and 59% had *not* revealed their sexual orientation to associates at work ("Results of Poll," 1989).

Anxiety, Suspicion, and Insecurity

The constant pressure to conceal their sexual orientations from families, friends, and coworkers often leaves gay, lesbian, and bisexual clients feeling guarded and vigilant in many social circumstances and situations. Accordingly, protective vigilance among sexual minority populations frequently results in generalized feelings of anxiety, suspicion, and insecurity, all of which may present in therapy as thought, mood, or personality disorders (see Chapter 8). In addition, lesbians and gay men may exhibit decreased control, life satisfaction, and a sense that life is difficult and unfair (Birt & Dion, 1987), as well as other depressive symptoms. For these clients, stigmatization amplifies the impact of life events and often results in sadness, as well as emotional and psychological distress (Dombrowski, Wodarski, Smokowski, & Bricout, 1995; Herek, 1991; Herek et al., 2000; Meyer, 1995; Rotheram-Borus, Rosario, Van Rossem, & Reid, 1995; Ross, 1990).

Denial of Minority Group Membership

Many gay men, lesbians, and bisexuals are skillful at talking around and away from their erotic and emotional attractions, masking the sex of their intimate partners and obscuring the quality of their social activities. This need to "pass" as heterosexual in order to avoid discrimination and rejection (Herek, 1991) has many sexual minority clients strategizing behaviors that are designed to mislead family, friends, and coworkers. These "passing" strategies may become so perfected that even therapists can be totally unaware of their clients' minority sexual orientations.

Bisexuals, lesbians, and gay men may personally and socially deny their sexual minority group membership when they assume the facade of heterosexuality. For some, the discrepancy between public and private identities is painful; they may feel inauthentic and as if they are living a lie (DiPlacido, 2000; Herek, 1991). Relationships with family and friends are strained "as lesbians and gay men create distance from others in order to avoid revealing their sexual orientation. When contact cannot be avoided, they may keep their interactions at a superficial level as a self-protective strategy" (p. 74). The anguish of this isolation ushers many clients into therapy.

Dominant Group Identification

In addition to the loneliness created by this isolation, many gay, lesbian, and bisexual clients who overvalue and idealize the heterosexual majority suffer from self-hatred and seek treatment to improve self-worth. This low self-esteem, or internalized homophobia, frequently results from their personalization of many negative societal attitudes toward lesbians and gay men. Such "self-hating dominant group identification" (Allport, 1954) often leads some sexual minorities to depreciate and devalue other gay men and lesbians, as well as additional minority groups. This harmful effect of heterosexism may never be seen in the counseling office or the consultation room, however, because discriminatory attitudes toward others rarely cause individuals to seek mental health services. Nonetheless, bisexuals, lesbians, and gay men often seek psychotherapy when oppressive external or internal forces finally compel them to address issues related to their own sexual minority condition.

CONCLUSION

The next chapter explores historical influences that have shaped contemporary perspectives on homosexuality, as well as current concepts and models of sexual orientation. These discussions aim to offer psychotherapists the expanded scope of understanding necessary to empower sexual minority clients through objectifying and reframing their socially constructed status.

2

Concepts of Sexual Orientation

Helping clients understand both historical and contemporary conceptualizations of sexual orientation often is an essential first step in their examining the personal meaning of their bisexuality or homosexuality. "The meanings and associations carried by sexual labels may vary tremendously, and self-labeling may serve different coping functions at different times" (Paul, 1996, p. 444). The goal of affirmative psychotherapy, then, is to reduce the negative connotations and "detoxify" culturally stigmatized identities, thereby "supporting and validating the client's inner experience" (Paul, 1996, p. 445).

Historical forces have formed contemporary approaches to understanding sexual orientation. Throughout the course of Western civilization, popular concepts of homosexuality have been constructed from the prevailing beliefs and mythologies of various cultures. Powerful civil, religious, and professional institutions within these societies often have attributed less than positive social constructions to intimate relationships between people of the same sex; in fact, these influential shaping forces have criminalized, condemned, and pathologized their inclinations and behaviors. Such negative conceptualizations have been further deconstructed and reconstructed over succeeding generations and centuries, resulting in diverse notions and opinions about homosexuality being held among bisexuals, lesbians, and gay men themselves. Psychotherapy often involves offering frames of reference and psychoeducation to clients so they can view their sexuality from a broader, more objective, and less personalized perspective. Ideally, the brief historical conceptualizations as well as current viewpoints discussed in this chapter will provide therapists with the frames of reference necessary to accomplish these tasks.

HISTORICAL PERSPECTIVES

Sociological phenomena in Western cultures have molded and changed mores and values, which, in turn, have determined attitudes toward bisexuals, lesbians, and gay men. Social tolerance of homosexuality, for example, was evident during the early Greco-Roman period, as same-sex love was sanctioned and even celebrated in ancient Greece. Likewise, neither the law nor the religion of imperial Rome discriminated against homosexual (as contrasted with heterosexual) eroticism; however, in other times and places distinctions clearly were made in terms of acceptability (Alyson Publications, 1993; Boswell, 1980, 1994). Subsequently, the alternating ebb and flow of social intolerance over the centuries has formed and modified a code of Judeo-Christian sexual ethics based more on coincidence, control, and conquest than on scriptural and theological moral principles (Boswell, 1980).

The Rise of Intolerance

Social prejudice toward people of same-sex orientation began to rise as the Roman state was falling during the third through the sixth centuries. As Rome was losing control of its vast empire, defending its borders and leaving its urban centers unprotected, one way to contain the people was by legislating and enforcing codes of ethics and conduct. During the early Middle Ages, meanwhile, the Western church neither initiated nor supported the governmental oppression of same-sex love. Because prominent bishops were the only persons known by name to have been punished for homosexual acts, politicians likely enacted anti-gay legislation to subdue and suppress powerful clerics. For reasons that defy linear explanation, however, religious as well as social intolerance toward ethnic, cultural, and sexual minorities increased during the later Middle Ages (Boswell, 1980, 1994).

By the 13th and 14th centuries, anti-homosexual attitudes and beliefs had become integrated into the social fabric of Christendom as well as into the moral theology of Christianity. In 1260 C.E., same-sex love between women, in addition to between men, was criminalized, condemned, and punished for one of the first times in European history (Alyson Publications, 1993). Beginning in 1479 and in 1542 C.E., respectively, the Spanish and Roman Inquisitions oppressed and expelled Jews, Muslims, and Protestants from Spain and many other parts of Europe. In addition, dissidents and nonconformists were tortured and executed (Boswell, 1980). Caught in this web of social and religious persecution, sexual minorities often were maimed and killed for violating some of the same legal and moral traditions that legitimize the oppression of bisexuals, lesbians, and gay men today.

Paralleling the rise of legalism and authoritarianism in Western Christendom, Muslim cultures similarly have established oppressive and intolerant positions toward gay and lesbian people (Blumenfeld & Raymond, 1998; Knopp, 1990). Death is the penalty for lesbian activity, for example, in Iran and Saudi Arabia (Richards, 1990). Nonetheless, some Middle Eastern, Asian, and other non-European civilizations have histories of tolerance toward same-sex relationships. Rich evidence of these associations exists in ancient Chinese literature, in the pre-Columbian civilizations of Mesoamerica, in African societies, and among the Japanese samurai (Alyson Publications, 1990, 1993; Boswell, 1980; Knopp, 1990; Potgieter, 1997). A separate and respected gay subculture, in fact, existed in Japan as late as the mid-1800s (Goode & Wagner, 1993). As in Western societies, however, discrimination and oppression currently predominate in these cultures; thus, both immigrant and second-generation clients are likely to carry with them the prejudice of their indigenous cultures regarding sexual minorities (Knopp, 1990).

Intolerance in North America

The extermination of homosexuality and "other indigenous Native American customs shocking to the Christian conscience was one early aspect of the Spanish and French mission in America" (Katz, 1983, p. 28). As early as the 1500s, Spanish and French explorers and missionaries discovered homosexual activity among Native American men in territories now known as Florida, Illinois, California, and Louisiana. As was necessary in Europe, regulating and restricting personal morality and sexual behavior was required in the North American colonies to establish conformity with the social order.

Similarly, the Dutch settlers arrived in the New World with their own biases against same-sex relations while the English imported to the American colonies their tradition of criminalizing sodomy. Historical records from 1607 to 1740 document nearly 20 legal cases involving charges of sodomy or other homosexual acts either between men or between women in the New England, mid-Atlantic, and southern territories. In 1649, Goodwife Sara Norman became the first woman in America known to be convicted of lesbian activity, found guilty, and forced to confess in public. The relatively light penalty imposed by the court against Sara Norman, however, suggests that her offense was not considered as serious as the more severely punished acts of sodomy between men (Alyson Publications, 1993; Katz, 1983). Colonial American laws imposing the death penalty for sodomy criminalized any male sexual act that deviated from the procreative function of sexual intercourse because nonreproductive sex threatened marriage and family, "institutions vital to a young society struggling to survive against difficult odds" (Goode & Wagner, 1993, p. 50). No one in early America, however, attributed homosexuality to a particular category of people.

THE CLASSIFICATION OF HOMOSEXUALITY

Prior to the mid-19th century, the moral and criminal codes of the church and the state heavily influenced popular opinion about same-sex eroticism. Thereafter, the fields of medicine and psychiatry became strong forces in shaping and changing social, cultural, and political attitudes and beliefs. Karl Heinrich Ulrichs was one of the first individuals to attribute same-sex attraction to a particular category of people, who would later become known as homosexuals. In 1863, he wrote two pamphlets in German within which he presented an impartial and scholarly explanation of homosexuality. Three years later, he spoke out in favor of gay rights before a conference of lawyers in Munich and, at this gathering, became the first known person in modern times to publicly declare himself a *Uranian*, his nonderogatory term describing people born with a homosexual orientation (Alyson Publications, 1993; McWhirter, Sanders, & Reinisch, 1990).

In 1869, a Hungarian physician named Karoly Maria Benkert (under the pseudonym Kertbeny) coined the term *homosexual* to designate a distinct category of people erotically attracted to others of their own sex (Alyson Publications, 1993; Blumenfeld & Raymond, 1988; Hansen, 1989; Katz, 1983; Weinrich & Williams, 1991). Prior to the 1860s, all individuals were assumed to be heterosexual and same-sex behaviors were considered violations of nature, morality, or law. The coining of this terminology created an identity for people that altered both the way they saw themselves and were seen by society. No longer was homosexuality applied to the specific acts but, rather, to the actors themselves.

A Natural Variation

Distinguishing a separate category of human beings based on their same-sex attractions was accompanied by controversies regarding the nature of those thus classified. Contrary to majority opinion, for example, Karl Heinrich Ulrichs considered the instincts of male and female Uranians (*urning* and *uringin*, respectively) inborn and therefore natural. To him, these individuals were *spiritual* hermaphrodites, with the mind and soul of one sex born into the body of the other (De Cecco, 1987). As such, they comprised a distinct species, a "third sex," who possessed the sex-specific physical attributes "but whose sexual instinct failed to correspond to their sexual organs, resulting in an inversion of sexual desires" (McWhirter et al., 1990, p. 10). The term *inversion* was later used by the 19th-century sexologist Havelock Ellis, who struggled in his writings to "escape the language of disease, suggesting that instead people think of homosexuality as an 'anomaly' or 'sport of nature' " (Blumenfeld & Raymond, 1988, p. 357). His coauthor, John Addington Symonds, also referred to same-sex attractions as sexual inversions and saw these inclinations as analogous to color-blindness, a harmless variation.

A Pathological Deviation

Unfortunately, the nonpathological views of Ulrichs, Ellis, and Symonds were replaced by many in the medical community who rendered homosexuals ill in order to treat their "congenital sexual inversion," an inborn "physical condition for which the individual was not 'responsible' " (Katz, 1983, p. 154). For them, "removing [homosexuality] from the realm of the criminal into what they saw as the kindlier province of medicine" (Goode & Wagner, 1993, p. 50) was a more humane approach because, by diagnosing pathology in these patients, they were able to treat their homoerotic impulses and instincts. Further, because they were not responsible for their physical condition, homosexuals were innocent patients in need of treatment rather than guilty criminals deserving of punishment.

The first of 12 editions of the best-selling textbook *Psychopathia Sexualis*, published in Germany in 1884, represented the sympathetic yet pathologizing mentality prevalent in the medical community of his era. In this work, Dr. Richard von Krafft-Ebing (1884/1965), an Austrian sex researcher and professor of psychiatry and neurology, discussed an anomaly that is "limited to the sexual life, and does not more deeply and seriously affect character and mental personality" (p. 240); at the same time, however, he referred to the "inverted" (p. 94) and "abnormal" (p. 258) sexual instincts of "sexually perverse" (p. 262) individuals. Beginning in the 1880s, the ideas of Krafft-Ebing and similar thinkers were exported to the United States and appeared in U.S. medical journals within which contributing physicians began referring to their homosexual patients as sexual perverts and inverts and to their behavior as sexual perversion and inversion (Katz, 1983). These discussions were confined largely to the realm of medicine until the 1920s, when " 'the homosexual' emerged into the sphere of the speakable" (Katz, 1983, p. 167) and the popular media began to discuss and differentiate "normal" heterosexuality from "abnormal" homosexuality.

This new media attention to sexual perversion also challenged the preexisting notion of Platonic, nonerotic same-sex intimacy (Katz, 1983) and sounded "the death knell of romantic friendship" (Faderman, 1991, p. 4). Friendships between men and between women now had become suspect. No longer were women seen as intimate friends but rather as lesbians or female sexual inverts. Walt Whitman's virtues of "manly love" and "fervent comradeships" became medical conditions demanding a cure. Amid this climate of fear and suspicion, "men and women still immersed in 19th century notions of romanticism and sentimental friendship" (Goode & Wagner, 1993, p. 51) became self-conscious and hypersensitive to sexual matters and to same-sex relationships.

In the end, however, the contributions of well-meaning sexologists such as Karl Heinrich Ulrichs, who attempted to liberate nonheterosexual people from the institutional forces that criminalized their sexual behaviors and pathologized their erotic attractions, were not taken as seriously as those of physicians such as Richard von Krafft-Ebing. Ironically, even the medical community's hopes of engendering compassion and legal clemency for patients born with sexual inversions were thwarted. Although the medical diagnosis of homosexuality originally offered the prospect of interpreting behaviors in a new way, it later became a focal point in the social oppression of lesbians and gay men (Hansen, 1989; C. Silverstein, 1996).

Depathologizing Homosexuality

This social oppression of nonheterosexuals reached its zenith during the McCarthy era of the early 1950s when homosexuals, along with communists, were the targets of pernicious witch hunts (Hooker, 1993). In 1952, *homosexuality* was officially classified as a mental illness (i.e., a sexual deviation) in the first edition of the *Diagnostic and Statistical Manual of Mental Disorders* (American Psychiatric Association, 1952) "although it is apparent that tradition rather than science was behind the inclusion of homosexuality in the diagnostic nomenclature" (Krajeski, 1996, p. 21). During the following year, however, the ongoing process of depathologizing same-sex eroticism was set in further motion when a professor of psychology at UCLA responded to the challenge of a former student to study gay men like himself. Although Dr. Evelyn Hooker had been taught to pathologize homosexuality, her associations with gay men contradicted her training and education. Thus, she applied for a grant from the National Institute of Mental Health to study nonpatient, nonprisoner samples of male homosexuals. In her scientific investigation, she administered the Rorschach and other psychological tests to 30 gay and 30 nongay men. None of the three psychologists, including Rorschach expert Brunner Klopfer, who interpreted the results were able distinguish homosexuals from heterosexuals. No differences in either adjustment or psychopathology were detected between the two populations.

In 1972, another psychologist, Dr. M. Siegelman, tested large numbers of lesbian and heterosexual women and, consequently, confirmed Dr. Hooker's research findings. These and other studies led the American Psychiatric Association, in 1973, to officially declassify and remove *homosexuality* from the diagnostic terminology of DSM-II. Two years later, the American Psychological Association endorsed the decision of the American Psychiatric Association and, furthermore, defined the "absence of psychopathology" as the term had been applied to same-sex attraction (Burr, 1993; Hooker, 1993).

Politicizing Homosexuality

While psychologists were challenging the illness model of homosexuality, lesbians and gay men were mobilizing to affirm themselves and their sexual orientation (Alyson Publications, 1993; C. Silverstein, 1991, 1996; M. Thompson, 1994). In 1950, Harry Hay, a political activist called for the "Androgynous Minority" to unite (Alyson Publications, 1993, p. 24). A small group of gay men responded to his call, gathered at his home in Los Angeles, and later formed the Mattachine Society (Blumenfeld & Raymond, 1988). Although not the first group to organize, Mattachine is thought to represent the foundation of the current gay (then known as *homophile*) rights movement. In 1955, Del Martin and Phyllis Lyon formed the Daughters of Bilitis, the first lesbian membership group in San Francisco, which later grew into a national organization with educational and political goals. By 1960, both organizations had chapters in cities on both coasts. This transcontinental expansion was helped by the rise of lesbian and gay publications during the mid 1950s. *ONE*, the first openly gay magazine to receive wide circulation, was published in 1953. Two years later, the *Mattachine Review* began circulation and, in 1956, the Daughters of Bilitis publication *The Ladder* became the first lesbian magazine.

By the mid-1960s, the national gay and lesbian movement was politically active and gaining momentum (Alyson Publications, 1993; M. Thompson, 1994). For example, state sodomy laws were being challenged and a handful of openly gay candidates were campaigning for elected office. Public demonstrations calling for civil rights were held at the Civil Service Commission, the Pentagon, the White House, and Independence Hall in Philadelphia. The first gay and lesbian organization was founded on a college campus, and the American Sociological Association became the first professional organization to take a stand against discrimination based on sexual orientation. On a broader front, the American Civil Liberties Union advocated a similar position. By 1968, the movement had grown such that representatives of 26 gay and lesbian groups attended the North American Conference of Homophile Organizations (NACHO). On June 28, 1969, a police raid on a gay bar in New York City met with intense opposition. The resistance has since been called the Stonewall Rebellion and has come to symbolize the fountainhead of modern gay and lesbian liberation. In a sense, then, the driving force of previous decades crested that evening, drawing the attention and commitment of many others to the movement.

Relabeling Homosexuality

While lesbians and gay men were mobilizing to affirm their sexual orientation, they were adopting new vocabularies to refer to themselves. Some heard the word *homosexual* echo "with implications of diagnosis and pathology" (Gonsiorek & Weinrich, 1991, p. 2) whereas others regarded the 19th-century medical terminology as derogatory, negative, and oppressive. Instead, many men and women adopted the word *gay* (which had been introduced in 1933) to refer to their emerging sociopolitical identities rather than to their sexual behaviors. For them, the term implied a positive self-image and way of being that transcended the narrow focus on homosexual acts (Donovan, 1992).

For some women, however, the word *gay* held frivolous and trivial connotations. Given their belief that affectional orientation and political perspective were central to self-definition (Gonsiorek & Weinrich, 1991), they contended that the term was too strongly associated with sexual behavior and fantasy. According to this perspective, sexual "identity is constructed both societally and psychologically; it is both a social and a personal process" (Golden, 1987, p. 31). The word *lesbian* first had been used in the late 19th century to highlight the mutual nurturing and egalitarian companionship that women can bring to each other when they live and work creatively together (Alyson Publications, 1993; Downing, 1991, 1995). The term was adopted from the women's community that flourished on the Greek isle of Lesbos in the 6th century B.C.E. where the members learned from the poet Sappho and "shared in the delight of the mind as well as the body" (Blumenfeld & Raymond, 1988, p. 78). Not all, however, elected to call themselves lesbians, preferring instead to be known as gay women (Faderman, 1991). Nonetheless, the word grew in popularity over years and, in October 1990, *The Advocate* changed its subtitle to the national gay *and lesbian* newsmagazine (M. Thompson, 1994). "This explicit inclusion by the community's flagship periodical perhaps marks the demise of *gay* as a nongender-marked term" (Donovan, 1992, p. 44).

As introduced in Chapter 1, the term *sexual minorities* is used interchangeably with *lesbians, bisexuals*, and *gay men* throughout this book. This vocabulary is preferred to *homosexual* and *homosexuality* in order to minimize the pathological implications of 19th-century medical terminology. These terms are used occasionally, however, when other word choices would be cumbersome. Similarly, *same-sex* will be favored over *homosexual* and used interchangeably with *gay and lesbian* to modify or describe relationships as well as attractions and behaviors. Rarely, if ever, is *homosexual* used as a noun to describe individuals; it used now and then as a modifier.

Repathologizing Homosexuality

In spite of the widespread efforts of lesbians and gay men to affirm their sociopolitical and sexual identities, by the late 1970s their voices only partially had reached the medical and psychiatric communities. Many had worked hard for public acceptance and social respectability and hoped that the U.S. public was coming to view them as nonpathological and well adjusted. The optimism they drew from the American Psychiatric Association's removal of *homosexuality* from DSM-II in 1973 was short-lived, however. The process of depathologizing same-sex attraction was undermined when, in 1980, the psychiatric diagnosis of *ego-dystonic homosexuality* replaced the category of *sexual orientation disturbance* in DSM-III (De Cecco, 1987; Krajeski, 1996). This new diagnostic category, then, pathologized psychological distress over same-sex attraction which, in essence, reclassified struggles with homosexuality as a mental disorder.

Although "persistent and marked distress about one's sexual orientation" still was listed as an example of *sexual disorder not otherwise specified*, in 1987 *ego-dystonic homosexuality* was eliminated as a diagnosis in DSM-III-R. What was remarkable about the removal, however, was that for the first time gay psychiatrists and psychologists played a significant role in bringing about changes in psychiatric diagnosis. In working for extraction of the "diagnostic relic" of *ego-dystonic homosexuality,* the arguments of Drs. Cabaj, Krajeski, Malyon, and T. S. Stein (whose works are cited in this book) noted "that empirical data do not support the diagnosis, that it is inappropriate to label culturally induced homophobia as a mental disorder, that the diagnosis was rarely used clinically, and that few articles in the scientific literature use the concept" (Krajeski, 1996, p. 26). Unfortunately, the retraction that resulted from this reasoning was insufficient to depathologize same-sex attraction entirely, given that the illness model of homosexuality reflected in former editions of the diagnostic manual remained in the minds of many. These impressions, combined with the physiologically based explanations currently being offered by the scientific community, seem to recreate a pathologically focused mindset. Accordingly, De Cecco (1987) believes that these emerging psychobiological explanations of sexual orientation repathologize homosexuality, represent "a misguided compassion"

(p. 106), and leave "the door . . . wide open to its being treated as a physical abnormality" (p. 107).

Three lines of psychobiological research have attempted to explain sexual orientation (Burr, 1993; De Cecco, 1987). The prenatal hormone theory hypothesizes that the endocrine system hormonally masculinizes or feminizes the brain of the developing fetus and influences the directionality of erotic attraction. Different levels of prenatal hormones, then, are thought to predispose individuals to diverse sexual inclinations (C. Silverstein, 1996). A second thread of inquiry suggests that sexual orientation can be studied at the molecular level of synapses and neurons and at basic sites of brain structural differences. These perspectives thus examine differences in neuroanatomy between homosexual and heterosexual individuals and the nature of the interaction between hormonalization patterns and anatomic organization (Byne, 1996). Finally, another line of research examines the role of genetics in determining sexual orientation. In these investigations, *heritability* is usually measured by studying monozygotic and dizygotic twins as well as biological and adopted siblings. One of the key premises of these studies is that if homosexuality is primarily genetic in origin, the more closely related that people are, the more similar their sexual orientations should be (Burr, 1993).

Depending on one's frame of reference, these hormonal, neuroanatomical, and genetic differences (see Chapter 3 for further discussions) can be considered either natural variations or pathological deviations from the norm of heterosexuality. Unfortunately, heterosexist bias additionally and frequently influences the interpretation of psychobiological research findings. The presumption that heterosexuality is normative resurrects 19th-century notions that lesbians and gay men belong to a third sex and, therefore, are "not ideal exemplars of their biological sexes, neither true females nor true males" (De Cecco, 1987, p. 107). From this perspective, gay and lesbian sexuality is repathologized and, once again, seen as abnormal.

CONTEMPORARY MODELS OF SEXUAL ORIENTATION

The diverse meanings of homosexuality described previously can be attributed not only to historical forces of social and political change but also to the complexity of sexual orientation itself. Currently, *sexual orientation* is understood as a multidimensional constellation of variables that defies precise definition but often is misconstrued as a singular concept, such as *sexual behavior*, *sexual desire*, or *sexual identity* (Michaels, 1996). Several theorists have developed models for understanding and assessing sexual orientation. After the traditional psychoanalytic dichotomy is discussed briefly, the more recent continuum and/or multidimensional formulations of Kinsey, Storms, Klein, and Coleman are described. This latter group of models allow for the measurement of bisexuality as an entity equal in legitimacy to homosexual or heterosexual orientations.

Psychoanalytic Model

Many psychotherapists are still strongly influenced by early psychoanalytic models of sexual orientation (Cabaj, 1996a; Glassgold & Iasenza, 1995; Krajeski, 1996; N. O'Connor & Ryan, 1993). These conceptualizations are based on Freud's theory of innate bisexuality and his dichotomous assumption about sexual object choice. Freud hypothesized that people are bisexually oriented from birth but normally learn to restrict these innate bisexual impulses by repressing their erotic desires for their own sex and redirecting them to the other. Thus, he assumed that heterosexuality is the outcome of normal psychosexual development which involves a process of repression and redirection with regard to same-sex eroticism (Fox, 1996a).

Homosexuality, the opposite end of this developmental course, results from an unsuccessful resolution of the Oedipal conflict. Conversely, the successful resolution of the Oedipal conflict leads to the establishment of a culturally appropriate masculine or feminine gender identity and, hence, heterosexual object choice. In other words, gender identity determines sexual object choice. Through a process of identification with the same-sex parent, children develop either a masculine or a feminine identity and, subsequently, choose a love object of the other sex. Masculine identity in girls and feminine identity in boys are considered masculinity and femininity "complexes," respectively, and prognostic indications of homosexual object choice in adulthood (Freud, 1905/1953, 1914/1957, 1924/1961a, 1925/1961b, 1917/1963, 1940/1964a, 1933/1964b).

Kinsey Scale

Prior to the pioneering research of Dr. Alfred C. Kinsey, sexual orientation was seen from the Freudian perspective which suggested mutually exclusive outcomes of psychosexual development. Although previously an individual was regarded as either a *homosexual* or a *heterosexual*, Kinsey and his associates introduced the idea of sexuality as a continuous variable (McWhirter et al., 1990). While preparing to teach a human sexuality course at the University of Indiana in the 1940s, Kinsey designed an extensive sexual behavior inventory and eventually his research team surveyed more than 10,000 people to gather data on the subject. Later, these data were published in two volumes, *Sexual Behavior in the Human Male* (Kinsey, Pomeroy, & Martin, 1948) and *Sexual Behavior in the Human Female* (Kinsey, Pomeroy, Martin, & Gebhard, 1953). The Kinsey studies published in 1948 and 1953 indicated that 37% of the male and 20% of the female population had some form of overt homosexual experience after puberty and that only 63% of males and 80% of females were exclusively heterosexual prior to the date of their interviews. To reflect the diverse range of sexual responses, "Kinsey developed the [heterosexuality–homosexuality] scale to stress sexuality as a continuum" (Udis-Kessler, 1992, p. 312). Whereas Freudians dichotomized heterosexual and homosexual persons into discrete categories, Kinsey and his associates plotted sexual behaviors along a 7-point continuum from exclusively heterosexual (0) to exclusively homosexual (6). The Kinsey scale, then, marked a paradigm shift away from a dichotomy toward a continuum model of sexual orientation (Fox, 1996a; M. S. Weinberg, Williams, & Pryor, 1994).

Though the Kinsey surveys are unsurpassed as sociological studies of sexual behavior (De Cecco, 1990), they were not designed to describe mutually exclusive categories of human beings. Perhaps because of the psychoanalytic tradition of discriminating between heterosexual and homosexual persons, "there was at least a little confusion even in the minds of the Kinsey investigators as to whether they were rating individuals or their sex histories" (pp. 376-377). As their purpose became clearer, however, they stressed that engaging in homosexual acts does not necessarily make an individual a *homosexual*. According to Kinsey and his associates, there is no such thing as a *homosexual* or *bisexual* but, rather, only people with various combinations of behaviors. Therefore, the classifications of persons on the Kinsey scale can best be understood as the extent to which they have engaged in erotic behaviors with members of the same or other sex (Gagnon, 1990; Paul, 1996). Hypothetically, then, individuals can reposition themselves on the continuum by adding new partners to their sexual histories.

In challenging the psychoanalytic illness model, the Kinsey investigators introduced a revolutionary view that emphasizes "biological normality" and "personal diversity" (Gagnon, 1990, p. 202). To the Kinsey team, sexual behaviors reflect the diversity of nature rather than deviations from biological or cultural norms for sexual propriety and protocol (Kinsey et al., 1948). Homosexual behaviors are not seen as defects in biology but, rather, as reflections of the natural evolution of the human species. In this regard, Kinsey and his associates shared with the Freudians the perspective that there existed "a severe tension between the offerings of nature and the strictures of culture" (Gagnon, 1990, p. 188).

Kinsey Expansions

Over the years, the Kinsey scale has been challenged for suggesting an inverse or reciprocal relationship between heterosexuality and homosexuality, and for measuring sexual orientation exclusively in terms of sexual behavior. A number of researchers have attempted to expand this model to compensate for perceived deficits. During the 1970s, Storms was among the first to dispute the notion of a directly converse relationship between homosexuality and heterosexuality in a given individual. Accordingly, he found from his studies of sexuality and erotic fantasies that bisexually oriented individuals fantasize about the other sex as much as heterosexuals and about the same sex as much as lesbians and gay men (Storms, 1980, 1981; Udis-Kessler, 1992). This discovery led him to question the Kinsey scale's bipolar assumption that "the more homosexual an individual is, the less heterosexual he or she must be" (S. A. Sanders, Reinisch, & McWhirter, 1990, p. xxiii). Storms's own findings suggested that bisexuality seemed to encompass the totality of heterosexuality and homosexuality in a way not indicated by the Kinsey scale which rated bisexuality between bipolar opposites. Therefore, in 1980, he proposed a new scale that measured heterosexual and homosexual eroticism on x–y axis, with high scores on both indicating bisexuality and low scores on both indicating asexuality. Although Storms's sample was quite small and his conceptual thesis untested, his model developed more fully the concept of bisexuality by directly countering the mutually exclusive polarities of Kinsey's heterosexuality–homosexuality scale (Udis-Kessler, 1992).

Although Storms questioned the Kinsey bipolar assumption of sexual orientation, others have challenged the Kinsey scale's rather singular concentration on sexual conduct by focusing on cognitive and affective components as well as behavioral variables. For example, McConaghy (1987) found that more than 40% of 346 Australian medical students surveyed acknowledged current awareness of some homosexual feelings. Likewise, in their survey of 428 adults, L. Ellis, Burke, and Ames (1987) found that about one-third of both men and women reported "at least occasionally fantasizing about sexually interacting with members of the same sex" (p. 523). As a result of these and similar findings, most current conceptualizations of sexual orientation consider feelings and fantasies along with sexual behavior and, thus, are more comprehensive indices than the earlier scales. The assessment instruments of Klein and Coleman discussed next illustrate the multidimensional nature of human sexual orientation as well as demonstrate the complexity of its measurement.

Variable	Past	Present	Ideal
Sexual Attraction*			
Sexual Behavior*			
Sexual Fantasies*			
Emotional Preference*			
Social Preference*			
Hetero/Homo Lifestyle**			
Self-Identification**			

People rate themselves on a 7-point scale from 1 to 7 as follows:

* 1 = other sex only
  2 = other sex mostly
  3 = other sex somewhat more
  4 = both sexes equally
  5 = same sex somewhat more
  6 = same sex mostly
  7 = same sex only

**1 = heterosexual only
  2 = heterosexual mostly
  3 = heterosexual somewhat more
  4 = heterosexual/gay–lesbian equally
  5 = gay–lesbian somewhat more
  6 = gay–lesbian mostly
  7 = gay–lesbian only

FIGURE 2.1. Klein Sexual Orientation Grid. From Klein (1993, p. 19). Copyright by Harrington Park Press, an imprint of The Haworth Press. Reprinted by permission.

Klein Sexual Orientation Grid

Psychiatrist Fritz Klein (Klein, 1990; Klein, Sepekoff, & Wolf, 1985) presumed that sexual orientation is comprised of both sexual and nonsexual elements that vary over time. Accordingly, he and his colleagues developed the Klein Sexual Orientation Grid (KSOG) (see Figure 2.1) to measure sexual orientation as a multivariate and dynamic process. To the single variable of sexual behavior measured on the Kinsey scale, Klein added six others: sexual attraction and fantasy, social and emotional preferences, self-identification, and lifestyle. These seven components of sexual orientation were then placed on the *x*-axis of a grid; three other measures (past, present, and ideal) that reflect the dynamic nature of these multiple components were placed on the grid's *y*-axis. The 21 cells on the 7-by-3 grid allow for numerical ratings from 1 to 7 which, similar to the Kinsey's ratings from 0 to 6, correspond to choices on a heterosexual–homosexual continuum. Klein (1990) noted that "the seven variables and three time frames eliminate the shortcoming of the Kinsey heterosexual/homosexual scale while taking into account the complexity of the sexual orientation concept" (p. 282).

Coleman's Assessment of Sexual Orientation

Like Klein, psychologist Eli Coleman (1988, 1990) sought to broaden or expand the concept of sexual orientation beyond that of measuring only sexual behavior, as well as to avoid the labeling implications of the Kinsey categories (Fox, 1996a; Paul, 1996). To assess in clinical interviews the intricacy of erotic attractions and experiences, Coleman constructed an instrument that incorporated nine dimensions from the related writings of other theorists. The following discussion describes these nine dimensions of Coleman's Assessment of Sexual Orientation and gives credit to those influential in developing these concepts.

Current Relationship Status

From their study of 1,000 lesbians and gay men, including monogamous and non-monogamous couples as well as sexually active and inactive singles, Bell and Weinberg (1978) concluded that psychological adjustment was correlated with lifestyle, or current relationship status. They found further that people who function in relationships were healthier psychologically and had a more integrated sexual orientation identity than did sexually inactive and dysfunctional singles. E. Coleman (1988) incorporated these findings of Bell and Weinberg (1978) on his scale by asking respondents to indicate which of seven possible relationship circumstances best described their situation. A somewhat similar variable can be found on the KSOG where it is described as *Heterosexual/Homosexual Lifestyle* and refers specifically to the group with whom individuals spend most of their time (Klein et al., 1985).

Self-Identification of Sexual Orientation

Given his beliefs that self-image strongly affects thoughts and actions and that sexual orientation changes over time, Klein et al. (1985) included past, present, and ideal ratings of self-identification on the KSOG. Coleman collapsed Klein's past and present measures and used only the *present* and *ideal* dimensions of sexual orientation self-identification on his Assessment of Sexual Orientation. These two chronological manifestations are Coleman's second and third (of nine) dimensions.

Comfort with Current Sexual Orientation Identity

From the findings of Bell and Weinberg (1978) regarding the integration of sexual orientation identity, E. Coleman (1990) concluded that "a person's self-acceptance about his or her identity is also an important qualitative descriptor" (p. 271). In addition, Cass (1979) and E. Coleman (1981/1982) recognized that self-acceptance precedes identity integration and maturity of self-concept. Thus, Coleman included a global measure of comfort with sexual orientation on his appraisal instrument.

Physical Identity

Shively and De Cecco (1977) divided sexual identity into four distinct parts: *biological sex*, *gender identity*, *sex role identity*, and *sexual orientation identity*. The first component, *biological sex*, refers to the genetic material encoded in chromosomes. Coleman refers to this fifth dimension as *physical identity* on his assessment instrument.

Gender Identity

The second of these components refers to a psychological sense or basic conviction of being male or female (Shively & De Cecco, 1977). E. Coleman (1988) contends that *gender identity* is different from *physical identity* and is not necessarily dependent on the person's biological sex, as in the case of transsexual individuals.

Sex Role Identity

Social sex role refers to compliance with culturally established norms for socially appropriate male and female attitudes and behaviors (Shively & De Cecco, 1977). Because cultural expectations about masculinity and femininity are so strong that entire identities are formed around them, Coleman refers to this component as *sex role identity* in his appraisal system.

Sexual Orientation Identity

Shively and De Cecco (1977) described *sexual orientation* as erotic and/or affectional inclination to the same and/or other sex and included this concept among their four components of sexual identity. Gonsiorek and Weinrich (1991) noted, however, that "the first three bear no necessary relationship to sexual orientation in any given individual" (p. 1). Therefore, the concepts of *physical identity, gender identity,* and *social sex role* are distinct variables that are measured separately in order not to confuse them with each other, or with the global concept of sexual orientation. Further, to refine the evaluation of *sexual orientation identity,* as well as to appraise the relationship between factors, Coleman included distinct measures of *sexual behavior, sexual fantasies,* and *emotional attachments* on his evaluation form (as suggested by Shively & De Cecco, 1977).

Ideal Sexual Identity

This measure of *ideal sexual identity* (Coleman's ninth dimension) incorporates the previously-discussed four components of *sexual orientation identity* (i.e., *physical, gender, sex role,* and *sexual orientation identities*) that were measured in the present (eighth dimension). Each of the four dimensions also is rated as a future ideal because, like Klein, E. Coleman believed in the fluidity and complexity of sexual identity. Coleman (1988) contended that "it is the comparison of the present to the future that yields the most valuable clinical information" because "with this method, the problem of permanence is addressed, as well as yielding an additional measure of self-acceptance (pp. 20, 23). On Coleman's Assessment of Sexual Orientation (see Figure 2.2), all ratings are made on pie charts rather than on bipolar scales to reflect the "integration of male and female aspects of sexual identity into a conceptual whole" (E. Coleman, 1990, p. 274).

BISEXUALITY

Each model of sexual orientation described previously considers the concept of bisexuality from its own perspective. For example, the psychoanalytic dichotomy presumes that individuals are born with bisexual orientations but normally learn to repress their homosexual impulses. The Kinsey scale rates sexual behavior on a 7-point heterosexual–homosexual continuum, with 0 reflecting exclusive heterosexuality and 6 reflecting exclusive homosexuality. Bisexuality, then, might be indicated in ratings anywhere from 1 to 5

What is your current relationship status? (check one)

☐ single; no sexual partners
☐ single; one committed partner (how long? _____)
☐ single; multiple partners
☐ coupled; living together (committed to an exclusive sexual relationship)
☐ coupled; living together (other partners permitted under certain ircumstances)
☐ coupled; living apart (committed to an exclusive sexual relationship)
☐ coupled; living apart (other partners permitted under certain circumstances)
☐ other (please specify) _____

In terms of my sexual orientation, I identify myself as. . .	In the future, I would like to identify myself as. . .
☐ exclusively lesbian/gay	☐ exclusively lesbian/gay
☐ predominantly lesbian/gay	☐ predominantly lesbian/gay
☐ bisexual	☐ bisexual
☐ predominantly heterosexual	☐ predominantly heterosexual
☐ exclusively heterosexual	☐ exclusively heterosexual
☐ uncertain	☐ uncertain

In terms of comfort with my current sexual orientation, I would say that I am. . .

☐ very comfortable	☐ not very comfortable
☐ mostly comfortable	☐ very uncomfortable
☐ comfortable	

Divide the circles into percentages or slices of a pie, indicating the degree to which your response is Male (M) or Female (F):

Physical Identity

I was born as a biological. . .   Ideally, I wish I had been born as a biological. . .

Gender Identity

I think of myself as a physical. . .   Ideally, I would like to think of myself as a physical. . .

In my sexual fantasies, I imagine myself as a physical. . .   In my sexual fantasies, I wish I could imagine myself as a physical. . .

Sex-Role Identity

My interests, attitudes, appearance, and behaviors would be considered to be female or male (as traditionally defined). . .   I wish my interests, attitudes, appearance, and behaviors would be considered to be female or male (as traditionally defined). . .

Sexual Orientation Identity

My sexual behavior has been with. . .   I wish my sexual behavior would be with. . .

My sexual fantasies have been with. . .   I wish my sexual fantasies would be with. . .

My emotional attachments (not necessarily sexual) have been with. . .   I wish my emotional attachments (not necessarily sexual) would be with. . .

FIGURE 2.2. Coleman's Assessment of Sexual Orientation. From E. Coleman (1990, pp. 272–273). Copyright by E. Coleman. Reprinted by permission.

on the scale depending on the criteria applied to the classification. The x–y axis proposed by Storms attempts to correct the Kinsey assumption that heterosexuality and homosexuality are inversely related bipolar opposites. To him, the heterosexual–homosexual trade-off of the Kinsey scale could potentially misrepresent bisexuality as a midrange compromise rather than as the ability to fully behave sexually with, and fantasize about, both sexes.

Similar to the Kinsey scale, the KSOG rates seven variables on a 7-point continuum, adding past and future dimensions to the present time frame. On the KSOG, 1 refers to heterosexual orientation and 7 refers to homosexual orientation. Bisexuality at the present time, then, might be indicated in a mean rating of 4 "even if in one case the 4 is made up of 4, 4, 4, 4, 4, 4, 4, and in another case the numbers are 3, 5, 2, 6, 1, 6, 5" (Klein, 1990, p. 281).

Rather than numerically rating people along a heterosexual–homosexual continuum, Coleman's Assessment of Sexual Orientation uses circles "that individuals can divide into percentages or slices of a pie" (E. Coleman, 1988, p. 23). Although these pie charts attempt to reflect the integration of orientation toward both sexes into the concept of sexual identity, some might misinterpret slices of a pie representing bisexuality as part heterosexuality/part homosexuality rather than as the capacity to fully eroticize both men and women, as Storms suggested.

Defining Bisexuality

Zinik (1985) refers to bisexuality as "a dual-gender sexual orientation and identity" and applies three criteria to define the concept (p. 8):

- Eroticizing or being sexually aroused by both females and males.
- Engaging in (or desiring) sexual activity with both.
- Adopting "bisexual" as a sexual identity label (as opposed to labeling one's self "heterosexual" or "homosexual").

Rather than using the three elements of arousal, activity, and identity to define bisexuality, M. S. Weinberg et al. (1994) adopted the dimensions of *sexual feelings* (sexual attractions as exemplified in fantasies, daydreams, unfulfilled desires, etc.), *sexual behavior* (i.e., actual engagement in activity), and *romantic feelings* (i.e., falling in love). They used these scales of attractions, behavior, and feelings in their study of a large sample (n = 800) of bisexual, homosexual, and heterosexual individuals. Their "use of these scales falls in the tradition of empirically assessing how the relevant dimensions combine and how this produces the variety of sexual profiles that people have who use the same label to describe their sexuality" (M. S. Weinberger et al., p. 43). In this regard, one of their purposes in conducting the research was to show what types of bisexualities exist and whether there is overlap with heterosexual and homosexual identities. Their investigation was the first to compare directly these three populations. According to the authors, "when we began our investigation ten years ago, almost nothing was known about bisexuality. Even today [1994], we are struck by the virtual absence of research on people attracted erotically to both sexes, especially in light of research that suggests that bisexuality is fairly widespread" (pp. 4–5).

Current thinking about bisexuality suggests that dimensions such as arousal (or attraction), behavior, and self-identification (or identity) are to some extent independent of each other (Firestein, 1996; Fox, 1996b). For example, several authors have concluded that the cognitive and affective dimensions of sexuality occur more frequently than do the behavioral components (Berkey, Perelman-Hall, & Kurdek, 1990; L. Ellis, Burke, & Ames, 1987; McConaghy, 1987). In other words, people think about sex and feel aroused more than they engage in erotic activity. Further, most individuals who are sexually active with both men and women do not describe themselves as bisexual. As a matter of fact, in a study of 6,982 men who admitted having had adult erotic experiences with both sexes, only 29% labeled themselves *bisexual* (Lever, Kanouse, Rogers, & Carson, 1992).

The bisexual identity is just emerging, and "its relative lack of clarity and lack of dissemination throughout our society mean that only a minority of persons who behave bisexually have adopted it" (M. S. Weinberg et al., 1994, p. 297). Hence, a definition of bisexuality based solely on identity would exclude a large number of men and fewer women with bisexual experience in adulthood (see discussion on gender differences later in this chapter). Consequently, Paul (1996) believes that "many researchers have moved away from describing individuals simply as 'bisexual' and instead are more explicit about whether people are bisexually active, self-identified bisexuals, etc." (p. 442).

Bisexual Types

Regarding self-definition of identity, M. S. Weinberg et al. (1994; discussed earlier in this chapter) were interested in how their three dimensions of *sexual feelings, sexual behaviors*, and *romantic* feelings "blend together to form a more complete sexual profile among people who define themselves as bisexual" (p. 46). The authors used Kinsey scale scores to measure the three dimensions and then focused their analysis on *groups* of respondents who had similar patterns. In accordance with current thinking, scores revealed a variety of bisexualities that are described herein in terms of four clusters conceptualized by M. S. Weinberg and his colleagues (see Figure 2.3).

The Pure Type and the Midtype

Few the self-defined bisexuals in the study fit the stereotype of being equally attracted to both sexes. Accordingly, only 2% of the men and 17% of the women fit the "pure" type, which is someone who is a perfect 3 on all three dimensions of the Kinsey scale. In contrast, the "midtype" of bisexual scored a 3 on at least one dimension and anywhere from a 2 to a 4 on the other dimensions. About a third of both men and women fit this pattern.

The Heterosexual-Leaning Type

This group of respondents scored themselves as more heterosexual than homosexual on all three dimensions, falling between 0 and 2 on each. More men (45%) fit this pattern than women (20%). The men in this cluster scored themselves as 1–2 when rating their sexual feelings and sexual activity with men but had few romantic attachments with individuals of their biological sex (0–1 on the Kinsey scale). On the other hand, *no* women assigned a 0 rating to their romantic feelings toward other women. The researchers believe that gender socialization plays an important role in these findings (see discussion later for their explanation).

Pure Type

	Heterosexual						Homosexual
Sexual Feelings	0	1	2	3	4	5	6
Sexual Behaviors	0	1	2	3	4	5	6
Romantic Feelings	0	1	2	3	4	5	6

Midtype(s)

	Heterosexual						Homosexual
Sexual Feelings	0	1	2	3	4	5	6
Sexual Behaviors	0	1	2	3	4	5	6
Romantic Feelings	0	1	2	3	4	5	6

	Heterosexual						Homosexual
Sexual Feelings	0	1	2	3	4	5	6
Sexual Behaviors	0	1	2	3	4	5	6
Romantic Feelings	0	1	2	3	4	5	6

	Heterosexual						Homosexual
Sexual Feelings	0	1	2	3	4	5	6
Sexual Behaviors	0	1	2	3	4	5	6
Romantic Feelings	0	1	2	3	4	5	6

Heterosexual-Leaning Type

	Heterosexual						Homosexual
Sexual Feelings	0	1	2	3	4	5	6
Sexual Behaviors	0	1	2	3	4	5	6
Romantic Feelings	0	1	2	3	4	5	6

Homosexual-Leaning Type

	Heterosexual						Homosexual
Sexual Feelings	0	1	2	3	4	5	6
Sexual Behaviors	0	1	2	3	4	5	6
Romantic Feelings	0	1	2	3	4	5	6

FIGURE 2.3. Bisexual types.

The Homosexual-Leaning Type

The respondents in this group rated themselves as more homosexual than heterosexual in attractions, behaviors, and romantic feelings (between 4 and 6 on each dimension). Fifteen percent of both women and men were found to be bisexuals of this type. For women, this is about the same percentage who were classified as heterosexual-leaning types. On the other hand, men were three times as likely to lean toward the heterosexual (45%), rather than the homosexual (15%), type. (Chapter 1 discussed the correlation of male attitudes with heterosexism was discussed.)

The Varied Type

M. S. Weinberg et al. (1994) found that some of the self-identified bisexuals were much more heterosexual on one dimension but considerably more homosexual on another. These individuals, as well as others who did not fit clearly into any of the type groups but had at least three Kinsey scale points between any two dimensions, were classified as the "varied type" (about 10% of both men and women). "The disjunction for the men was a greater degree of homosexual sexual activity than one might predict from their more heterosexual sexual feelings [i.e., attractions] or romantic feelings" (p. 47).

As indicated previously, gender socialization is thought to be influential in determining the patterns people reported. "Compared with women, men seem less likely to experience or explore homosexual love. Although other men may meet their needs for sex, it is women to whom they turn for romance" (M. S. Weinberg et al., 1994, p. 47). These men found it more difficult to fall in love with men than to have sex with them. For women, on the other hand, "it was easier to fall in love with other women than to have sex with them" (p. 7). Though the study found many behavioral, physical, and emotional differences between men and women, individuals of both sexes seemed to share the same traditional ideas about gender and believe that each gender had something different or unique to offer. This, apparently, "formed the basis of bisexuals' dual attractions" (p. 7).

Bisexual Patterns

The incidence of bisexuality reflected in the Kinsey research (1948, 1953) supports the belief that the capacity to respond erotically to both sexes seems to be a relatively common human characteristic (Fox, 1996a, 1996b; Toufexis, 1992; M. S. Weinberg et al., 1994). Although Kinsey and his associates found that 46% of the men and 12% of the women they interviewed reported erotic experiences with both sexes, Shuster (1987) contends that there is no bisexual standard and that bisexually oriented people have diverse sexual backgrounds. For example, studies have found that some individuals move from a heterosexual self-description to a bisexual identity, whereas others first define themselves as lesbian or gay before identifying as bisexual (Fox, 1995; Golden, 1987; Rust, 1993a, 1996). In any case, heterosexual development usually is established first, "suggesting that for the majority of bisexuals, homosexuality is an 'add on' to an already-developed heterosexuality" that does "not close the door to further development in a homosexual direction" (M. S. Weinberg et al., 1994, pp. 47 & 286). In other words, their "open gender schema" leaves unrepressed the ability to eroticize same-sex internal and external experiences. For such individuals, their bisexuality usually matures over time, depending on a range of sexual and cultural experiences; however, many do not define themselves as bisexual until years after their first dual attraction. Sexual attractions, fantasy, behavior, and self-identification thus may vary across the lifespan, not only for those with lesbian, gay, and heterosexual inclinations but for bisexual individuals as well (Fox, 1996a, 1996b).

For many bisexually-inclined people, their inclinations do not change significantly over time, but these attractions might not be expressed in actual behaviors or identities that may be constrained by the structure and dynamics of current relationships (Fox, 1996a). An example of the extent of this phenomenon is reflected in psychiatrist Judd Marmor's estimate that there are "26,943,000 married bisexual or homosexual persons living in the United States" (as cited in Hill, 1987, p. 260). Similarly, Rust (1996) conducted a study designed to examine the variety of bisexuals' relational forms. The first 577 completed questionnaires reflected that only 277 (48%) of the respondents described themselves as solely or primarily bisexual. Lesbian or gay was the self-description indicated by another 83, whereas 27 identified themselves as heterosexual. The remainder selected a variety of other self-portrayals. Rust (1996) described her data as "consistent with previous findings that many people with 'bisexual' feelings or experiences choose not to identify themselves as bisexual" (p. 134).

Bisexual Histories

Zinik (1985) identifies three general histories of simultaneous, concurrent, and serial bisexuality. *Simultaneous bisexuality* refers to conjoint erotic activity with at least one partner of both sexes during the same sexual episode. *Concurrent bisexuality* refers to parallel sexual experiences with men and with women during the same period. *Serial bisexuality* refers to alternating sexual activity with male and female sexual partners over the lifespan.

On the other hand, Klein (1993) describes four historical patterns of bisexuality: *transitional*, *historical*, *sequential*, and *concurrent*. *Transitional bisexuality* refers to the prevalent belief that all bisexuals are in a passing phase—typically from a heterosexual to a homosexual orientation. According to Klein's (1993) research and experience, however, only a small percentage of individuals use bisexuality as "a bridge to change their sexual orientation from one end of the continuum to the other" (p. 20). *Historical bisexuality* is illustrated by the person who lives a primarily heterosexual or homosexual way of life, but in whose history there are minimal to extensive bisexual experiences or fantasies. In addition, Klein's *sequential bisexuality* is similar conceptually to Zinik's *serial bisexuality*, in which a person's sexual relationships are limited to only one sex at any given phase of life. This pattern is thought to be quite common. Finally, *concurrent bisexuality* describes cases in which individuals have relationships with both men and women at the same time.

Multidimensional Sexuality Scale

The Multidimensional Sexuality Scale (MSS) developed by Berkey et al. (1990) measures various bisexual patterns and histories. Specifically, the MSS provides for the assessment of exclusively heterosexual, exclusively homosexual, and asexual orientations, as well as for distinguishing among the following six categories of bisexuality (p. 70):

- Homosexual orientation prior to exclusive heterosexual orientation.
- Heterosexual orientation prior to exclusive homosexual orientation.
- Predominant homosexual orientation with infrequent heterosexual desires and/or sexual contacts.
- Predominant heterosexual orientation with infrequent homosexual desires and/or sexual contacts.

- Equal orientation toward members of both sexes, where desires for, and/or sexual contact with members of both sexes occur on a fairly regular basis (concurrent bisexual).
- Equal orientation toward members of both sexes, where exclusive homosexual orientation is followed by exclusive heterosexual orientation (or vice versa), on an ongoing basis (sequential bisexual).

Similar to the other continuum models previously discussed, the MSS challenges dichotomous assumptions about sexual orientation, as well as validates bisexuality as a distinct sexual orientation and identity. By distinguishing among six categories of bisexuality, the scale accounts for changes in sexual orientation over time, thus generating potentially useful data in an area of bisexuality in which little research exists (Fox, 1995). Further, by including asexuality, exclusive homosexuality, and exclusive heterosexuality along with the six bisexual options, the MSS assesses the diversity, fluidity, and intricacy of bisexual orientations.

Clearly, then, bisexual identity formation cannot be conceptualized as a linear process with a fixed outcome as reflected in current models of lesbian and gay identity formation (Fox, 1996b) (see Chapter 5 for further discussion). In fact, "the development of bisexual identities has been viewed as a more complex and open-ended process in light of the necessity of considering patterns of homosexual *and* heterosexual attractions, fantasies, behaviors, and relationships that occur during any particular period of time and over time" (Fox, 1995, p. 57). In other words, shifts occur on a variety of levels and in a number of different time frames (Paul, 1996). Given the complex nature of these stressors, however, research has shown that similar to gay men and lesbians, bisexual women and men evidence no greater psychopathology or psychological maladjustment than individuals in the general population (Fox, 1996a, 1996b).

SOCIAL CONSTRUCTIONISM

Thus far, this chapter has discussed models that reflect the diversity, multidimensional nature, and fluidity of sexual orientation. As these discussions have progressed, the complexity of these formulations has increased in terms of the number of variables, patterns, and temporal dimensions considered. Psychotherapists are reminded that these current, as well as past, conceptualizations each reflect the thinking of a particular time, place, and culture. In essence, all models of sexual orientation are socially formulated within a cultural context. In fact, social constructionism implies that there is nothing essentially true about sexual orientation other than a given society's assumptions about it (Gonsiorek & Weinrich, 1991). As illustrated earlier, for example, the medical community in the late 1800s artificially created a diagnostic category of *homosexuality* in order to offer humane treatment for a condition that previous cultures had morally condemned or legally criminalized.

Gender Socialization and Identity Redefinition

In addition to models of sexual orientation, scripts for gender socialization and sexual behavior also vary between era and location (Udis-Kessler, 1990). These scripts include the gender roles and functions attached to being male or female (Nichols, 1990) which "in some way influence the development and expression of sexual orientation" (p. 352). Accordingly, gender-specific attributes may shape interpretations and manifestations of sexual orientation without necessarily altering erotic feelings and attractions. In other words, changing meanings and contexts determine the interpretation given to distinctly masculine or feminine elements of sexual attractions, behaviors, and identities but may not affect the ways in which these phenomena are experienced internally by individuals themselves.

Although the dimensions of sexual orientation are fluid and may change over time (Dworkin, 2000a, 2000b; Fox, 1996a, 1996b; Gonsiorek & Weinrich, 1991; D. Richardson, 1987; Rust, 1996; Weise, 1992), the variability of erotic and emotional attraction is not necessarily willfully chosen or intentional (Udis-Kessler, 1990). If a shift in some aspect of sexual orientation is experienced, individuals may need to redefine the way they identify sexually within the range of meanings constructed by the dominant culture, as well as those established by the sexual minority community or that exist within their ethnic or cultural group. In other words, the heterosexist majority, the gay, lesbian, and bisexual subcultures, and gender, social class, familial, and ethnic norms have created social constructs which sexual minority clients use to define themselves. (Part III further discusses this complex process of identity formation.)

Essentialism and Constructionism

Social constructionists contend that sexual orientation is not an entity in and of itself but, rather, exists only as a description of human lives and experiences. Others, conversely, describe sexuality as an essence, or ontological classification, and depict sexual orientation as an innate and fundamental component of the sexual self (Udis-Kessler, 1990). Namely, these essentialists believe that "there is a predetermined orientational 'core of truth' in any person, regardless of his or her sexual behavior" (p. 53) and that this trait is almost as immutable as height or skin color (Nichols, 1990). Not unexpectedly, social constructionists generally reject biological theories of sexual orientation (which is discussed in Chapter 3). Essentialists, however, often accept these physiological speculations. Nonetheless, their conceptualizations rarely rely exclusively on biological determinants and generally include psychological factors as well (Gonsiorek & Weinrich, 1991).

On one hand, constructionism addresses critical cultural, ethnic, social class, and political variables that govern the conceptualizations of sexual orientation and identity. On the other, minority group members often establish their social networks on the basis of perceived innate commonalities. Although constructionist interpretations may provide better explanations of human sexuality, the very components which empower sexual minorities and enable them to form communities are essentialist in nature (Udis-Kessler, 1990). Obviously, the debate is complex and ongoing. In the long run and apart from the politics, however, synthesized positions are the most likely to be empirically valid (Gonsiorek & Weinrich, 1991).

Just as clients tend to polarize sexual object choice (same vs. other sex), they also fail to grasp the difference between deterministic causations and societally influenced explanations of their sexuality. To comprehend and accept the nature of their own attractions, behaviors, and feelings, both essentialism and constructionism within the context of evolving cultural definitions must be offered for their consideration. The next chapter carries the discussion of essentialism and constructionism even further by addressing various past and current theories regarding the development of minority sexual orientations. Often by simply realizing the speculative nature of developmental influences on sexual orientation, clients can be helped further to separate the tentative opinions of others about their etiologies and formative experiences from their own truth about themselves.

CONCLUSION

This chapter discussed historical perspectives on homosexuality and contemporary models of sexual orientation, as well as bisexuality and social constructionism. These discussions offer clinicians the foundations for helping gay, lesbian, and bisexual clients develop a broader understanding and deeper appreciation of their complex sexual natures and dispositions. The biological, familial, psychosocial, and psychodynamic influences on sexual orientation discussed in the next chapter similarly provide therapists with theoretical and scientific frameworks for affirmative practice with sexual minorities.

3

Sexual Orientations: Origins and Influences

Whereas the previous chapter addressed historical and contemporary conceptualizations of heterosexual, homosexual, and bisexual orientations, this one extends the discussion further by focusing on possible developmental etiologies. Both chapters share the common purpose, though, of providing both clinicians and clients with the information and perspective necessary to view minority sexual orientations through the lens of theory and science rather than through the filter of folk wisdom and bias.

All human development involves the interaction of internal processes and environmental conditions. Thus, any application of developmental theory to sexual minority populations must consider the impact of heterosexism, racism, and sexism as well as psychobiological factors on change and growth (B. Greene, 1994a, 1994b, 1997a, 1997b). As discussed in Chapter 1, Allport (1954) was among the first to emphasize the effects of these sociocultural forces on the personality characteristics of oppressed minorities which he referred to as "traits due to victimization." Most research, however, tends to operate at the microlevel of individual and family, rather than at a macrolevel of culture and society, when examining the influence of heterosexist stigma on lifespan development (Gonsiorek & Rudolph, 1991). At the macrolevel, de Monteflores (1986) asserts that the establishment and maintenance of heterosexuality as a sociocultural norm compromises the developmental trajectory for sexual minorities as well having a great impact on their intrapsychic functioning.

According to Erikson (1963), positive identity formation is contingent upon the degree to which the previous stages of psychosocial development have been negotiated successfully. Favorable resolution of these earlier phases has been defined almost exclusively on the basis of heterosexist assumptions, and relatively little has been formulated about how bisexuals, lesbians, and gay men living in a heterosexually biased sociocultural matrix advance and transition across the lifespan (B. Greene, 1994a; Isay, 1989; Kimmel, 1978). Consequently, Gonsiorek (1994) reflects the opinion of numerous individuals whose work is described in this book that the task now is "to put our theories to empiri-

47

cal test; to engage in theoretical revision as necessary; and most important, to reconnect our theories and data to the main body of psychological theory, research, and practice" (p. ix).

Inasmuch as empirical investigation into gay, lesbian, and bisexual development lacks methodologically sound longitudinal inquiry into how sexual minorities evolve across the lifespan (D'Augelli, 1994b), the presentations in this chapter concentrate primarily on developmental variables related to minority sexual orientations rather than on empirically based theories of change and growth. This chapter considers current hypotheses and speculations regarding biological influences, familial factors, and psychosocial correlates. It also examines psychoanalytic reformulations of normative and nonpathological sexual minority development and describes reinterpretations from a self psychology perspective.

DEVELOPMENT AND MINORITY SEXUAL ORIENTATIONS

Human sexual orientations, including homosexuality, undoubtedly develop from a constellation of etiologies and involve a complex interaction of numerous forces operating in variable proportions. Some theorists have expanded on genetic–hormonal, pharmacological, maternal stress, immunological, and social experimental explanations for the entire spectrum of sexual attraction and behavior, whereas others have integrated perspectives from evolutionary biology, psychoanalysis, and social processes with various theories about the etiology of sexual orientation (L. Ellis & Ames, 1987; Gallagher, 1998; Savin-Williams, 1988; Silverman, 1990; Stoller, 1986).

Accordingly, survey results indicate that opinions of American Psychiatric Association members are moving away from the profession's singular psychosexual focus toward a more complex, interactive perspective (Vreeland, Gallagher, & McFalls, 1995). When asked their view of the etiological strength of 12 separate factors involved in male homosexuality, the two theories that received the most support were *prenatal hormone development* and *genetic inheritance*. The following discussions address these hypotheses as well as two additional developmental variables related to minority sexual orientations; they are clustered herein as biological influences, familial factors, and psychosocial correlates.

Biological Influences

Bailey (1995) believes that all behavior (including socially acquired traits) is "caused by brain states" (p. 104), and that the differences in these cerebral conditions result in behavioral variations. Because all brain states have a biological component, all behaviors therefore are "biologically determined" (p. 104). Similarly, Byne (1996) notes that "all psychological phenomena are dependent on the biological activity of the brain" (p. 130). In acknowledging the current scientific and popular interest in "biological" studies of homosexuality, Rosario (1996) notes that this attention is not as recent as some might think, but, rather, the concept has invited speculation since the term *homosexual* was coined in the late 19th century. Several excellent literature surveys relative to these biological influences on the etiology of sexual orientation are available (Bancroft, 1990;

Burr, 1993; Byne, 1994; Dickemann, 1995; Gladue, 1987, 1988; Gooren, 1990; Rosario, 1996), and summaries include descriptions of hormonal, neuroendocrine, and genetic studies, in addition to those involving offspring of hormone-treated pregnancies. A comprehensive treatment of this rapidly growing body of research is beyond the scope of this book, but brief summaries are provided in this section from the viewpoints introduced in Chapter 2. Prenatal hormonalization and neuroanatomical perspectives, however, are described under a heading titled *neuroendocrine influences*, while *genetic effects* are discussed separately.

Neuroendocrine Influences

According to Bailey (1995), the assumption behind neuroendocrine studies "is that the brains of gay men have something in common with those of heterosexual women, and similarly for lesbians and heterosexual men" (p. 107). These theories of prenatal hormonalization speculate that different levels of prenatal hormones, primarily androgens, establish brain structures that predispose individuals to diverse sexual inclinations (L. B. Silverstein, 1996), and that sexual differentiation of brain structures affects sexual orientation much as it brings about feminization or masculization of the internal sex organs and external genitalia (Byne & Parsons, 1993; Meyer-Bahlburg, 1984). In other words, the endocrine system hormonally masculinizes or feminizes the brain of the developing fetus by establishing organizing configurations that subsequently influence genital anatomy, as well as the directionality of erotic attractions. "Presumably, masculinization of the relevant brain structures in heterosexual men and homosexual women occurs because of relatively high levels of androgens, while development in a feminine direction requires a relative dearth of androgens (or relatively low sensitivity to androgens)" (Bailey, 1995, p. 109).

These neuroendocrine hypotheses make "rather strong predictions about the existence of relevant neural structures affecting sexual orientation in men and women" (Bailey, 1995, p. 109). Money (1988) maintains, however, that there is no evidence that sexual orientations are predetermined by prenatal hormones, absolutely and independently, apart from postnatal influences. Conversely, "when nature and nurture interact at critical developmental periods" (p. 50), the orientational outcomes may persist without change.

PRENATAL HORMONALIZATION

Because ethical guidelines prohibit hormonal manipulation on human fetuses, studies that have examined the effect of this orchestration on sexual behaviors have been conducted with animals. Prenatal (or even perinatal) administration of androgens, for example, has been found to increase rodent mounting behavior in both male and female rats (Bailey, 1995). On the other hand, surgical or chemical castration results in receptive "female" lordosis postures in both sexes. The question, however, is whether these rodent phenomena are directly relevant to humans as "homosexual men do not appear to show decreased mounting behavior, nor homosexual women an increase in mounting behavior, compared to their heterosexual counterparts" (p. 110). Others (Byne, 1996; Byne & Parsons, 1993) have argued, in addition, that some researchers have assumed too close a correspondence between the brain organization and sexual behavior of rats and *homo sapiens,* given that human homosexuals do not display a pattern of copulatory behavior typical of the opposite sex. Extending the argument further, Bancroft (1990) also rejects the "simplistic equation that masculinity in a man or femininity in a woman equals heterosexuality" even though the "evidence does strongly suggest that these dimensions of the human experience interact" (p. 103).

With regard to human beings, researchers have investigated the offspring of pregnancies therapeutically treated with estrogens and progestogens and the results have been inconclusive (Byne & Parsons, 1993). The findings, however, suggest that hormones do not actually determine, but may contribute to, the development of sexual orientation. Although positive correlations between prenatal sex steroid exposure and homosexuality have been found, analyses of *common* neuroendocrine functions and peripheral sex steroid (i.e., testosterone and estrogen) levels reveal no convincing differences between homosexuals and heterosexuals. Thus, it is highly improbable that further studies of these peripheral hormone values will produce clues to the nature of sexual orientation (Gooren, 1990).

On the other hand, Money (1988) contends that "there are only a few infrequently occurring clinical syndromes in which it is possible to reconstruct the prenatal and neonatal hormonal history and relate it to subsequent orientation as heterosexual, bisexual, or homosexual" (p. 50). Bailey (1995) refers to these conditions as "natural experiments" (p. 111) and sees them as helpful in understanding the effects of hormones on the development of sex-dimorphic behavior such as sexual orientation.

Two of these relatively rare hypo- and hyperandrogenizing prenatal endocrine disorders (i.e., *androgen insensitivity* and *congenital adrenal hyperplasia)* and their effects on sexuality have been studied. In androgen insensitivity syndrome, genetic males lack the gene needed to use the available androgens effectively, and, hence, aspects of feminine development occur. These males thus appear as typical females, both anatomically and psychologically, but without the internal reproductive organs characteristic of females (Money, 1988). Conversely, females affected by congenital adrenal hyperplasia (CAH) have been exposed to levels of androgens sufficient to cause a degree of genital masculinization such that the sex of the child often is ambiguous at birth (Bailey, 1995). Although most studies have found some homosexuality or bisexuality in women with CAH, the findings are inconclusive (Dittmann, Kappes, & Kappes, 1992; Money, Schwartz, & Lewis, 1984; Zucker et al., 1992).

Indirect support for a neuroendocrine theory of homosexuality, however, is provided by findings of gender atypicality in female children with CAH. Several studies of this nature are available (Bailey, 1995), one of which (Berenbaum & Hines, 1992) is considered to be the most rigorous methodologically. In this experiment, girls and boys with CAH and unaffected control boys were much more likely to play with "masculine" toys and less likely to play with "feminine" toys than were control girls, when all toys were equally available. Further, parents of both girls with CAH and nonaffected girls did not differ in their reports of behavior toward their daughters, a point which appears to neutralize the effects of postnatal socialization. To complicate the issue further, Berenbaum and Hines (1992) found that the degree of masculine toy preference in their girls with CAH was unrelated to the degree of genital virilization reported at diagnosis. Thus, toy selection and configuration of the external genitalia may be independent rather than interactive factors.

CHILDHOOD TEMPERAMENTS

One of the most probable explanations for the basis of sexual orientation lies in the belief that "certain sexually dimorphic traits or dispositions are laid down in the brain before birth" (Money & Ehrhardt, 1972, p. 244). Accordingly, these characteristics or temperaments may facilitate the development of erotic attraction "but are too strongly bivalent to be exclusive and invariant determinants of either homo- or heterosexuality, or of their shared bisexual state" (p. 244).

Bem (1996, 1997), a leading spokesperson for this line of thinking, has developed what he refers to as the *exotic-becomes-erotic* (EBE) theory of sexual orientation. He believes that the EBE theory accommodates and reconciles "the empirical evidence of the biological essentialists—who can point to correlations between sexual orientation and biological variables—and the cultural relativism of the social constructionists" (Bem, 1997, p. 1) who cite historical and anthropological evidence that the notion of sexual orientation itself is a social fabrication. In the EBE theory, biological variables (e.g., genes or prenatal hormones) provide codes for childhood temperaments rather than for sexual orientation per se. These temperaments then predispose individuals to enjoy certain kinds of activities more than others. For example, some children gravitate toward competitive sports and rough-and-tumble play (i.e., male-typical activities) or toward more social and quiet recreation, such as playing jacks, hopscotch, or dolls (female-typical activities). Bem refers to children who prefer sex-typical activities and same-sex playmates as *gender conforming*, and to those who gravitate toward sex-atypical activities and opposite-sex playmates as *gender nonconforming*. These latter individuals feel different from same-sex peers, whereas *gender conforming* youngsters feel different from opposite-sex peers.

Bem (1997) further speculates that "these feelings of being different produce heightened physiological arousal. . . . Regardless of the specific source or affective tone of the childhood arousal, it is subsequently transformed into erotic attraction" (p. 2). In other words, the gender nonconforming child feels heightened animation (e.g., anger, fear, timidity, and apprehension) around same-sex peers from whom he or she feels different (primarily in terms of interest in aggressive, rough-and-tumble play, and in general activity level), and this contrast or *exotic* is recreated into *erotic*. Bem (1997) cites extensive experimental evidence demonstrating that individuals who have been physiologically aroused will show heightened sexual responsiveness to target sources. Further, this excitement "gets eroticized when the maturational, cognitive, and situational factors coalesce to provide the defining attributional moment" (p. 4). Bem emphasizes that, while EBE theory is not an inevitable, universal trajectory to sexual orientation, it is the "modal path followed by most men and women in a gender-polarizing culture like ours" (p. 2).

MATERNAL STRESS

One specific line of biological research tests the theory that maternal stress during pregnancy temporarily blocks the synthesis and release of sex hormones which, in turn, influence the development of minority sexual orientations. For example, barbiturate and other drug use by expectant human and rodent mothers appears to have a demasculinizing influence on male offspring and a masculinizing effect on females (L. Ellis, 1996a; Money, 1988). Among nonhuman species, prenatal maternal stress also is known to have a demasculinizing effect on rat pups, but in the few studies involving human beings, the findings have been inconclusive (L. Ellis, 1996a). In one such study (L. Ellis, Ames, Peckham, & Burke, 1988), 285 women with adult children were asked to provide retrospective accounts of stressful experiences they had during the 21 months prior to giving birth. *Severely* stressful experiences helped to predict minority sexual orientation in male offspring but not in female children. Contradictory results were found by J. M. Bailey, Willerman, and Parks (1991), who obtained retrospective reports of stress during pregnancy from 215 mothers of male and female heterosexuals and bisexuals, as well as of lesbians and gay men. Data analyses revealed no maternal stress effect for either sexual orientation or overall childhood gender nonconformity, but effeminacy for boys and maternal recall of stress were linked significantly. Male homosexuality, however, was found to be strongly familial, leading the authors to suggest that genetic and systemic family influences likewise are involved.

Genetic Effects

As with temperament, Hamer and Copeland (1998) trace the connection between several large gene-linked traits, such as thrill seeking and anxiety, to specific sexual behaviors. Taking this a step farther, Hamer (according to Gallagher, 1998) believes that "a variety of genetic markers conspire in a complex manner to shape a person's tendency to be gay or straight" (Gallagher, 1998, p. 39). Likewise, Pillard (according to Gallagher, 1998) believes that the evidence favors a genetic explanation for traits, particularly sexual orientation. One method for researching biological influences on the development of sexual orientation is to study siblings and other family members (Burr, 1993). The most common genetic research methodology compares the concordance rates for sexual orientation between samples of monozygotic (MZ) and dizygotic (DZ) twins. Table 3.1 summarizes data from two of these twin studies. Claiming that their findings were consistent with those of Bailey and Pillard (1991), Whitam, Diamond, and Martin (1993) concluded that "in both studies the rates of concordance for MZ twins are sufficiently high as to suggest a strong biological basis for sexual orientation" (p. 202).

Numerous other twin studies have been conducted (Buhrich, Bailey, & Martin, 1991; Eckert, Bouchard, Bohlen, & Heston, 1986; King & McDonald, 1992), all of which point to a significant biological or genetic influence on sexual orientation. Further, this body of research suggests that genetic interactions are complex but insufficient to explain the development of erotic attraction and behavior. Beyond twins, researchers have studied other siblings of lesbians and gay men to search for biological influences. Bailey and Benishay (1993) found a higher proportion of lesbian sisters among the 84 lesbians than among the 79 heterosexual women whom they studied. They also detected a higher proportion of gay brothers among the lesbian cohort, although the difference between the two samples of women was not significant. Finally, 66 gay men with gay brothers, repre-

TABLE 3.1. Concordance Rates for Sexual Orientation between Samples of MZ and DZ Twins

Researchers	MZ	DZ
Bailey and Pillard (1991)	52% (*n* = 56)	22% (*n* = 54)
Whitam, Diamond, and Martin (1993)	65.8% (*n* = 38)	30.4% (*n* = 23)

senting 37 gay male sibling pairs, were surveyed to assess behavior of various measures (Dawood, Pillard, Horvath, Revelle, & Bailey, 2000). Consistent with studies using twins, the gay brothers were similar in their degree of childhood gender nonconfirmity. These findings and those of Bailey and Benishay (1993) seem to support the twin studies data that reflect a biological contribution to the development of a minority sexual orientation.

In addition to siblings, other family members have been studied, but with inconclusive results. For example, Zuger (1989) examined the extended families of 55 boys with "early effeminate (cross-gender) behavior." At the onset of the 30-year study, the children ranged from ages 6 to 16. The sexual orientations of 372 extended family members, including parents, siblings, aunts, and uncles, were determined. The findings indicated that boys who expressed childhood gender nonconformity (a psychosocial correlate discussed later in this chapter) were no more likely to have homosexual relatives than were boys from the general population.

Neuroanatomy

As introduced in Chapter 2, the third line of inquiry suggests that sexual orientation can be studied at the molecular level of synapses and neurons and thus examines differences in neuroanatomy between homosexuals and heterosexuals. Although sexually diverse people are thought by some to be biologically different and anatomically distinct, systematic searches for neuroanatomical correlates of human sexual orientation are "rare indeed" (Bailey, 1995, p. 116). Byne (1995, 1996), in particular, believes that studies based on measurements of human brain structures have a "dismal record of replicability" (Byne, 1996, p. 138) and that none have met the criterion of being replicated three times over. Nonetheless, a few of these investigations are discussed next.

In 1978, Gorski led a team of neurobiologists (Gorski, Gordon, Shryne, & Southam) who studied the brains of rats. These researchers located a small cluster of cells in the rodent hypothalamus which was five times larger in males than in females. Later, Gorski's colleague Laura Allen (cited in Burr, 1993, and in LeVay & Hamer, 1994) studied human brains and identified four small groups of interstitial neurons in the anterior portion of the hypothalamus, the second (INAH2) and third (INAH3) of which her research demonstrated to be significantly larger in men than in women. Swaab and Fliers (1985) reported that they, like Allen, had found evidence of neuroanatomical sex differences, or gender dimorphism in human brains. Swaab and Hofman (1990) presented research showing a suprachiasmatic nucleus dimorphic according to sexual orientation that was twice as large in gay men than in heterosexual males.

Following these researchers, LeVay (1991) hypothesized that INAH2 and INAH3 would be dimorphic according to sexual orientation as well as according to sex. In other words, he speculated that INAH2 and INAH3 would be larger in people sexually oriented toward women (heterosexual men and lesbians) and smaller in individuals sexually oriented to men (heterosexual women and gay men). Thus, LeVay dissected brain tissue obtained from routine autopsies of 19 gay men, 16 presumed heterosexual men, and 6 presumed heterosexual women. No brain tissue from lesbians was available, thus, rendering his initial hypothesis difficult to prove. Nonetheless, he not only found, like Allen and Gorski, that INAH3 was more than twice as large in the men than it was in the women but also that it was two to three times larger in heterosexual males than it was in gay men. "This finding suggests a difference related to male sexual orientation about as great as that related to sex" (LeVay & Hamer, 1994, p. 46). Unfortunately, women have not been included in genetic and/or neuroanatomical research populations in sufficient numbers to make similar statements in their regard (Gallagher, 1998).

Summary

Despite the earnest efforts of researchers, Gooren (1990) concludes that "up to the present day, solid evidence of biological correlates of homosexuality is lacking" (p. 85). Similarly, Bailey (1995) refers to the current state of research as "one of inconclusive complexity" (p. 129). Several rudimentary research trails are fragmentary and have yielded inconclusive results, leading LeVay (according to Gallagher, 1998) to comment about the lack of "huge breakthroughs" in the area of biology (Gallagher, 1998, p. 39). Further, numerous single-strand attempts to study a multivariate and dynamic concept like sexual orientation are bound to bump into other influences that likewise must be considered. Several of these familial factors are discussed next. Psychosocial correlates are presented in a following section.

Familial Factors

Prior to the 1980s, numerous articles exploring the relationship between family composition, family dynamics, and same-sex orientation appeared in professional journals. Seemingly, the main purpose of these studies and discussions was to identify etiological family correlates of homosexuality for the purpose of either preventing or curing a perceived developmental disorder. A much smaller amount of this literature has been published in recent years, and that which is available appears mainly in the psychiatric and psychoanalytic journals. Familial factors, nevertheless, must be considered when questioning the developmental derivations of minority sexual orientations. In the following section, two family-of-origin variables are addressed, namely, family composition and family dynamics. Although these concepts are presented as discrete elements, they likely interact with each other, as well as with the biological influences discussed previously.

Family Composition

In some of the pre-1980s studies dealing with lesbian family composition, "only child" status was examined and contradictory findings resulted. For example, the data from one study (Hogan, Fox, & Kirchner, 1977) indicated a high percentage of single offsprings in a sample of 205 lesbians, while those from another survey of 202 lesbians (Perkins, 1978) revealed no significant relationship between being an only child and developing a lesbian sexual orientation. In a later replication study (Hogan, Kirchner, Hogan, & Fox, 1980), however, significant differences were detected between the 137 lesbian women who were only children and the 68 who had siblings. The conclusion from these investigations suggests that single offspring status plays an etiological role in the formation of various attitudes in adult lesbians but not necessarily in the development of lesbianism itself.

Some research attention continues to focus on extended families. Comparison survey data from 193 gay men, 204 lesbians, and 273 heterosexual males (Blanchard & Sheridan, 1992), for example, reflected that lesbians had more siblings than do heterosexual males but not as many as gay men, who had more siblings, more brothers (131 brothers per 100 sisters), and a later birth order than the other two groups. In another study, Blanchard and Bogaert (1996a) administered questionnaires to 302 homosexual men and 302 age-matched heterosexual men. Results indicated that homosexuality was correlated positively with the number of *older* brothers but not with the number of younger brothers or with sisters of any birth order. Further, each older brother was found to increase the odds of homosexuality by 33% but older sisters neither enhanced nor counteracted this effect.

Another data set (i.e., survey interviews of 4,104 heterosexual and 844 homosexual White postpubertal males conducted by the Kinsey Institute from 1938 to 1963) provided the same investigators (Blanchard & Bogaert, 1996b) with results that extended previous findings. Accordingly, homosexual men were found to have a later birth order, and a greater number of *older* brothers, but not more older sisters, than heterosexual men. Bogaert (1997) also used the Kinsey database to examine birth order in lesbians ($n = 257$) and heterosexual women (5,008) and found no significant birth order effect. Finally, the two investigators (Blanchard & Bogaert, 1997) again replicated their findings after surveying 343 heterosexual and homosexual males over age 40 about the marital histories and heterosexual cohabitation patterns of their 717 siblings. Never-married male siblings (most of whom were thought to be homosexual) were more likely to come from the sibships of the homosexual probands, and they had a greater average number of older brothers. As expected, there were no significant findings for the female siblings.

Blanchard and his colleagues (Blanchard, Zucker, Siegelman, Dickey, & Klassen, 1998) continued their investigation when they surveyed 964 homosexual and heterosexual male and female volunteers and found that gay men have a higher mean birth order than do heterosexual men, primarily because they have a greater number of older brothers. They hypothesized that this phenomenon reflects the progressive immunization of certain mothers to H-Y antigen by succeeding male fetuses and the increasing effects of H-Y antibodies on sexual differentiation of the brain in succeeding male fetuses. Lesbians did not differ from the heterosexual women with regard to any class of sibling.

As to the frequency of homosexuality among siblings of lesbians and gay men, some research attention has been given to the investigation of this occurrence. Bailey and Benishay (1993), for example, recruited 79 heterosexual and 84 lesbian women plus 60% of their 395 siblings. Findings revealed that 15.4% of the sisters of the lesbian probands rated themselves as either lesbian or bisexual, whereas only 3.5% of the sisters of heterosexual women similarly described themselves. Pillard, Poumadere, and Carretta (1981) likewise examined the family trees of 80 "sex variant" subjects in an earlier study (Henry, 1941) and concluded that 10.6% of the brothers were gay and 7.7% of the sisters were lesbian. In this same literature review, the authors (Pillard et al., 1981) noted that Henry's subjects, as well as those of several other researchers, came from families with an aggregation of homosexual members that exceeded chance. In a later review, Pillard (1996) also cited several studies that detected this same phenomenon. He concluded this summary by noting that "powerful evidence exists that homosexuality runs in families and no evidence contradicts it" (p. 120).

Family Dynamics

As discussed previously, much of the early research that investigated the family dynamics of sexual minorities was designed to identify familial variables related to the development of homosexuality so that a cure or a prevention for this supposed disorder could be developed. The first studies focused on gay men, and only recently have the families of origin of lesbians been examined (Dancey, 1990; Moberly, 1986). In one of the older studies, Stephan (1973) compared survey data from a sample of 88 young gay male activists and a control group of 105 heterosexual men on variables relating to parental relationships and early social experiences. His findings revealed that the mothers of gay men were more dominant and affectionate than their fathers, that neither parent encouraged their gay sons to develop masculine role behaviors, and that positive masculine role models were less available for them than for their heterosexual counterparts. Similarly, Hendin (1978) reviewed anthropological studies and concluded that male homosexuality results from the confusion of parents about their own sexual identity and their collusion to stifle masculinity in their sons. In these families, anger is eroticized, whereas competition and envy surround the negotiation of gender roles.

From a potentially pathologizing similar perspective, Bieber and Bieber (1979) reported data from psychiatric interviews with over 1,000 Black, White, and Puerto Rican gay men and 100 pairs of their parents. After reviewing their findings, they contended that gay men have a basically masculine identification but that their sense of masculinity is impaired. The Biebers further concluded that unsatisfactory relationships between parents, overly close bonds between mothers and their gay sons that discourage assertiveness in the offspring, hostile and competitive fathers who did not counteract detrimental maternal influences, and disturbed sibling relationships induce the adaptation of sons to homosexuality.

The early thinking about lesbian development, though not based in empiricism, was comparable essentially to that describing the etiology of homosexuality in gay men (Magee & Miller, 1996); namely, lesbianism resulted from such dynamics as failed identification with the mother, object relations with the maternal caretaker that were disturbed to the point of inducing identification with the father, and failed separation–individuation from the mother. Accordingly, early physical or emotional separation from the same-sex parent was thought to produce a defensive reaction against positive identification in both sexes (Moberly, 1986). In other words, homosexuality was a developmental disorder in which incomplete gender identification resulted in the disidentification between boys and their fathers as well as girls and their mothers.

To base these kinds of speculations on accurate data, Dancey (1990) examined the influence of family attitudes and behaviors (i.e., parental affirmation, family protectiveness, gender role enforcement, and maternal supportiveness) on female sexual orientation in a sample of 88 women. Her findings subsequently indicated that no single element or constellation of variables significantly predicted heterosexuality or lesbianism within her population. After examining empirical investigations similar to the one conducted by Dancey, as well as numerous case studies, Magee and Miller (1996) concluded that "the . . . search for distinguishing etiology and distinguishing clinical characteristics of gay men and lesbian women has to date met with no more success than the similar search undertaken by sexologists or biological investigators" (p. 203). Bailey (1995) concurred that "these theories have generated remarkably little empirical support" (p. 108). Even in the instance of the one that has garnered the most advocates (i.e., that homosexual males appear to have poorer childhood relationships with their fathers than do male heterosexuals), "the direction of causation is ambiguous" (p. 108). For example, it is possible that the fathers are reacting to the effeminate childhood behaviors of their "prehomosexual" sons rather than causing their homosexuality (Bailey, 1995; L. Ellis, 1996b).

Psychosocial Correlates

In addition to biological influences and familial factors, psychosocial variables have been figured into the multiplex formula for understanding the development of sexual orientations, including homosexuality and bisexuality. The effect of early sexual experiences is discussed briefly in this regard. The ramifications of gender nonconformity, however, are considered in more detail because considerable speculation has arisen around this concept.

Early Sexual Experiences

During the initial stages of the identity formation process, many gay, lesbian, and bisexual clients wonder whether early sexual experiences, particularly negative ones, have influenced the development of their homosexuality. As mentioned previously, sexual minority youth have reported higher rates of parental beatings, physical and sexual abuse, rape, and incest than do heterosexual children and adolescents (Bradford et al., 1994; D'Augelli, 1998). Incidents such as these undoubtedly prompt individuals to question the relationship between these unpleasant events and their homosexuality.

Some studies have attempted to unravel the complexities of this question. Peters and Cantrell (1991), for example, examined differences between 134 lesbians and 105 heterosexual women to test the theory that lesbians would report more negative early sexual experiences with males and more positive early sexual experiences with females than did their heterosexual counterparts. Their findings, however, confirmed neither of these hypotheses and supported the conclusion that a lesbian orientation cannot be understood in terms of early sexual trauma or negative heterosexual encounters. On the other hand, Van Wyk and Giest (1984) sampled 7,669 adult men and found a correlation between being gay and positive same-sex experiences. Accordingly, men who disclosed that their first erotic encounters were with other males tended to be gay and to have developed differently from those who reported that their initial sexual experiences were with females. Though this imprinting theory appears to have some support particularly with regard to early maturing males (Storms, 1981; Wasserman & Storms, 1984), virtually all research that has attempted to demonstrate a causative relationship between early negative sexual experiences and homosexuality has failed to demonstrate significant findings.

Although it is widely recognized in scientific circles that correlation does not equal causation, the works of psychologist Paul Cameron and his colleagues nonetheless have had a considerable effect on state and national public opinion and policy regarding homosexuality (Herek, 1998a). By linking homosexuality to such causes as incest, child molestation, and gay or lesbian parenting (Cameron & Cameron, 1995, 1996a, 1996b), the Cameron group has promoted stigma and fostered "unfounded stereotypes of lesbians and gay men as predatory, dangerous, and diseased" (Herek, 1998a, p. 247). Herek (1998a) contends that serious researchers have virtually ignored their publications and findings, citing reasons such as sampling errors, low response rates, small subsamples, doubtful validity of questionnaire items, and bias during interviewing and data collection. Nonetheless, voters for statewide anti-gay amendments, members of Congress formulating policy for the military, and many citizens themselves have taken the biased and unfounded findings as fact and at face value. Likewise, although they probably have not heard of Cameron, many clients have formed their self-concepts by widespread misinformation promulgated by spokespeople such as Cameron.

Gender Nonconformity

As introduced in Chapter 1, nonconformity to the standards of gender role socialization stigmatize gender-discordant heterosexuals as well as homosexuals. For centuries, masculine women and feminine men have been perceived as sexually different. Further extending this stereotype, "students of human sexuality have observed, rightly or wrongly, that homosexual men often appear more 'feminine' than heterosexual men and homosexual women seem more 'masculine' than their heterosexual counterparts" (Pillard, 1991b, p. 32). Pioneers in the field of sex research discussed this issue extensively. For example, Richard von Krafft-Ebing (1894/1965), author of the text *Psychopathia Sexualis*, classified gay men according to either their loss of masculine personality traits or their acquisition of feminine characteristics. Karl Heinrich Ulrichs, who was introduced in the second chapter, believed that those who are now called lesbians and gay men were born with the mind and soul of one sex in the body of the other. Also in the 19th century, Havelock Ellis referred to this gender reversal as inversion and believed that some degree of boyishness was always present in inverted women (Pillard, 1991b). Over the years, the popularity of these theories have prompted research efforts aimed at establishing a link between gender nonconformity and same-sex orientation (Dawood et al., 2000).

CHILDHOOD GENDER NONCONFORMITY

Bailey and Zucker (1995) conducted a meta-analysis of 32 retrospective studies comparing childhood sex-typed behavior and adult sexual orientation and obtained a large effect size of approximately 1.3 for the comparison between gay and heterosexual men. According to their calculations, almost 90% of gay men exceeded the typical heterosexual man on scores of childhood feminine gender identity (e.g., cross-dressing, lack of interest in rough play or sports, preference for female peers, and interest in feminine activities and toys), whereas only 2% of the heterosexual men scored above the representative gay man. The investigators (Bailey & Zucker, 1995) also conducted a similar meta-analysis of 16 studies of women in order to examine the association between childhood gender nonconformity in girls and subsequent adult sexual orientation. Similar to their examination of the 32 studies involving males (described earlier), lesbian and bisexual women recalled significantly more childhood masculinity on most measures, and no study reported higher scores for heterosexual women on a masculinity measure. The effect size separating the lesbian and heterosexual women was large (1.0) but nevertheless was significantly smaller than that for Bailey and Zucker's (1995) meta-analysis of men (1.3). Accordingly, 81% of the lesbians exceeded the typical heterosexual woman on measures of childhood gender nonconformity, whereas only 12% of heterosexual women surpassed the characteristic lesbian.

As can be seen in Bailey and Zucker's (1995) two analyses, the majority of the earliest studies examining the relationship between childhood gender identity and adult sexual orientation focused on males. No prospective study has followed tomboys into adulthood, but the retrospective studies indicated that lesbians tended to be more tomboyish children than were girls who later became heterosexual women (Bailey, 1996). The findings, however, suggest "that masculine childhood gender identity is less predictive of homosexuality in women than is feminine childhood gender identity in men" (p. 78). In other words, there probably are "more tomboys who later identified as heterosexual women than feminine boys who become heterosexual men" (p. 78).

In one of the pre-1990s studies of women (R. Green, Williams, & Goodman, 1982), 49 tomboys were compared to 50 traditionally sex-typed girls. Findings reflected that the tomboys were significantly different from their peers with respect to their choice of toys, preference for male playmates, level of sports participation, the nature of the roles assumed in playing house, and the expressed wish to be a boy. Similarly, R. Green (1985, 1987) studied 66 boys whom he referred to as *feminine* (males ages 4–12 in whom several cross-gender behaviors were described by their parents as "frequently" present) and contrasted them with a more sex-typed matched comparison group (*n* = 56). Between 50% and 80% of the *feminine* boys, compared with between 5 and 10% of the control group, were reported to cross-dress, play with dolls, take female roles in games such as playing house, relate better to girls rather than boys as peers, and mention at least an occasional wish to be a girl. Parents noted that the nonmasculine behaviors emerged when their sons were quite young, with three-quarters of the boys described as cross-dressing before the age of 4; virtually all boys had begun by the age of 6. Approximately two-thirds of each sample remained in the study at its conclusion and were available for interviewing during the subjects' adolescence or early adulthood. In the final analysis, three-fourths of the *feminine* boys, compared to only one in the *masculine* cohort, were found to be homosexual or bisexual as measured by Kinsey ratings of sexual fantasies and patterns of sexual behavior.

Zuger (1984) similarly studied 55 feminine boys whose average age was 9. In his interviews with their parents, only two mothers dated the outset of their son's effeminate behavior after the age of 6. Forty-eight of the participants were available for follow-up when they were at an average age of 19.7 years. His findings were comparable to R. Green's (1985, 1987) in that 73% (35 of the 48) of the men were judged to have homosexual or bisexual orientations, 6% (*n* = 3) were heterosexual, and 21% (*n* = 10) could not be determined due to insufficient information (not surprising given the relative youth of the subjects [19.7 years] and the probable early stages of identity formation for those who would eventually identify as gay). Zuger (1988) also observed 57 boys who were formally admitted to his study around the age of 5 but whose effeminate behavior was identified as early as age 2. He concluded, after following the boys for 10 years, that differences in heterosexual and homosexual development become apparent at about 2 years of age and that early feminine behavior and later homosexuality are part of a consistent developmental sequence.

Whitam (1977) also found significant differences between gay (*n* = 206) and heterosexual (*n* = 780) subjects on the basis of six childhood indicators of male homosexuality: interest in dolls, cross-dressing, preference for playing with girls rather than boys, preference for the company of older women rather than older men, being seen by other boys as a sissy, and interest in sex play with boys rather than girls. He concluded that for males, the stronger the gay sexual orientation ratings, the greater the number of childhood indicators. Several years later, Whitam and Mathy (1991) replicated these findings with a cross-cultural sample of female subjects. Accordingly, they interviewed 225 heterosexual women and 222 lesbians from Brazil, Peru, the Philippines, and the United States regarding their childhood cross-gender behavior. Their data revealed statistically significant childhood differences in play, dress, and socialization between the lesbian and heterosexual women and significant cross-cultural consistency. The investigators consequently speculated that the concordant patterns of these differences may reflect universal aspects of sexual orientation and gender development.

Billingham and Hockenberry (1987) studied gender (non)conformity, objects of childhood infatuation and adolescent masturbation fantasies and found that all three of these variables could differentiate between heterosexual (n = 69) and gay (n = 106) men. They thus concluded that adult sexual orientation can be predicted from childhood behaviors and fantasies. In part from Whitam's (1977) six childhood indicators of homosexuality, as well as from a scale measuring feminine gender identity, Hockenberry and Billingham (1987) developed the Boyhood Gender Conformity Scale (BGCS). After evaluating 118 gay and 110 heterosexual men, they found that the BGCS significantly differentiated between the two adult male groups. In addition to substantiating the findings of similar studies, the research team discovered that the absence of masculine behaviors and traits (i.e., imagining oneself as sports figure and reading adventure and sports stories) was a stronger predictor of gay identification in adulthood than traditionally feminine or gender-discordant traits and behaviors.

CONTRADICTORY EVIDENCE?

In a study that appears to differ from the findings of Billingham and Hockenberry (1987), 139 male participants (54 heterosexuals, 24 bisexuals, and 61 gay men) were asked to recall on the BGCS the degree to which they had engaged in gender-conforming (masculine) and gender-discordant (feminine) behaviors during childhood (Phillips & Over, 1992). No significant differences were found in the potential of childhood memories to predict adult sexual orientation. In other words, recollections of childhood gender conformity and gender discordance did not differ in their ability to forecast heterosexual, bisexual, or gay identification in adulthood.

Just as memories have not been found to predict adult sexual orientation, neither have childhood photographs. Twenty judges in one study were unable to differentiate between 19 gay and 11 heterosexual men by comparing pictures of them when their ages ranged between 6 months and 6 years (Grellert, 1989). In a companion study, a factor analysis of personality characteristics observed by evaluators in these photographs delineated two traits associated with masculinity (i.e., extroversion and toughness). The two groups of men were found not to differ on these masculine attributes, however.

Carrier (1986) questions research that attempts to find a relationship between childhood cross-gender behavior and adult homosexuality. First, the limited amount of data from these studies precludes the generalization of these findings to larger populations. Further, differences among measures used to describe childhood behavior and the lack of generally accepted criteria for childhood cross-gender characteristics generate problems in interpreting the results. More important, however, Bailey (1996) contends that "retrospective studies have serious methodological limitations" since "memory is imperfect, especially for events that occurred years ago" (p. 77). He also believes that, because of traditional male gender role socialization, gay men may be more likely to remember or even exaggerate feminine childhood behaviors while heterosexual men could tend to deny or forget such actions. Despite these possible methodological biases, however, the preponderance of evidence from retrospective and prospective studies converge to suggest that "feminine boys become gay men at much higher rates than expected, . . . and a substantial percentage of gay men were somewhat feminine boys" (p. 77). Given the likelihood of alternative developmental routes to adult male homosexuality, some typically masculine boys consequently become gay men just as some gay men are stereotypically masculine. Regardless of the degree to which preadolescent gender discordance is associated with adult homoeroticism, Zucker and Bradley (1995) note that "there are simply no formal empirical studies demonstrating that therapeutic intervention in childhood alters the developmental path toward . . . homosexuality" (p. 270).

ADULT GENDER NONCONFORMITY

Gender nonconformity has been studied in adults as well as in children for the purpose of exploring its relationship to same-sex orientation. D. Hawkins, Herron, Gibson, and Hoban (1988), for example, administered six sex role scales, including the Bem Sex-Role Inventory, to a sample of 120 men and women representing both majority and minority sexual orientations. Results indicated that lesbians and gay men differed from heterosexuals in their responses on the subscales of the various instruments. The most consistent difference was the greater femininity of gay men compared with heterosexual men. Another study (Downey, Ehrhardt, Schiffman, & Dyrenfurth, 1987) found lesbians to be more physically active than heterosexual women.

In other research with female populations, however, Armon (1960) found that heterosexual and lesbian women differed very little on variables of dependency, perception of femininity, and perception of masculinity. Lesbians, in fact, viewed both masculinity and femininity in much the same way as did heterosexual women and were no less dependent than their nonlesbian counterparts. Dancey (1992) likewise found that masculine and feminine personality variables (instrumentality and expressivity, respectively) were unable to predict sexual orientation in 54 lesbians and 105 heterosexual women. The lesbians differed neither from the heterosexual women nor from the 161 control group members unless they were being compared to housewives who tended to score lower on masculine instrumentality. In other words, lesbians were found to be more instrumental (i.e., masculine) than housewives but no more instrumental than heterosexual women in general.

COGNITIVE DIFFERENCES

In addition to studies of gender nonconformity in childhood and adulthood, research efforts have been made to determine whether gender-atypical patterns of cognitive ability are associated with same-sex orientation. Theoretically, this particular line of inquiry is based on the notion of heterosexual/homosexual dimorphism in human neuroanatomy (as discussed earlier in this chapter), as well as on the hypothetical effects of cross-gender role socialization on sexual minority populations (e.g., the development of expressive language skills among gay men; see Willmott & Brierley, 1984).

One study in this body of research compared 20 gay men and 20 heterosexual males with 20 women of unspecified sexual orientation (Willmott & Brierley, 1984). After finding significant male group differences in Wechsler Adult Intelligence Scale (WAIS; Wechsler, 1955) verbal and performance IQs, the researchers concluded that superior verbal ability is linked with nonconforming gender-related interests characteristic of gay men. Similarly, G. Sanders and Ross-Field (1986) tested the hypothesis that gay men would resemble heterosexual females rather than heterosexual males in terms of cognitive ability. On two tasks of visuospatial ability, they found that the performances of gay men and heterosexual women did not differ significantly. On the other hand, Tuttle and Pillard (1991) found no differences on measures of cognitive ability between 49 gay men and 34 lesbians and their heterosexual comparison groups. They did find, however, that both lesbians and gay men were strongly gender-atypical on the Femininity/Masculinity scale (F/M) of the California Psychological Inventory relative to their heterosexual counterparts.

Psychodynamic Perspectives

The research summarized thus far in this chapter indicates that biological, familial and psychosocial factors influence the development of sexual orientation by interacting in multiple and complex patterns. Psychoanalysts and self psychologists also have provided their own explanations for the etiology of homosexuality, bisexuality, and heterosexuality. In this regard, both psychoanalytic reformulations for both gay men and lesbians, as well as self psychology reinterpretations are presented briefly herein.

Traditionally, psychoanalytic theory has asserted that familial factors influence many aspects of personality formation, including the development of sexual orientation. Psychoanalysts have conceptualized homosexuality as the consequence of unresolved conflicts experienced throughout the pre-Oedipal and Oedipal phases, during which insufficient identifications with same-sex parents predispose children to affectional and erotic orientations toward their own sex (Mills, 1990). Many analysts contend that these developmental disturbances and distortions imposed on the personality in early childhood are pathological conditions (R. M. Friedman, 1986; Leavy, 1985/1986).

Chodorow (1992, 1994), however, challenges the heterosexist assumptions that limit the applicability of a large amount of psychoanalytic theory to sexual minority populations. She believes that while traditional psychoanalysts have assumed heterosexuality to be the outcome of normal psychosexual development, they have neglected to describe its etiology with precision or an adequate degree of detail. Consequently, no normative model of heterosexual maturation against which to compare developmental accounts of homosexuality has been developed. Further, most psychoanalytic explanations of sexual orientation imply that heterosexuality and homosexuality are structurally similar in terms of defenses, drives, conflict resolution, and the role of object relations in ego development. Thus, distinguishing between heterosexuality and homosexuality according to any criteria other than a statistical standard of normalcy becomes a difficult task.

Like Chodorow, others question the widespread belief regarding the normative nature of heterosexuality (Blum & Pfetzing, 1997; Corbett, 1996, 1997; Glassgold & Iasenza, 1995; Gould, 1995; Isay, 1986; Morgenthaler, 1984/1988). Morgenthaler also contends that the influence of Judeo-Christian ethics and values permeates psychoanalysis and that ethnocentric psychoanalytic theory ignores important elements of non-Western cultures such as diverse mothering styles and gender delineations. From his ethnopsychoanalytic perspective, homosexuality is normally equivalent to heterosexuality and mutually exclusive sexual categories are false social constructs based on the prevailing conditions of society.

Psychoanalytic Reformulations

N. O'Connor and Ryan (1993) argue "that there should be theoretical and conceptual space in psychoanalytic theory for non-pathological possibilities in relation to homosexuality" (p. 10). In this regard, they contend that there are virtually no case histories available of lesbians and gay men who have been treated from anything other than the traditional approach that considers heterosexuality as normative. Respecting the significant diversity among sexual minority people, N. O'Connor and Ryan do not present an alternative or reformed theory of psychoanalysis but instead question traditional thinking. Finally, they find it "striking that hitherto the main challenges to the universality of the Oedipus complex have come either from a cross-cultural perspective [e.g., Morgenthaler], or from those speaking from a position of exclusion and marginality and not included within the mainstream of psychoanalytic positions" (p. 268).

Sohier (1986), as well, departs from traditional theory when she expands the Eriksonian concept of mutuality to include same-sex partnerships. Erikson believed that only heterosexual couples had the capacity for true mutuality and used the term *mutual narcissistic mirroring* to describe the interactive processes operating between same-sex partners. Sohier challenges his belief and contends that gay men and lesbians are equally capable of commitment, generativity, and true engagement with others. In other words, same-sex orientation does not correlate necessarily with narcissism, and sexual minorities are as capable as heterosexuals of close interpersonal relationships and personality integration.

Eisenbud (1986) discusses the patriarchal bias in psychoanalysis and the "chauvinistic nature of application of certain classic dynamics to explain primary Lesbian choice" (p. 216). Although a growing number of theorists believe that central aspects of traditional theories are inadequate to explain lesbian development (Glassgold, 1995; Glassgold & Iasenza, 1995; Wolfson, 1987), others suggest that the psychoanalytic model of male homosexuality is equally out of touch with contemporary research and with patient needs (R. M. Friedman, 1986). R. C. Friedman (1986, 1988) agrees and stresses the need for revising key ideas about gay men in light of current biosocial and psychoanalytic research findings in the area of sexual orientation. For example, he disputes the traditional idea that homosexual male adult fantasies are motivated by unconscious conflict.

GAY MEN

In recent years, theorists have attempted to formulate the psychosexual development of lesbians and gay men from a normative and nonpathological perspective (Isay, 1986). For example, psychiatrist Isay (1987, 1989) argues that paternal distancing is a reaction to, rather than the cause of, same-sex dispositions in little boys. In other words, detached fathers do not induce homosexual adaptations in their sons but distance themselves in response to their children's homoerotic attractions. Blum and Pfetzing (1997) likewise note the "uncomfortable (to put it mildly)" (pp. 430–431) reactions of many fathers to their son's sexual and affectional expressions. In fact, they maintain that the young boy's endearments, attachments, and behaviors disturb not only his father but many people in his world.

Isay (1987, 1989) further contends that the majority of gay men report having distant fathers, almost all of whom have been conditioned according to the norms of masculine gender role socialization. On the other hand, nearly all homosexually oriented little boys experience a developmental need for closeness with their dads. Consequently, a father's heterosexist conditioning often leaves him feeling threatened when he perceives his son's desire for same-sex intimacy. Isay further believes that, due to this early erotic attraction and attachment to their same-sex parents, little boys who later will identify with being gay sometimes acquire feminine characteristics through maternal modeling in order to charm their fathers as their mothers have. He proposes that if fathers, in particular, could be less rejecting and more affirming, then they could help facilitate, rather than frustrate, the passage of their homosexually oriented sons through the stages of gay identity development: the acquisition stage of childhood, the consolidation of adolescence, and the integration stage of adulthood.

Also attempting to counter traditional psychoanalytic theory, Malyon (1982) offered a psychodynamic model of affirmative psychotherapy for gay men. Accordingly, he believed that internalized homophobia biases their psychological development as it "becomes an aspect of the ego, functioning both as an unconscious introject, and as a conscious system of attitudes and accompanying affects. As a component of the ego, it influences identity formation, self-esteem, the elaboration of defenses, patterns of cognition, and object relations" (p. 60). This homophobia also influences superego functioning and contributes to a tendency for guilt and intropunitiveness among gay men. Further, the adolescent task of identity formation is affected negatively in that a false identity is developed in order to obtain peer group acceptance. "This adaptation is inherently conflictive. As a result, psychological defenses become highly elaborated to bind the accompanying chronic anxiety and to maintain a tenuous and brittle false identity" (p. 61). Similar to Grace's (1979, 1992) concept of developmental lag (see Chapter 5), Malyon (1982) believed that the intrapsychic consequences of this adaptation was an interruption of sometimes a decade or more in the processes of identity formation and ego integrity. This chronological disruption, however, is not essentially pathological.

Blum and Pfetzing (1997) similarly discussed the intrapsychic effects of the "relentless shaming" (p. 431) by society of gender-atypical behaviors in "proto-gay" boys. This intense disapproval and ridicule are managed, almost always alone, with varying degrees of consciousness and unconsciousness. In any case, the widespread dishonoring becomes a source of enduring interior conflict, guilt, shame, and fear, all of which are structured internally in the psyche. A splitting of consciousness or dissociation then occurs and "these traumatic experiences are laid down as unconsciousness memory traces (often somatic), powerfully influential, reactivated later in life" (p. 433). Hence, the task of psychotherapy becomes that of illuminating this undigested material so that the ego is finally given the opportunity to digest or organize the earlier occurrences and thereby correct the "memory of humiliation" (p. 432). If the gay male client was highly gender nonconforming in childhood, clinicians specifically might have to address the depression and anxiety that has been present for most of the individual's life (Weinrich, Atkinson, McCutchan, & Grant, 1995).

LESBIANS

Psychoanalytically trained clinicians also have written regarding a normative developmental trajectory leading to lesbian object choice. Eisenbud (1982, 1986), for example, suggests that little girls who later will identify as lesbian long for closeness with their mothers and try to engage them with behaviors such as wooing, pestering or clutching. Natural weaning grief often is experienced around 18 months as the mother is perceived as having withdrawn from the daughter. In later childhood, the girl may champion, rescue, and protect the mother as "a way in" (Eisenbud, 1982, p. 100). Sometimes she tries to escape an emotional double bind by creating a tomboy role in which she outwardly rejects dolls, girl play, and mothering, as her mother rejected her. If she is punished for her active and independent activity, the little girl becomes tough and reserved. Unlike the gay men whom Isay described, however, most lesbians contend that their parents were not rejecting of their cross-gender appearance and behavior in childhood and recall early experiences of support for their "tomboyism." These women further assert that only during adolescence do parents withdraw support for their daughter's "masculine mirroring" and insist that femininity be demonstrated in character and conduct (Pearlman, 1995, p. 311).

A love–hate affair between parent and child may develop if, during the process of the lesbian daughter's individuation, the mother attempts to bind her child close to herself and demands that she replicate and mirror her image in as many ways as possible. Naturally, the little girl needs an ally in negotiating these developmental tasks and often looks to her father for help. The nature of the father's role, however, depends on his ego strength and willingness to challenge the mother, as well as on his comfort level with his daughter's gender nonconformity and nonfeminine gender role socialization (Eisenbud, 1986; Pearlman, 1995). If, because of his conditioning, he is not able to respond to her request for assistance, she often feels alone, unsupported, and invalidated.

Eisenbud (1982) contends that "when the inner love affair with a female love object becomes actualized again in later contexts," this actuality should not be depicted as "energy regressing from sexual feelings to oral dependency or to a fixation due to early seduction but as a replay of primary, sexual, erotic feeling" (p. 67). In this sense, pre-Oedipal maternal attachments are neither secondary nor inferior to later paternal Oedipal attachments but normative. A lesbian object choice also is not defensive and reparative (as Freud contended); rather, it is developmentally equivalent to a heterosexual object choice based on the assumption that the love boys develop for their Oedipal mothers depends on and is determined by their pre-Oedipal maternal attachment (Deutsch, 1995).

Eisenbud (1986) also prefers to consider lesbian development as progressive, rather than regressive, and a "primary positive early forward choice" (p. 223). Similarly, Suchet (1995) alleges that lesbian love can be established on "mature oedipal mother–daughter (and father–daughter) relationships which include self–other differentiation," rather than on the assumption of "a preoedipally based relationship with elements of fusion, regression, and lack of differentiation" (p. 55). She notes that both boys and girls need to make similar developmental shifts and will relate differently to both parents as pre-Oedipal, Oedipal, or post-Oedipal figures. Hence, the resolution of the Oedipus complex (a shift from preoedipal to postoedipal parental object relations) is normative for all individuals, regardless of sexual orientation. Rather than the sex of the post-Oedipal object, successful accomplishment of that shift is the key issue.

Self Psychology Reinterpretations

In recent years, several writers have applied self psychology principles to sexual minority populations. Unlike Sohier (1986), who denies a necessary correlation between a minority sexual orientation and narcissism, these theorists (Beard & Glickauf-Hughes, 1994; de Monteflores, 1986; Gonsiorek & Rudolph, 1991; Isay, 1987, 1989; Moberly, 1986) believe that almost every gay, lesbian, and bisexual individual suffers from a narcissistic wound. Further, they attribute these narcissistic injuries to a lack of mirroring by heterosexual parents, as well as by society at large. Most people, regardless of sexual orientation, have experienced some feelings of rejection from their parents, but rarely do heterosexuals become targets for parental disapproval based on the nature of their attractions and behaviors relative to the same and to the other sex. For lesbians, bisexuals, and gay men, however, homosexuality becomes a focus for aspects of themselves that make them feel hated and hateful (Isay, 1989). The majority have been wounded at their essential core by a (sometimes subtle) lack of parental mirroring responsiveness to their early, emerging attachment and affectionate expressions. Having no empathic other to help them "modulate affect states, process information, and verbally encode particular 'experiences' " of shame and humiliation, memory traces of these occurrences are structured internally in their psyches (Blum & Pfetzing, 1997, p. 434).

Both the devaluation and the rejection of a fundamental aspect of the self are traumatic and "for the majority of gay and lesbian youth, the point of awareness of their differentness, and eventually, homosexuality . . . is an experience in narcissistic injury" which manifests itself in low self-esteem, reduced initiative, and a lack of legitimate entitlement (Gonsiorek & Rudolph, 1991, p. 170). Because the intrapsychic effects of this wound are extensive, "the self is prone to fragmentation, enfeeblement, and disharmony" and only coming out can heal the narcissistic injury and "restore integrity and functioning to the damaged self" (p. 171).

de Monteflores (1986) contends that the narcissistic disturbance which affects many lesbian and gay individuals can be distinguished from a diagnosable narcissistic personality disorder. Accordingly, she refers to "areas of difficulty within the large frame of a healthy ego" (p. 85) which were not mirrored by society and significant others. Her explanation of the narcissistic wound experienced by rejected individuals and groups is similar to the interpretation of Beard and Glickauf-Hughes (1994), who consider the injury an outcome of "the parent's inability to provide accurate empathy, mirroring, and acceptance for the gay child's 'true self' " (p. 35). Chapter 8 includes a discussion of this narcissistic-appearing characterological overlay to personality structure (Gonsiorek, 1982), as well as suggestions for distinguishing it from a true Axis II personality disorder.

All the self psychologists discussed previously believe that the mirroring of the client by the psychotherapist can heal this narcissistic injury. Accordingly, de Monteflores (1986) asserts that the clinician must embrace the universe of the client, "recreating a kind of omnipotent union" (p. 100). Similarly, Gonsiorek and Rudolph (1991) believe that the psychotherapist serves as a selfobject in "empathic intuneness with the client" and, through mirroring, facilitates the "delayed structuralization of the self" (p. 173). By providing "adequate narcissistic supplies" (Beard & Glickauf-Hughes, 1994, p. 35), clinicians offer clients a corrective emotional experience that was lacking in their families and missing from their childhoods. In the selfobject transference with the psychotherapist, developmental needs are reanimated and narcissistic injuries reassessed (Moberly, 1986).

CONCLUSION

This chapter addressed variables related to the development of sexual orientation. Scientific inquiries into three biological influences—neuroendocrine, genetic, and neuroanatomical—were reviewed. Some of these failed to differentiate between human and rodent sexual behavior and attraction, while others searched for simple biological determinants of culturally determined constructs (Paul, 1993). A discussion of familial factors included research on family composition and family dynamics. Studies that considered early sexual experiences and gender nonconformity comprised a summary of psychosocial correlates associated with the formation of erotic attachments and attractions.

Information from these investigations can be used to address the concerns of both sexual majority and minority clients, whose worst fears often are reflective of the heterosexism of the dominant culture. Many men, for example, automatically wonder whether they are gay when they are unable to form intimate relationships with women (Goff, 1990). Other individuals, both male and female, who are now or have been gender nonconforming, may experience same-sex attractions regardless of their sexual inclinations (McConaghy & Silove, 1991). In any case, psychotherapeutic perspective on the variables related to the development of sexual orientation often clarifies confusion and relieves anxiety in clients.

Not unlike some of the researchers cited on the previous pages, sexual minority clients often wonder how they developed affectional and erotic attractions to their own or both sexes. Further, many try to reduce the *cause* or *origin* of their sexual orientation to a single factor or set or variables. Although some compare their growth and change patterns to those of heterosexuals, others seek psychotherapy for answers to their etiological questions and developmental concerns. Before responding to these inquiries and issues, however, clinicians need to remind both themselves and their clients that even the questions and concerns *themselves* are laden with heterosexist assumptions. In other words, social and cultural influences on the development of oppressed populations, especially sexual minorities, must be explained to help clients see that they personally are not dishonored. Rather, *all* gay, lesbian, and bisexual development is compromised by heterosexism.

The dominant society has adopted many of the heterosexist assumptions of traditional psychoanalytic theory regarding the formation of sexual orientation. Sexual minority clients thus may benefit from psychoanalytic reformulations that depathologize and normalize gay, lesbian, and bisexual development. Likewise, affirming reinterpretations from a self psychology perspective may relieve some of the psychic pain inflicted by the lack of mirroring which led to their narcissistic injuries. The next chapter examines the status of sexual minorities under laws that often reflect and reinforce heterosexist suppositions. Ongoing efforts to maximize legal protection and minimize injustice are described for clients and their therapists.

4

Sexual Orientation and the Law

This chapter discusses the constitutional rights and numerous legal concerns of sexual minority clients and illustrates ongoing efforts to minimize their unequal protection under the law. As indicated in these discussions, the current legal status of gay, lesbian, and bisexual Americans varies from state to state and from city to city. These variances in legal standing reflect the ambivalence and reluctance of U.S. society, culture, and politics to recognize, guarantee, and defend the civil rights of sexual minority citizens. The legal inequities they encounter further reveal the social, cultural, and political heterosexism that has been cited throughout this book as a major source of psychosocial stress.

Sexual minority citizens often are treated differently under the law from their heterosexual counterparts. In fact, many of the very civil rights and liberties that most Americans take for granted are not available to lesbians, bisexuals, and gay men. Because sexual minorities are not protected to the same degree as other U.S. residents, they are legally vulnerable in numerous areas of their lives. Some of these legal issues involve the following:

- Discrimination based on sexual orientation
- Unfair employment practices
- Unequal access to housing and public accommodations
- Denial of marriage and family privileges and benefits
- Refusal of parental and custodial rights
- Lack of assurances of physical safety
- Restricted freedom of expression and association in the armed services
- Immigration restrictions

Although providing legal guidance is beyond the scope of psychotherapeutic practice, clinicians need to understand the potential legal ramifications of many of the issues that clients bring to therapy. Often their distress revolves around one or more of the concerns listed previously, yet they and sometimes their therapists are unaware of possible

68

avenues of legal resolution that may be available. Clinicians also may need a certain amount of contextual information to determine whether specific client dilemmas warrant a referral to appropriate legal counsel. Therefore, considerable illustration is provided in certain sections of this chapter with the understanding that readers may find certain portions of the discussion more relevant than others to their caseloads. Further, many of the issues reviewed below have been discussed in earlier chapters (e.g., adolescents [6], career and workplace [11], health concerns [12], families [14], couples [15], and parents and children [17]) and sometimes the discourse may have touched upon some of the related legal issues that are elucidated herein in more detail. Before beginning these explanations, however, this chapter presents foundations for legal arguments supporting the constitutional rights of sexual minorities.

CONSTITUTIONAL RIGHTS

Legal advocates who assert that laws breach the constitutional rights of lesbians and gay men commonly propose one of two legal arguments. In some instances, they contend that particular statutes transgress the fundamental right to privacy or right of self-determination. In other cases, they allege that the laws maliciously discriminate against lesbians and gay men as a group in violation of equal protection regulations. Both arguments are established firmly in the Fifth and Fourteenth amendments to the U.S. Constitution (Bersoff & Ogden, 1991).

In *Bowers v. Hardwick* (1986), the U.S. Supreme Court ruled on an appeal from the state of Georgia that the U.S. Constitution does not guarantee citizens a fundamental right to engage in homosexual behavior, thereby allowing states the freedom to criminalize intimate conduct between people of the same sex. In 2001 sodomy laws criminalizing certain private sexual acts between consenting adults remained on the books in 17 of the 50 states (with 12 of these prohibiting activity between *both* different-sex and same-sex partners and 5 singling out lesbians and gay men), but these statutes are being challenged continually and often are reversed. In 1998, for example, the Georgia Supreme Court struck down the state's sodomy law, declaring that private, consensual sexual behavior between adults of the same or other sex cannot be criminalized. Based on the constitutional right to privacy, the ruling nullified with regard to private conduct the very same Georgia statute that the U.S. Supreme Court upheld in *Bowers v. Hardwick* (1986). Sodomy laws also were overturned during the late 1990s in Georgia, Montana, Tennessee, and Kentucky, largely as a result of efforts by Lambda (Legal Defense and Education Fund) and other groups. In 1999, Lambda also appealed the conviction of a gay couple for having sex at home under the Texas Homosexual Conduct Law, as well as brought a case before the Arkansas Supreme Court. Attorneys argued in both instances that laws banning oral and anal sex by gay and lesbian couples violate the right to privacy and equal protection by unfairly criminalizing their intimate behaviors. The Texas Court of Appeals for the Fourteenth Circuit agreed and struck down the Homosexual Conduct Law in its Houston area jurisdiction. Ideally, the ruling can influence other courts across Texas.

"Equal protection" further provides a constitutional route to protecting lesbians and gay men against discrimination. Under this provision, a class of persons must be declared *suspect* to qualify for the highest level of protection. Accordingly, the group should demonstrate that the characteristic for which it is oppressed is *immutable* (R. Green, 1988; Rivera, 1991). As reviewed in Chapter 3, a growing body of research data suggests that sexual orientation may be influenced biologically. In Chapter 13, the low rate of sexual reorientation via psychotherapeutic or religious intervention is discussed. Aside from homosexuality's etiology, the inadequacy of treatment to affect sexual orientation change seems to satisfy the legal concept of *immutabilty*, thus rendering sexual minorities a *suspect class* of persons and meeting the Supreme court's criteria for applying strict scrutiny to laws that discriminate against lesbians and gay men (R. Green, 1988).

LEGAL CONCERNS OF SEXUAL MINORITY CLIENTS

Based on arguments similar to those described previously, numerous legal challenges have been advanced to further the constitutional rights of sexual minorities. A concise compendium of legal activity in several arenas is presented later. Although many of the cases described have been settled, new suits are being filed continuously in all the areas discussed. In numerous instances, *amicus curiae* ("friends of the court") briefs have been submitted or oral arguments have been heard and cases are awaiting appellate court decisions at the time of this writing. Given the increase in legal activity related to the concerns of disenfranchised sexual minority individuals, appeals assuredly will continue to be filed and findings of lower courts challenged until these citizens gain the same rights and privileges as heterosexuals.

Because numerous cases in various jurisdictions at different times have been condensed in these synopses, individual citations are used sparingly. Unless otherwise noted, all information used in these summaries was extracted from the most current American Civil Liberties Union (ACLU) publications; the Human Rights Campaign's *HRC Quarterly*; and the quarterly newsletter of the Lambda Legal Defense and Education Fund (Lambda), *The Lambda Update*. For ongoing synopses of legal issues and equal rights efforts, readers are referred to the Resources section for these publications, as well as for listings of organizations providing legal advice, support, and materials.

Discrimination Based on Sexual Orientation

Equal protection under the law is foundational for guaranteeing the civil rights of all citizens, sexual minorities included. Among these basic entitlements is right to a fair and impartial trial, which for many gay men and lesbians has been difficult to insure. Numerous instances of problematic judges, attorneys, and juries are cited throughout this chapter, but a 2000 case in Texas can be used as an example. In this instance, a prosecutor urged the jury to sentence a defendant to death rather than to prison because sending the gay male to the penitentiary with other men was not "a very bad punishment for a homosexual." The same prosecutor, in continuing to argue for the death sentence, also suggested that the defendant presented a danger to the community based on a 1971 conviction for consensual sodomy. The judge in the case set aside the gay man's conviction and death sentence because his court-appointed legal counsel slept through much of the trial. Civil rights organizations, therefore, did not need to use a brief they had filed arguing that the prosecutor's deliberate appeal to the anti-gay prejudice of the jury violated the defendant's civil rights under the Constitution.

California passed the nation's first law in 2000 banning discrimination against potential jurors because they are lesbian or gay. This new legislation added sexual orientation to an existing ban on dismissing jurors based on race, color, occupation, religion, sex, national origin, or economic status. Ideally, legislation similar to the California law can be passed in other states, thereby better ensuring sexual minorities and other defendants that their peers truly are included in jury pools.

In reference to equal protection under the law, a 1996 U.S. Supreme Court decision declared unconstitutional a Colorado voter-approved referendum (Amendment 2) that would have prohibited the enactment of legislation to protect homosexuals from discrimination. In the case of *Romer v. Evans* (1996), the nation's highest court held that no state may "deem a class of persons a stranger to its laws," and that Colorado had no legitimate government interest for violating the constitutional guarantee of equal protection. According to the majority ruling, "Amendment 2 classifies homosexuals not to further a proper legislative end, but to make them unequal to everyone else, " and that "animosity toward the class of persons affected" is not a legitimate reason for precluding all legislative, executive, or judicial action designed to protect individuals based on their sexual orientation. The decision neither forces states to offer new civil rights protections by enacting anti-discrimination legislation nor prohibits them from discriminating on the basis of sexual orientation. In fact, all state laws banning anti-gay legislation still stand.

The victory for lesbian, gay, and bisexual citizens in *Romer v. Evans* was supported by *amicus curiae* briefs filed by the ACLU and Lambda, in conjunction with 7 cities, 10 states and the District of Columbia, constitutional scholars, professional associations, labor unions, civil rights organizations, and religious groups. All these "friends of the court" are committed to what they see as a virtually endless series of future legal challenges in which plaintiffs will use the language and rationale of the historic decision for their protection and to adjudicate their rights.

In 1994, attempts were made in 10 states to place anti-gay propositions on local and state ballots. Although efforts succeeded in Idaho and Oregon, both measures were defeated. During the following year (1995), however, other bills and initiatives were proposed in 20 states and more were being drafted for future referenda when the *Romer v. Evans* decision was handed down by the U.S. Supreme Court. Immediately after that ruling, Oregon withdrew several anti-gay initiatives which had been slated for the 1996 ballot and other states retired similar proposals. Some of these propositions either expanded or limited existing civil rights legislation, while others focused specifically on issues relative to adoptions and marriage rights for same-sex couples, or on prevention programs (AIDS, violence, suicide) in schools for sexual minority youth. Several of these proposals were reintroduced in succeeding years at local and state levels but in forms that did not violate state and federal constitutions or the *Romer v. Evans* ruling.

The Human Rights Campaign (HRC) and the National Gay and Lesbian Task Force (NGLTF) have provided substantial training and assistance to states and local communities, both to promote the passage of gay-positive ordinances and to defeat statutes that would either permit discrimination based on sexual orientation or restrict information on homosexuality (see Resources section). As of June 2001, 12 states, the District of Columbia, and about 200 counties and municipalities banned discrimination against lesbians, bisexuals, and gay men in employment, housing and public accommodations. In most parts of the country, however, these civil rights remain legally vulnerable and questionable. To facilitate passage of favorable legislation, HRC assists state partners with the drafting of legislation, legal research, lobby preparation, registration of voters, training of volunteers, provision of campaign expertise to political candidates, and public education. NGLTF, through its annual Creating Change conference and numerous other efforts, is active in the formation of public policy as well as in local community building, statewide organizing, and legislative and congressional efforts. HRC and NGLTF both contend that their advocacy, legislative, and political efforts will continue until sexual minorities are free from discrimination in all parts of the country and in all areas of their lives.

Marriage

Because sexual minority couples and their families lack legal recognition and protection (e.g., legal and medical powers of attorney; tax equity; and rights of guardianship, survivorship, and inheritance), the concept of domestic partnership was developed as a basis for legitimizing same-sex relationships. As of mid-2001, 4,266 employers, including 146 Fortune 500 companies, 3,862 private companies, nonprofits and unions, 153 colleges and universities, and 111 state and local governments had implemented domestic partnership programs (Human Rights Campaign, 2001). Many companies have joined a list that includes American Express, Apple Computer, AT&T, Eastman Kodak, IBM, Marriott, Mattel, Walt Disney, Xerox, General Mills, Motorola, Boeing, Shell Oil, and American and United Airlines, but others have refused to do so. When Exxon and Mobil merged and formed Exxon Mobil Corporation, for example, the new company's executives decided to discontinue Mobil's nondiscrimination policy covering sexual orientation and domestic partner benefits.

On a more positive note, New York City in 1993 extended health benefits originally reserved for the spouses and children of heterosexually married workers to the domestic partners of all city employees (n = 230,000) and retirees. Similarly, municipal workers in Philadelphia, Minneapolis, and San Francisco and state employees in Massachusetts, Oregon, and California are eligible for domestic partner benefits. California's 2001 registered domestic partner law also guarantees about a dozen rights typically reserved for married couples, in areas such as medical decisions, lawsuits, adoption, unemployment benefits, inheritance, conservatorship, and sick leave. Hawaii extends health benefits, family leave, and joint auto insurance to registered "reciprocal beneficiaries." In 2000, General Motors, Ford, and Daimler-Chrysler's Chrysler division announced that they would offer medical, dental, and prescription drug benefits for same-sex partners of their 466,000 hourly and salaried employees in the United States. This offering was considered by groups such as the HRC to be the largest move yet by corporate America.

The American Center for Law and Justice (ACLJ), a group affiliated with politician and conservative minister, Pat Robertson, and the Christian Coalition has filed numerous suits in various parts of the country contending that cities lack the power to provide domestic partner benefits and to maintain a registry because state law ostensibly prevents local governments from doing anything related to family relationships that varies from the marriage laws, including the compensation of their own employees. The ACLJ won its suit in Boston but lost pleas against the City of New York and the California cities of San Francisco and Santa Barbara in 1999. ACLJ appealed both decisions but withdrew the Santa Barbara complaint after the passage of a bill that established the nation's first statewide domestic partner registry.

Hawaii has come closer than any other state in granting gay and lesbian couples the legal right to marry. In 1993, the Hawaii Supreme Court ruled that denying marriage licenses to same-sex pairs violates the state's constitutional guarantee of equal protection on the basis of sex. In November 1998, an amendment to the state constitution giving power to the legislature to limit marriage to opposite-sex couples was drafted and eventually passed by a vote of 69% to 29%. In late 1999, the Hawaii Supreme Court ruled that its hands were tied by this action, but it did not overrule is 1993 decision, nor did it rule on potential future claims or advocacy for the protections, benefits, and responsibilities that come with civil marriage. The passing of the amendment, however, was costly and generated intense debate on both sides of the issue.

As a result of the controversy in Hawaii, a backlash of legislation prohibiting same-sex marriages was introduced in numerous other jurisdictions. Thirty-five states had passed such legislation by June 2001, undoubtedly, according to a Lambda spokesperson (E. Wolfson, 1996), guaranteeing themselves costly future litigation. Bills preventing federal recognition of same-sex marriage were passed in both houses of Congress and signed into law by former President Clinton. Several organizations, such as Parents, Families and Friends of Lesbians and Gays (PFLAG), the NGLTF, the Gay and Lesbian Alliance Against Defamation (GLAAD), the HRC, and Lambda's Marriage Project, joined together to form the Freedom to Marry Coalition. Public education, including efforts directed toward lawmakers, religious leaders, parents, and nongay supporters, became a major focus of the Coalition's outreach efforts.

In late 1999, the Vermont Supreme Court ruled unanimously that the refusal to grant marriage licenses to same-sex couples unconstitutionally denies them the same rights and legal benefits extended to married heterosexuals. The court ordered Vermont legislators either to legalize same-sex marriage or to create a new status of domestic partnership that would entitle members to more than 300 legal benefits, including access to a partner's health, life and disability insurance, child custody and inheritance rights, spousal support, and pension and hospital visitation privileges. State representatives and senators spent early 2000 crafting an equivalent statutory domestic partnership system, while gay activists were protesting that the proposals did not go far enough in guaranteeing truly equal rights to same-sex couples and right-wing opponents were attempting to ensure that any bill did not cross the threshold of heterosexual marriage. The governor signed a bill creating marriage-like "civil unions" in April 2000, the farthest that any state has gone in giving same-sex couples a legal status approximating heterosexual marriage. Although the rights and privileges granted by Vermont civil unions do not extend beyond the borders of the state, the fact that there is no residency requirement in the law enables couples from other states to register their unions in Vermont. This fact alone undoubtedly will have ramifications in other jurisdictions when couples whose unions were acknowledged in Vermont will sue to have their partnerships recognized in the other 49 states. Further, when similar legislation is advanced in other states, advocates will be able to point to the Vermont precedent because "many states have constitutional provisions similar to the 'common benefits' and 'equal protection' clauses that motivated the Vermont supreme court to mandate benefits for gay and lesbian couples" (Dahir, 2000, p. 58). Years of costly legal challenges undoubtedly will result and Lambda and others expect that this issue eventually will reach the level of the U.S. Supreme Court.

Parental and Custodial Rights

Psychological studies are critical to winning custody and visitation cases because a handful of states still have per se precedents that guide all rulings and automatically assume sexual minorities to be incapable of fit parenting. Several states have *nexus* or detriment precedents and there is a trend toward this standard in many jurisdictions without previous rulings. In other words, the burden is shifting onto the opposing party of proving that a parent's homosexuality is affecting the child negatively; no longer can there be an automatic presumption of harm if a parent is gay or lesbian. Legal defense provided by groups such as Lambda, the National Center for Lesbian Rights (NCLR), and the ACLU continually challenge presumptions of harm to a child that are based exclusively on stereotypes, distortions in fact, ill-supported assumptions, undue focus on sexual orientation, and homophobic bias on the part of expert and other witnesses, trial judges, and the courts themselves. As a result of these arguments, gay and lesbian parents are becoming increasingly more successful at securing visitation and custody of their biological children, such as in 1999 victories in Maryland and Illinois. Far too often, however, custody still continues to be awarded or denied solely on the basis of sexual orientation and needless modifications in custody are common. Similarly, in situations in which visitation privileges are granted to gay and lesbian parents, artificial restrictions often are mandated, such as a biological parent's same-sex partner not being allowed in their home when the child is visiting (Baggett, 1992; Benkov, 1994; Gottsfield, 1985; Logue, 2000).

A case of this nature occurred in Georgia in 1999 when a county superior court refused to vacate extraordinary restrictions on a gay man's visits with his three daughters. The gag order forbade the father from discussing his sexual orientation with his offspring under any circumstances, and if the children asked any questions, he was ordered not to answer them but to refer the girls to their religiously conservative mother. He also was banned from having any gay or lesbian overnight houseguests when the three children were present. The judge noted that these directives furthered the best interests of the man's daughters.

When a gay father in Ohio lost custody of his son after raising him for 10 years, Lambda (together with the American Academy of Child and Adolescent Psychiatry, the Ohio Psychological Association, and the National Association of Social Workers [NASW]) filed an appellate brief with the Ohio Court of Appeals. In the challenge, Lambda contended that the case raised due process issues because there was no lower court testimony that the child had been harmed by the sexual orientation of his father. Further, the contested court decision appeared to have focused unduly on the issue of homosexuality, despite considerable evidence (including home studies and a psychological report) that the child was doing well living with his father, his father's partner, and his stepsister. As a result of the argument, temporary custody was regained pending the appeal. A somewhat parallel case occurred in North Carolina when a county court's decision led to the removal of two sons from a gay father's custody. The only home that the boys, ages 4 and 8, ever had known was one shared with their father and his partner. Lambda appealed the decision and noted in its brief that the custody ruling was replete with factual distortions, ill-supported assumptions, and homophobia. For example, the court allowed questions about the particulars of the men's sex lives while the biological mother's testimony about her sex life was deemed irrelevant. The court of appeals found no evidence of harm to the children caused by the father and ruled in favor of him.

Rather than giving the boys to their father, however, the biological mother appealed the decision to the North Carolina Supreme Court.

Coparenting and Biology

When a coparenting lesbian relationship dissolves or the birth mother dies, the custody or visitation rights of the nonbiological mother frequently are challenged by the biological father or grandparents. In these kinds of cases, biologically related individuals usually are granted custody of the child(ren), given the long-standing "legal bias toward recognizing a heterosexual procreative unit as family over other family forms" (Benkov, 1994, p. 246). Despite this "societal and legal tradition of relying on biological connection to determine parental status" (p. 246), however, victories for widowed nonbiological lesbian mothers do occasionally occur, but often at considerable financial and emotional cost. For example, two years after a nonbiological mother filed a lawsuit in the Brooklyn (New York) Family Court against relatives of her deceased partner's offspring, the trial court ruled in 1995 that she was the most appropriate person to be the child's guardian. In addition, the court acknowledged the two women's intention to parent the child together and that the sexual orientation of the surviving lesbian partner was irrelevant to determining the child's best interest.

A more common instance in which the rights of the nonbiological mother were denied transpired in Florida after the biological mother died and her parents (the child's biological grandparents) were granted guardianship of their granddaughter. Within 2 years, the older couple legally adopted the young girl and consequently acquired full parental rights. At this point the nonbiological mother appealed to a Florida circuit court for guardianship and custody of the daughter whom she and her late partner had coparented. The adoption was overturned and the nonbiological mother was awarded physical and legal custody of her daughter. The grandparents then challenged the ruling and the appeals court judge refused to give the nonbiological mother the opportunity to present evidence because she was seen by the court as a third party with less standing than the grandparents who were biologically related to the child. The standing in court also was not granted as, under Florida law, gay men and lesbians are not allowed to adopt children.

Results often are more favorable in cases involving the dissolution of lesbian relationships. For example, the New Jersey Supreme Court in 2000 awarded visitation rights to twin toddlers to a nonbiological mother. The woman had coparented the children from birth until 2 years later when the relationship with her former partner ended. The court's unanimous ruling granted the visitation rights based on the fact that the nonbiological parent had the status of a "psychological parent" to the children and thus had a right to share parenting duties. Similarly, in 1995, the Wisconsin Supreme Court ordered a lower court to reconsider its decision to disallow a nonbiological mother's requests for visits with her son after she and her former partner separated. The court reasoned in this case that if a parent allows another adult to establish a parent-like relationship with a child, it might not be in the child's best interest to sever that bond.

On a less positive note, a nonbiological mother's appeal for the right to visit with her daughter reached the level of the Florida Supreme Court in 2000. The woman and her partner had been in a committed relationship for several years before deciding to conceive the child through artificial insemination. They attended birthing classes and doctor's visits together, and the nonbiological mother was present in the delivery room during the birth and listed on the birth certificate as a parent. Because Florida law does not permit second-parent adoptions, the women executed a "delegation of parental authority" so the child's relationship with both mothers would be protected. When the couple separated, the biological mother sued for custody rights and refused to allow the other parent to see their daughter. Lower courts refused to grant the nonbiological mother the legal standing in court necessary to demonstrate that she was a de facto parent to the child because Florida law recognizes parental rights of custody only for biological or adoptive parents or grandparents. Thus, the woman was unable to present evidence in her behalf, including letters from her former partner attesting to her status as a mother to their child. An Illinois appellate court in 1999 and a Tennessee court of appeals in 2000 issued similar rulings that determined that three nonbiological lesbian mothers had no standing to seek contact with the children they had raised with their former partners.

The concept of *in loco parentis* describes a situation in which adults who are "like parents" have taken on parental rights and responsibilities in the absence of biological or adoptive parents. A related concept, de facto parent, likewise attempts to recognize the relational components of a parent–child relationship, apart from biology or legal contents. In spite of the logic inherent in these notions, most requests for parental rights for nonbiological parents have been stymied at a preliminary level because the coparents are deemed without standing to be heard in a court of law. Though civil rights organizations are committed to providing assistance in filing suits and appeals until the rights of nonbiological parents are established firmly, both clients and therapists can play a role in reducing the number of arguments between coparents that escalate to the point at which the courts are asked to adjudicate. A cooperative effort between Lambda, ACLU, NCLR, Family Pride Coalition, COLAGE (Children of Lesbians and Gays Everywhere), and GLAD (Gay and Lesbian Legal Advocates and Defenders), for example has attempted to educate separating same-sex parental couples about the dangers of resorting to desperate legal methods to solve disagreements. Accordingly, they have published a set of guidelines titled *Protecting Families: Standards for Child Custody Disputes in Same-Sex Relationships* (available from the Lambda website; see Resources section). Clinicians can cooperate in this endeavor through education and psychotherapy so that the process of resolving conflict can be less hurtful and destructive to both children and their parents.

Donor Insemination

In other situations related to biology, sperm donors are more often seeking and winning custody and visitation rights from both biological and nonbiological mothers. Lamentably, these kinds of disputes are arising more frequently. Given an ideology that prohibits women raising children without fathers, lesbians historically have been denied the right to anonymous donor insemination and usually have become pregnant with known donors. With the climate changing in recent years, a considerable number are opting for the use of sperm banks to induce pregnancy (not withstanding the rise in legislation proposed by conservative legislators forbidding lesbians and other "single women" from utilizing these services). Others, however, still continue to choose known donors in order to give their children "a sense of their biological roots" (Benkov, 1994, p. 242).

In selecting known donors, lesbian couples are usually quite careful and often choose long-time friends. Often these are gay men, who could never use the mothers' homosexuality against them in a potential custody battle. Others are gay male couples who often, likewise, have searched for ways to parent a child. In any case, donor arrangements depend on a considerable degree of trust between the lesbian couple and the man they select as a donor or the men with whom they choose to coparent. A considerable number of these alliances have been successful for many years.

Foster Parenting and Adoption

Legal battles abound in various states regarding the right of lesbians and gay men to serve as foster parents and to adopt children (Connolly, 1998). Many licenses to serve as a foster parent and petitions for adoption have been granted, although not always on the first request. Appeals are common, as in the Illinois case of a member of a lesbian couple who applied to serve as a foster parent. Although she submitted her request as an individual, she lived with her long-time partner. Her application was denied on the basis that only single persons or married couples are allowed to become foster parents in Illinois. Even though the applicant and her partner had participated in months of foster parent training and extensive background checks, the Department of Children and Family Services (DCFS) reasoned that the license was not granted because the applicant did not meet the criteria of being either single or married. With Lambda's assistance, the decision was appealed to the regional director of DCFS who reinvestigated the case and reversed the original decision. Subsequently, a license enabling the applicant to serve as a foster parent was issued. Although the situation was reconciled favorably without formal litigation, numerous others involving sexual minority adults and their rights to legally parent children take years to be resolved, often at considerable emotional (and usually financial) expense to the individuals challenging current statutes and regulations.

Because of these kinds of difficulties, many same-sex couples are applying to adopt children from other countries. Lesbians, in particular, have been adopting girls from China, which has an abundance of unwanted female infants and young girls (Rich, 2000). The increase in the international adoption rate by same-sex couples, often posing as single individuals in order to facilitate the process, has led the religious right to demand that these overseas adoptions by sexual minorities be restricted. An international adoption treaty brought before Congress was stalled for this reason.

The 47 state statutes that permit sexual minorities to adopt children vary considerably and often are quite specific regarding the circumstances under which this might occur. In Texas, for example, lesbian and gay couples cannot "adopt" children but can get "biological rights." The partners of biological parents can be "conservators." For individuals adopting unrelated children, there are few absolute legal barriers but numerous legal loopholes. Because of the difficulties involved with navigating these legalities, gay, bisexual, and lesbian individuals and same-sex couples who are considering the foster parenting or adoption process are advised to study their applicable state laws. They also are encouraged to consult an attorney before proceeding with a plan (A. Sullivan, 1995).

Second-Parent Adoption

Because nonbiological and nonadoptive parents have no legally sanctioned connections to their children, wills to stipulate guardianship and coparenting contracts are not adequate substitutes for the basic legal recognition of [heterosexual] family relationships. To legalize the child–parent relationship, second-parent adoption gradually is becoming an option for gay and lesbian parents, as it historically has been for heterosexual stepparents. The availability is somewhat limited, with slightly over 20 states and the District of Columbia permitting lesbian or gay coparents legally to adopt their partner's biological or adopted children. Each challenge to existing law is different, and favorable judgments are more difficult in some situations than in others.

Housing and Public Accommodations

Several court challenges to anti-discrimination legislation have been brought by landlords who claim that First Amendment protection of their religious beliefs permits them to deny housing to certain prospective renters. Some of these claims specifically involve a landlord's aversion to homosexuality, while others represent a moral opposition to acts of fornication by unmarried couples. In one such instance, the California Supreme Court ruled in 1996 that the state law prohibiting marital status discrimination in housing forbids bias against unmarried couples and that landlords renting to the general public have no constitutional or statutory exemption from that law. The court further noted that property owners could avoid any burden the law placed on their religious beliefs by simply selling the houses or apartments and placing their capitol in another investment. The landlord subsequently filed a petition for *certiorari* with the U.S. Supreme Court. Because similar free exercise of religion claims seeking to justify the violation of numerous anti-discrimination statutes are becoming increasingly common, the California Supreme Court ruling is expected to have a significant impact on the enforceability of equal rights ordinances nationwide.

Sexual minority plaintiffs and their attorneys are finding that statutes prohibiting discrimination on the basis of marital status can be used to support diverse claims of bias. These laws have been particularly helpful in a few cases involving the transfer of ownership shares in cooperative apartment buildings to former or deceased partners. They also might be useful in cases initiated by lesbians, bisexuals, and gay men involving the denial of various benefits to same-sex couples otherwise provided to legally married partners. Some of these complaints brought before the courts and before governmental boards/commissions concern advantages granted to legally married spouses relative to a range of issues, including the following:

- Social security benefits
- State and federal income tax reductions
- Family illness and bereavement leaves
- Health insurance packages
- Shared private rooms in a hospital or care facility
- Association and organizational memberships
- Family memberships in pools and recreation facilities
- Spousal frequent flyer programs benefits
- Automobile insurance reductions
- Jointly held credit cards
- Child custody and guardianship
- Privileges for survivors relative to:
  - Estate tax marital deductions
  - Inheritance
  - Home ownership

– Rent control
– Workers' compensation
– Pension plans
– The Veterans Administration

Discrimination in public accommodation suits also encompass a range of issues, including whether a dental or medical office qualifies as such and, hence, must comply with state civil rights legislation. Most challenges, however, center around the right of sexual minorities to rent houses, apartments, or hotel (or motel) rooms with same-sex partners; to dance with a person of the same-sex at businesses open to the public (i.e., bars and clubs); or to eat in restaurants and shop in stores. With the aging of the "out" gay and lesbian population, issues such as the right to be treated fairly in nursing homes or long-term care facilities and other concerns of the elderly will assume a more prominent position in litigation.

Recent discrimination cases involve the right to join organizations engaging in commercial transactions with nonmembers, such as the Boy Scouts of America (BSA). The U.S. Supreme Court, for example, has determined that *truly private* organizations have First Amendment protection even to discriminate. The Court, in fact, ruled that forcing the BSA to accept gay leaders would violate the organization's right of "expressive association" under the First Amendment. The Justices issued this ruling despite the fact that the BSA is chartered by Congress and receives benefits and special access from the military, state and municipal agencies, police and fire departments, and public schools (which sponsor about 20% of the troops). At the time of the Supreme Court ruling, the ACLU and others had filed ongoing lawsuits or threatened legal action against several government entities to force the BSA to abandon discrimination or to decline support from those agencies. Numerous other suits undoubtedly will ensue in order to force courts to rule on various nuances of the Supreme Court decision.

Employment

The employment section (Title VII) of the Civil Rights Act of 1964 does not protect workers from workplace discrimination based on sexual orientation. The Department of Justice (including the FBI) and the Office of Personnel Management (which governs all federal employees), however, cannot discriminate on the basis of sexual orientation, make inferences regarding an applicant's or employee's susceptibility to coercion, or deny the issuance of security clearances. Further, almost all national labor unions at least nominally protect their gay, lesbian, and bisexual members. Federal laws, unfortunately, provide no security for sexual minority employees who work for school districts, local and state governments, or private employers. The Employment Non-Discrimination Act (ENDA), the first federal legislation to provide employment protection to people on the basis of sexual orientation, was first defeated in the U.S. Senate by one vote (49 to 50) in 1996. Bills similar to the ENDA were introduced in each Congress for several years and were supported by numerous corporate endorsements, as well as by organizations such as the HRC, the AFL-CIO, NAACP, and PFLAG. Conservative members of Congress strongly opposed the introduction of each bill patterned after the ENDA, with their arguments usually confounding the difference between affirmative action and anti-discrimination.

Government Workers

As of June 2001, only 12 states and the District of Columbia offered civil rights legal protection, including employment security, on the basis of sexual orientation. In the rest of the country, employees fired for being lesbian or gay have no legal recourse unless they work in a locality with its own anti-discrimination ordinance. Although less than 200 municipalities also have protective ordinances, these statutes do not carry the weight of the law. Numerous challenges demanding full enforcement of laws have been initiated in several jurisdictions, and lawsuits alleging bias have been filed in other states without explicit legislation safeguarding employment. The territories of the United States also have experienced problems with first amendment employment rights. In a case litigated in Puerto Rico on behalf of the Gay Officers Action League (GOAL), the Puerto Rico Police Department's disciplinary rule forbidding officers from "associating with homosexuals" was contested. The court judged that the rule violated the rights of employees and prohibited the police commissioner from ever punishing officers who associated with homosexuals.

Military

Armed services procedures subject lesbians, bisexuals, and gay men to different standards of speech, conduct, and status than their heterosexual comrades while the U.S. military continues to prosecute and discharge sexual minorities under its "don't ask, don't tell" policy (Zeeland, 1993, 1995, 1996, 1999). When this procedure was first implemented in 1994, 617 service members were discharged for homosexuality, compared with 1,145 in 1998. By 2000, 6 years after the policy's implementation, dismissals for sexual orientation rose 73%. Witch hunts and criminal prosecutions declined slightly from February 1999 to February 2000 (968), however, as commanders simply chose to discharge sexual minorities instead. Women, who comprised 14% of military personnel, constituted 31% of the expulsions (Wildman, 2000).

In a challenge to the "don't ask, don't tell" policy, six service personnel (one lesbian and five gay men) sued for their constitutional right to serve in the armed forces under the same rules that apply to their heterosexual counterparts. In its closing argument, the government admitted that "the proscription on service has nothing to do with unjustified assumptions that homosexuals are not just as capable physically, mentally, and psychologically to serve in the U.S. military as heterosexuals" (Dohrn, 1995, p. 1). According to Lambda legal director Beatrice Dohrn, this acknowledgment clearly exposed the ban as a means to accommodate prejudice. The judge in the case appeared to agree when he ruled that the military ban against lesbians and gay men violated the First Amendment and equal protection clause of the Constitution. The government, in spite of its own prejudicial acknowledgment, appealed the lower court's decision to the U.S. Court of Appeals for the Second Circuit. Lambda and the ACLU presented the case, *Able v. U.S.A* (1996) on behalf of the six plaintiffs. In 1996, the appellate court required the lower court to consider the constitutional question of whether the military may subject lesbian and gay service members to entirely different rules of conduct than it applies to their heterosexual associates.

The beating to death with a baseball bat of an army private at Fort Campbell, Kentucky, in 1999 led to the speculation that the "don't ask, don't tell" policy created a dangerous atmosphere in the military by treating one group of individuals differently from the others. After two army personnel were convicted of the murder, the President of the United States admitted that the policy was not working as intended. In response to a public outcry and strong statements by the Servicemembers Legal Defense Network, the Pentagon finally in 2000 released policy guidelines first prepared 3 years previously but not released to field officers. These guidelines mandated sensitivity training for troops regarding anti-gay aggravation, implemented policies for investigations of harassment or threats to personnel, and required any inquiry into a service member's perceived sexual orientation to involve senior-level officers in the military justice system. The Army's inspector general conducted an investigation into whether officers at Fort Campbell tolerated or overlooked anti-gay slurs and taunting in the months before Private Barry Winchell's murder. The Army reassigned the commander of the military base to the Pentagon staff before the investigation was complete.

Public School Employees

Specifically in regard to public school teachers, several advocacy organizations (e.g., the ACLU, Lambda, the American Federation of Teachers [AFT], and the National Education Association [NEA]) are committed to protecting the rights of educators to free speech, equal protection, job security, and freedom from harassment. In addition to the assistance provided by groups such as those listed previously, teachers also have the protection of *MarcMorrison v. State Board of Education* (1969). In this decision, the California Supreme Court determined that the status of homosexuality was insufficient grounds for dismissal unless it is coupled with some related misbehavior. The court further called for an extensive analysis of the employee's behavior in relation to the responsibilities of the job before employment dismissal is possible. Consequently, the *Morrison* judgment, which held that a relationship must exist between private action and job-related criteria, is considered the landmark decision in employment restrictions within any profession (Harbeck, 1992).

The precedence of the *Morrison* decision is reflected in a 1999 ruling of the California Labor Commission that ordered the Rio Bravo–Greeley Union School District to stop removing students from a science instructor's class simply because he is gay or perceived to be so. The biology teacher, Dr. Jim Merrick, disclosed his sexual orientation to the local media in May 1998 when commenting about anti-gay statements made by a commissioner during a public meeting of the county Human Relations Commission (*Merrick v. Rio Bravo–Greeley Union School District*, 1999). Merrick filed his complaint in October after school administrators transferred the first of 15 students from his classroom at the request of their parents. The Labor Commission ruling also mandated that discrimination or harassment of students or staff based on actual or perceived sexual orientation would not be tolerated, and that the district was to develop a tolerance training program for employees. Merrick was awarded the Colin Higgins Courage Award for his action.

Based on her research, Harbeck (1992) concludes that, generally, school boards are willing to look the other way if the only issue is a teacher, administrator, or counselor's minority sexual orientation but may attempt to dismiss or demote a homosexual employee if some indiscretion, scandal, or community controversy (as in the *Merrick* case) occurs. Although tenure and the fear of expensive litigation costs often prevent outright job discrimination and termination on the part of school boards, "there remains, however, the real possibility of insidious incidents relating to limited advancement, ungranted tenure, mundane duty assignments, and undesirable teaching loads" (p. 131).

Immigration

Although the Immigration and Naturalization Service (INS) prohibits discrimination based on sexual orientation, a foreigner either must be sponsored by a heterosexual legal spouse or fiancée, a family member, or an employer or must be granted political asylum in order to enter the United States. Currently, spousal or family sponsorship does not apply to gay and lesbian binational couples who are treated as legal strangers to one another. Ten countries in the world, including Canada, England, and Australia, recognize same-sex relationships for immigration purposes, but the United States is not included among them. This policy causes intense distress to thousands of binational couples, many of whom met while studying, working, or traveling in each other's countries. The INS also bars HIV-infected immigrants from entering the United States and numerous suits challenging this policy have been brought before the courts. Lambda court challenges, however, have forced the INS to authorize the issuance of orphan visa petitions to applicants who intend to coparent a foreign-born child with their same-sex domestic partners.

Regarding asylum, the INS has granted sanctuary to about 40 sexual minority immigrants out of thousands who have applied. Most of the applications have come from individuals holding citizenship in Central and South American, Asian, or Middle Eastern countries. The granting of asylum is based on a specific set of standards, one of which is that applicants must have a well-established fear of persecution. This includes showing proof of human rights violations against sexual minorities in their country. Using these criteria, the INS has rejected several petitions contending persecution based on sexual orientation filed by clearly endangered immigrants, despite United Nations Convention and Protocol opposition to returning refugees to countries where they may be harmed.

Public Safety

Herek (1989) defined hate crimes as "words or actions intended to harm or intimidate an individual because of her or his membership in a minority group" (p. 948). When individuals are harmed, others in their group are intimidated; not only is the victim's identity assailed but an entire class of people also is victimized. This brutality or cruelty motivated by prejudice against the minority group with which a victim is identified has been referred to as *ethnoviolence* (Ehrlich, 1990) and often includes physical attacks, homicide, sexual assault, and property damage, as well as violent threats and other intimidating acts (Finn & McNeil, 1987; Herek & Berrill, 1991).

Only in recent years have injuries against sexual minorities been recognized as hate crimes. Throughout the 1980s, the Anti-Violence Project of the NGLTF documented the extent of the problem and lobbied Congress to pass corrective legislation. Passage in 1990 of the Hate Crimes Statistics Act recognized that the status of lesbians and gay men, like that of ethnic minorities, requires special protection against hate-motivated crimes (Klinger & Stein, 1996). As of June 2001, 27 states and the District of Columbia had passed hate crimes laws that included sexual orientation. Sixteen other states had hate crimes legislation that did not include offenses based on sexual orientation, and the remaining 7 states (largely in the South and Southwest) did not have hate crime laws that included misdemeanors or felonies based on any characteristics (see the website for the National Gay and Lesbian Task Force noted in the Resources section).

A large number of lesbians and gay men have experienced violence as a result of their sexual orientation, but precise figures are unknown because most victims never report anti-gay hate crimes, partially due to their dread of losing jobs or child custody or to their fear of becoming the subjects of hostility, harassment, or rejection if their homosexuality becomes known (Herek, 1989, 1996). In fact, "more incidents of violence against lesbians, gay men, and bisexual individuals are believed to go unreported than reported" (Klinger & Stein, 1996, p. 803). Hundreds of violent events, nonetheless, are reported each year by or on behalf of sexual minorities and include murders, assaults, police abuse, arson, vandalism, threats, harassment, and campus and HIV-related violence. Information from the FBI reflected that in 1999, 17% of all hate crimes reported were based on the victim's sexual orientation (1,300 out of 7,549) (Quick Facts: Hate Crimes, 2001). According to a survey by the National Coalition of Anti-Violence Programs, reports of physical attacks on gay men and lesbians in 1998 increased significantly over the year before (Bull, 1999a), and FBI data indicated a 14.3% rise for 1998 (Doyle, 2000). According to Bull (1999a), a spokesman for the Southern Poverty Law Center further noted that "in ordinary crimes people are beaten or shot. That doesn't seen to be enough for these killers of homosexuals. They have to break every bone in their face or stab them 30 times" (p. 24).

In addition to violence and other hate crimes, murders of gay men and lesbians continue to occur (Bull, 1999c). An Oregon lesbian couple, for example, was found in 1995 shot to death in the head, execution style. The women had helped form a PFLAG chapter in their community and had been active in the statewide fight for sexual minority civil rights. Eleven gay and transgendered people were beheaded or shot, strangled, or stabbed to death from October 1998 to March 1999. An Alabama man, Billy Jack Gaither, was beaten to death with an ax handle and thrown into a pyre of burning tires by two men, one of whom pleaded guilty to participating in the killing because Gaither had allegedly made a pass at him. The other was convicted of murder and given a life sentence in prison, after providing evidence in his defense that his accomplice recently had been intimately involved with another man. Matthew Shepard, a 21-year-old University of Wyoming student, was robbed, tortured, tied to a fence in freezing temperatures, and left to die. He was found the next morning and succumbed to his injuries 4 days later. Both of his killers, one of whom attempted to use a "gay panic" defense which has no standing in Wyoming law, were convicted of murder.

The Matthew Shepard Foundation (e-mail: MatthewShepard@wyoming.com) was created by his parents after his death to support causes related to gay men and lesbians, as well as educational programs on international human rights issues. Judy Shepard, his mother, has become a nationally recognized hate crimes spokeswoman and also has joined with key civil rights, religious, labor, and nearly 100 other organizations to encourage the passage by Congress of a Hate Crimes Prevention Act (HCPA). This act would expand federal jurisdiction to investigate and prosecute bias-related crimes committed on the basis of race, color, religion, or national origin, as well as widen the definition of those crimes to include victimization based on real or perceived sexual orientation, gender, or disability.

LEGAL PROTECTION FOR SEXUAL MINORITY CLIENTS

As evident from the overview just presented, sexual minorities are legally vulnerable in all aspects of their lives and need to protect themselves and their families as much as possible (Curry, Clifford, Hertz, & Leonard, 1999; Ettelbrick, 1991; Gewirtzman, 2000). The following sections, using sources such as those cited earlier, describe some strategies for protecting personal investments, relationships, and property so individuals can establish a degree of freedom and autonomy within the context of existing law. These synopses are intended to familiarize clinicians with the kinds of documents that gay, lesbian, and bisexual clients can develop, with the help of appropriate legal counsel, to put their personal affairs in order. Legal resources are outlined further in the Resources section.

Last Will and Testament

Because same-sex relationships legally cannot be recognized through marriage, gay and lesbian partners are guaranteed none of the rights and privileges that the law offers to heterosexually married couples. If either party wants someone other than a parent, sibling, or child to inherit property; serve as a legal guardian or as an executor of the estate; outline burial arrangements, or care for pets, then executing a last will and testament to specify these intentions is imperative. Because wills provide for the expression of personal wishes on a range of matters, they are necessary whether or not an individual has a significant relationship or owns property of a substantial value. Without a legal will, statutes known as intestacy laws automatically dictate that a biological family inherit all property and possessions even though the deceased may have had other priorities.

Joint Property

According to Ettelbrick (1991), same-sex spouses may be wise to own joint property because a surviving partner often needs immediate resources in order to satisfy debts or expenses payable during the costly and lengthy process of probating a will. If, for example, two women or men bought their home as *joint tenants with a right of survivorship*, the survivor would be allowed to assume full ownership of the property immediately upon the death of the other partner. Conversely, if they purchased their home as *tenants in common*, each would own an equal share of the property. In this case, their wills would need to provide for distributing their half in order to prevent a biological next of kin from inheriting 50% of the surviving partner's house. Many lawyers recommend owning, or holding, homes, bank accounts, and many other financial investments jointly with rights of survivorship. Both partners must recognize, however, that mutual trust is essential because either person may withdraw all the funds from a joint account at any time.

Cohabitation Contracts

When same-sex partners share most expenses and buy household items together, or when one is financially supporting the relationship more than the other, gay and lesbian couples are wise to consider negotiating cohabitation contracts. These agreements are designed to address each partner's rights and responsibilities regarding property distribution, income(s), and expenses. In addition, they may outline individual responsibilities toward funding or providing care for children or dependent adults, as applicable and appropriate. For these contracts to be lawfully binding, however, the intention of the agreement must be legal and a negotiated exchange must be documented (Ettelbrick, 1991).

Durable Power of Attorney

Although conservators may be assigned to manage personal care (i.e., medical treatment and hospitalization) for someone who has been debilitated, the durable power of attorney is the preferable document for more ordinary concerns. This legal authorization enables a designated agent to act as a representative in legal and financial matters on behalf of another. Because the power may expire upon incapacitation, individuals are advised to make their wishes clear in this regard when signing the document. In certain states, *Durable Power of Attorney for Health Care* laws have been passed specifically allowing individuals to appoint others to make their health care decisions. These determinations may include the authority to visit loved ones in intensive care units, gain access to their medical records, transport them to other hospitals, and replace their physicians. Because of the differences in state laws, the advice of an attorney familiar with the issues of sexual minorities is essential.

Living Wills

Although medical technology enables physicians to prolong life, most states have enacted legislation permitting patients to instruct doctors ahead of time to withhold or withdraw artificial life support if their conditions become terminal or irreversible. These contractual agreements are called living wills and, to be legitimate, must conform exactly to the guideline specified in state law. In other words, the patient's meaning and purpose must be outlined clearly. Individuals coordinating primary care for their partners or friends with illnesses that require frequent hospitalization are advised to file photocopies of the their durable power of attorney for health care, along with the living will, in the patient medical record upon each admission. Personal physicians should be given copies as well. These actions ensure compliance with the directives and make certain that biological relatives do not have legal and medical decision-making power if that is not the wish of the patient.

CONCLUSION

Until equal protection under the law is established firmly and fully, sexual minority individuals will continue to develop their identities, relationships, and careers in environments of questionable support, if not obvious discrimination. Consequently, they are likely to seek psychotherapy in order to reverse the psychological effects of stigma. It is hoped that this book can inform and sustain clinicians who treat these negative consequences of oppression, as well as assist them in considering *both* the external forces *and* internal dynamics that shape client development. Finally, therapists are encouraged to promote positive change in both domains.

Part II

IDENTITY FORMATION AND PSYCHOLOGICAL DEVELOPMENT

5

Theories of Gay, Lesbian, and Bisexual Identity Formation

The Kinsey, Storms, Klein, and Coleman models discussed in Chapter 2 challenge the Freudian dichotomy between heterosexuality and homosexuality and reflect the natural diversity of erotic and emotional attractions. These formulations are useful for helping clients *describe* the dynamic and multidimensional nature of their sexual orientation. They are too ambiguous or complicated, however, to be practical for helping them *define* themselves in reference to social constructions based on their thoughts, feelings, fantasies, and behaviors. In other words, "Kinsey 3's" and "Klein 3-5-2-6-1-6-5's" must identify at some point with being gay/lesbian, bisexual, or heterosexual in order to establish a stable sense of self.

Without this stability of selfhood, people find it difficult to locate a community with which to affiliate. As introduced in the first chapter, minority groups come together because of characteristic features that are devalued by dominant segments of society (Herek, 1991). In such a group, the common traits and similarities reflected among the members reinforce individual as well as communal identity. Within a heterosexist majority culture, then, the process of identity formation becomes a critical undertaking for developing the self-concept and facilitating a sense of belonging for sexual minority clients.

Though the foundations of sexual orientation probably are established prenatally or early in life (Bailey, 1995; Bem, 1996, 1997; Burr, 1993; Gallagher, 1998; Hamer & Copeland, 1998; see Chapter 3), sexual identity clearly is a social construct based on historical changes and perspectives. In a sense, the formation of a gay, lesbian, or bisexual identity is an achieved rather than an acquired status (Garnets & Kimmel, 1991). People achieve their sexual identities in idiosyncratic ways based on how they reconcile their personal scripts and meanings with socially constructed roles and functions. The process of blending *essential characteristics* of the self with *social constructs* of the community to form a sexual minority identity is often lifelong and evolving. Numerous theories have been proposed as to how this identity development occurs. This chapter discusses four models of gay and lesbian identity formation and some of their limitations, as well as bisexual variations. Chapter 9 focuses on psychotherapeutic applications of these formulations, sex differences, and other factors associated with the sexual minority identification process.

LESBIAN AND GAY IDENTITY DEVELOPMENT MODELS

Many theorists have proposed models for describing the process of gay and lesbian identity development. Most of these formulations refer only to lesbians and gay men without incorporating an identity formation trajectory for bisexual individuals. As discussed in Chapter 2, recent research and speculation indicate that bisexual identity formation is characterized by its own inherent complexity (Fox, 1993, 1995; G. D. Morrow, 1989; Paul, 1996; Zinik, 1985), although the basic process for sexual minority populations is essentially similar. To remain true to the original models, the following discussion refers primarily to gay men and lesbians. Bisexual variations are presented later in this chapter.

The four models described herein are selected for discussion because they are believed to represent current mainstream thinking about lesbian and gay identity formation. Table 5.1 outlines parallels between these formulations and their developmental stages are outlined. In some instances, these comparisons reflect references that the theorists themselves have made to the each other's models. In most cases, however, the relationships drawn in Table 5.1 are inferential and included only to assist clinicians in assessing approximate levels of identity development among their sexual minority clients.

The Cass Model

During several years of clinical work with gay and lesbian clients, Australian psychologist Vivienne Cass (1979, 1983/1984) generated a theoretical model of identity formation that she applied to both men and women of homosexual orientation. Cass (1979) assumed that "identity is acquired through a developmental process" (p. 219) and that "stability and change in human behavior are dependent on the congruency or incongruency that exists within an individual's interpersonal environment" (p. 220). In other words, she asserted that consistency or inconsistency between how individuals see them-

TABLE 5.1. Models of Gay and Lesbian Identity Formation

Cass (1979, 1984)	Troiden (1979, 1989)	Coleman (1981/1982)	Grace (1979, 1992)
	Sensitization	Pre-Coming Out	Emergence
Identity Confusion Identity Comparison	Identity Confusion	Coming Out	Acknowledgment
Identity Tolerance	Identity Assumption	Exploration	Finding Community (men) First Relationships (women)
Identity Acceptance	Commitment	First Relationships	First Relationships (men) Finding Community (women)
Identity Pride Identity Synthesis		Integration	Self-Definition and Reintegration

selves and the way they perceive others seeing them shapes the course of identity formation. Thus, she proposed six stages of development through which sexual minorities pass on the way to fully integrating a gay or lesbian identity within an overall self-concept.

A process of socialization, however, precedes these stages of identity development. Most families and communities assume that their children are either born heterosexual or will develop erotic and emotional attractions to the other sex. Consequently, children internalize these heterosexist assumptions about their sexual orientations. For gay, lesbian, and bisexual youth, these introjects are discordant and fail to describe their subjective experiences. These clients, then, usually have conformed to identities prescribed for them by the heterosexual majority and thus have limited awareness of their attractions to their same sex.

Stage 1: Identity Confusion

For people attracted to members of their own sex, the actual process of identity formation begins when they become consciously aware that information regarding homosexuality acquired directly or indirectly somehow applies to them. As they continue to personalize this information, the heterosexual identities they have assumed for themselves and to which they have attempted to conform begin to feel discordant. This incongruency results in emotional tension, often in the form of anxiety, confusion, or both (Cass, 1990). While experiencing these unpleasant emotions, individuals are privately labeling their thoughts, feelings and fantasies as *possibly* gay or lesbian. Publicly, however, they are maintaining heterosexual images of themselves which they assume others perceive as well. Cass (1979) described three different ways in which people evaluate the accuracy/ acceptability of defining themselves and their experiences as gay or lesbian, relieve their internal conflict, and resolve this crisis (pp. 223–224):

1. *Correct and acceptable.* People for whom homosexuality is a *correct and acceptable* self-definition begin to question a heterosexual identity and ask themselves, "Am I gay or lesbian?" (Cass, 1979). According to psychotherapist Betty Berzon (1988), these individuals are likely to adopt an "information-seeking strategy" (p. 48) in order to address this question and proceed to the second stage of identity development.

2. *Correct but undesirable.* To reject a *correct but undesirable* self-definition (Cass, 1979), individuals may adopt an "inhibition strategy" (Berzon, 1988, p. 46) and take one or more of the following courses of action outlined by Cass and described by Berzon:

- Restrict information regarding homosexuality
- Deny its personal relevance
- Inhibit romantic or erotic behavior with same-sex partners
- Become hypersexual with members of the other sex
- Become celibate
- Seek a "cure"
- Morally crusade against lesbians and gay men

3. *Incorrect and undesirable.* People for whom homosexuality is an *incorrect and undesirable* self-definition may adopt a "personal innocence strategy" (Berzon, 1988, p. 46) in order to redefine the meaning or the context of their experiences. Cass (1979) observed a difference between how men and women restructure cognitions about their

same-sex attractions and behaviors. Accordingly, many men perceive male-to-male geni-tal contact as not being "gay" as long as they refrain from exposing their feelings, kissing on the mouth, or having sex with the same person more than once. Conversely, many women consider intense emotional involvements with other females as not being "les-bian" as long as they abstain from genital contact.

To disclaim responsibility for their nonheterosexual behavior, individuals may reframe the context in which their same-sex contacts occur (Berzon, 1988; Cass, 1979):

- "I was only experimenting."
- "I was very drunk."
- "I only did it for the money."
- "I was doing my friend a favor."
- "It happened by accident."
- "(S)he took advantage of me."

To succeed at using the "inhibition and personal innocence strategies," individuals must be able "to avoid provocative situations and to employ the psychological defense of denial" (Berzon, 1988, p. 48). If these efforts to restructure confusing and otherwise threatening cognitions are successful, the potential for being gay or lesbian is rejected and sexual minorities thus foreclose on the process of identity formation (Cass, 1979). Con-versely, those who seek information about homosexuality in order to reduce confusion inadvertently enhance the discordance between their previously assumed and emerging identities. This increasing cognitive and affective dissonance often motivates them to pro-ceed to the next stage of identity development.

Stage 2: Identity Comparison

The second stage of the process occurs when people attracted to members of their own sex can accept the possibility that they might *not* be heterosexual after all. Their ability to admit that they may be gay or lesbian reflects a significant decrease in the confusion they sought to reduce during the first stage of identity formation and marks an initial step to-ward committing to a lesbian or gay self-image (Cass, 1979, 1990). While feeling less confused about themselves and their experiences, this rising commitment leads them to feel more alienated from others. Accordingly, they develop "a sense of 'not belonging' to society at large as well as to specific subgroups such as family and peers" (Cass, 1979, p. 225). These feelings of alienation may be intensified when individuals are geographi-cally and socially isolated, assume that they are unique in their same-sex attractions, or belong to religious groups which condemn homosexuality.

Accepting the possibility of being gay or lesbian eventually leads many individuals "to realize that all the guidelines for behavior, ideals, and expectations for the future that accompany a heterosexual identity are no longer relevant . . . and, most impor-tantly, have not been replaced by others" (Cass, 1979, p. 225). According to Berzon (1988), "grieving the loss of that heterosexual blueprint for life is an inescapable part" (p. 49) of identity formation. For many, transforming the loss of a heterosexual life im-age and developing a positive gay or lesbian identity are parallel processes (O'Neill & Ritter, 1992).

Cass (1979) identified four approaches or paths that people adopt to "reduce the feelings of alienation evident at Stage 2" (p. 226). The path chosen will depend on their images of themselves, as well as the degree to which they perceive being lesbian or gay as desirable (Cass, 1990).

1. *Devalue the importance of others and present a public image of heterosexuality.* Cass (1979) identified three groups of people who react positively to the notion of being different and are thus able to *devalue the importance of others* (p. 226):

- *Those who sense that they have always been different because of their thoughts, feelings, and fantasies about members of their own sex.* During the early stages of the identity formation process, these same-sex attractions are identified and validated. Consequently, individuals are led to an awareness that there is a group of people (lesbians and gay men) to which they rightfully belong. This social category "provides them with a label for their difference . . . and diminishes their sense of isolation" (Troiden, 1989, p. 58).
- *Those who attribute their feelings of being different to their noncompliance with heterosexist socialization.* For example, some people resist the conditioning that automatically assumes heterosexual marriage to be the only option for adulthood. For these individuals, a gay or lesbian identity may legitimize their nonconformity in a favorable manner and justify their choice to remain unmarried to a person of the other sex.
- *Those who consider being different exciting, extraordinary, or special.* "As with the other two groups, the felt difference between themselves and others is given a positive evaluation" (Cass, 1979, p. 226).

While discounting the significance of others, many of these individuals continue to present a public image of heterosexuality. Passing as heterosexual enables them to avoid negative reactions from others regarding homosexuality and allows them additional time to adjust to a gay or lesbian identity. "Passing can be a relatively easy task because it entails simply continuing in old patterns of behavior" (Cass, 1979, pp. 226–227).

Cass (1979) identified four ways that many people attracted to members of their own sex successfully use the "passing strategy" (p. 227):

- By avoiding situations that threaten to expose their lack of commitment to heterosexist social and gender roles (i.e., social gatherings where guests are expected to bring a date of the other sex)
- By controlling information about themselves (i.e., adopting behavioral patterns and clothing styles that contradict gay or lesbian stereotypes)
- By intentionally exaggerating and flaunting the image of heterosexuality or celibacy
- By role distancing, detaching, or dissociating from behaviors commonly associated with lesbians and gay men

2. *Reduce the importance of a gay or lesbian self-image.* Cass (1979) identified four strategies that allow individuals to redefine the meaning of their same-sex experiences while rejecting a gay or lesbian identity:

- *Special case strategy.* People who adopt this approach consider their same-sex experience as "an isolated case, a one-time occurrence, part of a special, never-to-be-repeated relationship" (Troiden, 1989, p. 57). For example, a woman's explanation might be expressed as "I'm not a lesbian; I'm just in love with

Marion," while a man's interpretation might be verbalized as "If it were not for Carlos, I would be straight."

- *Ambisexual strategy.* People who adopt this common strategy perceive themselves as attracted and oriented to both sexes. As long as they acknowledge their personal potential for heterosexual behavior, they can excuse themselves from heterosexual relationships. Further, by applying the bisexual label to well-known public figures and focusing on theories of universal bisexuality, they reduce their feelings of alienation and enhance their identification with others.

- *Temporary identity strategy.* People who adopt this approach explain their same-sex experiences as temporary stages or phases of development (Cass, 1979; Troiden, 1989). In one study of 164 men (Troiden, 1979), 54% of those surveyed did not label their sexual attractions as definitely gay "because they were interpreted as a phase of development that would eventually pass" (pp. 366–367). Thus, by viewing feelings as temporary, they leave open the option to behave or identify as heterosexual in the future.

- *Personal innocence strategy.* Frequently, people who negatively view being gay or lesbian acknowledge their erotic attractions but deny personal responsibility for their same-sex experiences. While many self-affirming lesbians and gay men *attribute* their sexual orientations to biological origins, some self-deprecating individuals *blame* their homosexuality on biology (i.e., "I can't help it; I was born this way"). Others blame a sexual assault for their same-sex inclinations (i.e., "If I hadn't been raped, I wouldn't be lesbian," or, "If I hadn't been molested, I wouldn't be gay"). Others attribute their sexual orientation to a seduction ("If [s]he hadn't led me on, I would be straight"). Still others accuse one or both parents for the conditions that led to their homosexuality.

3. *Reduce the fear of others' negative reactions.* People who are attracted to members of their own sex often anticipate strong negative reactions from their families, peers, or religious groups. In these cases, individuals are likely to adopt strategies to conceal or inhibit their sexual behavior. Fear of these disapproving responses often motivates some of them to move to another city or to leave their church or synagogue. Others seek professional help to repress their same-sex impulses. The process of curbing homoerotic attractions, however, frequently suppresses all sexual arousal and feeling. This inhibition of sexual awareness and behaviors, nonetheless, allows some to assume an asexual role and self-image. Hence, a pretense of asexuality removes them from potentially provocative situations and thus reinforces the inhibition strategy. Unfortunately, "successful inhibition [of homosexual self-perception] leads to identity foreclosure" (Cass, 1979, p. 229).

4. *Inhibit same-sex behavior; devalue homosexuality, and esteem heterosexuality.* People who feel extremely alienated from significant others because of their same-sex feelings frequently wish to change their attractions, behaviors, and self-images. While some seek psychotherapy to redirect their homosexual impulses, others seek religious conversion to heterosexuality (see Chapter 13). By attempting to rechannel their sexual urges from the same to the other sex, they reject the possibility of being gay or lesbian and thus foreclose on the process of identity formation. When efforts to inhibit same-sex attraction and behavior are unsuccessful, self-hatred is often intensified.

The second stage of identity formation can result in several possible outcomes. As with every stage in the process, individuals may foreclose on developing a positive identity. Some people entertain the possibility of bisexuality, whereas others conclude that their same-sex attractions are only temporary or specific to a certain person. Still others complete this phase perceiving themselves as *probably* gay or lesbian. Of these individuals, some view this probable identity as positive while others see it as negative.

Stage 3: Identity Tolerance

The third stage of the process occurs when people attracted to members of their own sex can admit that they *probably* are lesbian or gay. Although they only tolerate (rather than fully accept) a gay or lesbian self-image, this greater level of commitment nonetheless alleviates some of the confusion about their identities. The partial relief of this uncertainty enables them to acknowledge their social, emotional, and sexual needs. On the other hand, this increased commitment highlights the discrepancy between the way they see themselves (i.e., probably gay or lesbian) and the way they perceive others seeing them (i.e., probably heterosexual). As their feelings of alienation increase, they seek out gay and lesbian individuals and communities in order to reduce their isolation.

More critical for identity formation than establishing contact with other lesbians and gay men is the emotional quality of these first encounters. In other words, perceiving these initial experiences as favorable is essential for positive identity development. Many variables, however, may contribute to an individual's negative perceptions of these contacts: "poor social skills; shyness; low self-esteem; and fear of exposure" (Cass, 1979, p. 230). When these encounters are perceived as negative, the gay and lesbian subculture is devalued, contacts with lesbians and gay men are minimized or ceased, and self-esteem is lowered.

When these experiences are seen as positive, however, further identification with the gay and lesbian community is intensified, self-esteem is raised, and ongoing contact with lesbians and gay men is reinforced. "Socialization with homosexuals, at whatever level, allows for the rehearsal of the homosexual role, which then encourages others to identify the individual as a homosexual" (Cass, 1990, p. 249). Further, socializing with the gay and lesbian community provides people with opportunities to meet potential partners, find positive role models, learn better identity management strategies, practice feeling more comfortable with the subculture, and access ready-made support groups.

Stage 4: Identity Acceptance

The fourth stage of identity formation is characterized by ongoing and additional contacts with other lesbians and gay men. These validating and "normalizing" encounters lead individuals to accept (rather than tolerate) a gay or lesbian self-image. As their contacts with others increase in frequency and regularity, individuals discover preferences for same-sex social contexts and start to form friendships within them. The kinds of gay and lesbian community subgroups within which they socialize, however, strongly influence the way they progress through the remaining stages of the process. Whereas some groups espouse attitudes or beliefs that fully legitimize a same-sex orientation (i.e., being gay or lesbian is valid both publicly and privately), others advocate only a partial legitimization philosophy (i.e., a gay or lesbian self-image is valid as a private identity but should not be exposed to the rest of society, or is "nobody else's business").

Attitudes or beliefs that only partially legitimize homosexuality emphasize "fitting in" and thus relieve or prevent feelings of incongruency with the heterosexual majority.

Cass (1979) identified three strategies for maintaining a partial legitimization philosophy (p. 232):

1. *Passing.* By Stage 4, passing has become a habitual maneuver for compartmentalizing a gay or lesbian way of life and decreasing the possibility of being confronted with negative reactions from heterosexual others. If passing as heterosexual is an acceptable strategy, "the developmental path will lead to foreclosure at a stage that is relatively peaceful and fulfilling" (Cass, 1990, p. 249).

2. *Limited contact.* Along with passing, limiting contacts with heterosexuals diminishes feelings of difference from the majority culture.

3. *Selective disclosure.* To alleviate feelings of incongruency with the dominant group, individuals may selectively self-disclose their gay or lesbian identity to significant heterosexual others, who, in turn, function to protect and keep the secret.

When these strategies are applied successfully, inner tension is either held to a manageable level or reduced and identity foreclosure results. If these tactics fail to relieve the turmoil, individuals may either reapply them or reject the partial legitimization philosophy by adopting a fully legitimate perspective.

A philosophy of full legitimization validates and "normalizes" the newly formed identities of lesbians and gay men. Socializing with affirming peers has helped them to clarify a more positive self-image and to feel greater security with being gay or lesbian. This affirmation, however, also accentuates the difference between how individuals see themselves (i.e., positively) and how they perceive society as seeing them (i.e., negatively). With newfound friends fully legitimizing their gay or lesbian identities, prejudiced attitudes toward sexual minorities become particularly incongruent and offensive. This "incongruity of being acceptable in some places and not in others" (Cass, 1990, p. 88) frequently leads them to reject angrily the secrecy and negative status that passing for heterosexual carries with it. These individuals, then, proceed to the fifth stage of identity development in order to resolve these feelings of anger toward a homophobic and heterosexist society (Berzon, 1988; Cass, 1979, 1990; Falco, 1991).

Stage 5: Identity Pride

Gay and lesbian individuals enter the fifth stage of identity formation with a strong sense of the incongruency between the positive way they have come to accept themselves and society's devaluation of their identities. To manage these discordant feelings, they tend to discriminate between people based on sexual orientation and identification. In other words, they apply strategies that depreciate the significance of heterosexuals and appreciate, if not exaggerate, the importance of other lesbians and gay men. Thus, they now not only *accept* but also *prefer* their new identities to a heterosexual self-image. A strong commitment to the gay and lesbian community generates feelings of group identity, belonging, and pride. This immersion in the subculture is often characterized by what Cass (1979) refers to as *voracious consumption* of gay and lesbian media and services.

While these dichotomizing strategies relieve internal conflicts for newly identified lesbians and gay men, daily encounters with a heterosexist, if not homophobic, outer world generate "feelings of anger born of frustration and alienation" (Cass, 1979, p. 233). This anger combines with feelings of pride and energizes individuals into becoming activists for the gay and lesbian community. Because this kind of militancy often leads individuals to confront the heterosexual establishment, activists put themselves in positions in which passing strategies are no longer practical. Instead, they adopt disclosure as a coping response.

According to Cass (1979), disclosure has two possible positive outcomes, depending on its nature and circumstances. First, the more that others know about an individual's same-sex orientation, the more that person's gay or lesbian self-image potentially is reflected and reinforced. Second, disclosure allows public and private identities to converge and consolidate into a single self-concept. While disclosure naturally evokes reactions from others, an individual's perception of those responses often determines whether or not identity development proceeds. When derogatory attitudes or behaviors are aroused in others, the person's expectations are confirmed and the "them versus us" dichotomy is fortified. In these instances, individuals potentially foreclose on their identities, particularly if they are especially fearful of rejection or excessively ashamed. On the other hand, if negative reactions are anticipated and positive responses from others are received, the outcomes are unexpected. This effect often results in gay men and lesbians feeling a sense of discordance or cognitive dissonance. To relieve this inconsistency, some individuals move to the sixth stage of identity formation (Berzon, 1988; Cass, 1979, 1990; Falco, 1991).

Stage 6: Identity Synthesis

People enter this final phase of identity development with a sense that the formerly adopted "them versus us" philosophy no longer applies. As this "heterosexual versus homosexual" dichotomy is relinquished, feelings of anger and pride become less overwhelming. Lesbians and gay men now discriminate on the basis of perceived support rather than focusing exclusively on the sexual orientation of another. While greater trust is placed in sensitive and sympathetic heterosexuals (Cass, 1979), "unsupportive heterosexuals are further devalued" (p. 234). Sexual minority individuals are now able to acknowledge potential similarities between themselves and their heterosexual counterparts, as well as possible differences between themselves and members of their own community. Public and private aspects of self become synthesized into an integrated identity which includes sexual orientation along with many other dimensions. As they feel greater security in their integrated identities, gay men and lesbians self-disclose almost automatically. Finally, at peace with themselves, they are free to proceed with the typical developmental tasks of adulthood (Berzon, 1988; Cass, 1979, 1990).

In the process of identity formation, however, Cass (1990) observed individual differences in "the rate of progression through the stages, the final stage of development reached, the paths of development taken within each stage, and strategies adopted to cope with the tasks of each stage" (p. 247). Further, she anticipated sex differences resulting from gender role socialization and variances among age groups based on changing social attitudes and assumptions.

The Troiden Model

Sociologist Richard Troiden elaborated on his previous work (1979) with which he synthesized the works of Cass (1979, 1984), Plummer (1975), and Ponse (1978) in order to formulate his four-stage model of gay and lesbian identity development. Like other conceptualizations, Troiden's (1989) model views identity formation as "taking place against a backdrop of stigma" (p. 47), developing over an extended period, including a number of critical transitions, and involving eventual self-labeling as gay or lesbian. His model further assumes that recurrent themes recalled by lesbians and gay men cluster according to developmental phases in their life histories. These age-specific themes thus "provide the content and characteristics of each stage" (p. 47) of identity development. Because these stages are not linear, they build on one another, sometimes recur, and often overlap. He names them *Sensitization*, *Identity Confusion*, *Identity Assumption*, and *Commitment*.

Stage 1: Sensitization

According to Troiden (1989), "the *sensitization* stage occurs before puberty" (p. 50) and is characterized by childhood feelings of difference from same-sex peers. Young girls sometimes describe themselves as different by not being interested in boys; feeling unfeminine, ungraceful, and not very pretty; and considering themselves more masculine, independent, and aggressive than other girls. Some young boys, on the other hand, describe themselves as being more interested in the arts than their male peers and less interested in sports and boys' games. Echoing the discussion in Chapter 3, Troiden's study of 150 gay men (1979) reflected these childhood themes of marginality, alienation, and estrangement from other males. In particular, those interviewed remembered feeling *socially different* prior to age 13. Further, 99% of these men recalled feeling *sexually different* from ages 13 to 17, with 40% indicating less interest in girls than their peers and 25% reporting sexual interest or activity with other males. These adolescent differences stemmed primarily from the *erotic* as well as *emotional* domain.

As explained in Chapters 3 and 6, feeling *socially different* during childhood for gender-inappropriate interests sensitizes "prehomosexuals" for subsequently defining themselves as lesbian or gay (Troiden, 1979, 1989). The meanings attributed to these childhood experiences of social difference are later reinterpreted as indicating a homosexual potential. In fact, Troiden contends that these reinterpretations are necessary conditions for the eventual adoption of a gay or lesbian identity. Thus, rather than the experiences themselves, the meanings attached to them become critical variables in the process of identity development.

Stage 2: Identity Confusion

Troiden's second stage of identity formation bears the same name as, and borrows insights from, the first stage of the model Cass outlined. Further, many concepts and strategies from her second stage, *Identity Comparison*, are adopted, as well. Both models allege that by middle to late adolescence, people attracted to their own sex come to suspect that they might be gay or lesbian (Schäfer, 1976, Troiden & Goode, 1980). During these teenage years, "childhood perceptions of self as different crystallize into perceptions of self as sexually different" and lead to identity disturbance (Troiden, 1989, p. 53). While the stigma surrounding homosexuality further creates problems of shame and secrecy, the societal emphasis on gender roles alienates and isolates those who do not conform. These conditions, combined with ignorance and inaccurate knowledge about a homosexual orientation, intensify the identity confusion.

Troiden (1989) contends that people respond to this disorientation by adopting a number of possible strategies (pp. 52–58), many of which are similar to those described in the previous discussion of the Cass model. Following is a brief outline of Troiden's strategies (see his original sources [1979, 1984/1985, 1988, 1989; Troiden & Goode, 1980] and Cass's descriptions for further detail):

1. *Denial.* This method involves rejecting the personal relevance of same-sex feelings, fantasies, or behaviors.

2. *Repair.* This process involves seeking professional help to eliminate same-sex feelings, fantasies, or behaviors.

3. *Avoidance.* This strategy involves the following:

- Inhibiting behaviors or interests associated with being gay or lesbian and adopting those associated with being heterosexual
- Concealing their lack of heterosexual responsiveness from family and friends by limiting their exposure to the other sex
- Avoiding exposure to information about homosexuality that may confirm their fears and suspicions about themselves
- Adopting anti-homosexual stances and distancing themselves from their own homoerotic feelings, often by attacking and ridiculing lesbians and gay men
- Immersing themselves in heterosexual relationships in order to eliminate same-sex attractions
- Escaping homoerotic feelings through substance abuse to temporarily relieve pain and confusion over their emerging identities

4. *Redefinition.* This method involves the following (see the foregoing Cass discussion):

- Applying a *special case* strategy
- Adopting an *ambisexual* strategy
- Assuming a *temporary identity* strategy
- Using a situational redefinitional (*personal innocence*) strategy

5. *Acceptance.* Having acknowledged and accepted their same-sex fantasies, feelings, and behaviors, many individuals seek information to learn more about their sexuality. The process of labeling themselves as belonging to a social category diminishes their sense of isolation and moves them to a third stage of identity formation.

Stage 3: Identity Assumption

During or after late adolescence, individuals who have moved thus far along Troiden's (1989) trajectory begin a process of *Identity Assumption*. Accordingly, this level of development incorporates the phases of *Identity Tolerance* and *Identity Acceptance* outlined in the Cass model. Tolerating and accepting a new identity, associating with other lesbians and gay men, experimenting sexually, and exploring of a new subculture are the tasks of this stage.

A gay or lesbian identity initially is tolerated and only later accepted. Due to factors related to gender role socialization, "lesbians and gay males typically define themselves as homosexual at different ages and in different contexts" (Troiden, 1989, p. 59). Between the ages of 19 and 21, the average man defines himself as gay within the context of sexual experimentation. On the other hand, the typical woman is between the ages of 21 and 23 when she begins to perceive herself as lesbian while involved in an intense emotional or romantic relationship. Only a small percentage of individuals achieve a lesbian or gay self-definition without direct contact with others oriented sexually like themselves. Ponse (1978) refers to this solitary phenomenon of identity development as *disembodied affiliation*. Most people, however, seem to need the presence of others like themselves in order to self-identify. If these contacts are positive, the process of identity formation is facilitated.

With the assumption of a gay or lesbian identity, individuals are confronted with the need to manage the societal stigma associated with homosexuality. Troiden borrowed from Humphreys (1972) four possible stigma-evasion strategies:

1. *Capitulation.* Internalizing and acquiescing to negative views of homosexuality, and avoiding same-sex behavior.
2. *Minstrelization.* Expressing a homosexual orientation according to popular cultural stereotypes (i.e., dressing like a "drag queen," becoming a "motorcycle dyke," or "camping" with other gay men).
3. *Passing.* Polarizing and compartmentalizing the social universe into gay/lesbian versus heterosexual worlds, and leading "double lives."
4. *Group alignment.* Immersing the self completely in the lesbian/gay subculture, and avoiding all stigmatizing heterosexual contexts.

Capitulation clearly leads to identity foreclosure. Minstrelization involves adopting a popular caricature of homosexuality and thus inhibits the process of authentic identity formation. On the other hand, passing and group alignment may well be developmentally appropriate survival tactics that facilitate identity consolidation. Passing strategies acknowledge and incorporate the gay or lesbian dimension of an individual's identity, and group alignment potentially counteracts years of heterosexual socialization. This resistance of the dominant group and immersion in the subculture lead many to accept, assume, and eventually commit themselves to their positive gay and lesbian identities.

Stage 4: Commitment

For the committed lesbian or gay man, functioning as a heterosexual eventually becomes difficult and unattractive. Commitment itself has a variety of both internal and external indicators, and following is a list of those outlined by Troiden (1979, 1989):

Internal indicators

- Sexuality and emotionality fuse into a significant whole, thus legitimizing the same sex as a source of both love and romance as well as of sexual gratification.
- The meanings attached to being gay or lesbian shift from a form of behavior or sexual orientation to an "essential" identity, a "state of being" and "way of life."
- The gay or lesbian identity is reconceptualized as natural, normal, and valid for the self.
- Satisfaction with being gay or lesbian is expressed as reluctance to abandon the new identity.

- Happiness increases as people gain and crystallize a sense of identity and clarify their sexual desires and emotional needs.

External indicators

- Entering a same-sex love relationships often marks the onset of commitment to a gay or lesbian identity and reflects the fusion of sexuality and emotionality occurring internally.
- The desire to disclose to heterosexual others increases as the lesbian or gay identity is reconceptualized and crystallized.
- Stigma-management strategies shift from passing and group alignment to the following:
  - *Covering*. Painstaking assimilation with the heterosexual majority in order to maintain respectability, while self-disclosing to selected heterosexuals.
  - *Blending*. Neither announcing nor denying being gay or lesbian, perceiving sexual orientation to be irrelevant to their activities with heterosexuals.
  - *Converting*. Transforming the gay or lesbian identity from a vice or mark of shame to a virtue or mark of self-respect (which parallels the Cass stages of *Identity Pride* and *Identity Synthesis*).

As a gay or lesbian identity develops and solidifies, it is manifested in a wider range of contexts. Troiden (1989) contends that the identity itself "is emergent: never fully determined in a fixed or absolute sense, but always subject to modification and further change" (p. 68). Because commitment may vary across time and place, gay and lesbian identity formation is an ongoing, lifelong process.

The Coleman Model

Psychologist Eli Coleman (1981/1982) proposed a five-stage model of identity development. His model assumes that people enter the identity formation process at different stages and that not everyone passes through every phase. Further, Coleman believes that some individuals are challenged by developmental tasks of more than one stage at a time and that identity synthesis depends on mastery of tasks at all previous levels. However, some people "become locked into one stage or another and never experience identity integration" (p. 32).

Stage 1: Pre-Coming Out

Coleman's first level of identity development is similar to Troiden's initial stage of *Sensitization* (discussed previously) during which young boys and girls, even in early childhood, know they are different from their peers. Because of this difference, then, these children feel alienated and alone, and often develop low self-esteem. They keep their thoughts and feelings private because they sense, consciously or preconsciously, that admitting their same-sex attractions would mean rejection and ridicule, and perhaps even precipitate a family crisis.

Although such young people rarely are able to describe their confusion, they almost intuitively protect themselves from awareness though various defense mechanisms, such as denial, repression, reaction formation, sublimation, and rationalization (E. Coleman, 1981/1982). In many cases, "they can only communicate their conflict through behavioral problems, psychosomatic illnesses, suicidal attempts, or various other symptoms" (p. 33). In other instances, they suffer from dysthymic and depressive disorders. If, per chance, awareness breaks through their protective defenses and same-sex attractions surface to the level of consciousness, these individuals are ready to move into the second stage.

Stage 2: Coming Out

The first developmental task of Coleman's second stage of identity formation involves acknowledging thoughts, feelings, or fantasies that indicate same-sex attractions. During this phase, people do not necessarily have a clear understanding of what it means to be gay or lesbian and, therefore, often feel confused (Cass, 1979). Although they are now aware of strong feelings toward their own sex, they often are not yet ready to label them lesbian or gay. E. Coleman (1981/1982) believes that most individuals are unable to verbalize these feelings, even to a psychotherapist, unless the clinician initiates the discussion. Once, however, the attractions have been acknowledged and identified, the next developmental task involves telling others about them. This first step of "coming out" to significant others is risky. Negative responses can reinforce low self-esteem and therefore forestall identity development. If the reactions are positive, however, "the existential crisis begins to resolve in a positive direction" (p. 34).

Because acceptance (or rejection) from close friends or family members usually means more than those from strangers and because heterosexuality is still the more valued orientation, acceptance by significant heterosexual others is validating to an individual's new and precarious identity. Conversely, the perceived societal status of other lesbians and gay men is typically low at this stage of development; hence, acceptance by them frequently has little value. Those individuals who first find acceptance from heterosexual significant others, in addition to gay and lesbian associates, generally are able to withstand negative responses from family members.

Stage 3: Exploration

Positive reactions from significant others motivate individuals to experiment with their new sexual identities. According to E. Coleman (1981/1982), this stage marks "the first major experience of sexual and social activity with others" (p. 35). Although previous same-sex behavior may have occurred, gay or lesbian meaning was not attributed to these episodes. Now, however, these experiences "are definitely understood to be homosexual" (p. 36).

E. Coleman (1981/1982) has identified three developmental tasks that individuals face during this stage of exploration (pp. 36–37):

1. *To develop interpersonal skills.* Having been socialized to behave heterosexually both with their own and the other sex, people need to learn the skills necessary for establishing intimate same-sex relationships.

2. *To develop a sense of personal attractiveness and sexual competence.* Prior to this stage of exploration, most lesbians and gay men have not been developmentally ready to experiment sexually with the sex they eroticize. Therefore, they need to learn to feel at-

tractive to their own sex and to "develop a sense of mastery and competence with regard to being sexual with others" (p. 36).

3. *To develop positive self-concepts.* During this stage of interpersonal skill acquisition and sexual experimentation, some people view their activities as immature, immoral, or promiscuous. If these individuals can be helped to see their behaviors within a developmental framework, they can complete this stage and proceed to the next with positive, rather than negative, images of themselves.

Stage 4: First Relationships

As people develop interpersonal skills, sexual competence, and self-esteem, their needs for intimacy increase. Hence, they search for intimate relationships that include emotional as well as physical attractions. E. Coleman (1981/1982) describes these first relationships as being "characterized by intensity, possessiveness, and lack of trust. The intense need for intimacy can easily create desperation" (p. 38). This desperation often compels people to form partnerships before consolidating their own gay or lesbian identity. Because they lack same-sex couple experience, individuals often bring idealistic and unrealistic expectations to these first relationships, as well. Many thus end in turbulence. These self-perceived disasters cause many to return to the exploration stage or to abandon future attempts to form committed partnerships altogether. Learning how to function in a same-sex relationship, on the other hand, often prepares people for the final stage of identity development.

Stage 5: Integration

E. Coleman (1981/1982) likens his final stage of *Integration* to the Cass stage of *Identity Synthesis*. "Here individuals incorporate their public and private identities into one self-image" (p. 39). Although many people with integrated identities choose to remain uncoupled, others commit to relationships that are now characterized by mutual trust and psychological health. Regardless of relationship status, all are better prepared to handle the tasks of midlife and maturity than those expending their energies working through earlier stages of gay and lesbian identity development.

The Grace Model

John Grace (1992), a social worker, proposed another five-stage model of gay and lesbian identity formation. His competence-based model examines "major life tasks and common developmental obstacles that retard or arrest positive stage movement" (p. 33). According to Grace, the concept of homophobia (or heterosexism) must be understood before the developmental dilemmas faced by lesbians and gay men can be explained. To facilitate such an understanding, Grace identified extrinsic impediments to self-identification among four specific categories of homophobia: personal/active, personal/passive, institutional/active and institutional/passive (p. 34):

- *Personal*: includes both intrapersonal experiences and interpersonal interactions.
- *Institutional*: involves a relationship between an individual and a societal institution (e.g., family, school, church, business, or government).

- *Active*: expressed through physical assault, verbal abuse, hostile stereotypes, and pressure to conform to heterosexist norms.
- *Passive*: appears as heterosexist assumptions, ignorance about the experience of lesbians and gay men, and neglect toward their basic human rights and needs.

These four homophobic external barriers negatively and harmfully affect the pace and quality of both personality development and identity formation. Thus, Grace believes that a nonpejorative theory of motivation which emphasizes the oppressive effects of the environment is essential for understanding lesbians and gay men. Such a theory explains not only their difficulties in proceeding with identity development but also the homophobia-induced developmental lag experienced by many of these individuals. For example, from early childhood, a significant number recall feeling threatened and fearful of physical injury, verbal humiliation, abandonment, or rejection. "This chronic sense of danger" (p. 37) results in the developmental lag which Grace (1992) defines as "significant and problematic discrepancies between chronological age and physical maturity that impedes successful identification and mastery of essential psychosocial milestones" (p. 33). Personal, institutional, active, and passive homophobia thus influence personality development as well as identity formation, and have the following "very serious consequences" (p. 37) for lesbians and gay men:

- Large amounts of time and energy are devoted to survival and defense rather than to intimacy and growth.
- A generalized view of the world as threatening and dangerous is developed.
- Two selves are created: a public self that disguises and armors a private self which is alienated from the rest of the world.
- A sense of shame about core identity and basic needs is fostered by isolation.

Consequently, people feel deeply ashamed and work to conceal at all costs the private self that is seen as defective, worthless, bad, and unlovable. In other words, societal heterosexism instills shame in individuals who, in turn, develop defenses to manage their feelings of inferiority. Fearing exposure, they become either competent liars or competent frauds, building barriers rather bridges between themselves and others. These shame-based defenses "protect against additional shame from the world outside, and to contain internalized shame and prevent it from being reactivated by exposure to others" (p. 40). In this climate, individuals begin the process of identity formation outlined by Grace.

Stage 1: Emergence

Grace's (1992) first level of identity development (*Emergence*) is similar to the initial stages of Troiden (*Sensitization*) and Coleman (*Pre-Coming Out*), during which children sense they are different from their agemates. Although same-sex attractions are ambiguous, they are sufficiently shameful to cause social and performance anxiety. Sensing strong heterosexist and gender-specific norms to which they must conform, people often "experience a double-binding fear of being noticed if they don't behave 'correctly' and being noticed if they don't try at all" (pp. 40–41). This approach–avoidance conflict frequently results in anxiety-impaired performance, or in passing for heterosexual—which only further splits the public and private selves.

Stage 2: Acknowledgment

As ambiguous same-sex attractions crystallize into explicit homoerotic fantasies, feelings of shame and fear may intensify. This second stage of identity formation typically occurs during adolescence, generally earlier for boys than for girls (Jay & Young, 1977; Troiden & Goode, 1980), and within a teenage social context that is extremely heterosexist and shaming of sexual minorities. Fear of acknowledging their same-sex feelings leads many to deny, rationalize, or bargain in order to limit conscious awareness of their emerging sexual identities. These responses are quite similar to strategies outlined by Cass and Troiden for managing the stage of *Identity Confusion* (described earlier in this chapter).

Because shame is frequently disguised as perfectionism, "homophobic bargaining often takes on perfectionist proportions" (Grace, 1992, p. 41). One of Grace's clients described this process as learning to look good while feeling bad. Some perform so well that they are able to assimilate into heterosexual peer groups and thus avoid stigmatization and social exclusion. At some level, nonetheless, they know they are deceiving others and depreciating themselves. Intense distress often accompanies self-hatred and frequently sexual minorities engage in both healthy and unhealthy activities that provide relief "from the pain of chronic isolation and self-disgust" (p. 42). During the *Emergence* and *Acknowledgment* stages, these cumulative effects of homophobia can impair the willingness or ability of individuals to proceed further with identity formation. In such cases, identity foreclosure (Cass, 1979) occurs and same-sex attractions are either denied or repressed. If the process has not been arrested, however, people are positioned to move the next developmental stage.

Stage 3: Finding Community

Once lesbians and gay men have acknowledged their sexual identities, the next step is to find a peer group or community where they can publicly share their private selves. Grace (1992) refers to the stage of *Finding Community* as "gay and lesbian adolescence" during which time people often feel an urgency to make up for the teenage era they spent living as a "pseudo-heterosexual" (p. 43). Depending on the number of years devoted to passing for heterosexual, this emotional adolescence may occur anytime during adulthood and is particularly unsettling for adults who have otherwise matured financially, vocationally, and intellectually (Grace, 1979). Lacking experience in initiating and maintaining relationships with the sex they eroticize, individuals often feel inadequate about how to behave and how to manage new and unfamiliar feelings. As with the chronological teenage years, gay and lesbian adolescence is a period filled with awkwardness, uncertainty, and pain (Grace, 1992).

Some adults compound the problem by "crashing out" during this coming-out process (Grace, 1979). Sensing the "developmental lag" or the loss of a chronological adolescence, they feel the pinch of time and are compelled to move beyond this painful stage of identity development as soon as possible. As they rush through a process that best unfolds naturally, some lesbians and gay men behave in ways they otherwise would consider inappropriate for people their age. Consequently, they often judge themselves unfairly as immature, immoral, or less than honorable. This self-criticism activates the internalized shame that has been accumulating over a lifetime, as well as reinforces their pervasive sense of badness or differentness. For some, unfortunately, this shame continues as a lifelong pattern and further operates to foreclose identity development. Others are affirmed in their emerging identities, however, and continue along a favorable developmental trajectory in spite of the barriers and obstacles to finding community with other lesbians and gay men.

Stage 4: First Relationships

Although Grace developed his model from clinical work with gay men, he acknowledged that there may be sex differences in the stage sequencing of the identity development process. Specifically, he credits Feigal (1983) for corroborating "the model's applicability for women with the reversal of finding community and first relationship stages to reflect different socialization patterns" (Grace, 1992, p. 35). In order not to detract from the discussion of the Grace model, though, Chapter 9 addresses these and other sex differences.

Whether first relationships precede or follow finding community, they typically include a number of stages which Grace (1992) adopted from Schroeder (1980):

1. *The dream world stage.* Partners idealize each other and their relationship and emphasize only positive characteristics of both.
2. *The disillusionment stage.* As unrealistic expectations are not met, dislikes and differences begin to be noticed.
3. *Misery.* At this transition stage, internalized shame can destroy a relationship and foreclose further identity development.
4. *Enlightenment.* Partners assume personal responsibility for the success of their relationship.
5. *Mutual respect.* Truthfully admitting their strengths and weaknesses as well as their similarities and differences, partners decide mindfully about the permanence of their relationship.

First relationships have the potential to be seriously damaging or intensely healing to the psyches of the individuals involved. As basic needs for affirmation, physical and sexual contact, and emotional nurturance are met during the dream world stage, the "psychic armor" (Grace, 1992, p. 45) built over the years to protect the private self begins to soften. As a result, people are extremely vulnerable to their partners, their own feelings, and the emotional impact of the relationship. In this newfound state of openness and receptivity, however, lifelong shame sometimes contaminates the partnership. If so, misery may escalate "into rage and violence or despair and depression" (p. 46). Such a negative experience often leads individuals to foreclose on further growth. If, however, the new vulnerability results in a positive attachment, then the authentic lesbian or gay self is validated and consolidated.

Stage Five: Self-Definition and Reintegration

Grace (1979, 1992) describes this final stage of identity development as an open-ended, ongoing, and lifelong process. As the gay and lesbian identity continues to be affirmed and solidified, new images and concepts of the self evolve which allow for new social networks and relationships. Mastering the tasks of all five stages provides individuals with a reservoir of skills and resources for coping with the situational demands of life. For example, when relationships end or when circumstances require yet another "coming out," people at Stage 5 have a repertoire of previous experiences from which to draw. Having defined themselves as lesbian or gay, individuals are now free to engage in the process of integrating this identity within the totality of their being. With this self-consolidation comes the ego strength necessary for proceeding with other important developmental tasks of adulthood.

Limitations of Identity Development Models

Now that four models of identity development have been summarized, a few comments about these formulations are in order. The following observations are provided not to discredit these models but, rather, to frame them within a realistic perspective. First, the samples from which data were drawn to develop these formulations are not necessarily representative of all sexual minority individuals. This sampling problem, however, exists with any studies involving hidden, oppressed, or stigmatized populations. First and foremost, participants must be identifiable and available for research purposes, which often results in investigators relying on those who frequent homosexually oriented establishments and organizations. Consequently, individuals in the first stages of identity formation often are underrepresented in research which attempts to validate the identity development models because they do not yet see themselves as gay, lesbian, or bisexual (Brady & Busse, 1994).

Further, most studies of gay men appear to underrepresent those 45 years of age or older who are relatively inactive in the subculture (Harry, 1986). Given the lack of a visible and validating gay and lesbian community when they were young adults, these men are likely to have come out later in life. A description of the 26 White, suburban, middle-class gay men whom F. R. Lynch (1987) studied might characterize this population. These individualistic men primarily were oriented to their work and career building, to suburban home ownership, and to establishing a long-term same-sex love relationship. Because they were well integrated into the majority culture, these men were unlikely to be easily identifiable and readily located within the gay community for research purposes. Most readers can either identify or imagine similar lesbian populations that fit this description. In any case, respondents who are recruited for study from the gay and lesbian community or from psychotherapy clients may be different from those acquired through the general media or from invisible, but more representative, samples (Harry, 1986).

In addition, those who come out earlier as opposed to later are more likely to be included in research involving sexual minority populations. Generally, these individuals are more educated and come from families with higher levels of parental education (Harry, 1986); only recently have people of color been included in the research pools. Finally, the definition of sexual orientation is problematic with different researchers assessing the construct in various ways (e.g., by sexual behavior, self-definition, or membership in gay organizations; Krajeski, 1986; Rothblum, 1994). After reviewing the 144 studies published in the *Journal of Homosexuality* from 1974 to 1993, for example, Chung and Katayama (1996) concluded that the most typical method for assessing sexual orientation was self-definition. Participants' sexual orientations were assumed, rather than assessed, in about one-third of the studies. As noted previously, those in the early stages of identity development who have not yet self-labeled are not represented in the any of the samples, regardless of how sexual orientation is measured.

Psychotherapists are encouraged, therefore, to keep in mind that the generalizability of any research finding or identity formation model is limited by the demographics of the individuals from whose dynamics the conclusion were drawn and formulations constructed. When using studies or models for psychoeducation purposes or to guide their work with clients, clinicians must consider factors such as age, gender, ethnicity, socioeconomic status, educational level, and religious background, as well as the definition of sexual orientation used in the design.

BISEXUAL IDENTITY FORMATION

The final phases of the identity formation models discussed thus far in this chapter generally assume that sexual orientation is a stable core trait. Further, these models outline a set sequence of stages that culminate in some sort of an integration of, and a commitment to, a gay or lesbian identity that an individual comes to "own" and that "can guide and direct one's emotional and erotic preferences rather than simply describe them" (Paul, 1996, p. 443). Given the multifaceted and fluid nature of bisexuality and the complexity of identifying oneself as bisexual (described in Chapter 2), some (M. S. Weinberg et al., 1994) question the extent of overlap with the process of defining oneself as gay or lesbian.

To the knowledge of M. S. Weinberg et al., for example, no previous model of bisexual identity formation existed at the time of the completion of their investigation. They, nevertheless, were able to construct an explanatory framework based on information gathered from fieldwork and interviews related to their comparative study of 800 self-identified bisexuals, lesbians, heterosexuals, and gay men (see Chapter 2). Accordingly, the three researchers found four stages that captured their bisexual respondents' most common experiences related to the evolution of their identities. M. S. Weinberg et al. (1994) noted, however, that the phases of their model "are very broad and somewhat simplified," but that their conjectures "can form the basis for the development of more sophisticated models of bisexual identity formation" (p. 37). Further, they caution against generalizing their stages to bisexual individuals in all circumstances, given that the respondents in their study already had self-labeled and were members of a bisexual social organization in San Francisco. The vast majority of bisexually-oriented people in other locations and situations undoubtedly move through the early phases of the bisexual identity process with a great deal more difficulty given the lack of information and support. In fact, "many probably never reach the later stages" (p. 37).

While descriptive in nature and presently lacking empirical support, the pioneering work of Weinberg and his associates can serve nonetheless as a framework for describing common experiences of those who eventually identify as bisexual. These phases necessarily are quite expansive and potentially inclusive, given the number of bisexual types (M. S. Weinberg et al., 1994) and the wide range of patterns and histories of bisexually identified individuals (see Chapter 2). Their first three stages (*Initial Confusion, Finding and Applying the Label*, and *Settling into the Identity*) are mentioned only briefly because they are similar to those phases that describe the difficulties faced by gay men and lesbians as they move through the identity formation process (see previous discussions of the models of Cass, Troiden, Coleman, and Grace). Most of the attention in the following discussion, then, is focused on Weinberg's last stage, *Continued Uncertainty*, as the ongoing nature of the dilemma makes this stage unique to bisexually oriented individuals.

Initial Confusion

Most individuals are quite confused when the reality of their attractions to members of two sexes becomes conscious. Because long-term denial is common in bisexual people, few have dared to inform themselves about the nature of their situation. Rarely do they know, for example, that in recent years bisexuality has come to be seen as a legitimate sexual orientation. The majority probably hold the (prevalent) dichotomized view of erotic directionality and thus see their only orientation options as being either heterosexual or homosexual. Having ruled out heterosexuality as completely valid for them, there appears only the lesbian or gay option as a sexual identity (Fox. 1995).

Most bisexually oriented individuals at this stage have spent their lives viewing themselves as heterosexual and are extremely frightened of the notion of being even somewhat homosexually oriented. Others who have struggled to consolidate a lesbian or gay identity are disconcerted severely by this new awareness. Fox (1996b) summarizes many of their reactions:

> uncertainty about how to interpret concurrent sexual attractions to both women and men; alienation, feeling different from heterosexuals and from gay men and lesbians; isolation, not knowing other bisexual women or men and feeling the lack of a sense of community; self-acceptance, dealing with external and internalized homophobia and biphobia; and apprehension about the impact of disclosing bisexual attractions, behavior, and identity in existing or new relationships. (p. 29)

The majority, even those who reside in many urban areas, see no visible bisexuality community and are convinced there are no others like themselves anywhere (Fox, 1995).

The tasks for psychotherapists at this phase include providing psychoeducation and helping clients come to grips with internalized homophobia and biphobia (Paul, 1996). Information regarding of the most current thinking about bisexuality is essential for these individuals because their confusion often is only adding to their distress and torment (Dworkin, 2000a; Rust, 1996). Internalized heterosexism and homophobia must be addressed directly as clients undertake the painful process of acknowledging their same-sex attractions. Generally speaking, men may find this experience more troublesome than do women, given the nature of male attitudes toward homosexuality (see Chapter 1). Most important, however, all clients need to have their experience affirmed as legitimate.

Finding and Applying the Label

Just as in the process of gay and lesbian identity formation, bisexual individuals at some point must decide whether to undertake the arduous process of testing out their bisexual inclinations with others. Many decide not to press the matter further after they conclude that the risks are greater than they are willing to assume. Individuals in heterosexual or same-sex committed relationships usually are particularly anguished at this phase as they struggle with issues of loyalty to their partners. For those who choose to pursue their bisexual attractions, the experiences they encounter are essentially similar to those of most gay and lesbians as they explore new relationships, attempt to find community, and engage in the unceasing process of coming out.

Clinicians at this phase should continue to provide corrective information on human sexuality "that allows the individual to integrate his or her varying affectional feelings, sexual impulses, and desires" (Paul, 1996, p. 446). The presence of existing and seemingly competing loyalties (such as to partners, children and to family unity), combined with the virtual absence of a visible community, makes this integration of a bisexual identity extremely complex and difficult. In addition, the stressors unique to bisexuality are compounded by those related to the client's religious, ethnic, biracial or bicultural backgrounds, social class, and age (Dworkin, 2000b). Encouragement and support from therapists often are crucial elements in terms of identity development.

Settling into the Identity

It often takes years after first sexual attractions or behaviors to identify as bisexual. In spite of the name given to this phase by M. S. Weinberg and his associates, few individuals truly seem to "settle" into a bisexual identity. In fact, after comparing the experiences of their bisexual subjects with those characteristic of homosexuals (study described previously and in Chapter 2), M. S. Weinberg et al. (1994) "were struck by the absence of closure that characterized our bisexual respondents—even those who appeared most committed to the identity" (p. 34). Unlike many lesbians and gay men who eventually achieve a sense of identity consolidation, the investigators found that ongoing doubts about their identities were present in most of their bisexual subjects. These uncertainties of identity appeared to be especially intense when they were in an exclusive sexual relationship with a partner of one biological sex and found themselves attracted to a person of the other. Because of the persisting nature of this incertitude, Weinberg and his associates thus offered a fourth stage of identity formation of identity that seemed unique to bisexuals.

Continued Uncertainty

Two issues seem to sustain the continued uncertainty of identity described by many bisexual individuals. The first has to do with the severe lack of accurate information about bisexuality. Although those in the general public may be excused for simply being misinformed, the judgment and prejudice demonstrated by some lesbians and gay men toward them are extremely alienating to bisexuals struggling for acceptance, understanding, and validation. The second source of ongoing stress has to do with intimate relationships and the continual need to negotiate and redefine them. The fear of rejection frequently is present, as well as the jealousy and misunderstanding of significant (or potentially significant) others. The following sections discuss these and related issues.

Judgment and Prejudice

Most individuals who come to accept the bisexual label for themselves find a lack of social validation and support for their bisexual identity. Few heterosexuals seem to understand their dilemma. Needing companionship and with little community of their own, many affiliate themselves with lesbians and gay men. Often, however, they encounter prejudice, lack of understanding, and pressure to conform. For example, many gay and lesbian individuals believe there is no such thing as a bisexual identity and, hence, do not see one as crystallized or complete. To them, bisexuals are in transition to homosexuality but are afraid of stigma if they identity as gay or lesbian. To avoid this negativity by members of the only community that they see as available to them, bisexuals are less likely to be "out" than homosexuals and secrecy continues to play a greater role in their lives (Paul, 1996).

In lesbian and feminist communities, bisexuality often is viewed as a phase and a "cop-out," with bisexual women seen as shirkers who want all the good of being with women "without taking the heat it brings on" (Weise, 1992, p. ix). Bisexuals also are considered by some as individuals who cannot make up their minds or are afraid to face the stigma of homosexuality. Many lesbians, in fact, have been found to perceive bisexual women as a threat and untrustworthy (Paul, 1996). Rust (1993b) tested this empirically by administering questionnaires to 346 self-identified lesbians and found several generalizations. These included viewpoints that bisexual women are in transition to lesbianism and are in denial of their core homosexuality, they are more likely to desert their female friends than lesbians, and they cannot be trusted as political allies because they will abandon lesbian political struggles under pressure to conform to heterosexual norms. M. S. Weinberg et al. (1994) likewise found in their study that "lesbians were especially negative toward bisexual women" (p. 293).

Though not as vocal in the literature, many gay men also are disapproving and judgmental toward bisexual individuals. In fact, "the illusion that bisexuality is usually a 'way station' to avoid facing one's homosexuality is so strong in gay culture that men who have acknowledged their gay identity are surprised when they meet a woman they find sexually exciting" (Matteson, 1996, p. 439). On a more positive note, however, M. S. Weinberg et al. (1994) found greater acceptance of bisexuality by younger homosexuals than older ones who tended more "to emphasize exclusivity of same-sex partners as the basis of a homosexual identity, since this is the identity they had to fight for" (p. 299).

Relationships

There are numerous practical concerns involved in living as an identified bisexual, including the meaning of new and existing relationships on a social and personal level. Coming out to both current and potential partners is stressful and the possibly of rejection continually is present. Many people, regardless of sexual orientation, are reluctant to stay in, or to enter into, intimate relationships with bisexual individuals given the known fluidity of their attractions. These individuals usually desire monogamous relationships and refuse to share their partners with another now or in the future. Some indicate that they would like to avoid the distress that would occur should their bisexual mate attempt to negotiate an open relationship with them, have secret encounters after having promised monogamy, or become infected with HIV.

Once individuals disclose their bisexuality to others, considerable renegotiation and reinvention of primary and other existing relationships are essential, even if they have been struggling privately with their identities for some time (Paul, 1996). Matteson (1996) maintains that this honest acknowledgment usually leads to significant changes in heterosexual marriages, but many of the issues and dynamics he discusses also occur in same-sex relationships. In any case, a revelation of bisexuality usually destabilizes the balance in a relationship, and it often is this destabilization that brings couples to therapy.

If the two people wish to continue in the partnership, new contracts and agreements need to be negotiated. The possibility, or reality, of other mates must be discussed openly and "the values—and risks—of triangulation in a lifestyle with dual or multiple relationships need to be understood for effective counseling" (Matteson, 1996, p. 443). The difficulty of managing multiple partners and the intricate "balancing act" this entails should be talked about candidly. Matteson contends that various living arrangements are possible, including three people sharing the same household and open relationships outside the dyad, but all parties involved must be clear on the agreements and consent to participate. Often these are workable only if the original couple agrees that their relationship will remain primary, because fear of losing their couplehood is the main source of the jealousy that usually accompanies sharing one's significant other.

Rust (1996) discusses the concept of *polyamory* in reference to various forms of relationships outside a primary relationship. She explains selecting this term in favor of one such as *nonmonogamy* in order to avoid the inherent negative implications. Also, bisexual clients can better be assisted in making healthy relationship choices if the parameters of possibilities are broadened and neutralized and the cultural idealization of monogamy is rejected. Because many bisexuals desire some form of polyamorous relationship, Rust stresses the importance of establishing ground rules for the conduct of romantic or sexual encounters outside the primary relationship in order to protect the principal alliance from potential threat, ease the feelings of jealousy, and promote greater honesty. She suggests helping couples discuss what kinds of activities are permissible; if sexual activity is allowed, what kinds and how frequently; with whom these outside liaisons may take place; whether or not to disclose to each other outside encounters; if disclosure is expected, whether it should happen before or after the involvements; and how the primary relationship is to be presented to others.

Even with the best intentions, conflict, misunderstandings, and jealousies are inevitable for couples with at least one bisexual member and ongoing support is essential. Because lifelong therapy often is neither feasible nor desirable, support groups frequently are the best option for these pairs. Most of these are held in larger cities, however, so many clients will have to travel some distance to avail themselves of such opportunities. Fortunately, online and printed resources are gradually becoming available for bisexual couples and individuals, and the Resources section contains several recommendations and resources to assist clients through a process involving continual uncertainty.

CONCLUSION

This chapter outlined four models (Cass, Coleman, Troiden, and Grace) to help psychotherapists chart a course for helping their sexual minority clients form positive identities. Table 5.1 provides a visual image of how these models may compare to one another. Helping clients recognize their own dynamics within the specific stages of identity development is frequently an extremely useful first step in affirmative psychotherapy with lesbians and gay men. This knowledge can assist individuals by reducing confusion and increasing perspective related to their own feelings and behaviors, thus helping them to feel (maybe for the first time in their lives) less isolated and different, and more like others.

The unique process of bisexual identity formation was discussed, with particular emphasis on the continual uncertainty that many bisexually oriented individuals experience as they struggle to achieve and integration of their identities. The social alienation and relationship difficulties associated with this process also were described and interventions for therapists were suggested.

A later chapter (Chapter 9) addresses psychotherapeutic applications of a paradigm adapted from the four models of gay and lesbian identity formation discussed in this chapter. First, however, it is important to explore the impact of oppression and stigmatization on the other issues involved in the assessment process. Hence, Chapters 6 and 7, respectively, explore the psychological development of adolescents and adults, and Chapter 8 examines psychodiagnostic concerns. separate from sexual minority identity formation. Chapter 9 then offers clinicians phase-specific interventions for moving their clients along a developmental trajectory leading to the integration of a sexual minority identity and describes several additional factors that might modify or impede this passage toward identity crystallization. These factors include variations due to bisexual and gender role socialization, fluidity in patterns of sexual attraction, extent of psychosocial adjustment, and the social and relational environments of clients.

6

Issues for Sexual
Minority Adolescents

Gay, lesbian, and bisexual adolescents are at high risk both personally and so-cially for serious developmental problems, not necessarily because of their sexual orienta-tion but primarily because of oppression, prejudice, and stigmatization (Cook & Pawlowski, 1991; Fergusson, Horwood, & Beautrais, 1999; Garofalo, Wolf, Kessel, Pal-frey, & DuRant, 1998; Gonsiorek, 1988; A. D. Martin, 1982; Rosario, Rotheram-Borus, & Reid, 1996; Savin-Williams, 1994; Unks, 1995). Growing up in a culture that devalues minority sexual orientations not only affects mental health but also disrupts important milestones of psychosocial development. "By the time they reach early adolescence, chil-dren have been deeply enculturated in the sexual attitudes and values of their family, the larger culture, and their particular subcultures" (Cook & Pawlowski, 1991, p. 3). Virtu-ally all young people, including those developing minority sexual orientations, are bom-barded from early childhood with rigid notions of gender-appropriate behavior, as well as with heterosexist images and messages. Upon entering kindergarten, children who are gender nonconforming already know that being a "sissy" or a "tomboy" is highly unde-sirable and may bring ridicule from other students, neglect from teachers, and chastise-ment from parents. Further, they hear adults joking about "fags" and "dykes" and see controversial stories about lesbians and gay men on television. By the onset of puberty, then, sexual minority youth have internalized the negative intra- and interpersonal effects of this oppression (Mallet, Apostolidis, & Paty, 1997; see also Chapter 1) and thus are sensitive and vulnerable to heterosexist peer perceptions and pressures.

"Prehomosexual" children feel socially different from their peers and usually experi-ence childhoods characterized by themes of marginality, alienation, and estrangement (Troiden, 1979, 1989). Although their feelings of social difference do not become con-sciously sexualized until adolescence, ambiguous same-sex attractions frequently cause shame, anxiety, secrecy, low self-esteem, denial of feelings, and excessive efforts to pass as heterosexual (Bozett & Sussman, 1989; Grace, 1992; Martin & Hetrick, 1988; Rad-owsky & Siegel, 1997). Secrecy is a matter of psychological survival to these youth, as often they are excruciatingly careful about their public images and usually live in a "nightmare of self-consciousness" (Hersch, 1991, p. 38). The teens, in a sense, are victims of a stigmatizing societal process that produces a variety of physical, social, and mental health problems. Their secrecy leads to invisibility and isolates them to suffer in silence without adequate social support for their developmental needs. This cognitive, social, and emotional isolation often extends into adulthood and manifests itself in mental health problems, such as anxiety, depression, self-hatred, demoralization, and loneliness (D'Augelli, 1994a; Hetrick & Martin, 1987; Lock & Steiner, 1999; Martin & Hetrick, 1988; M. F. O'Connor, 1992; G. J. Remafedi, 1985; Savin-Williams, 1989b, 1990; Zera, 1992).

GAY, LESBIAN, AND BISEXUAL ADOLESCENT ISSUES

Ordinarily, teenagers ought to be dealing with several formidable responsibilities, including individuating from parents, socializing with peers, forming an identity, exploring intimate relationships, and orienting themselves to the future (E. Coleman & Remafedi, 1989; Gibson, 1989; G. H. Herdt, 1992; Sullivan & Schneider, 1987). Clinicians working with sexual minority teens, in addition, must consider the issues that prevent these clients from mastering the developmental tasks that are assumed to be normative for all adolescents. Regrettably, the primary task for gay, lesbian, and bisexual youth is entry into a stigmatized role and the major developmental issues of their lives revolve around passage into that social identity (Bridget & Lucille, 1996; Hetrick & Martin, 1987). Because so much of their psychic energies are consumed with stigma management, many have difficulty with normative developmental concerns of adolescence, such as building self-esteem, developing social skills, and maintaining a sense of identity (N. Evans & Levine, 1990).

Along with feeling ambivalent about their sexual orientations, gay, lesbian, and bisexual adolescents often lose friends, as well as abandon personal, academic, and career goals. Remafedi (1987a, 1987b) interviewed 137 sexual minority males and reported deteriorating academic performance and serious substance abuse among the majority of these teens. Nearly half of the boys described having run away from home, being arrested, or having a sexually transmitted disease. A significant minority had attempted suicide, traded sex for money, or been sexually victimized. They reported strong homophobic attitudes from their parents (43%) and friends (41%). Thirty percent had been assaulted physically (with half of these attacks occurring on school property), 37% discriminated against, and 58% abused verbally because of their sexual orientation. Numerous additional authors have focused on these and other related dynamics and have reported similar histories among lesbian teens. For example, some writers have discussed homelessness; lack of vocational and educational training; rejection by families, friends, and communities; substance abuse; and HIV distress among lesbian as well as gay and bisexual adolescents (Bass & Kaufman, 1996; E. Coleman & Remafedi, 1989; Due, 1995; Ghindia & Kola, 1996; L. Meyer, 1999; Remafedi, 1987b; Rotheram-Borus, Murphy, Reid, & Coleman, 1996; Ryan & Futterman, 1998; Savin-Williams, 1994, 1998; Unks, 1995; Winters, Remafedi, & Chan, 1996).

Without an extensive research base, any comprehensive attempt to describe a population-specific developmental process for sexual minority girls and boys is inadequate. Unfortunately, the validity of many fundamental assumptions about gay, lesbian, and bisexual youth and their development is questionable given that most studies have focused on gay men and their adult recollections of childhood and adolescent experiences (Boxer & Cohler, 1989; Zera, 1992). Gender bias, the cohort-bound nature of the research, and the virtual absence of longitudinal studies also limits the applicability of the findings. On a more positive note, however, numerous authors are now describing the lives of sexual minority adolescents as they are living them (Bass & Kaufman, 1996; Due, 1995; Savin-Williams, 1998), and teens increasingly are telling their own stories (Bull, 2000a; Kirby, 2000a). As a result of these narratives and available empirical data, there appears to be considerable consensus regarding some of the salient issues that prevent sexual minority teens from mastering the normative developmental tasks of adolescence. Several of these are discussed in separate sections herein.

Emotional Problems

In Heron's (1983) edited collection *One Teenager in Ten: Writings by Gay and Lesbian Youth*, sexual minority adolescents report their emotional reactions to discovering their same-sex orientations:

- "I walked around like a shell shock victim for days" (p. 9–10).
- "My feelings are turning into gnawing monsters trying to clamber out" (p. 10).
- "When I realized I was homosexual, the first thing I did was sit down and cry" (p. 15).
- "Every day I lived in fear that there was nothing else, that I would never know anyone who could understand me and my feelings" (p. 39).
- "At first the word 'lesbian' sounded negative to me" and "I also was very confused by the stereotypes of lesbians" (p. 102).

As mentioned previously, these profound feelings of pain, anguish, and loneliness follow many gay, lesbian, and bisexual teens throughout adolescence, and the widespread contempt for lesbians and gay men can wound deeply. In other words, "the despair of homosexual adolescents in a culture that teaches them to hate themselves is intense" (Hersch, 1991, p. 38). Not surprisingly, sexual minority teens often feel negatively about themselves, isolated from family and friends, and depressed and confused about their sexual identities (Hunter & Schaecher, 1987; Lock & Steiner, 1999; B. S. Newman & Muzzonigro, 1993; M. Schneider, 1989; M. Schneider & Tremble, 1985/1986; Teague, 1992). Data from a New Zealand longitudinal study of a birth cohort of 1,265 children (of which 1,007 were available at sampling when the group was 21 years old), indicated that 28 were classified as being gay, lesbian, or bisexual. Results also reflected that these sexual minority individuals were at increased risk for major depression, generalized anxiety disorder, conduct disorder, nicotine or other substance abuse dependence, suicidal ideation, and suicide attempts (Fergusson et al., 1999).

Many lesbian, bisexual, and gay adolescents live as prisoners of their own fears, becoming alienated both socially and emotionally as their dread of discovery motivates them to decrease their involvement in school and peer group activities. Isolated from heterosexual peers and unaware of other homosexual teens, they often feel alone and afraid (Paroski, 1990; Zera, 1992). While other adolescents might turn to their parents for emotional support, sexual minority youth generally keep the most distressing and significant parts of their lives secret from their parents. They do so to shield their families from the pain of having a gay or lesbian member, as well as to protect themselves from being rejected (D'Augelli & Herschberger, 1993; Hersch, 1991).

Suicide

Alienation and isolation from peer groups and families are among the many stresses experienced by gay, lesbian, and bisexual adolescents. These teens often internalize the homophobia of others, develop a self-loathing that mirrors heterosexist society's disgust with lesbians and gay men (Hersch, 1991), and form what Goffman (1963) referred to as a spoiled identity. Feeling alienated and isolated, their depression and self-hatred frequently leads to suicidal symptoms (Cochran & Mays, 2000a; Kourany, 1987; Safren, 1998). Accordingly, suicide attempt rates among gay, lesbian, and bisexual youth have been found to range as high as 39% to 42% (Anhalt & Morris, 1998; D'Augelli & Herschberger, 1993 [n = 194]; Garofalo, Wolf, Wissow, Woods, & Goodman, 1999 [n = 3,365]; Rotheram-Borus, Hunter, & Rosario, 1994 [n = 138 males]. Data from interviews with 137 gay and bisexual males (ages 17–21) similarly revealed that nearly 30% had attempted suicide and roughly 15% had done so more than once (Remafedi, Farrow, & Deisher, 1991). One-third of the first attempts occurred during the same year that these young men had self-identified as gay or bisexual. Over half used moderately to highly lethal methods and 62% were only moderately to minimally within reach of crisis intervention services. These percentages support an earlier survey of the concerns of 66 psychiatrists treating gay and lesbian adolescents (Kourany, 1987) who considered their patients' suicide attempts more severe and their risks higher than those of other teens.

The actual rates of suicide attempts and completions among sexual minorities are unknown (Remafedi, 1999). One report on youth suicide for the U.S. Department of Health and Human Services (DHHS) (Gibson, 1989) summarizes existing studies and estimates that gay and lesbian adolescents attempt suicide two to three times more frequently than other teens and comprise up to 30% of completed youth suicides annually. These estimates have received considerable attention, but the DHHS report has been criticized severely for having reached these conclusions without substantiating research data to support them (Bull, 1994; Muehrer, 1995).

In this regard, some writers allege that the numerous methodological limitations in most studies preclude accurate conclusions about the relationship between sexual orientation and suicidal behavior (Anhalt & Morris, 1998; Muehrer; 1995; Remafedi, 1999). Muehrer (1995), in particular, advocates a community sampling strategy in which relatives and friends of suicide victims are interviewed and other characteristics of the deceased are assessed in a psychological autopsy. Using this kind of a technique, two studies (C. L. Rich, Fowler, Young, & Blenkush, 1986; Shaffer, Fisher, Hicks, Parides, & Gould, 1995) found that only 2.5% to 5% of the suicides investigated were believed to be gay or lesbian.

Even this approach has its critics, however. According to Bull(1994), for example, two suicide experts (Herbert Hendin and Gary Remafedi) were interviewed regarding prepublished investigation findings (Shaffer et al., 1995) of 120 teenage suicides in New York City. During this interview, Hendin and Remafedi discussed methodological flaws in the study then being conducted by Shaffer and his colleagues. They particularly questioned the assumption that family members and friends freely and honestly disclose the sexual orientation of a deceased loved one, especially as many family survivors of suicide feel guilty, ashamed, or both, whereas others remain unaware of the victim's sexual orientation. According to Remafedi (cited in Bull, 1994), "the youths who are at the greatest risk for suicide are the ones who are least likely to reveal their sexual orientation to anyone;" in other words, "suicide may be a way of making sure that no one ever knows" (p. 38).

Rarely is sexual orientation the sole factor involved in suicide attempts (Bull, 1994; Remafedi, 1994). In one of the studies discussed previously (Remafedi et al., 1991), for example, gender nonconformity and precocious psychosexual development were predictive of suicide attempts. Perhaps more important, however, was the fact that most of the young gay and bisexual men who attempted suicide were more likely than their peers to have abused drugs (85%) and to have been sexually abused (61%). The researchers noted that drug and sexual abuse, along with high levels of family discord and dysfunction, commonly are reported correlates of completed youth suicide. Survey data based on a sample of 52 men in gay and lesbian college organizations and 56 men in gay discussion groups similarly reflected associations between familial and suicidal behavior (S. G. Schneider, Farberow, & Kruks, 1989). Accordingly, family backgrounds of alcoholism and physical abuse, along with gay-rejecting social supports, were found among the 55% of the participants who reported histories of suicidal ideation and in the 20% who had attempted suicide. Gender differences also may play at part. Sexual orientation was found to have an independent association with suicide attempts for males, but for females the association of sexual orientation with suicidality was mediated by drug use and violence or victimization in 3,365 Massachusetts teen respondents (Garofalo et al., 1999).

Several of the factors described previously also were found in a study of 200 lesbian, gay, and bisexual youth, ranging in age from 15 to 21 years (D'Augelli, 1994a). Although 40% denied ever having thought about killing themselves, 30% admitted that they sometimes or often did. In fact, 42% had one or more suicide attempts and 24% had two or more. Compared with nonattempters, those who had tried to take their own lives acknowledged their sexual orientation earlier, demonstrated lower self-worth, and reported more drug and alcohol problems. In addition, 50% reported histories of depression, anxiety, and worry, and more than half disclosed having sought professional counseling.

Similarly, Hammelman (1993) studied 48 gay and lesbian youth and identified contributing factors to their serious attempts (29%) or considerations (48%) of suicide: alcohol or drug problems, family rejection, and physical or emotional abuse. Hunter (1990) also found that suicide attempters often were victims of violence. In reviewing records on 500 adolescents (ages 14–21; predominantly people of color; approximately 80% male) seeking services at a facility serving gay and lesbian youth, she found that of the 205 (41%) youth with recorded histories of violence (from family members, peers, or strangers), 41% of the females and 34% of the males reported having attempted suicide.

In summary, the foregoing studies of sexual minority youth suicide appear to support the general conclusions in the literature, namely, that mental disorders and substance abuse consistently have been associated with suicide and suicide attempts (Fergusson et al., 1999; Muehrer, 1995; Safren, 1998). Specifically, the San Diego study of 283 suicides discussed previously (C. L. Rich et al., 1986) found that each of the 13 gay men who killed himself had at least one psychiatric diagnosis in his medical record. In other words, these data support the general findings that most individuals who commit or attempt suicide have a history of mental illness. Nonetheless, given the degree to which gay men, lesbians, and bisexuals are oppressed by heterosexism, it is probably safe to assume that struggles with sexual orientation in some way exacerbate or contribute to the mental disorders that are related to suicidality.

Physical and Sexual Abuse

Thus far in this chapter, several studies have reported high rates of physical abuse among gay, lesbian, and bisexual adolescents in general (G. Remafedi, 1987a, 1987b), and among those sexual minority teens who had either considered or attempted suicide in particular (Hammelman, 1993; Hunter, 1990; S. G. Schneider et al., 1989). Other studies and writings also have documented the high rates of abuse and violence directed toward gay, lesbian, and bisexual youth (J. Barrett, 2000; Hunter & Schaecher, 1990; Martin & Hetrick, 1988; Rotheram-Borus, Rosario, & Koopman, 1991; Savin-Williams & Cohen, 1996). Hunter (1990), for example, reviewed charts for the first 500 adolescents seeking services in 1988 at an agency serving sexual minority youth in order to study violence against gay and lesbian teens. Of these young people (ages 14–21; 35% Black, 46% Hispanic; 80% male, 20% female), 41% reported having suffered violence from families, peers, or strangers. Further, 46% of the victimization reported was said to be gay related.

Two studies (D'Augelli, 1989c, 1992) surveyed gay, lesbian, and bisexual undergraduates (n's = 125 and 121). Of those polled, approximately 75% in both investigations had been verbally abused, 26–27% had been threatened with physical violence, and 13–17% had experienced personal property damage. Based on his analysis of data also collected from college students, Harry (1989) concluded that his gay participants were significantly more abused by their parents during adolescence than their heterosexual counterparts. His interpretation of the literature on child abuse provided a succinct explanation for this conclusion. Accordingly, certain types of children seem to be singled out for abuse, specifically those "who depart from parental expectations in a manner to disappoint the parents" (p. 252). Because gay and lesbian offspring are often what he referred to as *different* children, they are a frequent disappointment to their parents and consequently at high risk for ill treatment. This *difference* in many of the gay male college students he studied was a history of childhood femininity that may have sensitized the fathers of his subjects to their sons' possible homosexuality. When the fathers' suspicions were confirmed by their sons' adolescent sexual behavior, physical punishment resulted.

In some cases, young males exhibiting stereotypically feminine characteristics are at the highest risk for sexual abuse as well as for nonsexual physical abuse. For example, 1,001 gay or bisexual men (age 18 years or older) were assessed for histories of childhood or adolescence sexual exploitation (Doll, Joy, Bartholow, & Harrison, 1992). Those who were gender nonconforming were found to be at greater risk than their more-masculine-appearing peers, given that more than one-third (37%) of these men reported that they had been seduced or pressured into sexual contact before the age of 19 with an older or more coercive partner, 94% of whom were men. Force was used in 51% of these sexual encounters, 33% of which involved anal sex. The victims were generally young (median age at first assault = 10 years), tended to be Black or Hispanic, and often lacked pronounced secondary sex characteristics.

In their review of pertinent research findings, Genuis, Thomlison, and Bagley (1991) likely referred to these *gender-discordant traits* as homosexual tendencies and also found them to be associated with child sexual abuse. Other related characteristics included low self-esteem, depression, learned helplessness, guilt, alienation, and distrust. Victims often were children from alcoholic or otherwise disrupted homes, or young people who excessively were punished physically or neglected emotionally.

As mentioned earlier in this chapter, feelings of difference negatively affect the self-esteem of "prehomosexual" children. Accordingly, these young people frequently feel anxious, depressed, alienated, isolated, helpless, and unsupported and are often quite vulnerable to external forces. When these children come from chaotic and disorganized families, they are even more susceptible to physical and sexual assaults. Though most remain in their homes until late adolescence and simply endure the pain, some teens run away to prevent further abuse. Others are thrown out of their homes because of their sexual orientation.

Homelessness, Prostitution, and Substance Abuse

According to Gibson (1989), 26% of gay and lesbian youth are forced to leave home due to conflicts over their sexual orientation. In fact, "gay male, lesbian, bisexual, and transsexual youth comprise as many as 25 percent of all youth living on the streets in this country" (p. 3-114), and in at least one major metropolitan area (Los Angeles), 30% of young runaways have been thought to be sexual minority (J. W. Peterson, 1989). Many run away to escape unpleasant, if not intolerable, living situations, and some do so repeatedly (Remafedi, 1987a). In Los Angeles, for example, many of the adolescents seeking services at the Gay and Lesbian Community Services Center are runaways who have had arguments with their parents (Brownsworth, 1992; see Resources section for runaway services.) After coming out to parents, many teens are "rejected, mistreated, or become the focus of the family's dysfunction" (Gonsiorek, 1988, p. 116). The intense fear that many gay, lesbian, and bisexual teens feel toward the reactions of their fathers (D'Augelli, 1991) are well-justified in some cases, as nearly 1 in 10 who come out to their fathers are thrown out of their homes (Boxer, Cook, & Herdt, 1991).

Once sexual minority youth hit the streets, either because they run away or are kicked out, their loneliness, isolation, and vulnerability intensify. If they are unable to locate services that meet their needs within a couple of weeks, they often fall victim to prostitution, HIV infection, pregnancy, or substance abuse (Cates, 1989; E. Coleman, 1989; Jordan, 2000; Kruks, 1991; J. W. Peterson, 1989; Rotheram-Borus et al., 1991; Ryan & Futterman, 1998; Savin-Williams & Cohen, 1996; T. R. Sullivan, 1996). In one study involving 60 teens attending a community agency for gay and bisexual youth, for example, 23% of the participants traded money and drugs for sexual acts (Rotheram-Borus et al., 1992). Both sexes thus are highly susceptible to sexually transmitted diseases, while homeless girls who trade sex for money also increase their risks of becoming pregnant (Paroski, 1990). Further, gay and lesbian teens are highly likely to be counted among an estimated 12% to 20% of all homeless youth who are HIV-infected or who are at extremely high risk for HIV transmission (General Accounting Office, 1990; National Coalition for the Homeless, 1990).

Another unfortunate consequence for many sexual minority youth, whether living in their homes or on the streets, is the abuse of alcohol or drugs to seek relief for feelings of depression and loneliness (E. Coleman, 1989; Jordan, 2000; J. W. Peterson, 1989; Rotheram-Borus et al., 1991). In a study cited previously (Remafedi, 1987a), 60% of the

137 gay and bisexual male adolescents in the sample met DSM-III-R (American Psychiatric Association, 1987) diagnostic criteria for substance abuse. Frequently, the anguish of isolation and alienation are so intense that gay, lesbian, and bisexual teens rely on chemicals to numb their pain; others enter the turbulent world of drinking and partying to hide from their families and peers and to escape their feelings of being sexually different (Ziebold & Mongeon, 1985). Finally, as discussed earlier in this chapter, the drugs and alcohol taken to manage the stigma and secrecy often are associated with suicide in this teenage population (D'Augelli, 1994a; Hammelman, 1993; Remafedi et al., 1991; Safren, 1998).

Dating Dilemmas

Exploring sexuality and consolidating a sexual identity are normal developmental tasks of adolescence. Mastery of these tasks becomes extremely difficult, if not impossible, for sexual minority youth in a culture "uncomfortable about adult sex, worried about adolescent sex, and downright hostile about homosexual sex" (Hersch, 1991, p. 38). Many of these teens attempt to deny or inhibit their same-sex feelings and desires by conforming to heterosexist norms of dating the opposite sex, while others experiment heterosexually in order to test the relative strength of their hetero- and homoerotic attractions (Rosario, Meyer-Bahlburg, Hunter, & Exner, 1996). In two different studies, over half of gay and bisexual male youths reported heterosexual experiences, while an even greater percentage (75% to 80%) of lesbian and bisexual young women had engaged in sex with young men (Savin-Williams, 1990; Sears, 1991b). These girls frequently behave heterosexually, "ranging from simple experimentation to heterosexual promiscuity" (Hetrick & Martin, 1988, p. 33), and some even become pregnant to "pass as straight" (Paroski, 1990, p. 168). Despite their fears of parental reactions, an unwanted pregnancy often is more acceptable in their families than having a lesbian daughter.

For some adolescents who are active sexually with the opposite sex, heterosexual experiences feel pleasurable but lack emotional intensity. For others, they feel unnatural. One young man (described by Heron, 1983) concluded that he was incapable of human love because he never felt emotionally intimate with any of his female sexual partners during high school. On the other hand, initial same-sex experiences frequently feel natural, emotionally intense, and intimately satisfying for many gay and lesbian teens, and thus they are able to experience personal confirmation and sexual validation for the first time. While feeling affirmed on one level, however, a second set of emotions often is infected with internalized heterosexism and social stigma. Another young man (also quoted by Heron, 1983) summarized this discordance: "It was a shock to discover that my impassioned, if unarticulated, love affairs with fellow schoolboys which had held so much poignant beauty carried that weighty word *homosexual*" (p. 104).

Nonetheless, some teens persist in spite of extremely negative social climates and continue to date beyond these first encounters. In fact, Sears (1991b) found that 25% of the southern sexual minority youth he surveyed dated a member of the same sex during high school. Guilt and secrecy often contaminated their romances, however, and shortened the duration of many of these relationships. These and other gay, lesbian, and bisexual teens frequently feel like "sexual outlaws" in a society that assumes heterosexuality and live in hidden and mysterious worlds, spinning lies to protect their secrets (Savin-Williams & Rodriguez, 1993).

Educational Concerns

To protect themselves as well as their secrets, some sexual minority youth isolate themselves not only from their families but also from their teachers and classmates. According to Hetrick and Martin (1987), "the young person avoids school to escape the pressures of hiding, the taunts of classmates, or humiliations within the classroom and goes where [s/he needs to hide" (p. 33). Other writers also note that many gay, lesbian, and bisexual youth are absent, truant, fail classes, and drop out of school because they are harassed, and sometimes even violently attacked, by their peers (Bass & Kaufman, 1996; Hunter, 1990; Hunter & Schaecher, 1990; Price & Telljohann, 1991; Rivers, 2000). In this regard, G. Remafedi (1987a, 1987b) found that over two-thirds of the 137 gay and bisexual male adolescents he studied reported experiencing school-related problems, with 40% cutting classes and 28% quitting school.

Student Experiences

Sears (1991a, 1991b) interviewed 36 southern gay, lesbian, and bisexual individuals and asked them to describe or recall their high school experiences. Of the three dozen interviewed, 97% remembered negative attitudes by classmates toward homosexuality. Most feared potential harassment and chose not to "come out" during high school. Only 2 of the 36 found a supportive group of friends. Most reported that the topic of homosexuality simply was avoided by school administrators, counselors, and teachers and few reported accounts of supportive educators who influenced their teenage lives. Because the interviewees generally saw these adults to be misinformed and uncaring, most felt uncomfortable talking to them and only a handful reported speaking about their sexual orientation to a guidance counselor or teacher. Similarly, Mercier and Berger (1989) explored the psychosocial problems of 49 gay and lesbian adolescents (ages 15 to 21) and found that relatively few had sought help from adults outside the family, such as teachers, counselors, therapists, and other school personnel. Unfortunately, then, although many sexual minority youth feel anxious, depressed and suicidal, few discuss their feelings and concerns with professionals (Gay, Lesbian and Straight Education Network, 1999; M. R. White, 1991).

The Massachusetts Department of Education, with funding from the Centers for Disease Control, administers the Massachusetts Youth Risk Behavior Survey (MYRBS) every 2 years. In 1995, for example, a total of 4,159 high school students were surveyed (Garofalo et al., 1998). As outlined in Table 6.1, lesbian, gay, and bisexual (LGB) students were more than four times more likely than their peers to have attempted suicide in the past year and five times more likely to have skipped school in the past month because of feeling unsafe en route to or at school, to have been threatened with a weapon at school in the past year, and to have used cocaine in their life.

A total of 3,982 students from 58 public high schools participated in the 1997 MYRBS. Participants were considered LGB on the basis of self-identification, same-sex behavior, or both. Accordingly, students meeting both of these criteria were 6.44 to 7.95 times more likely than their non-LGB counterparts to have tried taking their lives, felt unsafe and cut class, experienced armed threats on campus, and used cocaine (Goodenow & Hack, 1998). The results of two other studies conducted by the Minnesota Attorney General and the Vermont Department of Education in 1997 revealed similar findings rel-

TABLE 6.1. Massachusetts Youth Risk Behavior Survey

Reported behaviors	1995 students (n = 4,159)		1997 students (n = 3,982)			
	LGB	Other	LGB-identified only (n = 44)	Same-sex behavior only (n = 81)	LGB-identified with same-sex behavior (n = 36)	Other
Attempted suicide in past year	36.5	8.9	38.6	27.2	54.1	8.4
Felt unsafe and skipped school in past month	20.1	4.5	14.8	13.8	31.8	4.0
Threatened with weapon at school in past year	28.8	6.7	18.7	24.9	47.8	6.6
Used cocaine in life	31.0	6.8	23.6	26.3	45.5	6.1

ative to violence, being threatened or injured by a weapon, or having attempted suicide (Buckel, 1999).

The Gay, Lesbian and Straight Education Network (1999) conducted a survey of 496 adolescents from 32 states and grouped the findings into three categories: Homophobic Remarks in School, Harassment, and Overall Comfort in School. More than 90% reported sometimes or frequently hearing homophobic remarks in the educational setting. Almost all (99.4%) heard them from other students, and 36.6% heard them from faculty and staff. Nearly 40% (39.2%) of respondents reported that no one ever intervened in these circumstances. If someone did intercede, it was more often another student (82.4%) rather than a faculty member (66.5%). The majority of youth reported experiencing some form of harassment or violence (69%). Of the 61.1% describing verbal aggravation, 45.9% said it occurred almost daily. A large number (27.6%) reported being shoved or pushed, and 13.7% were physically assaulted by being beaten, punched, or kicked. Not surprisingly, a high percentage (41.7%; $n = 191$) of the reporting students indicated that they did not feel safe in their schools because of their sexual orientation or gender identity. Paradoxically, the majority of those who reported feeling safe did so *despite* hearing homophobic remarks sometimes or frequently. The authors of the survey noted that perceptions of safety can be subjective. In this study, the assumption could be made that 58.3% of students felt reasonably safe in their school, given that they did not report feeling unsafe. The fact that this many ($n = 305$) felt fairly secure, in spite of the fact that 86.7% of them had heard negative remarks and experienced harassment, might be reflective of their older age (mean = 17) or the fact that 87.5% indicated a certainty regarding their gay, lesbian, or bisexual identity. (On the other hand, 12.5% checked Unknown or Questioning when asked about their sexual orientation.) If this speculation is accurate, support can be provided to those studies reporting that having a higher level of identity formation is protective of self-esteem, even in the face of oppressive social circumstances.

Faculty and Staff Attitudes

To validate the fairly negative perceptions of sexual minority youth toward school personnel, Sears (1991a) surveyed 142 school counselors and 191 prospective teachers, mostly White women from South Carolina, using the Attitudes Toward Homosexuality (ATH) and Index of Homophobia (IH) scales. Based on their experience in the public schools, the counselors completed an additional questionnaire. According to Sears (1991a), most of the future teachers "expressed negative attitudes about homosexuality and harbored homophobic feelings toward lesbians and gay men. In comparison with other populations, these prospective teachers held much more negative feelings" (p. 53), and 8 of 10 of them harbored nonaffirmative feelings toward sexual minorities. Of these 80%, fully one-third scored as "high grade homophobics" on the IH scale. Somewhat similarly, nearly two-thirds of the school counselors surveyed by Sears expressed negative attitudes and feelings about both gay and lesbian individuals, as well as toward homosexuality itself. They were, however, slightly less homophobic and critical when compared with the prospective teachers. Sears concluded that many educators are reluctant to assume proactive roles in helping to create school atmospheres that foster the intellectual and social development of at-risk sexual minority students, and that their benign neglect reinforces heterosexism in the classroom and curriculum.

Likewise, several studies, articles, and reports also have indicated that school personnel often fall short of meeting the needs of LGB students and of opposing harassment due to a lack of awareness, knowledge, resources, or even the courage to face the consequences (Fontaine & Hammond, 1996; Freiberg, 1987; Gibson, 1989; Gay, Lesbian and Straight Education Network, 1999; Kirby, 2000a; Newton & Risch, 1981; I. W. Peterson, 1989; Rivers, 2000; Savin-Williams & Cohen, 1996). Further, by neglecting to educate youth about homosexuality and ignoring the subject in all curricula, teachers, counselors, and administrators do little to improve the self-esteem of gay and lesbian adolescents. In addition, the failure to protect these adolescents from verbal harassment and physical assault reflects the negative and critical attitudes of some staff members and students (Gibson, 1989).

Sometimes, unfortunately, those school personnel who are sensitive to the struggles of sexual minority students experience difficulty themselves. A Brookfield, Connecticut, English teacher, Veronica Berrill, placed on her classroom door a "Safe Zone" sticker, letting lesbian, gay, bisexual, and transgendered (LGBT) students know that her teaching area was a place where they would not face intolerance or harassment and could feel safe and supported. A parent of one of her students accused the teacher of "homosexual recruiting" and wrote several letters to the editor of the local newspaper and to the school board. Other parents joined the protestor and high school officials capitulated and discontinued the "Safe Spaces" program. Ms. Berrill, decided to fight the accusers and filed a libel suit against them, in spite of the fact that she was 70 years old, retiring from teaching, and taking care of her dying husband. Fortunately, GLSEN members and others from the community supported her during her stressful 3-year fight. The parties eventually settled out of court, the teacher received a financial settlement, and the parents retracted some of their previous remarks about Ms. Berrill.

Affirmative Responses

Not all educational institutions and systems have perpetuated the neglect of sexual minority students, and there appear to be a growing number of efforts designed to make schools safe for these students (J. Barrett, 2000; Bass & Kaufman, 1996; Kirby, 2000a).

As early as 1984, for example, school districts on both the Pacific and Atlantic coasts began to respond positively to the needs of LGB youth. At Fairfax High School, the Los Angeles Unified School District established Project Ten as a dropout prevention program for sexual minority adolescents. Since then, Project Ten also has educated teachers and counselors about gay and lesbian concerns, as well as infused these issues into other local student retention programs. The project also has spearheaded codes of discipline designed to protect the safety of sexual minority youth on campus, while working to enhance their lives off campus by connecting them to community resources. As of 2000, at least 40 of Los Angeles's 47 high schools and several alternative schools had some form of gay groups on campus. As Project Ten was being developed in California, the Harvey Milk alternative high school was established in New York City to provide a safe learning environment for distressed gay and lesbian students. Operated by the Hetrick–Martin Institute, the school is one of many alternative academic programs that the New York City school district runs in conjunction with community-based organizations. (Directory listings for both Project Ten and the Hetrick–Martin Institute can be found in the Resources section.)

On February 10, 1992, Massachusetts became the first state to respond officially to the problems of sexual minority teens when Governor William F. Weld and Lieutenant Governor Paul Cellucci issued an executive order creating the Governor's Commission on Gay and Lesbian Youth. Governor Weld was extremely concerned about the high rate of suicide among gay and lesbian youth and formed the Commission to prevent violence against, as well as suicide within, this population. Ninety people testified at five public hearings, and virtually every student questioned told stories of violence, abuse, and harassment from both adults and peers. In addition to these hearings, the Commission conducted a survey of 398 high school students, the data of which indicated that nearly all (97.5%) had heard anti-gay comments in their schools, with almost half (49%) having heard them very often.

The Governor's Commission on Gay and Lesbian Youth (1993) concluded that "parents, family, peers, and teachers are generally ignorant of what it means to be gay or lesbian" and that sexual minority youth "have little chance of talking with a knowledgeable or understanding person concerning his or her gay or lesbian identity" (p. 6). Based on the Commission's conclusion, the Massachusetts Department of Education established the nation's first program to train teachers and guidance counselors in violence and suicide prevention, and worked with the families of lesbian and gay students to keep the young people in the home and from running away ("Gov. Weld Asks Schools," 1993; Atkinson, 1993).

In step with the Commission Report, the endeavors of a small volunteer group from Boston and the efforts of several hundred high school students who campaigned, held candlelight vigils, and lobbied their legislators helped influence Massachusetts to become the first state to ban discrimination against gay and lesbian students in its public schools ("Anti-gay Bias," 1993; Rimer, 1993). This small volunteer group from Boston later became known as the Gay, Lesbian and Straight Education Network (GLSEN). Since 1994, GLSEN has grown into a national organization of more than 400 four hundred local chapters and groups that bring together teachers, parents, students, and concerned citizens to work together to end homophobia in their schools (see Resources section). These groups are being organized "at an astonishing rate" and in some of the more conservative areas of the country, including Orange County, California, and Baton Rouge, Louisiana (Kirby, 2000a, p. 29).

Numerous other positive responses to the plight of sexual minority children and adolescents can be found. For example, in 1999 GLSEN sent a booklet, *Just the Facts About Sexual Orientation and Youth* (see Resources section) to all 15,000 school superintendents across the nation. The 12-page publication was created and endorsed by 10 national organizations, including the American Psychological Association, the American Counseling Association, the American Federation of Teachers, and the National Education Association, to help school personnel understand sexual orientation and improve the educational and health needs of LGB students. Right-wing reaction was intense and the Family Research Council immediately released two publications designed to protect children "from pro-homosexuality propaganda in the schools." At approximately the same time, the Centers for Disease Control (CDC) supported an American Psychological Association proposal designed to increase the health of sexual minority students. This 5-year collaboration was aimed at the training in 2003 of school psychologists, nurses, counselors, and social workers to better serve LGB adolescents. A project designed especially to train educators interested in combating heterosexism in K–12 schools, "The Lunchbox: A Comprehensive Anti-Homophobia Training Kit" was produced by GLSEN in 2000 (available from GLSEN; see Resources section). The Lunchbox gave potential trainers a manual, exercises, visual aids, and videos designed to teach teachers and other school personnel how to create an understanding climate and safe conditions for all students.

To deal directly with safety issues and indirectly to address health concerns, the Massachusetts Department of Education began encouraging schools to offer campus-based support groups for gay, lesbian, and heterosexual students. Gay/Straight Alliances (GSAs), as these groups have become known, are thought to help reduce anti-gay violence, harassment, and discrimination by educating the school community about homophobia and by encouraging a greater degree of understanding from students and school personnel (see Resources section and Chapter 4). More than 700 GSAs have formed in all parts of the United States, giving students a safe place to discuss their feelings and fears related to sexual orientation, some of which might otherwise be quelled through suicide or medicated with drugs and alcohol.

PSYCHOTHERAPEUTIC CONSIDERATIONS

LGB youth who do consult counselors and psychotherapists during adolescence seek assistance for many of the personal, familial, and social stressors and problems discussed in this chapter (American Medical Association, 1996; Fontaine & Hammond, 1996; Rosario, Rotheram-Borus, & Reid, 1996). According to E. Coleman and Remafedi (1989), these stressors commonly include "efforts to clarify or change sexual orientation; family conflict regarding sexuality; anxiety; attempted suicide; grief over the dissolution of a first relationship; substance abuse; and other disorders of conduct" (p. 68). As discussed in the previous chapter, however, many adolescents have yet to explicitly identify their sexual orientation. Thus, the degree to which their erotic and emotional attractions are contributing to their presenting problems often is ambiguous.

Consequently, therapists frequently are caught in a bind. If they focus too closely on sexuality issues or urge their young clients to resolve prematurely questions of sexual orientation, they might either compound or complicate problems arising from same-sex feelings and attractions. Further, they may endanger any rapport established with these clients or their parents if they intervene too hastily. On the other hand, if clinicians consider the same-sex feelings of LGB adolescents illegitimate or irrelevant, they may likewise do harm to their teen clients. Broaching the subject, then, is a delicate process, and the lines are thin between intervening too strongly, too soon, too late, or not at all. Unfortunately, many clinicians resolve this dilemma by avoiding the issue of sexual orientation altogether (E. Coleman & Remafedi, 1989).

Many adolescents are frightened and reluctant to introduce the subject of homosexuality themselves, so opening the door for discussion becomes the therapist's intervention. Inclusive language which is free of heterosexist assumptions often invites sexual minority clients to disclose their homoerotic feelings. For example, gender-neutral references to their romantic interests, such as "date" or "partner" rather than "girlfriend" or "boyfriend," give clients permission to express attractions other than heterosexual. In addition, gay and lesbian affirming pamphlets in the waiting room or books on treatment room shelves might also open doors to disclosure. Posting certificates of membership in organizations such as GLSEN or PFLAG (Parents, Families and Friends of Lesbians and Gays) would be another inviting gesture. In other words, creating an atmosphere in which clients can discuss their most personal and frightening feelings in a nonthreatening, supportive environment is crucial for therapists working with these adolescents (Bass & Kaufman, 1996; E. Coleman & Remafedi, 1989; Fontaine & Hammond, 1996; Hetrick & Martin, 1987; J. A. Nelson, 1997).

Socialization

Another critical task for clinicians working with LGB adolescents is helping them identify and maximize opportunities for "dual socialization" (Gerstel, Feraios, & Herdt, 1989). Given that these individuals have been socialized as members of the heterosexual majority, they require immersion in the sexual minority culture in order to develop a positive gay or lesbian identity. Accordingly, M. Schneider (1991) surveyed 60 self-identified lesbian and gay teens and found that the most important milestone in their identity formation was the establishment of contact with people like themselves. Hetrick and Martin (1987) likewise were convinced that sexual minority adolescents needed "to socialize in a healthy environment" as well as have "opportunities for socialization with their peers in other than sexual settings" (p. 41). Hence, they formed the Institute for the Protection of Lesbian and Gay Youth (IPLGY) in New York City in order to create a setting where this peer social support and other assistance could be offered to teens.

Similarly, other advocates have created Gay and Lesbian Adolescent Social Services (GLASS) in West Hollywood, California, as a safe space for sexual minority teens, as well as to provide them and the community with education and referral sources. In addition to IPLGY and GLASS, the Resources section includes the Sexual Minority Youth Assistance League (SMYAL) in Washington, DC. Other similar projects exist in several US cities. Unfortunately, however, several teen-focused organizations have opened and been forced to close due to the lack of community or financial support to remain operative. Therapists, therefore, are advised to verify the addresses and telephone numbers of local, regional, and national directory listings before referring clients to any of these programs.

Family and Community Interventions

In addition to needing integration into the LGB community, sexual minority adolescents equally are isolated from the majority culture. Another therapeutic task, then, is to assist these teens in weaving themselves "into the social fabric" of their families, schools and communities, and to "become fully functioning members of society" (E. Coleman & Remafedi, 1989, p. 38). In this regard, a potential obstacle for clinicians working with sexual minority youth is the fact that adolescent clients under age 18 usually are regarded as minors unless legally emancipated from their parents. Thus, they neither hold their own legal privilege nor can afford to pay their own fees for services. Due to these legal and financial considerations, then, parents often feel entitled to participate in their children's therapy and even to influence the course of treatment with their own agendas.

The forces of sociocultural oppression frequently compel parents to seek heterosexual outcomes from therapy for their children who are struggling with issues of sexual identity. Sometimes, well-meaning mothers and fathers simply wish to protect their daughters and sons from discrimination and prejudice. Some parents, however, want to preserve their reputations from the disgrace of having a gay or lesbian child. Others hope to save their offspring from the "fires of hell" through conversion to heterosexuality. Clinicians thus are faced with a dilemma. On one hand, they must treat the parents respectfully without allowing their expectations to compromise the therapeutic process. On the other, they must protect the confidentiality of minor clients by not disclosing privileged information, as well as uphold their right of choice regarding the circumstances of their lives. The expectations of some parents can be modified by educating them and other family members about human sexuality, sexual orientation, and the difficult struggles their loved ones experience. Providing accurate information to dispel cultural myths and popular stereotypes is an essential component of this therapeutic work, as is helping families manage the stigma of having a gay, lesbian, or bisexual member and adapting to that reality (E. Coleman & Remafedi, 1989; Saltzburg, 1996). Further considerations for working with parents and families of sexual minority clients, including to referral to groups such as PFLAG and GLSEN, are beyond the scope of this section but are discussed later in Chapters 14 and 17.

Finally, clinicians indirectly can have an impact on LGB youth and their family members by educating the public through seminars on human sexuality that confront fears and ignorance with facts and information (Bass & Kaufman, 1996; E. Coleman & Remafedi, 1989; Radkowsky & Siegel, 1997). Subsequent studies based on suicidologist Durkheim's (1951) theory clearly indicate that there is a direct relationship between suicide rates and the outcast status of gay men and lesbians in society (Rotheram-Borus et al., 1994), and until social attitudes change significantly and homophobic attitudes decrease, "suicide will continue to plague lesbians and gay men" (Rofes, 1983, p. 118). Therefore, therapists are encouraged to consider their obligation to influence the entire sociocultural matrix in which their clients live.

CONCLUSION

This chapter addressed many of the issues lesbian, gay, and bisexual youth experience during adolescence that impact their psychosocial development and mental health. A sense of alienation and isolation from families and friends, for example, frequently exacerbates feelings of depression, anxiety, confusion, fear, and guilt. Additionally, these emotional problems often result in suicidal ideation, substance abuse, and psychiatric hospitalization. Verbal and physical abuse in hostile home and school environments may further complicate identity formation, interpersonal adjustment, academic achievement, and vocational ambition. Finally, the discussion of psychotherapeutic and systemic approaches offers clinicians strategies for fostering socialization and facilitating family and community support for sexual minority teens. The next chapter similarly addresses many of the issues lesbian, gay, and bisexual adults experience during midlife and maturity.

7

Midlife and Later-Life Issues for Sexual Minority Adults

If normative descriptions of sexual minority adolescent maturation are severely lacking (as discussed in the previous chapter), standard accounts of adult development for bisexuals, lesbians, and gay men are nearly impossible to find in the behavioral and social science literature. Because sexual orientation rarely was assessed by early researchers or indicated by their respondents, virtually every major developmental theory of adulthood has been constructed on the basis of the participants' assumed heterosexuality (Kimmel, 1978). The one exception was Vaillant's (1977) 30-year study of adult men and their lives, during which only one subject openly identified himself as gay. At the end of the investigation, both he and Vaillant agreed that neither understood the other very well. Further, these examiners investigated men more than women (Friend, 1987), with studies on women's development beginning in the late 1970s and progressing slowly due to funding problems. According to Tully (1992), sample sizes throughout the first 10 years of this research were so small that by the late 1980s, the knowledge base regarding older lesbians was built on data gathered from a total of only 183 women. As was discussed in Chapter 3 (this volume), then, developmental theory and longitudinal research designed specifically to explain or examine the lives of lesbians and gay men has yet to advance (D'Augelli, 1994b).

In addition to this scarcity of theoretical consideration, studies that primarily address even the developmental *issues* of older gay and lesbian adults have been declining. For example, only 17.25% (*n* = 358) of the professional journal articles published on gay, lesbian, and bisexual *adulthood* and *adult development* since 1990 (*n* = 2,075) have appeared since 1995 (PsycINFO, 1997). Of all 2,075 publications, only *10* specifically relate to *adult development*, whereas the remaining 2,065 submissions deal with various other concerns of adult life. Further, a review of the references cited in chapters on midlife and older sexual minority adults (Berger & Kelly, 1996; Ehrenberg, 1996; Jacobson & Grossman, 1996; Kertzner & Sved, 1996; Kimmel & Sang, 1995; Reid, 1995) from four contemporary edited collections indicate that most of the references in these volumes were published in the 1970s and 1980s. The few citations published since 1992 generally address healthcare-related issues or simply refer to other edited collections. Thus, even this cursory examination of available literature supports the notion that research on sexual minority adult development and related issues is in its infancy and clearly lacks a unified theory.

Once the search for a pathogenic etiology of homosexuality was virtually abandoned by everyone except psychoanalysts, researchers were left to investigate lesbians and gay men from any number of diverse, and often contradictory, perspectives. Although speaking of women's studies in particular, Tully's (1992) quote seems to apply to the majority of research on gay men, as well: "By studying issues that evolve from a variety of theoretical concepts, researchers investigate any number of seemingly unrelated topics" (p. 246). Like the literature, then, this chapter covers a range of topics, cites few recent empirical studies, is particularly contextual in scope, and is primarily atheoretical in nature (with the exception of two examples provided directly next).

MIDLIFE

Two sets of researchers (Cornett & Hudson, 1987; Kimmel, 1978) examined the lives of gay men from a developmental perspective by comparing them to the theories of Erikson (1963; Erikson & Erikson, 1981) and Levinson (1978), both of which were derived primarily from the study of heterosexual men. The discussion of midlife in the following section uses the conceptualizations provided by these theorists, at the same time incorporating supporting research and viewpoints from other individuals. Although research on lesbian-specific adult development is limited, information on older lesbians (over 65) is still more available than current data on midlife lesbians (ages 35–60) (Sang, 1992). Nevertheless, extra care has been taken to include findings related to women in the Levinson and Erikson discussions, as well as in those throughout the remainder of this chapter.

Levinson

Levinson (1978) studied 40 married, presumably heterosexual, men in four different occupations. They were primarily middle class and college educated and all were born in the United States in the 1930s and 1940s. After intensive interviews with the men regarding their experiences over the years, Levinson proposed that the following stages describe the lives of these individuals:

- The early adult transition (17–22)
- Entering the adult world (22–28)
- Age-30 transition (28–32)
- Settling down (33–40)
- Midlife transition (40–45)
- Age-50 transition (50–55)
- Late adult transition (60–65)

In an attempt to determine whether Levinson's stages applied to nonheterosexual males, Kimmel (1978) studied 14 New York City, White, well-educated, middle-class gay men over 55 years of age and observed considerable "coming-out" activity among his subjects. Developmental changes continued for most of them throughout their lifetime, and several made significant shifts in their 40s and 50s. Perhaps the developmental lag described in Chapter 5 (Grace, 1992) might best characterize their lives given that the adolescent task of identity development appeared to be a major task of their adulthood. Transitions did seem to occur, but a certain "off-timeness" was evident when compared with heterosexuals.

Charbonneau and Lander (1991) found a similar pattern of developmental variance when they studied 30 women of diverse ethnic, religious, and class backgrounds who were in their mid-30s to their mid-50s when they self-identified as lesbian. All except one had been married heterosexually for 1 to 32 years, and 17 had been married for more than 10 years. Two dozen women had children and, of the six who did not, four had tried unsuccessfully to conceive. In commenting on this study, Sang (1992) reminds psychotherapists that "coming out as lesbian is not restricted to earlier periods of development" (p. 39). Midlife women, just as those who are much younger, can feel attractions to their own sex for the first time or can choose to act on emotions they have been feeling for many years. When compared with heterosexual women, then, Kirkpatrick (1989) believes that lesbians have "a different middle age."

In addition to different *midlife transitions,* they also might have off-time *late adult transitions.* As at least 24 to 50% of lesbians have been married heterosexually, coming out, identifying as lesbian, or both, can occur at any stage in the lifespan (Ettore, 1980; Kehoe, 1986b; D. F. Morrow, 1996). For example, Buffy Dunker (1987), a teacher and therapist, married directly out of college, had three children, taught, retired, and came out to her children, grandchildren, friends, and relatives when she was over 65 years of age. She noted that women of her era were socialized for marriage and family life and that few of her 1926 college classmates chose not to marry. Further, the social upheavals following the events of the late 1960s regarding changing definitions of homosexuality gave many married lesbians (and undoubtedly gay men, as well) permission and courage to "come out" and define themselves in more self-congruent ways. Jensen's (1999) study of 25 women who married men and later came out as lesbian or bisexual provides insight into the cultural restraints that prevented these women from making different sexual choices earlier in their lives.

Hopcke (1992) contends that coming out is a more important developmental milestone for bisexuals, lesbians, and gay men than most other life events. For some, it begins in adolescence or young adulthood, whereas for others the precipitating events may occur later in life. In any event, the crisis of coming out "may be one of the most significant a gay person will face" (Kimmel, 1978, p. 117) and, accordingly, often instills a *crisis competence* that provides a buffer against later life adversities. This crisis competence is accompanied by an increased perspective on unfavorable circumstances which, according to Kimmel, precludes the occurrence of what frequently is referred to as the midlife crisis for some individuals. "The 'coming out crisis,' and the competency developing from it, may prepare the gay man [or lesbian woman] to be better able to objectively survey his [or her] life, and using the crisis as a focal point, balance the pros and cons for more accurate appraisal and much more accessible satisfaction" (Cornett & Hudson, 1987, p. 67). Clinicians should keep in mind, however, that whether or not such a singular midlife event occurs with sexual minority clients, their adult life trajectories, including *settling down* and other adult transition experiences, at least will be different from those of heterosexual clients given the coming-out experience and the lifelong process of identity formation.

Erikson

When applying Erikson's developmental stages to the lives of gay men, Cornett and Hudson (1987) focus particularly on the years of middle adulthood (40–60) when the major psychological crisis of this period focuses on *generativity versus stagnation*. They stress that with sexual minority clients, more so than for heterosexuals, the earlier Eriksonian stages of *identity versus role confusion* (adolescence) and *intimacy versus isolation* (young adulthood) may be operating concurrently with the stages of later life. In other words, therapists treating these individuals may need to provide assistance with negotiating the tasks of several life stages simultaneously.

Intimacy versus Isolation

Just as the process of gay, lesbian, or bisexual identity formation may be occurring during later-life transitions, so also might the quest for interpersonal intimacy. Hence, due to the effects of stigma and developmental lag, many middle-age and older sexual minority individuals are not involved in primary relationships. When interviewing single lesbians, for example, Coos (1991) found that the younger women (ages 24 to 37) anticipated being in a relationship at some time in the future, whereas women over 40 "didn't come out or come of age with the expectation that they would be part of a long-term committed couple sharing a home together" (p.132). Accordingly, half of the 50 lesbians (ages 65 to 85) whom Kehoe (1986b) questioned had no significant other.

Similarly, Berger (1982a, 1995) found that 65% of the 112 Caucasian gay men (ages 41 to 77) he studied had no current primary relationship, although many had a history of being a part of a couple. In contrast, the majority of heterosexual men in that age group are married and, in the course of midlife development, often shift investment from their careers to their intimate relationships. This change of focus, however, does not seem to be an option for many gay men. The very fact that most are uncoupled makes Levinson's *settling down* and three subsequent *transition* stages, as well as Erikson's young adult stage of *intimacy versus isolation*, different for sexual minority men. A similar point may be made for lesbians as well.

Further, a considerable number of sexual minority adults lose some form of connection with their families of origin in the coming-out process, but the formation of intentional families gives them life-giving emotional and social support (Cornett & Hudson, 1987; Kurdek, 1988b; Rothblum, 1990). It is through and within these families of creation that many gay, lesbian, and bisexual individuals deal with the developmental issues of intimacy, trust, and love. Being separated from their birth families, whether geographically, physically, or emotionally, also leads a considerable number of lesbians to establish deep and supportive friendships (Adelman, 1986; Sang, 1992; Tully, 1989; Weinstock & Rothblum, 1996). Similarly, Friend (1980) found that most of the 43 gay men he studied had many intimate friendships, and 86% had at least three close friends.

Generativity versus Stagnation

Not only do the lives of lesbians, bisexuals, and gay men differ from those of heterosexuals, but considerable variation can be observed among sexual minority subpopulations, as well. For example, Kimmel (1978) identified six adult social–sexual life patterns for lesbians and gay men:

1. Heterosexual marriage
    • with periodic homosexual relations
    • without periodic homosexual relations
    • following a gay lifestyle
    • followed by a gay lifestyle

2. Celibacy with homosexual affectional orientation
3. Raising biological or adopted children
4. Long-term same-sex relationship
5. Gay lifestyle with no long-term relationship
6. Bisexual lifestyle without marriage

Sometimes children are included within these various lifestyle choices, with lesbians more than gay men tending to have offspring. This tendency might be due to the previously discussed socialization of women in regard to marriage and family, combined with the phenomenon of later-life lesbian identification. On the other hand, 70 to 90% of gay men over 40 have been reported as having no biological or adopted children, but many of them are thought to meet their generativity needs by sharing their life experience with succeeding generations through their work (Cornett & Hudson, 1987). Erikson and Erikson (1981) propose that negotiating the polarities of *generativity versus stagnation* is one of the primary tasks of midlife, and that generativity has three major aspects: procreation, productivity, and creativity. With procreation not an avenue of task negotiation for many gay men and lesbians, careers and other productive and creative pursuits become important vehicles for life satisfaction and generativity (Terndrup, 1998).

Accelerated Aging

Along with heterosexism, sexual minority group members internalize the ageism of the broader society. For example, younger bisexuals, lesbians, and gay men seem reluctant to reach out to the elders of their communities (Lee, 1991). Although the AIDS crisis undoubtedly contributes to this intergenerational isolation, an internalized assumption among gay men that aging accelerates at midlife also may exacerbate this avoidance. In this context, *accelerated aging* refers to experiencing oneself as old at a time before one's chronological peers define themselves as aged (Friend, 1980, 1987).

Accordingly, J. J. Kelly (1977) interviewed 241 gay men in Los Angeles (ages 16 to 79) who themselves identified a mean age of 50 as marking the end of middle age and the beginning of old age, a milestone event they anticipated about 15 years earlier than did heterosexual males. Friend (1980, 1987) similarly reported that the mean age for nonheterosexual males to see themselves as "old" is 48, compared with a mean age of 65 for men in general (the age at which American men commonly have been "old" enough to retire). Harry (1982b) further found that the gay men in their early 40s he studied were more concerned about growing old and looking youthful than his younger or older respondents. These anxieties particularly were salient among the men without partners and prompted a midlife crisis of meaning for many of these individuals. Harry concluded that these men seem to have internalized the youth that parts of the gay world values, "which sets the stage for an aging crisis and defines what is to be considered a crisis" (p. 226).

On the other hand, not all research supports a theory of accelerated aging.

Minnigerode (1976), for example, distributed questionnaires to 95 gay men (ages 25 to 68) and asked whether they saw themselves as "young," "middle age," or "old." He found that the chronological means given for the onsets of middle age and old age were roughly the averages assigned by the general population of the United States (41.29 and 64.78 years, respectively). Minnigerode's data reveal that individuals in poorer physical or psychological health tend to anticipate an early onset of old age, but the findings also appear to contradict the prevailing thinking that "homosexual men enter middle and old age earlier than heterosexual men and that homosexual men experience accelerated aging" (p. 275). Kertzner (1999) questioned 30 gay men, ages 40 to 51 years, and likewise found that many of the men noted the absence of socially defined markers to delineate the aging process but most did not report psychological distress associated with entering middle age. He also concluded that the degree to which the subjects experienced a sense of reconciliation with past difficulties was related to psychological adjustment and attitudes toward growing older.

Whatever the final outcome of this debate, attractiveness seems to be more important to gay men than to lesbian women. Lesbians generally do not attribute attractiveness to youth (Almvig, 1982; Laner, 1979; Prime Timers Worldwide, 1997), but a youth orientation in the gay male community makes aging more stressful for its members than for sexual minority women (A. L. Ellis, 2000; Friend, 1987; Gutierrez, 1992). As is true for all humans, midlife lesbians do have concerns, but these concerns generally are not as related to the loss of attractiveness with aging as are the issues of gay men. In fact, Kehoe (1989) speculates that, possibly because they had escaped the expectations frequently imposed on wives, mothers, and grandmothers that could accelerate aging, some of the 100 lesbians over 60 whom she studied reported feeling more youthful than did their heterosexual counterparts. Noting this same comparative youthfulness, Cruikshank (1991) cites physical activity as a possible reason: "old lesbians may be more physically active than heterosexual women, from lifelong habit, partly because some of them held nontraditional jobs requiring physical labor" (p. 85).

Friend (1987) notes that the accelerated aging frequently seen in heterosexual women is comparable to that found in gay males. Given their common attraction to men, he believes that the key variable possibly is not sexual orientation per se but, rather, an expression of gender role socialization. Thus socialized, gay men are led to adopt a social construction of masculinity which values youth and beauty or which "assumes a future of singlehood necessitating retaining one's physical appearance" (p. 325). Whether accelerated aging is attributed to these factors or is universal, such internalized assumptions nevertheless create a stressful middle age for some heterosexual women and gay men but not necessarily for lesbians.

LATER LIFE

Paralleling the evolving social construction of homosexuality, the lives of contemporary sexual minorities, for the most part, have become dramatically different from those of their counterparts at the beginning of the 20th century (Cruikshank, 1991; Rosenfeld, 1999). When treating midlife and older gay, lesbian, and bisexual clients, clinicians must remember to consider the effects of historical events and changing societal conditions on their development; that is, the "tremendous economic, scientific, social, and political changes" they have experienced (Dunker, 1987, p. 73). For example, gay men and lesbians over 60 are the last generation to have lived most of their lives before the social, cultural, and political changes initiated by the 1969 Stonewall rebellion (Adelman, 1990).

Previously, compartmentalization was the norm and much effort was expended keeping the various aspects of their work and relationships separate from one another (Friend, 1990). The consequences of not doing so were often serious and included being fired from jobs; denied security clearances; discharged from the military; rejected by family, church, and friends; and being arrested for their actual or suspected sexual orientation. Further, the witch hunts of the McCarthy era particularly were frightening, and events such as these resulted in lesbians and gay men spending most of their adult lives in secrecy and small groups (Dunker, 1987). To many of these older individuals, "queer" was a negative slur to fearfully avoid rather than a positive label to proudly adopt as do many of today's younger gay, lesbian, bisexual, and transgender activists.

To examine the construction of the meaning of homosexuality, Rosenfeld (1999) conducted in-depth interviews with 17 gay men and 20 lesbian women over 65. She identified two specific "identity cohorts" among her subjects: those who considered themselves homosexual before the liberationist movements of the late 1960s and those who self-identified during later periods when some activists considered homosexuality as a source of status. Rosenfeld found that each identity cohort developed extremely different understandings of what it meant to be homosexual, the nature of the threat posed by the heterosexual society, and the appropriate response to that intimidation. What many in the earlier cohort considered a pragmatically sensible response to oppressive societal conditions was considered by others in the later cohort as a morally repugnant way to deal with subjugation.

Isolation

Sexual minority subcultures were unavailable when older lesbians and gay men were growing up and, in fact, did not begin to form until after World War II. Even then, if individuals had not served in the military or did not live in large or coastal cities, they usually were unaware that such communities existed. Most lived isolated, compartmentalized, or secret lives and did not know that there were many others like themselves. They often felt very much alone, with few opportunities for positive identification with other gay, lesbian, and bisexual individuals. An affirming social construct of homosexuality was not available to them; therefore, they formed their identities according to self-concepts largely influenced by popular opinions and heterosexist assumptions.

> A history of managing heterosexism is a significant factor which has influenced the ways in which the identities of older lesbian and gay people have been constructed. Some of these people have internalized these negative ideologies; others have accommodated to them, while still others have shaped their lives around a reconstructed set of positive and affirmative beliefs. (Friend, 1990, p. 116)

In any case, all have lived through extremely difficult times because of their sexual orientation. Yet now, as they age, many find that an additional stigma presents itself. Unfortunately, for these gay, lesbian, and bisexual elders, the dual oppression of heterosexism and ageism is a reality (Clunis & Green, 1988; Friend, 1987).

Self-Acceptance and Life Satisfaction

Because of stigma, oppression, and discrimination, life often has been perilous for older lesbian, gay, and bisexual individuals (Berger, 1992b). Nevertheless, many have weathered the turbulence of their times. For example, all of the 112 gay men whom Berger (1982a, 1995) studied (who were discussed earlier in this chapter) said the road to accepting themselves had been long and tortuous. In spite of this difficult journey, however, the life satisfaction of 72.1% of his respondents was rated as "high," whereas that of only 5.4% was scored as "low." Berger thus concluded that the levels of life satisfaction for his subjects were as high or higher than those of older men and women in the general population.

In addition to Berger's research, a few other assessments of psychological adjustment among older sexual minority persons were conducted during the 1970s and 1980s and those findings also refuted the stereotype of the poorly adapted elderly gay or lesbian individual. Unfortunately, no more recent empirical studies seem to be available beyond those described in the next paragraph (Berger & Kelly, 1996; Ehrenberg, 1996; Reid, 1995). Given the fact that each generation essentially lives in different historical eras, generalizing these basically favorable findings to contemporary older lesbians, bisexuals, and gay men is problematic.

In one of the first (and probably most extensive) surveys ever conducted, M. S. Weinberg and Williams (1975) distributed questionnaires to 2,500 gay men in the United States and Europe and found that the older respondents were psychologically "healthier" than their younger counterparts. Similarly, Berger's (1980, 1982a, 1995) 112 subjects (described previously) reported relatively high levels of self-acceptance and low levels of depression, and he contended that they matched or showed higher scores on these items than the M. S. Weinberg and Williams (1975) sample of adult homosexual males. Finally, Minnigerode, Adelman, and Fox (1980) compared the psychological, social, personal, and sexual adjustment of heterosexual, gay, and lesbian individuals over 60 years of age. Their results detected few and no differences between the populations in psychological adjustment as measured by the Life Satisfaction Index, the Self-Criticism Scale, and the Symptoms Index, even though all of the nonheterosexuals in the study reported reaching self-acceptance after a lifelong struggle.

On the other hand, Lee (1991) directed remarks toward the gerontologists whom he believed tended to overcompensate for "stereotypes of the miserable, lonely old dyke and faggot" by describing older lesbians and gay men as "not only happy, self-fulfilled people, but even more satisfied with their lives than their heterosexual counterparts" (p. xiv). He questioned not only the helpfulness but also the accuracy of such "Panglossian views" and contended that although most people of same-sex orientation are satisfied with their lives, there *are* unhappy and lonely lesbian and gay seniors. Clinicians, then, need to keep Lee's caveat in mind when individuals who do not fit the "new mythology" (p. xiv) of sexual minority aging present themselves for treatment.

Invisibility

Like J. A. Lee (1991), Cruikshank (1991) cautioned readers to interpret recent findings contradicting the stereotype of general unhappiness in "old homosexuals" from a realistic perspective. She surveyed the field of lesbian and gay studies on aging, which she observed was in its infancy, and concluded that the older lesbian and gay population "is still so hidden that those few who come forward to describe their lives are quite likely to be the most robust specimens of their group and are more likely to have a gay political consciousness" (p. 86).

Others also have written of this invisibility (Almvig, 1982; Clunis & Green 1988; Friend, 1987; Kimmel, 1978). H. B. McDonald and Steinhorn (1993), for example, believe it to be so pervasive that the majority of helping professionals rarely consider sexual orientation when taking a family history of a older person, or when planning nursing-home or day-treatment care for that individual. To hear what deeply may be disguised, they suggest that clinicians listen carefully to the language of their clients in order to detect possible euphemisms for their lovers, such as *friend*, *dear friend*, or *roommate*. Like others of their generation, many older clients rarely speak of their sexuality, let alone their sexual orientation (Dunker, 1987; Tully, 1992). Further, the language they use to describe themselves, if they do so at all, might be that of another era, such as *homosexual* (for both sexes) or as *gay* rather than *lesbian* (for women).

Due to the hostile social conditions described earlier, many older sexual minority adults spent their youth and middle age feeling extremely fearful of discovery, and continue to feel so even today. Others are like many of their younger counterparts and regard their sexual orientation as a personal issue, one not related to a broader political community, or even to a research agenda (Bradford & Ryan, 1991; Slusher, Mayer, & Dunkle, 1996). Still others have been waiting a lifetime for the kind of openness that is emerging in many segments of the United States today. These individuals welcome the occasion to be a part of a liberation movement and to speak publicly about their lives and experiences. As more individuals take advantage of this opportunity for generativity and identify as members of a sexual minority group, facts can be separated from myths and a more comprehensive profile of aging gay, lesbian, and bisexual populations may be developed.

Variables Related to Adjustment

A considerable diversity exists among the experiences of lesbians and gay men in later adulthood, and there appears to be a search for some common factors related to successful aging in these individuals. This trend corresponds to one in gerontological studies of the general population and undoubtedly is fueled by the fact that more people are living longer than ever before. The quest for those variables that correlate with satisfaction and adjustment in the later years of life, then, is providing an impetus for a number of researchers in gay and lesbian gerontology.

Some elements of a contented life are common to all humans, and needs for companionship, commitment, intimacy, ego enhancement, and fulfillment are no different for sexual minorities than for heterosexuals. In fact, these needs are so strong that they transcend sexual orientation (Lipman, 1986). As discussed previously, older lesbians and gay men typically live within a self-created, supportive network of friends, sometimes have long-time companions, and often have special roles in their biological families that reflect their unique social position (Grossman, D'Augelli, & Hershberger, 2000; Kimmel, 1992). Contrary to stereotypes, not all sexual minority adults are cut off from their families of origin and some even occupy roles such as a favorite aunt or uncle, or the caretaker of a widowed mother. As a matter of fact, in many families this latter responsibility may fall to lesbian or gay members because they are supposedly "single" and therefore not burdened with family responsibilities of their own (Berger, 1982a, 1995). Sang's (1991) mostly White, lesbian, professional sample (*n* = 110; ages 40 to 59) reflected this phenomena in reporting struggles to balance work, relationships, personal interests, child care, community, spirituality, and care of aging parents.

Social Support

Along with crisis competence and gender role flexibility, broad family and community support is one of three factors that facilitate adjustment for gay men and lesbians in later life (Friend, 1987; Grossman et al., 2000). In regard to social involvement, Quam and Whitford (1992) administered questionnaires to 80 lesbians and gay men (ages 50 to 73) who were quite active in the sexual minority community. The respondents reported a generally high level of life satisfaction and an acceptance of the aging process, despite predictable problems with aging and sexual orientation. Being active in the lesbian and gay community was found to be an asset to acceptance of growing older. Similarly, Cruikshank (1991) asserts that having a gay political consciousness is a source of high self-esteem at any age.

Not all older sexual minority individuals, however, would agree with this contention. Having grown up in extremely antagonistic circumstances and surrounded by negative societal evaluations of a minority sexual orientation, some have had few opportunities to develop a positive association with being gay, lesbian, or bisexual. Hence, many learned "to keep to themselves" and not risk socializing with anyone who might lead others to suspect that they might be homosexual. According to Adelman (1990), "the closets of the pre-Stonewall era provided comfort in a hostile environment by allowing one to have a positive self-image" (p. 30). Not surprising, then, are the findings that more "closeted" individuals prefer a mainstream heterosexual setting wherein they can assimilate and not be identified with the stigma attached to a sexual minority identity (Cruikshank, 1991; Friend, 1990). These people tend to distance themselves from anything stereotypically associated with homosexuality and often spend much energy passing as heterosexual. They have few gay, lesbian, or bisexual friends (Slusher et al., 1996).

Having thus survived by developing coping styles of isolation and compartmentalization, many (if not most) sexual minority seniors perpetuate these patterns today (Clunis & Green, 1988; Frost, 1997; Kehoe, 1986a, 1986b). This phenomenon might explain Adelman's (1990) findings that high life satisfaction among the 27 older gay men and 25 lesbians whom she studied was related to low involvement with other gays, and that low life satisfaction correlated with high involvement. Similarly, Kehoe (1986b) administered a questionnaire to the 50 lesbians (ages 65 to 85) discussed earlier in this chapter and found the profile of a woman with a "balanced, stable personality" (p. 148), who neither went to women's bars nor belonged to any social or professional lesbian groups. Her subjects did not see themselves as closeted and some occasionally attended lesbian functions. One-half of the women indicated they currently were "unattached." Despite normal problems associated with aging (i.e., health, finances, isolation, and loneliness), those without partners did not appear to be as unhappy with their lives as might be predicted. Nonetheless, Lipman (1986) found that older closed-couple lesbians and gay men with a strong commitment to the dyadic relationship were shown to be the happiest and best adjusted of the various older sexual minority subpopulations.

Crisis Competence

In addition to a supportive friendship network, however it is individually defined, Friend (1987) believes that the sense of competence that develops from having weathered the coming-out crisis successfully is another factor related to adjustment in later life. As discussed earlier in this chapter (Cornett & Hudson, 1987; Kimmel, 1978), several writers see this event and its related experiences as so developmentally influential that most other life crises virtually pale by comparison. A lifetime of managing issues and losses related to their sexual orientation, in a sense, prepares individuals for losses in their old age. As a result, many older sexual minority persons have developed the psychological skills necessary for coping with the difficult issues that confront people in the last years of their lives (Friend, 1990).

Another factor closely related to crisis competence that influences the way that some gay men and lesbians age is the fact that some are less involved in the developmental crises within families that typically affect the patterns of aging for heterosexuals (Kimmel, 1978). As suggested earlier in this chapter, some have no biological offspring and others are alienated from their families of origin. Even though these phenomena have their own pains and tribulations, the crises surrounding them customarily have occurred prior to the onset of old age and thus allow gay, lesbian, or bisexual individuals to face them before having to deal with issues of their own aging.

Kimmel also contends that, having been forced by society and circumstances to take care of themselves rather than to rely on others, sexual minority individuals often are better prepared emotionally and physically for self-reliance in their later years. Maintaining their own homes and creating their own social and support networks have provided many with a trust in their ability to weather hardship and adversity and has given them confidence in their skills to somehow manage life as they age. They have had to look to their own resources rather than to biological or nuclear families for financial and emotional support and, thus, are more likely than heterosexuals to have planned for their own future security. Difficult as this often lonely struggle has been, it has given them an important attribute in their old age (Berger, 1982a, 1995; Friend, 1987; H. B. McDonald & Steinhorn, 1993).

Conversely, after following 47 gay men (ages 50 to 80) for 4 years, J. A. Lee (1987) disputes the notion of crisis competence or that various crises equip sexual minority adults to age well. Instead, he contends that happiness in old age is more likely to result from people having had the good fortune or sufficient skill to avoid stressful outcomes. He concludes that older gay and heterosexual men are more similar than different and that generational class conflict is the major problem facing all older persons. J. A. Lee (1991) also believes that trying to convince unhappy and lonely gay and lesbian seniors "that they have superior capacities for adapting to old age (such as 'crisis competence') does a disservice" (p. xiv). For those who have not adjusted well, this notion has them blaming themselves for their misfortunes or wondering what is wrong with them. As a result, he cautions gerontologists (and likewise psychotherapists) to be realistic even at the risk of seeming homophobic and heterosexist.

Few would dispute Lee's cautionary advice regarding the practical application of crisis competence. His objections, however, do not seem to address themselves sufficiently to the issue of why certain lesbians, gay men, and bisexuals *have* been able to navigate successfully through oppressive and often hostile societal conditions while others have not. In spite of essentially similar historical and sociocultural events, some have developed the skills and ability to lead a satisfying life in their later years while others are distressed and dissatisfied. In other words, not all have developed the crisis competence necessary to lead gratifying lives in their old age.

Gender Flexibility

Along with social support and crisis competence, Friend (1987) believes that the gender role flexibility of many sexual minority individuals facilitates adaptation to aging. Accordingly, he contends that, because their concept of gender roles often is more flexible than that of their heterosexual counterparts, older gay men and lesbians are able to develop ways of taking care of themselves that feel comfortable and appropriate to them, as opposed to adopting those defined by society. In this regard, "challenging the social construction of gender roles may not pose a significant threat to the sexual identity of older homosexuals in ways that it might for older heterosexuals" (p. 311). Because of the kinds of circumstances described throughout this book, many have been forced during their lifetimes to do what was necessary to survive. Thus, Friend assumes that managing issues such as society's notions of sexual orientation and gender have been addressed earlier in life, and believes that lesbian and gay seniors often have developed a flexibility to engage in nontraditional gender role behaviors. Consequently, they may have a wider repertoire of available coping tools and responses at their disposal as they age.

Because they have had to support themselves all their lives, most older gay men and lesbians have been employed from the time they were young adults. Often they have worked in careers or jobs considered nontraditional for their sex. Simply because they were gay or lesbian, many have felt a need to work hard and achieve more than a comparison group of heterosexuals. (Incidentally, Goffman [1963] describes this as a common adaptational style among stigmatized groups.) As a result of this increased effort, however, some have been successful vocationally and financially. Unfortunately, many others (especially lesbians, but often gay men as well) have the same experience as women in the United States in that they have lower incomes than presumably heterosexual men relative to their level of education and experience (Sang, 1992). (See Chapter 11 for additional discussion of career issues.)

Regardless of income, however, the fact remains that gender role flexibility (whether innate or acquired by necessity) generally has increased the adaptability of lesbians, bisexuals, and gay men. For example, unlike many married heterosexual women, lesbians have had to prepare their own income taxes, maintain homes and automobiles, and otherwise make all minor and major decisions regarding their lives. Similarly, gay men have had to undertake the domestic tasks that heterosexually married men often rely on their wives to do, such as cooking, cleaning, shopping, and serving as the social and familial contact person for their households. In other words, greater flexibility in self-definition of gender roles has assisted many sexual minority individuals in adapting personally and professionally to stigmatizing conditions. Consequently, this flexibility frequently increases their ability to adapt to the universally difficult circumstances of old age (Berger & Kelly, 1986; Friend, 1990; H. B. McDonald & Steinhorn, 1993).

Identity Formation

As discussed previously, the formation of an affirmative and integrated lesbian, gay, or bisexual identity is a lifelong process. Like their younger counterparts, many older sexual minority adults live daily with the oppressive effects of heterosexism and thus struggle to either maintain or develop their sense of positive self-definition. In this regard, from her study of older gay men and lesbians, Adelman (1980) concluded that later life development was not as much affected by sexual orientation per se as by the social stigma attached to same-sex attraction and identification. In addition, both she and Berger (1982a, 1995) discovered that those subjects who were experiencing less life satisfaction likewise were less content with their gay or lesbian identities and also had more psychosomatic complaints than did individuals with a more favorable outlook on life. Although positive identity formation indeed can provide an enhanced ability for managing social stigma (Berger & Kelly, 1986), it neither relieves completely the natural anger and frustration sexual minorities feel toward unrelenting societal discrimination nor compensates for their ensuing need to maintain secrecy (Adelman, 1980).

Adelman (1990) interviewed 27 gay men (mean age = 65.63) and 25 lesbians (mean age = 64.48) in order to determine the relationship between their patterns of adjustment to later life and the sequence of their early developmental events. After reviewing related studies, she noted that her findings support research indicating that same-sex experimentation before self-definition (rather than vice versa) is associated with adaptation in the later years. In other words, the pattern with the more favorable long-range prognosis appeared to be one in which individuals withdrew and internally acclimatized *after* experimentation and *before* committing themselves further to a way of life which required continual adaptation to stigmatizing conditions. According to Adelman (1990), "the contingencies of stigma and the conditions of internal readjustment are manifested in the relationship between adjustment and delaying self-definition until after experimentation" (p. 21). Adelman's findings, then, seem to imply that a period of withdrawal and internal consolidation after experimenting with the same sex somehow fortifies and strengthens people for the lifelong battle against oppression.

Although this information could be helpful to psychotherapists working with clients of any age who have yet to either experiment sexually or label their sexual orientation, it probably is useful only for theoretical or clinical perspective regarding older lesbians and gay men who "came out" many years earlier and were frightened back into the closet in later life. Regardless of the sequence of early developmental events, however, clinicians should continue working for identity consolidation and enhancement with all older sexual minority adults, even those who experimented first and then self-identified, because the conditions that contributed to the devaluing of their identities continue to persist.

Granted, lifelong situational irritations and regrets are still present for sexual minority clients as they mature in identity development, but these negative external conditions no longer need result in internalized homophobia or heterosexism. In this regard, Friend (1990) proposes a three-stage theory of successful aging wherein, during the first stage, society's negative messages about same-sex orientation are internalized and considerably damage self-esteem. Those people in the midrange of his stage model accept some aspects of being lesbian or gay but continue to believe on some level that heterosexuality is better. Finally, sexual minority individuals who age successfully have an ability to evaluate critically the norms of society and arrive at a state of increased perspective regarding the social constructionistic elements in both homosexuality and heterosexuality. From this vantage point, they can evaluate societal standards more objectively and can reconstruct or reframe the meaning of being gay, lesbian, or bisexual into something positive. "Older gay and lesbian people who have had experience in reconstructing the arbitrary definitions of what homosexuality and gender mean are also more likely to be able to transfer these affirmative processes to their identities as older people" (p. 111). According to Friend (1989), this challenging of heterosexist assumptions is an important ingredient in successful aging.

Psychosocial Stressors

Many of later-life experiences are inherently difficult, regardless of sexual orientation. Although gay, bisexual, and lesbian seniors seek psychotherapy for primarily the same reasons as heterosexuals (i.e., adjustment to retirement, depression, isolation, financial concerns, declining health, and bereavement) (Kimmel, 1977), old age for sexual minority individuals adds its own unique stressors. Frost (1997), speaking specifically of gay men, notes that "aging . . . is a complex phenomenon involving identity, self-esteem, internalized homophobia, stereotypes about older gay men, and the paucity of positive gay male images or role models to help direct their development" (p. 267). Further, those without children or supportive family often worry about who will care for them in their later years, especially if their partners (if they have one) become disabled or precede them in death. In a closeted couple, the death of a lover is especially traumatic because an entire support network frequently is lost in the passing of the significant other (Clunis & Green, 1988; Friend, 1987; Kimmel, 1978; H. B. McDonald & Steinhorn, 1993; Rothblum, 1990). The grief is sometimes intensified if the survivor is excluded by the family of origin in health care, funeral, or estate matters.

Older sexual minority individuals who avail themselves of psychotherapy at arduous times such as these often respond well, particularly if clinicians see the circumstances of their lives and not their sexual orientation as the basic problem (P. P. Smith, 1992). Frost (1997) contends that group psychotherapy is the treatment of choice for numerous aging gay males, primarily because the format itself forces them to address a number of their significant issues. Because clients in his groups contract to "stay until the work is done" (p. 275), a new experience is created for those members whose customary pattern of managing their interpersonal anxiety is to leave stressful situations. He further contends that group psychotherapy can help gay men to increase their sense of self-worth as they learn new, nonsexual, and more satisfying ways to relate with other men. For many, the shame and anxiety associated with intimacy and vulnerability can be overcome, a sense of trust and connection can be developed, and relationships can begin "to feel real" (p. 281)—possibly for the first time.

Psychotherapists should be especially alert to the potential or actual legal difficulties of their older lesbian, gay, or bisexual clients. If individuals have not adequately prepared for their old age, they should be referred to competent and sympathetic legal counsel for estate planning, the drafting of a will, designating legal and medical powers of attorney, and arranging for their health care should the need arise (see Chapter 4). In addition, older gay, lesbian, and bisexual people often are extremely apprehensive about institutionalization in heterosexist nursing homes, which they should be helped to avoid if at all possible (Clunis & Green, 1988; Dunker, 1987; Friend, 1987; Kimmel, 1978; Rothblum,

1990). For many, living in such environments is reminiscent of the years they spent in the closet. Some fear not being allowed to share a room with their partner, and others dread having to deny their relationship or to negate their sexual orientation in order to receive fair and responsible treatment in surroundings relatively free of prejudice.

In one study (Lucco, 1987), most of the 57 lesbians and 399 gay men surveyed indicated an interest in planned retirement housing which would be sensitive to their needs and include a continuum of services. Many have been willing to relocate significant distances in order to live in such a community. The reality, however, is that most of these facilities exist in a small number of larger cities and accept only those individuals who can afford to pay the fees. The majority of older sexual minority clients, thus, will need assistance in planning for alternatives that are as affirming as possible of their orientations.

Some supportive alternatives already are being promoted and provided by various groups (see Resources section for listings and websites with links to numerous others). The 9,500-member American Society on Aging, for example, has established a Lesbian and Gay Aging Issues Network (LGAIN) to advance programs, policies, and educational opportunities which improve the quality of life for older lesbians and gay men. Further, the Gay and Lesbian Association of Retiring Persons (GLARP) is a non-profit corporation designed to enhance the aging experience of sexual minorities. In addition, several advocacy organizations have been formed to provide direct assistance to older gay, lesbian, and bisexual adults. Senior Action in a Gay Environment (SAGE) in New York City and Project Rainbow: Society for Senior Gay and Lesbian Citizens (SSGLC) in Los Angeles are examples of two such organizations. These latter two, in particular, are designed to contribute expertise regarding problems associated with aging, such as securing adequate health care, transportation, housing, household help, and legal consultation. Unfortunately, the few similar groups that currently exist are too geographically distant from most individuals who need direct resources. Several organizations, however, have developed websites that can be accessed at home by technologically literate seniors or from the office by psychotherapists.

Sometimes the people who require the foregoing kinds of information, support, or services are reluctant to seek help. As mentioned previously, many older gay, lesbian, and bisexual individuals have spent a lifetime hiding their sexual orientation. Thus, requesting assistance for information or for a problem associated with sexual minority stigmatization would mean taking a step in their later years that heretofore had been unthinkable. Therapeutically, then, the issue can be seen as one of identity formation and of helping clients manage the fear of having to disclose their sexual orientation, or at least their life circumstances (such as the existence of a same-sex partner), in order to secure the aid they need. This fear often can stimulate identity development in that some aging individuals might be more motivated to protect their health or financial security, or that of a loved one, than in continuing to hide their homosexuality. Dunker (1987) contends that sexual minorities "will have to confront some oppressive regulations even if it means coming out of the closet" (p. 80).

In this regard, the drastic social changes in recent decades brought about by the gay and lesbian liberation movement have served as an impetus to many seniors who "are tired of hiding their lifestyle and are no longer willing to tolerate the degree of persecution and oppression they experienced in the past" (Kimmel, 1977, p. 391). Several studies have shown that many older lesbians and gay men are less concerned with exposure than are their younger counterparts (Berger, 1982a, 1995; M. S. Weinberg & Williams, 1974).

In fact, Berger (1982a, 1995) found that 37% of his 112 gay male subjects neither cared nor worried about who knew of their same-sex orientation. Further, exposure was not an issue because many of their family, friends, and colleagues were aware of their sexual minority status. If their parents were alive, they were quite older and often relied on their children, regardless of sexual orientation, for assistance. Several years later (1992b), Berger also speculated that older individuals are sometimes less fearful of discovery either because they are more secure in their jobs or "because they are more likely to be retired and therefore freed from the worries of employment discrimination that keep many working gays in the closet" (p. 225). In any case, psychotherapeutic work is enhanced if any of these processes which may facilitate disclosure are operating in older gay, lesbian, and bisexual clients. If not, clinicians will need to proceed slowly and sequentially as they would normally, use multiple formats, and attempt the best possible balance between the needs of clients and their level of comfort (Frost, 1997).

CONCLUSION

This chapter considered several issues bisexuals, lesbians, and gay men experience during middle and later adulthood that affect their psychological maturity and vitality. Theories of adult development, for example, were discussed with reference to sexual minority clients in order to help clinicians further facilitate their identity formation across the lifespan and mature transition from youth to old age. In sum, Parts I and II of this book established the sociopolitical contexts and developmental concerns that must be assessed and addressed in the clinical practice of affirmative psychotherapy with gay, lesbian, and bisexual populations that will be described in Part III.

Part III

AFFIRMATIVE PRACTICE

8

Psychodiagnostic Considerations

Ethical practice calls clinicians to consider the heterosexist bias in specific diagnostic categories historically used to classify sexual minority populations. The American Psychiatric Association, for example, declassified and removed *homosexuality* from DSM-II (American Psychiatric Association, 1968) in 1973. In 1980, however, *persistent and marked distress* about sexual orientation was classified and introduced as *ego-dystonic homosexuality* in DSM-III. Though this new classification technically did not survive the manual's revision, its diagnostic criteria were reassigned to *sexual disorder not otherwise specified* (302.90) in DSM-III-R (American Psychiatric Association, 1987). The Diagnostic Index of the revised text further instructed readers searching for "homosexuality, ego-dystonic" to "See sexual disorder not otherwise specified" (p. 561). Although this cross-reference was deleted from DSM-IV (American Psychiatric Association, 1994), the *persistent and marked distress* criteria for a 302.90 diagnosis remained unchanged. Given the number of lenses through which same-sex orientation has been seen, diagnostic categories for psychiatric disorders appear to be "arbitrary constructions" and "reflections of cultural values that change over time" (Gould, 1995, p. 10). As these social constructions reflect the evolving heterosexist perspectives and values of society, some of the diagnostic categories of DSM mirror the bias of the macroculture (C. Silverstein, 1991, 1996; J. Smith, 1988).

Cultural heterosexism, nonetheless, often evokes persistent and marked distress about sexual orientation (or sexual *differentness* in those not yet aware of their homosexuality) that can contribute to various psychiatric disorders. Several presentations, including those of dysthymia or endogenous depression in highly closeted clients, can be manifestations of underlying distress about gender or sexual identity that lift dramatically when these individuals come out (Gonsiorek, 1982; J. Smith, 1988). The literature is replete with single-subject case studies of homosexual patients that either fail to consider or neglect to mention sociocultural influences on the diagnosed disorder. This lack of attribution tends to reinforce the association between homosexuality and various psychopathologies, such as borderline personality disorders, dysthymia, hypomania, homosex-

149

ual panic, and homosexual erotomania (Baptiste, 1990; Eminson, Gillett, & Hassanyeh, 1989; Issroff, 1988; Jafri & Greenberg, 1991; Signer, 1989).

This chapter discusses the influence of heterosexist bias on diagnosis. Emphasis is placed on the need for clinicians to understand common psychological and behavioral manifestations of psychically embedded heterosexism during the coming-out process. Guidelines are provided to assist in formulating a diagnosis that is clinically accurate but nonetheless accounts for the effects of this internalization. Paranoia, hypomania, borderline personality disorder, three characterological-appearing overlays to personality structures, and gender identity disorder are illustrated specifically in this regard. Accordingly, diagnostic criteria for these disorders or syndromes are compared with features manifested when otherwise functional individuals present with a sexual identity crisis or with atypical developmental differences.

HETEROSEXIST BIAS IN DIAGNOSIS

A growing body of research describes gender, ethnicity, and class bias in diagnosis (McGrath, Keita, Strickland, & Russo, 1990; Roades, Weber, & Biaggio, 1998; D. Russell, 1985, 1986). Examples include:

- perceiving clients as more disturbed and requiring more treatment based on sexist, racist, and classist assumptions (overpathologizing)
- attributing symptomology to group membership rather than to psychopathology (minimizing)
- overdiagnosing or underdiagnosing as a function of group membership

Although these examples are thought to apply further to sexual orientation bias in diagnosis (Committee on Lesbian and Gay Concerns, 1991; Gonsiorek, 1982; McHenry & Johnson, 1991), there is little empirical research that has examined the relationship between homosexuality and certain diagnostic categories. There also are no studies available that investigate how *perceptions* of this association influence specific diagnostic assignments. Finally, there has not been a systematic investigation of possible clinician bias with respect to assignment of diagnosis and judgment of psychological functioning (Biaggio, Rhodes, McCaffery, Cardinali, & Duffy, 1996).

One extensive survey, however, was conducted by a task force of the Committee on Lesbian and Gay Concerns (1991) of the American Psychological Association. After 2,544 psychologists responded to a questionnaire, the Committee published a report on bias in psychotherapy with lesbians and gay men. Key themes and examples of biased, inadequate, or inappropriate assessment were summarized, including:

- the belief that "homosexuality per se is a form of psychopathology, developmental arrest, or other psychological disorders" (p. 10)
- the automatic attribution of client problems to sexual orientation without corresponding evidence

Further, the Committee on Lesbian and Gay Concerns (1991) provided illustrations of exemplary assessment practice, including:

- the recognition of "the multiple ways that social prejudice and discrimination can create problems that lesbians and gay men may seek to address in therapy"
- the consideration of "sexual orientation as one of the many important attributes that characterize a client" without the assumption that "it is necessarily relevant to the client's problems" (Garnets et al., 1991, p. 968)

Exemplary practice thus incorporates consideration of relevant sociocultural variables, including the role of heterosexist influences on mental health, when conducting evaluations (Bieschke & Matthews, 1996; Cabaj, 1988b; McHenry & Johnson, 1991).

Data from additional surveys regarding therapist bias reveal inconsistent findings depending on the clinician population being studied. Rubinstein (1995) sampled 417 Israeli clinicians and found that they rated a hypothetical homosexual client's mental state more severely than that of a heterosexual client with the same diagnosis. Similarly, another study (Lilling & Friedman, 1995) examined the relationship between the attitudes of 82 psychoanalysts toward gay patients and their clinical assessments of these individuals on three measures. Results indicated that the clinicians held a subtle but significant negative bias toward homosexual patients, especially those with serious psychopathology.

The findings are far more affirmative, however, in studies in which the therapists surveyed are from more diverse backgrounds (i.e., not exclusively or predominately psychiatrically or psychoanalytically trained). For example, 422 members of the Psychotherapy Division (29) of the American Psychological Association were randomly selected and surveyed to assess clinician bias with respect to judgments of disturbance as a function of client sexual orientation (Biaggio et al., 1996). Using a hypothetical client with varying demographic characteristics, results indicated that clinicians displayed no strong evidence of bias against gay men and lesbians and made few significant differentiations of disturbance between sexual orientation groups. Similarly, Liddle (1999a) surveyed 366 gay and lesbian clients of counselors, psychologists, psychiatrists, and social workers and asked them to rate the helpfulness of their therapists. She also adapted from Garnets et al. (1991, described previously) a 12-item checklist of both inadequate and exemplary therapist practices and asked respondents to indicate whether their therapist had exhibited these practices. Clients of counselors, psychologists, and social workers were quite positive in their ratings; an average of 70% perceived their therapists as *very helpful,* 22% as *fairly helpful,* 5% as *not at all helpful,* and 3% as *destructive.* Ratings of psychiatrists were somewhat less favorable; 50% considered their psychiatrists *very helpful,* 26% *fairly helpful,* 9% *not at all helpful,* and 15% *destructive.* Although these ratings reflect far less clinician bias than in the earlier eras (see Chapter 2), psychodiagnostic considerations continue to warrant attention (Liddle, 1999b).

STIGMA, STRESS, OR PSYCHOPATHOLOGY?

As introduced in Chapter 1, Allport (1954) asserted that (1) no one can remain unaffected by the degradation of others, and (2) self-protectiveness often is encountered among members of groups that are stereotyped and stigmatized. Accordingly, people who are discriminated against and disparaged frequently experience extensive intrapsychic and interpersonal consequences. Among the "traits due to victimization" or "persecution-produced traits" to which Allport (1954) referred, these adverse effects include social withdrawal and passivity as well as obsessive anxiety, suspicion, and insecurity. Many of these characteristics describe lesbians, bisexuals, and gay men living without the support of family and community in a heterosexist and homophobic society.

Specifically, the association between internalized homophobia and psychological distress was assessed in 738 gay men (I. H. Meyer, 1995; I. H. Meyer & Dean, 1998). Separate multiple regression analyses revealed that the degree to which the men had internalized societal heterosexism was correlated with demoralization (a generalized measure of distress that includes symptoms of anxiety and depression), guilt feelings, and suicidal ideation. The authors, in fact, noted that "internalized homophobia is associated with a two- to threefold increase in risk for high levels of psychological distress" (I. H. Meyer & Dean, 1998, p. 173).

Chapters 3 and 15 extend this discussion further by considering the effects of internalized homophobia on superego functioning, elaboration of defenses, patterns of cognition, and object relations (Malyon, 1982), along with other consequences of oppression such as ego fragmentation and intense anxiety (Forstein, 1986; Malyon, 1982). These and other prevalent reactions to heterosexist bias, as well as the emotional and behavioral manifestations of a sexual identity crisis (Chapter 9), frequently resemble psychiatric symptomatology (Dworkin, 2000a; Gonsiorek, 1982, 1991; Gonsiorek & Rudolph, 1991).

Gonsiorek (1982) contends that the coming-out process often generates elaborate symptoms that appropriately are perceived as frightening, ego alien, and contributing to significant subjective distress. He believes that although equilibrium usually returns with time, many individuals do respond in "temporarily dramatic ways" consistent with their styles (p. 15). He maintains that unbiased clinical practice (Committee on Gay and Lesbian Concerns, 1991) mandates the ability of clinicians to distinguish among sexual minority clients:

- With clinically significant psychiatric disorders
- Who experience a particularly difficult time coming to terms with their sexuality but in whom serious underlying psychopathology is not present
- For whom the coming-out crisis serves as a precipitating event for the manifestations of serious underlying problems

Table 8.1 outlines these three possibilities and Gonsiorek's (1982) differential diagnoses between a sexual identity crisis and psychopathology, particularly paranoia and hypomania. He selected paranoia for discussion because of the traditional Freudian belief that it represents a defense against homosexual impulses. He contends that *any* serious threat to core sexual identity *may* elicit paranoid defenses, but the association between homosexuality and paranoia continues to persist. J. Smith (1988) believes similarly that although psychotic disorders do not occur with any greater frequency among sexual minorities, paranoia is particularly prone to be overdiagnosed and should be considered only if it is clear that the hypersensitivity, restricted affect, and pervasive suspiciousness are completely unwarranted given the degree of danger. Gonsiorek (1982) also choose to focus on hypomania because of the frequent differential diagnostic problems that exist between affective disorders and the mood swings, hyperactivity, and impulsive behaviors sometimes exhibited during a sexual identity crisis. Hypomania and paranoia, along with borderline personality disorder and characterological-appearing overlays of the personal-

TABLE 8.1. Sexual Identity Crisis, Paranoia, and Hypomania

	Paranoid disorders	Hypomanic episodes
Serious psychopathology may be mistaken for a sexual identity crisis.	During a psychotic episode, clients who are paranoid and thought-disordered may have persecutory delusions and ideas of reference about homosexuality, regardless of their sexual orientation.	During a hypomanic episode, clients may engage in sexual behavior that is otherwise indiscriminant and atypical for them, regardless of their sexual orientation.
A sexual identity crisis may be mistaken for serious psychopathology.	During a sexual identity crisis, homosexually oriented clients who are fearful, hypervigilant, suspicious, and confused may appear paranoid and thought-disordered.	During a sexual identity crisis, homosexually oriented clients may respond with mood swings, hyperactivity, and impulsive behaviors which are suggestive of hypomania.
A sexual identity crisis may either exacerbate or precipitate the onset of serious psychopathology.	Psychotic clients who are homosexually oriented may decompensate during a sexual identity crisis and become delusional and paranoid.	Hypomanic clients who are homosexually oriented may decompensate during a sexual identity crisis and become hypersexual, impulsive, or indiscriminant.

Note. Summarized from Gonsiorek (1982).

ity structure are discussed separately later. The chapter concludes with a consideration of gender identity disorder and the high potential for bias inherent in this diagnostic category.

Paranoia

During a psychotic episode, thought-disordered clients of any sexual orientation may be distressed considerably by delusions or ideas of reference about homosexuality. Similarly, sexual minority individuals who are having a difficult time accepting their homosexuality can experience panic and may appear thought-disordered and paranoid. Finally, gay, lesbian, or bisexual clients who are psychotic may decompensate during a sexual identity crisis and become delusional and paranoid (see Table 8.1). Figure 8.1 outlines Gonsiorek's (1982) conceptualization for differentiating among these three possibilities. He believes that clinicians must first determine the orientation of a client's sexual desires (i.e., to the same sex, other sex, or both) in order to rule out delusions which are "cerebral, ruminative ideas with little or no component of homosexual *desire*, either in the present or past, as determined by history" (p. 11).

Once the present sexual orientation of a client is determined as clearly as possible, the nature of the paranoid (or paranoid-appearing) ideation must be examined. Delusions of reference about homosexuality tend to lack a base in reality, and the connections between the fantasies and same-sex orientation often are more tenuous and idiosyncratic. On the other hand, the suspicions of gay men and lesbians during a sexual identity crisis are more likely to be reality based and to result from such experiences as severe interpersonal rejection, physical or sexual assault, or impending job loss. A detailed history, then, is essential in making this differential diagnosis. Finally, both homosexuality and para-

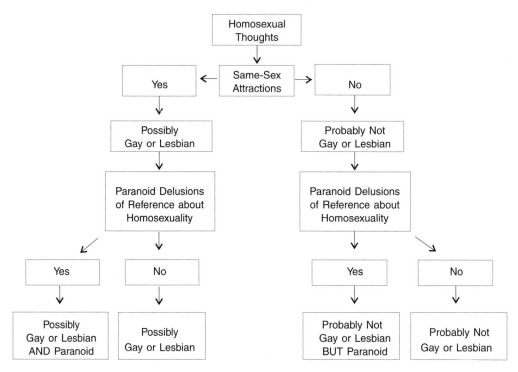

FIGURE 8.1. Differential diagnosis: Paranoia versus sexual orientation.

noid schizophrenia may be present. This combination may be seen particularly in individuals whose functioning was marginal prior to the sexual identity crisis and for whom the emergence of homosexual desire, behavior, or both precipitates a psychotic episode. In any case, if true psychopathology is determined to be present in clients of any sexual orientation, ethical practice dictates that the psychosis be treated.

Hypomania

Hypomanic clients, regardless of sexual orientation, often engage in indiscriminate behavior that is otherwise atypical for them (see Table 8.1). Further, they frequently manifest extensive denial about their behavior. This refusal to acknowledge a truth about themselves may appear similar to the denial of a minority sexual orientation in lesbian and gay individuals prior to or during the coming-out process. However, Gonsiorek (1982) contends that hypomanic denial "has a rigid, brittle quality" and that, when confronted, hypomanic clients usually become irritable, hostile, or flee "into euphoria" (p. 13). During a sexual identity crisis, on the other hand, individuals experience an increase in anxiety when confronted, and feel more "panicky" and stressed than hypomanic clients.

In addition, many homosexually oriented clients may exhibit impulsivity, mood swings, and other "hypomanic-like symptoms" during the coming-out process; nonetheless, "few will exhibit the symptom pattern and intensity of full blown hypomania"

(Gonsiorek, 1982, p. 13). A careful history can help clinicians to determine either previous same-sex interests or prior affective problems. Finally, the symptoms of hypomanic clients typically decrease dramatically after the prescription of a lithium compound (or one of the newer medications used to treat bipolar disorders), whereas the hypomanic-like manifestations exhibited during a sexual identity crisis remain relatively unaffected by pharmacotherapy. For those individuals who are *both* hypomanic and homosexually oriented, "determination of the latter must await stabilization of medication for the affective disorder" (p. 13).

Figure 8.2 is designed to assist clinicians further in making these differential diagnoses by listing the seven DSM-IV (American Psychiatric Association, 1994) subcriteria (listed under Criterion B) for an hypomanic episode (p. 338). A shaded box circumscribing those symptoms frequently displayed during a sexual identity crisis as well as during an hypomanic episode has been superimposed on these seven DSM-IV (American Psychiatric Association, 1994) subcriteria. If clients present symptoms listed outside of the shaded box, however, clinicians reasonably can be assured that a hypomanic episode is occurring. For example, rarely do individuals experience inflated self-esteem or feelings of grandiosity during the coming-out process, nor does the purposefulness of their activity increase. Rather, psychomotor agitation is more random and lacks directionality. Further, they often report that their thoughts are racing, but rarely do their verbalizations and ideations display the loose or tangential associations characteristics of true hypomanic episodes. As indicated previously, a positive response to medication also might be needed to confirm the presence of a true bipolar disorder; conversely, the absence of

CRITERION B FOR HYPOMANIC EPISODE
(see American Psychiatric Association, 1994, p. 338)

During the period of mood disturbance (elevated, expansive, or irritable mood), three (or more) of the following symptoms have persisted (four if the mood is only irritable) and have been present to a significant degree:

(1) inflated self-esteem or grandiosity.

(2) decreased need for sleep.

(3) more talkative than usual or . . .   pressure to keep talking.

(4) flight of ideas or . . .   subjective experience that thoughts are racing.

(5) distractibility.

(6) increase in goal-directed activity or . . .   psychomotor agitiation.

(7) excessive involvement in pleasurable activities that have a high potential for painful consequences.

SEXUAL IDENTITY CRISIS
(see Gonsiorek, 1982)

FIGURE 8.2. Differential diagnosis: Hypomanic episode versus sexual identity crisis.

response (or continuation of symptoms) after medication might be necessary to rule out hypomania.

Gonsiorek (1982) notes that the term *homosexual panic* sometimes has been used to refer to all three of the conditions described in Table 8.1 but that it is neither a DSM diagnostic category nor a diagnostic criteria. Studies, nonetheless, continue to describe clients with this condition. Chuang and Addington (1988) contend that the term historically has been used to indicate repressed and latent homosexuality but question its appropriateness and its heterosexist implications. While it is still used to describe anxiety reactions to a sexual identity crisis (both with and without psychopathology), Gonsiorek (1982) suggests that, due to pathologizing inferences, "the term 'homosexual panic' be permanently assigned to the junkyard of obsolete psychiatric terminology" (p. 11).

Borderline Personality Disorder

In addition to the classifications discussed previously, coming-out "behaviors may be misdiagnosed as narcissistic, borderline, or unstable personality at best instead of being seen as normal within a stage of development akin to delayed adolescence" (McHenry & Johnson, 1991, p. 19). When sexual minorities with serious psychopathology present for treatment, they often are perceived as clients with disorders of sexual object choice rather than as lesbians, bisexuals, and gay men with other problems (Marmor, 1980; Suchet, 1995). Because of these two factors, the over- and misdiagnosis of personality disorders among sexual minority populations is significant (Falco, 1991; C. Silverstein, 1988; J. Smith, 1988; Struzzo, 1989).

Diagnostic Bias

Various researchers claim to have found strong associations between homosexuality and borderline personality disorder (BPD) (Dulit, Fyer, Miller, Sacks, & Frances, 1993; Paris, Zwieg-Frank, & Guzder, 1995; Zubenko, George, Soloff, & Schulz, 1987), but only recently has the question of diagnostic bias been raised (Dworkin, 2000a; Zucker, 1996). Two of these studies are discussed here in some detail. In the first investigation, 12 (57%) of the 21 males diagnosed with BPD who presented for psychiatric outpatient treatment were predominately or exclusively homosexual (Zubenko et al., 1987). To replicate and extend these findings, the researchers generated a second set of data that they compared with those described previously. Accordingly, 80 psychiatric inpatients presumed to have a personality disorder were administered the Diagnostic Interview for Borderline Patients (DIBP) scale. Their sexual histories were "obtained by review of the impulse/action patterns and interpersonal relations sections" (p. 749) of the DIBP scale, by chart audit, and from clinical interviews. Of the 19 men who met criteria for BPD, 10 (53%) were considered homosexual, compared with 7 (11%) of the 61 women. One of the men and three of the women were considered bisexual. The researchers summarized their two sets of findings by concluding that "homosexuality was ten times more common among the men and six times more common among the women with borderline personality disorder than in the general population or in a depressed control group" (p. 748).

In a another study, researchers examined gender differences, demographic characteristics, and comorbid psychiatric diagnoses in a sample of 137 inpatients given a discharge diagnosis of BPD (Dulit et al., 1993). Data were obtained from systematic chart review of patients admitted between December 1981 and February 1984. Of the 137 patients whose charts were examined, 20% (*n* = 27) were male and 80% (*n* = 110) were female. A larger percentage of males (22%; 6 of 27) than females (3%; 3 of 110) were determined to be homosexual. Further, 26% (*n* = 7) of the men and 11% (*n* = 12) of the women were considered bisexual. Substance abuse was found to be "nearly universal" in the male borderline population (p. 184). Given the extent of assumed homosexuality and bisexuality among the male patients (48% combined), the researchers concluded that their findings support those of Zubenko et al. (1987, described earlier) that "homosexual behavior is more common among borderline males than among males in the general population" (p. 184). They also admitted a possibility of gender bias in the application of the borderline diagnosis to the female patients but did not mention the possibility of sexual orientation bias in regard to the gay and bisexual men in the study. Similarly, no indication was mentioned of a potential diagnostic bias given that all the chart notations were made using DSM-III which included *sexual impulsivity* and *disturbances of gender identity* among the diagnostic criteria for BPD.

In both of these studies, therefore, a strong possibility of diagnostic bias in regard to homosexuality and BPD exists. Both investigations used imprecise definitions of same-sex orientation, and only in their second round of data collection did Zubenko et al. (1987) eventually ask patients directly about the nature of their sexuality. All other data regarding homosexual or bisexual orientations were gathered by inference, primarily from retrospective chart inspection. Although meanings attributed to the social construct of homosexuality have altered considerably in the past decade, the possibility of bias in the recording of chart information seemingly was not considered in these studies. Readers are reminded of the discussion in Chapter 2 regarding the multivariate dimensions of both sexual identities and sexual orientations, as well as the associated difficulty with definition and measurement (E. Coleman, 1988, 1990; Gonsiorek & Weinrich, 1991; Klein et al., 1985; Shively & DeCecco, 1977). Given the complexity of assessing sexual orientation (Gonsiorek, Sell, & Weinrich, 1995), then, investigations which claim to have found an association between homosexuality and a particular psychiatric condition must be viewed with skepticism.

Differential Diagnosis

Because many manifestations of a sexual identity crisis resemble borderline symptomology, the possibility further exists for both overdiagnosis and misdiagnosis. Falco (1991), for example, contends that individuals who are "having a particularly difficult time coming out can look quite borderline temporarily, fitting the diagnostic criteria of impulsivity, intense anger, intense emotional relationships, and affective instability" (p. 63). In Figure 8.3, these criteria, as well as several others that are sometimes present during a sexual identity crisis, have been circumscribed in the shaded box from the remainder of the DSM-IV criteria for borderline personality disorder. Gonsiorek (1982) believes that the key to differentiating between the two conditions entails "a careful examination of ego functioning and object relations *prior* to the current crisis over same-sex feelings and behavior" (p. 14). In other words, an accurate history will detect a "relatively severe, chronic and characterologically based lack of ego differentiation and

301.83 BORDERLINE PERSONALITY DISORDER
(see American Psychiatric Association, 1994, p. 654)

A pervasive pattern of instability of interpersonal relationships, self-image, and affects, and marked impulsivity beginning by early adulthood and present in a variety of contexts, as indicated by five (or more) of the following:

(1) frantic	efforts to avoid real or imagined abandonment.	
(2) a pattern of	unstable and intense relationships . . .	characterized by alternating extremes of idealization and devaluation.
(3) marked and persistently	unstable self-image or sense of self.	
(4)	impulsivity in at least two areas that are potentially self-damaging.	
(5) recurrent	suicidal behavior, gestures, or threats, . . .	or self-mutilating behavior.
(6)	affective instability . . .	due to a marked reactivity of mood.
(7) chronic	feelings of emptiness.	
(8) inappropriate,	intense anger or difficulty controlling anger.	
(9)	transient, stress-related paranoid ideation . . .	or severe dissociative symptoms.

SEXUAL IDENTITY CRISIS
(see Gonsiorek, 1982)

FIGURE 8.3. Differential diagnosis: Borderline personality disorder versus sexual identity crisis.

boundaries" (p. 14) in clients with borderline personality. These individuals often are unable to distinguish between acquaintanceship, friendship, affection, love, and sexuality; have relatively primitive object relations; and exhibit splitting operations in a number of conflict areas.

On the other hand, individuals undergoing a sexual identity crisis (and who are *not* concurrently borderline) rarely self-mutilate, alternate between extremes of idealization and devaluation, or display dissociative symptoms. They may, however, experience a period in which boundary differentiations are poorly made, and "where splitting operations may temporarily occur in response to a stressful situation for which more typical coping styles are ineffective" (Gonsiorek, 1982, p. 14). Some clients are extremely frightened and symptomatic, especially those whose otherwise firm ego boundaries and clear differentiations in object relations are compromised by coming out. Because their new behaviors and feelings are ego alien when compared with their previously high level of performance, the contrast itself may exacerbate the stress and panic. Given the number of overlapping criteria between a true BPD and the "production of florid symptoms" (p. 15) often manifested by sexual minorities during existential crises of identity and self, the importance of a careful and accurate differential diagnosis cannot be overemphasized. On one hand, overpathologizing and misdiagnosis must be avoided; on the other, Axis II disorders can be neither minimized nor ignored without providing a disservice to clients.

Characterological-Appearing Overlays

Gonsiorek (1982) uses this designation to specify a range of reactions that various personality structures produce under stressful conditions. As examples, he refers to common response patterns displayed by individuals after engaging in combat, while being held in concentration camps, and during cataclysmic events such as floods, earthquakes, and airplane disasters. He also cites the typical reactions of gay men and lesbians who are in "situations where severe repercussions to disclosure realistically exist" (e.g., being married and closeted, feeling fearful of job termination, and feeling threatened with physical assault) and who develop paranoid-appearing overlays "characterized by hypervigilance, rumination, ideas of reference, hypersensitivity, etc." (p. 18). (Earlier in this chapter, clinically significant paranoia was differentiated from protective vigilance in sexual minorities [see Figure 8.1]).

To further complicate the issue, Gonsiorek (1982) notes that if an overlay remains a part of a person's functioning for a prolonged period of time, it "may begin to set down increasingly deep roots and begin to dwarf the pre-existing personality structure" (p. 19). In fact, "some victims may be scarred psychologically with the marks of social oppression of homosexuality as indelibly as some concentration camp victims retain their tattooed numbers" (p. 19). In any case, only a careful assessment can determine whether certain response patterns are truly diagnosable mental disorders that clearly differ from the coping mechanism overlays produced during stressful situations.

Gonsiorek (1982) discusses three other examples of characterological-appearing overlays to personality structures that are confused commonly with psychopathology in sexual minorities. The first involves the development of borderline-appearing personality features, including splitting mechanisms, in response to anonymous sexual behavior. The second entails the distinction between endogenous/chronic depression (dysthymia) and reactive depression (adjustment disorders) seen in most bisexual, lesbian, and gay clients during a sexual identity crisis. Finally, he cites the example of a narcissistic-appearing characterological overlay which often is confused with a narcissistic personality disorder in homosexually oriented clients.

Borderline-Appearing

As discussed in Chapter 16, the hostile environments in which sexual minorities reside leads some individuals to split apart their affectional and sexual feelings and to isolate both from the rest of their personalities. In particular, married or rural gay men may turn to anonymous sexual behaviors if they perceive that few other social, sexual, or intimate outlets are available. Others find that these kinds of encounters meet a variety of needs, including boosting self-esteem that has been deeply wounded by heterosexist society. Repeated anonymous sexual behaviors, however, may produce negative emotions (including guilt and self-recrimination) along with positive feelings (such as validation and excitement). Both sets of these intense affects, nonetheless, profoundly mobilize questions of self-esteem, body image, and safety, as well as other deep psychological concerns. In any case, highly charged and poorly differentiated feelings concurrently are generated and split off from each other and from the rest of the personality (Gonsiorek, 1982).

This splitting defense tends to disrupt healthy ego functioning and thus may increase the probability that splitting operations are performed in other situations (Gonsiorek, 1982). Splitting, in combination with behaviors that some would label "acting out," frequently leads to a diagnosis of BPD. These defenses often are personality overlays, however, rather than symptoms of a Axis II disorder (R. L. Hawkins, 1992), or "an overlay of borderline-appearing personality functions on a variety of preexisting personality styles" (Gonsiorek, 1982, p. 17). Therapy commonly begins with working through the particular overlay and its issues. Once this is accomplished, preexisting personality dynamics may emerge and thus enable psychotherapists to formulate appropriate differential diagnoses. Clinicians are referred to the discussion of BPD earlier in this chapter for additional considerations.

Depressive-Appearing

Depression is common in gay men and lesbians and, in fact, is the predominant reason that sexual minority women seek psychotherapy (Cochran & Mays, 2000a, 2000b; Markovic & Aaron, 2000; National Institute of Mental Health, 1987; Razzano et al., 2000). Frequently, the strain of dealing with a heterosexist macroculture and of living double lives, particularly for undisclosed and unsupported individuals, results in depression (Falco, 1991; Rothblum, 1990; J. Smith, 1988). Depression also may be related to unresolved identity issues, fear of being labeled homosexual, or relationship difficulties. Further, sadness is an intricate part of the coming-out process because clients are grieving the loss of a heterosexual identity (McHenry & Johnson, 1991; O'Neill & Ritter, 1992; Ritter & O'Neill, 1989; Stein & Cohen, 1984).

During a sexual identity crisis, homosexually oriented clients may develop "clinically significant emotional or behavioral symptoms in response to an identifiable psychosocial stressor or stressors" (American Psychiatric Association, 1994, p. 623), such as primary support group, social environment, or occupational problems (see Axis IV). Because predominant symptomology may include depressed mood, tearfulness, or feelings of hopelessness, a reactive depression (i.e., adjustment disorder with depressed mood) may be mistaken for endogenous or chronic depression (i.e., a major depressive or dysthymic disorder).

Gonsiorek (1982) believes that gay men and lesbians who have experienced a series of unresolved stressors without the benefit of an adequate support system may present the appearance of a depressive-appearing characterological overlay. Once the stressors are addressed in therapy and a support system is established, however, the depression frequently lifts. If the sadness persists, a careful history, including an evaluation of psychosocial and environmental problems, may determine that a chronic or dysthymic depression exists. Similarly, a multiaxial assessment may indicate the presence of a major depression, and symptomatic relief may require medication, a longer course of therapy, or both. Clinicians, nonetheless, should first consider a personality overlay (and, hence, a less severe diagnosis) with closeted sexual minority clients or those experiencing a sexual identity crisis before assuming that the depression is endogenous or chronic.

Narcissistic-Appearing

Since the time of Freud, homosexuality and narcissism have been related in the psychological literature (Beard & Glickauf-Hughes, 1994). Gonsiorek (1982) believes that individuals with narcissistic-appearing personality overlays frequently are raised in environments with extreme intolerance and harshness toward homosexuality. Because many neither have ever known nor interacted with another lesbian, gay, or bisexual person prior to acknowledging their own same-sex attractions, they often postpone acting on their own homosexual desires for a prolonged period after admitting these feelings to themselves. When they finally come out, they frequently "crash out" (Grace, 1979, 1992; see Chapter 5) with intense passion, indiscriminant disclosure, and radical changes in locale of residence, employment, clothing, body language, and speech. A considerable number adopt attitudes that conform to stereotypical perceptions of gay and lesbian community standards, overidentify with the most visible sexual minority groups and organizations, and immerse themselves in the alternating trends in lesbian and gay fashion and society. Clearly, then, in virtually every arena of their lives a dramatic difference may be seen between the present and their previous pre-coming-out personality, lifestyle, and environment. Having internalized many of the heterosexist and homophobic attitudes of their early surroundings, these individuals have elevated needs for validation and affirmation and, thus, are highly prone to develop narcissistic defenses (R. L. Hawkins, 1992). Hence, on the bases of their grandiosity, fantasy, needs for admiration, sense of entitlement, arrogance, superficiality, or shallowness, clinicians often automatically diagnose them as having a narcissistic personality disorder (D. Clark, 1987; Gonsiorek, 1982; Mass, 1983).

Another reason for this misdiagnosis is the presence of the previously discussed (see Chapter 3) narcissistic disturbance, injury, or wound seen in the majority of sexual minority clients. Many authors (Beard & Glickauf-Hughes, 1994; Blum & Pfetzing, 1997; de Monteflores, 1986; Gonsiorek & Rudolph, 1991; Isay, 1987, 1989; Malyon, 1982; Moberly, 1986) attribute this trauma to the lack of mirroring of the homosexually oriented child by parents and by the broader society. In the absence of parental acceptance and affirmative mirroring, children learn to split off the "different" parts of themselves and to approach others through a "false self" (Beard & Glickauf-Hughes, 1994). Narcissistic dynamics then result from the suppression of differentness and the superimposition of a false self on top of the "true self."

This insult to the personality core affects all gay, lesbian, and bisexual individuals to some degree as narcissistic difficulties occur when "any part of the self which is different is vulnerable to rejection by self-objects, whether parents or the larger social group" (de Monteflores, 1986, p. 85). If, however, sexual minorities arrive "at the coming out stage not otherwise psychologically crippled or severely traumatized (e.g., from prolonged involvement with pathological parents, or other toxic childhood experiences), the narcissistic injury is a temporary, albeit nontrivial, wound; a developmental challenge to be mastered" (Gonsiorek & Rudolph, 1991, p. 171). As discussed in Chapter 3, de Monteflores (1986) considers this condition a problem area "within the large frame of a healthy ego" (p. 85) and therefore should be distinguished from an Axis II narcissistic personality disorder. Likewise, Gonsiorek (1982) refers to it as a narcissistic overlay to a personality structure rather than a true characterological condition.

Clinically significant narcissistic personality disorders *do* exist in sexual minority individuals, however, and should be considered legitimately *after* accounting for the influences of heterosexist culture and the trauma of coming out on clients. As mentioned earlier (Beard & Glickauf-Hughes, 1994; Blum & Pfetzing, 1997; de Monteflores, 1986; Gonsiorek, 1982, 1991; Gonsiorek & Rudolph, 1991; Moberly, 1986; see Chapter 3), individuals first should be given the opportunity in psychotherapy to heal the narcissistic injuries inflicted by family and society. Only if the support and affirmation provided by therapists serving as mirroring self-objects fails to reduce the narcissistic symptomology should an Axis II diagnosis be assigned.

GENDER IDENTITY DISORDER

The diagnostic category of gender identity disorder (GID) has a high potential for heterosexist bias (Rottnek, 1999). Accordingly, Shannon Minter, an attorney for the National Center for Lesbian Rights (NCR), investigated several reported cases of the systematic abuse of sexual minority youth by the mental health industry and discovered DSM diagnostic categories and criteria that she contended "are 'tailor-made' for adolescents who exhibit gay, lesbian, or transgender tendencies" (Ricks, 1993, p. 39). Minter further reported that the adolescents who have contacted her for legal assistance have been hospitalized for displaying same-sex inclinations "under 'vaguely defined' disorders, such as gender identity disorder and borderline personality disorder" (p. 39).

Patterns, Disorders, and Sexual Orientation

As discussed in Chapter 3, several studies have found significant relationships between childhood gender nonconformity and adult homosexual orientation (Bailey & Zucker, 1995; Billingham & Hockenberry, 1987; R. Green, 1985, 1987; R. Green et al., 1982; Pleak, 1999; Whitam, 1977; Whitam & Mathy, 1991; Zucker, 1997; Zuger, 1984, 1988). Based on such studies, DSM-IV (American Psychiatric Association, 1994) course description of GID notes that, "by late adolescence or adulthood, about three-quarters of boys who had a childhood history of Gender Identity Disorder report a homosexual or bisexual orientation, but without concurrent Gender Identity Disorder," and that "the corresponding percentages for sexual orientation in girls are not known" (p. 536).

    Zucker and Bradley (1995) challenge the legitimacy of a discrete diagnostic category constructed from behavioral criteria and address two distinct questions: "(1) Is gender identity disorder of childhood really nothing more than homosexuality? and (2) What constitutes a disorder?" (p. 53). In this regard, they assert that "even if it can be agreed that gender identity disorder should be conceptually and empirically distinguished from a homosexual sexual orientation, one still needs to make the case that the behavioral pattern itself is a 'disorder' and not just a cluster of behaviors that go together" (p. 54). In other words, is childhood (or adolescent) cross-gender identification a diagnosable mental disorder or simply evidence of gender *atypical* (as opposed to *abnormal*) development?

    Isay (1989) and Pleak (1999) concur with current research that has found atypical gender behavior to be one early manifestation of bisexuality or homosexuality, but Isay sees homosexuality as "a nonpathological variant of human sexuality" (p. 15). Pleak, likewise, comments that "gender-typical and atypical behaviors should not be seen as dichotomies, but rather as being on a continuum or spectrum" (p. 37). Although the majority of the population has a preponderance of gender-typical behaviors, some people have a combination of typical and atypical practices and responses. A small minority of individuals has extensive cross-gender behavior and, for these clients, clinicians might consider the diagnosis of GID. Pleak himself notes that he does not use the GID diagnosis for child or adolescent patients because diagnoses written in clinical records or on insurance bills could result in discrimination later in life. Accordingly, "almost always, when a gender-dysphoric child is brought in to see a psychiatrist or other therapist, there are other issues or problems which can be diagnosed on record. If such a child has ADHD [attention-deficit/hyperactivity disorder] or a parent–child relational problem, either will suffice as the diagnosis of record" (p. 37).

Differential Diagnosis

Figure 8.4 indicates the criteria for the DSM-IV diagnosis of gender identity disorder in children (302.6). Criterion A reflects the child's cross-gender identification, indexed by a total of five behavioral characteristics, of which at least four must be manifested. The shaded box indicates behaviors that are *uncustomary* for the majority of children. The diagnostic question is whether these indicators can be seen as "simple nonconformity to stereotypical sex role behavior" (American Psychiatric Association, 1994, p. 536) rather than diagnosable psychopathology should four or more be present.

Those behaviors placed outside the shaded box distinctly reflect an insistence that the client *is* a member of the other sex or is preoccupied with the wish to *be* one. In adolescents and adults, DSM-IV appears to indicate that this latter set of indicators *must* be present for a diagnosis, but in children, these symptoms are only one of several (including the previously mentioned pattern of gender-atypical behaviors) that *may* be present. In other words, the criteria for a 302.6 diagnosis seems to be more variable for children than for adolescents and adults. Hence, the likelihood increases for mistaking *nonpathological* childhood gender nonconformity for a diagnosable mental disorder.

Although DSM-IV (American Psychiatric Association, 1994) notes that "this disorder [302.6] is not meant to describe a child's nonconformity to stereotypic sex-role behavior as, for example in 'tomboyishness' in girls or 'sissyish' behavior in boys" (p. 536), the symptoms of GID circumscribed within the shaded box *appear* to represent popular descriptions of "tomboys" and "sissies." The diagnostic manual thus seems to complicate (rather than clarify) Criterion A for a clinically significant 302.6 disorder, thereby increasing the possibility of over- or misdiagnosis.

Similarly, the Criterion B indicators are equally as dubious because the two indicators within the shaded box also could reflect "simple nonconformity to stereo-typical sex role behavior" (American Psychiatric Association, 1994, p. 536) rather than diagnosable psychopathology. The two specifiers outside the shaded box, however, clearly are symptoms that meet criteria for a diagnosis of gender identity disorder. As stated previously, DSM-IV makes no distinction between the two sets of examples when diagnosing children (as opposed to adolescents and adults), thus creating a high likelihood for confusion between the clinically significant disorder and atypical sex role socialization.

Diagnostic and Treatment Considerations

The following discussion demonstrates the sensitivity required to differentiate childhood gender nonconformity from a diagnosable GID. There appears to be little question that

302.6 GENDER IDENTITY DISORDER IN CHILDREN
(see American Psychiatric Association, 1994, p. 537)

CRITERION A

In children, the disturbance is manifested by four (or more) of the following:

- repeatedly stated desire to be . . . the other sex.
- in boys, preference for cross-dressing or simulating female attire;
- in girls, insistence on wearing only stereotypical masculine clothing.
- strong and persistent preferences for cross-sex roles in make believe play . . .
- intense desire to participate in the stereotypical games and pastimes of the other sex.
- strong preference for playmates of the other sex.

- insistence that he or she is the other sex.

- persistent fantasies of being the other sex.

CRITERION B

In children, the disturbance is manifested by any of the following:

- in boys, aversion toward rough-and-tumble play and rejection of male stereotypical toys
- in girls, marked aversion toward normative feminine clothing

- in boys, assertion that his penis or testes are disgusting or will disappear or assertion that it would be better not to have a penis;
- in girls, rejection of urinating in a sitting position, assertion that she has or will grow a penis, or assertion that she does not want to grow breasts or menstruate.

CHILDHOOD GENDER
NONCONFORMITY
(see Isay, 1989; Pleak, 1999;
Zucker & Bradley, 1995)

FIGURE 8.4. Differential diagnosis: Gender identity disorder in children versus childhood gender nonconformity.

the cross-gender interests, preferences, and behaviors of some children are qualitatively different from those of their peers and siblings (R. C. Friedman, 1997; Zucker, 1997). For example, Zucker (1997) and his team followed 253 boys and 40 girls who were referred to the Clarke Institute's Child and Adolescent Gender Identity Clinic (discussed earlier in this section) between 1978 and 1996. During this time, they observed numerous atypical behaviors in these children, such as relatively high activity levels in the girls and reduced activity levels in the boys, and concluded that these youngsters differed dramatically from control groups of their peers.

Difference, however, is not equivalent to a disorder and DSM-IV specifies that to be diagnosable, the disturbance must cause "clinically significant distress or impairment in social, occupational, or other important areas of functioning" (p. 538; Criterion D) and be apparent "by the extent and pervasiveness of the cross-gender wishes, interests, and activities" (p. 536). For those children for whom gender is not merely an area of idiosyncrasy but one of distress and confusion, J. Richardson (1996) stresses the need for extreme care during the assessment process. Accordingly, he recommends considering behavior along three phenomenological axes when evaluating for GID: the extremeness of the cross-gendered behavior, the presence of gender dysphoria, and the impairment in psychosocial functioning of the child. Each of these areas carries difficulties in definition and assessment, however, and Richardson notes that the line between atypicality and pathology remains controversial, even among mainstream clinicians. R. C. Friedman (1997), however, believes that informed psychiatrists, including those who created DSM-IV, "do not trivialize the question of whether a piece of behavior is simply uncommon or should in fact be considered pathological" and that "decisions about these matters are not set in stone, but subject to modification based on new data as it emerges" (p. 491).

R. C. Friedman (1997) further notes that "clinically significant gender identity disturbances of childhood" are not a "unitary entity" (pp. 491–492) and that certain differences between these children "are possibly caused by influences other than social prejudice" (p. 488). For example, the cross-gender experiences and activities for some boys ages 3–6 are associated with diverse symptomology such as intense separation anxiety. Pleak (1999), on the other hand, observes that children with less extensive gender-atypical behavior may not present with separation anxiety or other "internalizing" disorders, but may manifest their distress by exhibiting more disruptive or "externalizing" types of actions, such as attention-deficit/hyperactivity disorder or oppositional defiant disorder. Many times the family system is clinically disturbed and the systemic dysfunction is manifested in the symptomatic child. In another group of older boys, however, family psychopathology is relatively absent and the most common influence contributing to their suffering is "homophobia and heterosexism occurring among those in their social network" (R. C. Friedman, 1997, p. 493). Clinicians thus must take extra care in distinguishing between these two groups of boys because, in the first instance, the differences between these boys and their peers are caused by influences other than social prejudice.

Effects of Negative Labeling

Even if those children who manifest atypical sex role socialization are never technically diagnosed with GID, the long-term outcome for these individuals is not always favorable and many have lifetime symptoms of depression and anxiety (Weinrich et al., 1995). For example, after examining 77 boys (ages 4–16) referred for gender identity problems, Zucker (1990) concluded that negative social labeling (i.e., being called a "sissy") was the best predictor of psychopathology and had the most direct impact on the degree of psychopathology in middle to late childhood. Specifically, Zucker and his colleagues (Zucker & Bradley, 1995) at the Clarke Institute of Psychiatry's Child and Adolescent Gender Identity Clinic assessed the degree of psychopathology observed in 161 gender-referred boys compared with 90 of their male siblings, and in 24 gender-referred girls and 76 of their female siblings. Parent-report data obtained via the Child Behavior Checklist (CBCL) was used to measure the extent of disturbance. Teacher ratings on the CBCL also were obtained for 67 of the gender-referred boys. A wide range in the extent of CBCL psychopathology was detected in these boys, but in general they were found to be more disturbed than their male siblings. In fact, "the boys ages 6–11 with GID had significantly higher T scores than did male siblings on seven of the nine narrow-band scales: Schizoid–Anxious, Depressed, Uncommunicative, Obsessive–Compulsive, Social Withdrawal, Hyperactive, and Aggressive" (p. 82). Likewise, the girls diagnosed with GID had significantly higher scores than did their female siblings on four of the scales: Schizoid–Obsessive, Hyperactive, Delinquent, and Cruel. Younger (ages 4–5) gender-referred children of both sexes were not found to be any more disturbed than their siblings, however. "Multiple factors, including social ostracism and familial risk variables, appear to account for the associated psychopathology" in the latency-age population (p. 123).

Therapeutic Focus

Zucker and Bradley (1995) contend that exclusion by peers can be extremely intense and "often results in alienation, social isolation, and associated behavioral and emotional difficulties" (p. 266). R. C. Friedman (1997) also notes this frequent ostracization and victimization of children, particularly boys by other boys and men, for their cross-gender interests and behaviors. With these patients, he advocates addressing the immediate social prejudice that causes distress in order to help them to become less isolated, less lonely, and more secure, as well as to "assist those in the boy's social network to become less homophobic-heterosexist and less preoccupied with rigid, stereotypic standards for assessing masculine adequacy" (p. 493). Corbett (1997) agrees "that when a child is at risk of pain and humiliation, a certain degree of redirection and assistance, including the possibility of environmental change" (p. 504) must be provided.

Controversy appears to arise, however, even among clinicians who see gender nonconformity and homosexuality as normative developmental trajectories for many individuals, regarding how specifically to alleviate distress without creating additional difficulties for the client (Corbett, 1999; Isay, 1989; Pleak, 1999). For example, in attempting to redirect a boy's behavior in ways that reduce ostracization by family and peers, further repression of unacceptable sex-atypical feelings, attractions, and behaviors could occur. In other words, the client might learn to adopt enough masculine behaviors to reduce the cruelty and ridicule of others, while inducing the "symptoms, inhibitions, and character (disorders) that follow upon repression" (Corbett, 1997, p. 504).

Some clinicians believe that working with the parents of gender-atypical children is essential. Isay (1989), for example, believes that fathers of these male children could be helped to nourish their sons' interests and share common activities rather than withdrawing from them as so many do. "Mothers would be counseled to encourage these boys to spend more time with their fathers" (p. 131). By thus influencing the child's interactions with his parents, he can learn to see his interests and same-sex object choice as normal aspects of his development and will grow up loving himself in spite of being "different" from other boys. Pleak (1999) advocates informed consent with parents relative to a clear identification of their goals for treatment and an open discussion of the therapist's treatment approach, biases, theoretical orientation, and goals. He also advocates parent education about the natural history of extensive childhood cross-gender behaviors; the known associations between childhood gender identity and adult orientations and identities; the evidence for the proposed treatment modality to affect cross-gender behavior and identification; the lack of evidence for any treatment effect on later sexual orientation, "despite claims they may hear to the contrary" (p. 48); and nonpathology status of homosexuality and bisexuality. Pleak also helps parents to deal with any hostility or unfavorable treatment the child receives because of atypical gender behaviors and supports them in accepting and loving their child regardless of future sexual orientation or gender identification. He acknowledges that this latter ideal often is difficult for many parents.

CONCLUSION

Psychotherapists are encouraged to assume a systemic approach when assessing the presenting problems of gay, lesbian, and bisexual clients and to evaluate the influence of heterosexually biased psychosocial stressors on symptomology, personality structure, and current levels of functioning. Intrapersonal or familiar psychopathology must not be minimized or overlooked, but neither should treatment be so narrowly focused that the negative psychic effects living in an oppressive environment are considered inconsequential in the etiology of the presenting manifestations.

9

Psychotherapeutic Applications
for Identity Formation

The primary purpose of this chapter is to guide psychotherapists as they assist sexual minority clients in integrating their erotic and emotional attractions with a socially constructed formulation of a positive gay, lesbian, or bisexual identity. The discussion in Chapter 5 referred to this process as one of identity formation or development, which clients simply may describe as "coming out." Accordingly, four gay and lesbian developmental stage models (Cass, Coleman, Troiden, and Grace) were presented and sampling limitations discussed. The intermediate three chapters discussed developmental issues of adolescence and adulthood, as well as psychodiagnostic concerns. With this body of information in mind, clinicians now can turn their attentions to psychotherapeutic application and intervention.

Knowledge of normative bisexual identity formation is in its infancy and Chapter 5 also described the only known formulation of this trajectory (M. S. Weinberg et al., 1994). Because so little empirical data have been generated validating this or any other developmental model of bisexuality, specific psychotherapeutic interventions were suggested along with the four stages postulated by Weinberg and his associates. The discourse that follows, therefore, does not repeat this material but, rather, uses a five-phase consolidated outline of the four models of lesbian and gay identity formation (from Chapter 5) and then adds implications for bisexual individuals when appropriate. Because the final phase of the Weinberg et al. formulation (*Continued Uncertainty*) has no parallel stage for lesbians and gay men, the following overlay is only partially accurate for bisexuals. The client dynamics and suggestions for clinicians during the earlier phases seem to apply rather well, however. For information (in addition to what was summarized in Chapter 5) about treating bisexual clients who experience the ongoing incertitude described by M. S. Weinberg et al. (1994), psychotherapists are urged to refer to the growing body of new literature in this area.

After psychotherapeutic applications across the five phases are presented in the commentary that follows, this chapter articulates several factors that might influence the movement of clients through the trajectory. These include issues that are unique to bisexuals and lesbians, the fluidity of some sexual attractions, as well as variables related to the psychosocial adjustment and to the social and relational dynamics of certain individuals. Suggestions are offered for modifying clinical interventions such that these factors can be taken into consideration when attempting to provide maximum assistance to clients in their identity development.

PHASE-SPECIFIC PSYCHOTHERAPEUTIC INTERVENTIONS

To facilitate identity formation in gay, lesbian, and bisexual clients, psychotherapists must meet them at their level of development and intervene appropriately. In Tables 9.1–9.5, the four stage models outlined in Chapter 5 are reconfigured into five phases that integrate the concepts of Cass, Troiden, Coleman, and Grace into a singular paradigm. The left-hand column represents a summary of the client behaviors described by these theorists. In the right-hand column, phase-specific psychotherapeutic interventions are suggested for meeting the developmental needs of clients. The discussions following the five charts relate these interventions to the client behaviors and then elaborate on the recommended strategies.

Phase 1

During the first phase of the process, clients feel *socially* different, alienated, alone, and afraid. At this point, their same-sex attractions are preconscious, if not unconscious; hence they are unlikely to seek psychotherapy to address concerns about their sexual orientation. Rather, they often present with feelings of estrangement, isolation, loneliness, and fear. Depression is common in these clients, illnesses are frequent, and suicidal idea-

TABLE 9.1. Gay and Lesbian Identity Formation: Phase 1-Specific Client Behaviors and Psychotherapeutic Interventions

First phase: Sensitization (Troiden); Pre-Coming Out (Coleman); Emergence (Grace)	
Client behaviors	Psychotherapeutic interventions
• Feels *socially* different during childhood • Feels alienated and alone • Has ambiguous same-sex attractions • Senses strong heterosexist and gender-specific norms • Fears being noticed for both behaving incorrectly and for not trying • Keeps thoughts and feelings private • Protects self from awareness through various defense mechanisms • Feels depressed • Communicates conflict through behavioral problems, psychosomatic illnesses, suicidal attempts, etc.	• Empathize with client's feelings of alienation and fear • Destigmatize feeling *socially* different • Treat client's depression • Address behavioral problems • Refer for medical consultation • Intervene to prevent suicide • Rule out serious psychopathology

tion is not unusual. The defense structures that protect and inhibit their emotions and impulses often are rigid and impermeable, resulting in flattened affect, low energy, and diminished vitality. If their defenses are weak and fail to serve, these clients' protective functions, acting-out behaviors, and even suicidal gesturing may occur.

Initial Interventions

As with all depressed clients, the first therapeutic task is to assess actual suicide potential and intervene accordingly. Although same-sex attractions are ambiguous at this phase of identity development, substance abuse and mental disorders nearly always are correlated with attempted and completed suicides (Muehrer, 1995). These conditions, in other words, are more likely to reflect increased suicide risk than undifferentiated sexual orientation at this developmental level. Regardless of the predisposing factors, however, the first step of the counseling process is to preserve and provide professional support to maintain the client's life. Psychotherapists may need to solicit medical consultation for medication assessment and management, or for assistance with inpatient hospitalization. Serious psychopathology must be ruled out at this time and throughout the course of therapy (Gonsiorek, 1982; Hanley-Hackenbruck, 1989). Once life is stabilized, a medical examination may be indicated to update the status of the client's physical health; medical records can be requested so that the nature and frequency of any repeated or questionable illnesses can be ascertained.

Alleviating Isolation and Depression

From the onset of treatment, clinicians must be especially sensitive and careful not to underestimate these clients' feelings of fear and loneliness. Empathic responses can help individuals identify and verbalize heretofore unarticulated emotions, and once these feelings are expressed, the depth of their depression may become more apparent. Conventional approaches for treating depression then may be used with minimal modification at this phase of identity formation. Distorted and self-defeating cognitions should be challenged and replaced with more realistic and self-affirming thoughts. Daily activities may need to be structured incrementally to reduce social isolation, increase energy levels, and overcome lethargy. Exercise and bodywork may be helpful for such purposes, as well as for decreasing the physical rigidity so common among these clients. Because they have often kept to themselves for fear of being noticed, social and communication skills development may be essential for reducing loneliness and increasing socialization. Antidepressant medications might be necessary for mobilizing those with treatment-resistant dysphoric moods.

Addressing Behavioral Problems

For clients with weak or fluid defenses, behavioral problems may emerge. Lacking necessary ego strength and adequate defense mechanisms, these individuals often experience difficulties with impulse control. This impulsivity, combined with impaired judgment and reality testing, frequently results in school, social, sexual, legal, relationship, and vocational problems. Therapeutic interventions, thus, may include addressing school failure and truancy, providing safer-sex information, or referring to legal assistance for problems

TABLE 9.2. Gay and Lesbian Identity Formation: Phase 2-Specific Client Behaviors and Psychotherapeutic Interventions

Second phase: Identity Confusion (Cass, Troiden); Identity Comparison (Cass); Coming Out (Coleman); Acknowledgment (Grace)	
Client behaviors	Psychotherapeutic interventions
• Feels *sexually* different during adolescence • Realizes homosexuality has personal meaning • Privately labels feelings as *possibly* gay or lesbian • Distances self from own homoerotic feelings • Denies, rationalizes, or bargains to limit self-awareness • Acknowledges but fears same-gender feelings • Maintains but questions a heterosexual identity • Asks self, "Am I gay (or lesbian)?" • Feels more alienated from others • Avoids information about homosexuality • Inhibits behaviors associated with being gay or lesbian and adopts those associated with being heterosexual • Assimilates into heterosexual peer groups • Limits exposure to members of the other sex • Becomes an anti-gay/lesbian crusader • Immerses self in heterosexual relationships • Escapes homoerotic feelings through substances • Seeks professional help to change orientation • Seeks information to learn about being gay or lesbian • Initially self-discloses to others • Overvalues approval from heterosexuals • Realizes that heterosexual guidelines for behavior and expectations for future are no longer relevant • Grieves the loss of heterosexual blueprint for life	• Empathize with client's confusion • Explore personal meaning of confusing information • Discourage premature self-labeling • Help client identify and acknowledge same-sex feelings • Explore client's fears and anxieties • Mirror client's intrinsic worth • Provide accurate information upon client's request • Dispel myths and stereotypes about lesbians/gay men • Affirm client's ability to admit same-sex feelings • Challenge client's critical and punitive superego • Reframe being gay or lesbian as positive • Empathize with loss and facilitate grieving process • Reflect and gently challenge inhibition strategies • Encourage and support client to move beyond fear • Expose client to positive role models • Help client identify receptive supporters • Refer to affirming clergy, if necessary • Assess for substance abuse; intervene or refer

related to theft, drug activity and abuse, or physical aggression. Teaching anger management and decision making is often indicated.

Phase 2

When clients encounter information regarding homosexuality or bisexuality that potentially has personal meaning, they shift to the second phase of identity formation. Whether this message comes from newspapers, magazines, television, movies, family, friends, or even strangers, it seems intimately relevant. For the first time, individuals no longer automatically assume that they are entirely heterosexual (or homosexual, in the case of some bisexual clients) and they begin to challenge the heterosexist assumptions that others hold for them. This discrepancy leads them to privately label their feelings as possibly lesbian, gay, or bisexual, but most feel extremely confused and some seek psychotherapy to resolve their emotional turmoil (Cass, 1979).

Empathic Exploration

Psychotherapists must be careful to empathize with the confusion of clients about their possible sexual orientation, rather than to reflect and reinforce their fear that exclusive heterosexuality (or homosexuality, for some bisexual clients) no longer applies to them. Empathic interventions, in other words, should target primarily the confusion of clients without either magnifying or isolating their fear, which can be intensified further by clinicians taking a proactive stance regarding the benefits or liabilities of being bisexual, gay, or lesbian. Psychotherapists usually need to slow the pace of therapy for both themselves and their clients early in this second phase because individuals often are anxious to resolve their confusion and clinicians are eager to facilitate this resolution. Premature self-labeling should be discouraged and care taken to explore the meaning of the information that confuses clients and challenges their previous assumptions about their sexual orientations. Meanwhile, unspoken thoughts and feelings are given language and anxieties explored (E. Coleman, 1981/1982; Sophie, 1987).

Ideally, when psychotherapists are able to foster an impartial sense of curiosity in their clients, these individuals are eager to learn more about themselves (regardless of where the exploration leads). In reality, however, most clients are driven by pain to explore their sexuality—an extremely personal matter about which they are far from neutral—and request more information about being gay, lesbian, or bisexual in order to alleviate their intense fear and apprehension.

Superego Modification

Providing worried and distressed clients with accurate material about homosexuality or bisexuality, as requested, is essential because misinformation usually breeds the stereotypes that shape their frequently judgmental and condemning superegos. Hanley-Hackenbruck (1989) believes that "a major task of the coming out process is superego modification" (p. 26) that "proceeds from the critical or even punitive position through ambivalence to a positive, accepting position" (p. 27). In other words, the psychotherapeutic goal is to affect a change in the conscience structure such that clients can be more accepting of themselves and of their possible sexual orientation. Through the mirroring provided by the therapist, the client's superego is modified, ego functioning strengthened, and an authentic sense of self affirmed (Hanley-Hackenbruck, 1988, 1989; Sophie, 1987).

Facilitating Grief and Loss

In addition to accurate information, affirmative mirroring by clinicians assists clients in superego modification and in reframing being gay, lesbian, or bisexual as positive. A deep sense of loss usually results, however, as clients come to a deeper awareness of their minority sexual orientation. Like most people, sexual minority clients have been socialized with a heterosexual life image (O'Neill & Ritter, 1992) and thus have assumed a heterosexual identity (Hanley-Hackenbruck, 1989; C. A. Thompson, 1992). This blueprint for life, along with its dreams and privileges, must be grieved and eventually abandoned for a gay, lesbian, or bisexual identity. In other words, a new ego ideal can be formed only after the heterosexual life image has been relinquished.

"Grieving the losses which come with this major shift in interpersonal life frees the individual for new internal and external attachments and greater individuation" (Hanley-Hackenbruck, 1989, p. 29). One of the major psychotherapeutic tasks during the second phase of identity formation, therefore, is to facilitate client progress through this grieving process.

Challenging Inhibition Strategies

Individuals often complicate their grief and subsequent identity development by inhibiting awareness of their bisexual, gay, or lesbian inclinations. What traditionally have been called immature defenses (denial, rationalization, intellectualization, dissociation, etc.) should be seen as tactics to block awareness of same-sex feelings (or opposite-sex attractions for bisexuals questioning their exclusive homosexuality) and the losses associated with identifying with a new sexual orientation. These inhibition strategies should be gently challenged and clients invited to risk disclosure first to self and eventually to others (E. Coleman, 1981/1982). Psychotherapists, thus, must sensitively encourage individuals to face the new truth about themselves. Until this reality is accepted, clients are expending psychic energy containing painful information rather than mobilizing that momentum to surmount fear and overcome loss.

Using Referrals and Adjuncts

In addition to employing defense mechanisms and other strategies to limit self-awareness, many clients struggling with a minority sexual orientation medicate the pain of reality by abusing drugs and alcohol. Because substance abuse only compounds their shame, these individuals cannot proceed along the path to self-acceptance without first establishing sobriety. All clients, then, must be assessed for chemical dependency and those meeting the criteria be treated for substance abuse or referred for specialized treatment, if necessary. Likewise, clients with rigid religious introjects also may feel ashamed and guilty and, thus, have intense difficulty accepting a gay, lesbian, or bisexual identity. These internalizations usually hinder the intrapsychic process of superego modification as well as future identity development. A referral, therefore, to receptive, sensitive, and affirming clergy may be warranted to moderate a critical or punitive voice of conscience (Hanley-Hackenbruck, 1988, 1989; Sophie, 1987).

Clients need secure gay, lesbian, and bisexual examples with whom to identify in order to overcome their shame, as well as to find the courage to disclose their attractions beyond the sanctuary of the therapy room. Coming out, then, is an interpersonal as well as intrapsychic process. Providing clients with positive role models can be achieved in a number of ways, depending on the availability of community and regional resources. Descriptions or images of individuals with whom clients might identify can be found in books and magazines, or on educational videotapes available in gay and lesbian or feminist bookstores. Many communities have phone lines that people might call for support. Finally, with the client's permission, clinicians may invite to a therapy session a self-affirming gay, lesbian, or bisexual person to share a coming out story. Therapists must exercise extreme care and discretion in selecting this individual, however, in order to prevent client exploitation as well as to maximize therapeutic outcome.

Identifying Receptive Supporters

Once positive identification with gay, lesbian, or bisexual others is established, the next task is for clients to begin telling others of the newly acknowledged sexual orientation. Psychotherapists, in this regard, may assist clients in the development of a plan for selective self-disclosure, as well as in the selection of supportive receptors of this information. Although they often feel terrified, many clients initially want to tell their immediate family members from whom they seek the greatest approval. These clients frequently need to be redirected from coming out to their parents and significant others *first* and steered in the direction of telling more distant relatives or others with whom the stakes are lower. In other words, they need first to practice sharing their sexual orientation with people who are emotionally safe before disclosing to those with whom they are most personally invested.

Phase 3

Clients enter the third phase of identity development once they admit to themselves that they are *probably* rather than *possibly* gay, lesbian, or bisexual and then find the

TABLE 9.3. Gay and Lesbian Identity Formation: Phase 3-Specific Client Behaviors and Psychotherapeutic Interventions

Third phase: Identity Tolerance (Cass); Identity Assumption (Troiden); Exploration (Coleman); Finding Community (Grace)	
Client behaviors	Psychotherapeutic interventions
• Admits *probability* of being lesbian or gay	• Validate client's self perception of *probable* identity
• *Tolerates* a new identity	• Provide insight on identity formation
• Acknowledges social, emotional, and sexual needs	• Offer community resource information and references
• Seeks out gay and lesbian individuals and communities in order to overcome isolation	• Facilitate decision making about self-disclosures
• Explores the gay and lesbian subculture	• Rehearse self-disclosures in therapy
• Experiments sexually with same-sex partners (men)	• Foster interpersonal skill development
• Forms intense emotional relationships (women)	• Provide human sexuality education
• Attaches gay or lesbian meaning to sexual and social encounters with other members of the same sex	• Offer perspectives on first relationships
• Selectively self-discloses or "crashes out"	• Recast feelings and behaviors as "developmental lag"
• Experiences a "developmental lag"	• Assist completion of adolescent tasks
• Experiences gay or lesbian adolescence	• Continue to facilitate individuation from parents
• Feels inadequate about how to behave and how to manage new and unfamiliar feelings	• Facilitate further superego modification
• Behaves in ways otherwise considered inappropriate	• Help client build new personal and social identity
• Judges self unfairly as immature or immoral	• Reframe potential rejection as external problem
• Develops interpersonal skills, sense of attractiveness, sexual competence, and positive self-concept	
• Finds peer group or community where private self can be publicly shared	

courage to risk telling others. These events enable individuals to tolerate their new identity and acknowledge their personal needs, one of which is to conceptualize themselves as members of a particular sexual minority subculture. In the process of experimentation with a different way of being, they begin to socialize with members of their own sex (or other sex if they had earlier identified as lesbian or gay and are struggling with bisexuality). Often these relationships become either sexual or intensely emotional, and for the first time, they are able to attach either homosexual or bisexual meaning to these encounters. This identification with the *bisexual, gay,* or *lesbian* label allows them to experience belonging; consequently, they no longer feel the isolation of the previous two phases.

Therapeutic Continuity

Several of the clinical interventions at this third phase are continuations of those begun during Phase 2. Psychotherapists keep on providing information, but now are permitted by clients to add community resources and references to previous material related to a sexual minority orientation. With clients beginning to experiment sexually, offering gay/ lesbian/bisexual-specific education on human sexuality becomes essential (E. Coleman, 1981/1982). Facilitating decision making about self-disclosures also remains an important psychotherapeutic task. Clients may need additional help ascertaining the views of those on the receiving end of their self-revelations, judging the reality of their perceptions, and overcoming their fears of rejection (Wells & Kline, 1987). Some of the more difficult disclosures can be rehearsed in therapy, with best- and worst-case scenarios simulated in an empty-chair format (Sophie, 1987).

Reframing Developmental Lag

As mentioned previously, many sexual minority clients experience a developmental lag, or discrepancy between their chronological and developmental ages (Grace, 1979). They sometimes liken themselves to adolescents as they disclose feelings of inadequacy related to not knowing how to behave in dating or other social situations. Given the fact that many of these individuals spent their chronological adolescence identified as heterosexual, therapists can explain to them that these emotions are perfectly normal because they are now a gay, bisexual, or lesbian "teenager" for the first time. Along with providing this perspective on identity formation, clinicians may need to help their clients develop the interpersonal and social skills necessary for relating to the biological sex of those to whom they are acknowledging attractions.

Clients may experience intense anguish in their initial attempts to establish these new romantic relationships. Some report confusion over the rules and roles for various encounters and situations; others question the maturity or morality of their social and sexual behavior. Psychotherapists, again, might remind them that they are proceeding through bisexual, lesbian, or gay adolescence and that they consider recasting their experiences as the first efforts, and sometimes the false starts, of a teenager in love. This cognitive restructuring often can be successful in furthering superego modification and increasing client self-concept.

Finishing Adolescence

Hanley-Hackenbruck (1989) suggests that clinicians assist gay, lesbian, or bisexual clients with completing or renegotiating several adolescent tasks (p. 36):

- The defining of new values and standards contrary to one's upbringing
- The emergence of a new sexual self
- The development of a new social identity and peer group

If progress has been made toward the attainment of these goals, clients can become more individuated, less governed by parental expectations (Browning, 1987), and more capable of experiencing an internal locus of control. In other words, their sense of self will be hardier and more solid. The reframing of potential rejection, heterosexism, and homophobia as problems external to themselves can greatly reduce their shame (Sophie, 1987). And, finally, with increased social skills and enhanced sexual competence, clients can be better able to locate and join peer groups and communities where their sexual minority status can be shared and affirmed. Groups designed to help individuals "come out" exist in many communities and can be used to enhance the identity development process (D. F. Morrow, 1996).

Phase 4

The transition to the fourth phase of identity development depends on the quality of contacts with the sexual minority subculture established during Phase 3. When these encounters are positive, individuals begin to *accept*, rather than merely *tolerate*, their new identity and desire to socialize with others like themselves as much as possible. Clinicians should support their clients' active participation in these communities, because having a reference group can further the consolidation of a healthier new identity. During this phase, psychotherapists may now refer to their clients as gay, lesbian, or bisexual and encourage them to do the same (Sophie, 1987).

Couple Counseling

A major developmental task for many clients during this fourth phase is establishing a romantic relationship involving emotional as well as sexual attractions. Following years of loneliness and isolation, individuals often feel a desperate need for the closeness and intimacy these partnerships provide. Frequently, then, they enter relationships in an emotional state of extreme vulnerability, bringing with them idealistic, if not unrealistic, expectations of how this couplehood can satisfy their deepest desires. Further, a backlog of these unmet needs often compels gay, lesbian, and bisexual clients into intense partnerships before they have consolidated a new sexual minority identity. Any one or a combination of these issues can bring an individual or couple into counseling at this phase.

The primary psychotherapeutic objective with coupled clients is to assist them in functioning more effectively in their intimate relationships. Providing perspective on these partnerships is important in this regard so they can learn to view their situations more ra-

TABLE 9.4. Gay and Lesbian Identity Formation: Phase 4-Specific Client Behaviors and Psychotherapeutic Interventions

Fourth phase:

Identity Acceptance (Cass); Commitment (Troiden); First Relationships (Coleman, Grace)

Client behaviors	Psychotherapeutic interventions
• *Accepts* rather than *tolerates* a gay or lesbian self-image • Increases the frequency and regularity of contacts with other lesbians and gay men • Discovers preferences for same-sex social contexts • Starts to make gay and lesbian friends • Clarifies sexual desires and emotional needs • Feels intense need for intimacy • Searches for an intimate relationship that includes emotional as well as physical attraction • Enters a same-sex love relationship • Frequently "couples" before consolidating identity • Often has unrealistic expectations for first relationships • Feels extremely vulnerable to partner, feelings, and emotional impact of relationship • Learns to function in a same-sex love relationship • Meets basic needs for affirmation, physical and sexual contact, and emotional nurturance • Legitimizes the same sex as a source of love and romance as well as of sexual gratification • Reconceptualizes identity as natural, normal, and valid • Expresses satisfaction with being gay or lesbian and a reluctance to abandon new identity • Increasingly desires to disclose to heterosexual others • Applies passing strategies and selectively self-discloses • Adopts philosophy of full or partial legitimization	• Encourage client to adopt temporary identity label • Refer to client as gay, lesbian, or bisexual • Support active involvement in gay and lesbian community • Reframe kinship concept to include intentional family • Refine client's decision making about self-disclosures • Facilitate communication and relationship skill acquisition • Provide couple counseling, if requested • Facilitate a balance between merger and individuation • Clarify mindful choices for full and partial legitimization • Assist with conscious selection of passing strategies • Recast vocational goals, if necessary • Enhance client's discomfort with a dual identity

tionally and with less emotionality. Explaining the dynamics commonly involved in these first gay, bisexual, and lesbian relationships can help clients in attributing typical problems to "developmental lag" rather than interpreting them as personal failures. Further, after so many years in the closet, individuals often see themselves as relationally impaired and incapable of giving and receiving love. Objective discussions, then, can help counter their negative self-references. In addition, clinicians should assist each member of a couple in clarifying his or her sexual desires and emotional needs and in communicating them to the significant other. Partners also may need assistance in examining their personal and mutual expectations for the relationship, as well as in attending to unfinished individual developmental needs and tasks (E. Coleman, 1981/1982). Finally, successful therapy might require direct attention to improving couple communication skills, furthering understanding of the other, and facilitating a more complementary balance between merger and separation.

Even "good-enough" first relationships can serve a number of important developmental functions. Besides contributing to a sense of attractiveness and sexual competence, these partnerships can help clients legitimize the same sex (or the other sex, for bisexuals who identified previously as lesbian or gay) as an authentic source of romantic love and erotic passion. Further, such bondings can assist individuals in reformulating being lesbian, bisexual, or gay as both normative and satisfying for themselves. With this newfound enthusiasm, some clients will want to proclaim their identity to the world, whereas others will simply want those closest to them to know.

Disclosure and Decision Making

Learning selectivity about self-disclosures is a crucial skill to develop and clinicians can assist clients in making conscious decisions about revealing their new identities to others and under what circumstances. Until clients are ready to disclose their minority sexual orientation to their parents, siblings, and friends, psychotherapists may find it helpful to introduce the idea of an "intentional" family comprised of gay, lesbian, and bisexual brothers and sisters. Likewise, even individuals who have already revealed their homosexuality or bisexuality to members of their families of origin usually find that having an extended or intentional kinship network is comforting and supportive. Individuals at this crucial phase of identity formation need the sustenance and understanding provided by like-minded others and these chosen families can aid in the integration of their newly formed sexual minority identities.

Mindful choices to come out or to "pass" also can affect daily life in the workplace, as well as long-term vocational choices, and addressing these issues should be an integral part of the decision making around disclosure of minority sexual orientation (Browning, 1987). More important, however, clinicians should assist clients in examining their philosophical assumptions about full or partial legitimization, both in specific workplace situations and across the spectrum of their lives, because individuals frequently either apply or abandon passing strategies indiscriminantly, without deliberately considering the rationale underlying their actions. Psychotherapists, therefore, can help clients be more mindful in their choices by supporting the clients as they consciously select between those situations in which they opt to assimilate or "pass" and those others in which they choose to disclose. Each of these decisions can be evaluated in terms of whether the option either enhances or compromises their new gay, lesbian, or bisexual identity. By engaging in this process, clinicians thus can serve as "devil's advocates," in challenging clients to behave in ways that are congruent with their own integrity.

Phase 5

Clients enter the fifth phase of identity development expressing various forms of dissatisfaction with heterosexist oppression. Some virtually sever all ties with the sexual majority and completely immerse themselves in the sexual minority community. These individuals tend to reject all identification with the majority culture and consider any form of assimilation a violation of their principles. To them, the dichotomous distinctions based on sex-

TABLE 9.5. Gay and Lesbian Identity Formation: Phase 5-Specific Client Behaviors and Psychotherapeutic Interventions

Fifth phase:
Identity Pride/Synthesis (Cass); Integration (Coleman); Self-Definition and Reintegration (Grace)

Client behaviors	Psychotherapeutic interventions
• Dichotomizes between people based on sexual orientation and identification • Depreciates the significance of heterosexuals • Exaggerates the importance of other lesbians/gay men • *Prefers* the new identity to a heterosexual self-image • Immerses self in gay and lesbian subculture • Ravenously consumes lesbian and gay media and services • Becomes an activist for gay and lesbian community • Abandons previously applied passing strategies • Recognizes potential similarities between self and heterosexual counterparts • Acknowledges possible differences between self and members of gay and lesbian community • Abandons "them vs. us" philosophy • Feels less overwhelmed by anger and pride • Discriminates not on the basis of sexual orientation but on the basis of perceived support • Places greater trust in sensitive heterosexuals • Self-discloses almost automatically • Feels greater security in integrated identity • Incorporates and integrates public and private • identities into one self-image • Draws from reservoir of skills and resources from previous phases to meet situational demands of life • Proceeds with normal tasks of adult development	• Validate client's pride in being lesbian or gay • Encourage client to celebrate new identity • Legitimize the reality of heterosexist oppression • Empathize with client's rage • Explore negative outcomes of refusing to "pass" • Address client conflicts with heterosexist environment • Discuss consequences of isolation in gay or lesbian ghetto • Challenge dichotomous thinking • Increase client's identification with marginalized others • Help client explore differences as well as similarities between self and gay and lesbian subculture • Examine other dimensions of client's personality • Promote client's integrated view of self • Facilitate reintegration into dominant culture • Assist client with reframing his or her past to maintain continuity of life • Help client redefine former relationships • Resume superego modification when client • regresses • Advance to issues of authentic intimacy and generativity • Address normal developmental issues of adult life

ual orientation categorize heterosexuals as perpetrators of oppression and gay, lesbian, and bisexual people as victims of homophobia or biphobia.

Validating Anger at Oppression

Some Phase 5 clients seek counseling to resolve their unrelenting anger and self-consuming rage at social injustices aimed at themselves and their gay, lesbian, and bisexual sisters and brothers. Negative outcomes of refusing to pass also bring some clients to psychotherapy at this phase of the process. In both instances, acknowledging the reality of heterosexist oppression and empathizing with the legitimacy of client rage are important interventions (Hanley-Hackenbruck, 1988, 1989). Also essential is the validation of client pride in identifying as gay, lesbian, or bisexual and the willingness to help individuals celebrate their new identities (C. A. Thompson, 1992).

Unless these clients feel "heard" from the beginning of treatment, many will not tolerate psychotherapeutic interventions aimed at challenging their "them versus us" thinking. Nor will they accept a clinician's identification of the attitudes and behaviors that could be perpetuating conflict with the heterosexist environment. Some clients, particularly those who are politically sensitive, are extremely wary of psychotherapists who appear to espouse assimilationism. To them, these providers seemingly fail to comprehend the extent of oppression, blame sexual minorities for fueling the fire of homophobic backlash, or try to reduce rage by convincing clients to be diplomatic rather than to "rock the boat." Although there may be some validity to these positions, clients *first* must experience the counselor's empathic understanding of the magnitude of social injustice before they can trust that psychotherapeutic challenges are not coming from an assimilationist, naïve, or heterosexist stance.

Challenging Dichotomies

Eventually, however, most clients need to be strongly encouraged to see beyond their dichotomous thinking and isolation. Some individuals will facilitate their own psychotherapy in this regard by disclosing a growing sense alienation from mainstream society and a feeling of being separated from the majority and segregated in a ghetto. They may report missing their families and former friends, or feeling oppressed by pressures to conform to subcultural standards of dress, behavior, and lifestyle. These clients, then, are beginning to acknowledge possible differences between themselves and other gay, lesbian, and bisexual individuals, as well as potential similarities between themselves, other ghettoized minority groups, and their heterosexual friends and families of origin. From this frame of reference, they provide clinicians with opportunities for psychotherapeutic impact because they are less rigid and defended and more amenable to intervention. Clients who maintain inflexible delineations between themselves and the heterosexual majority, on the other hand, still can be challenged to reconsider the unpleasant consequences of their polarized (and potentially polarizing) attitudes and behaviors. The therapist, obviously, has some additional leverage if client actions have resulted in some form of negative backlash from family, friends, society, or coworkers. If, however, individuals describe few dissatisfactions with the sexual minority community or an absence of negative repercussions from others, clinicians, nevertheless, can still point out potentially distasteful aftereffects of their isolationist positions.

Reintegration

In any case, as clients relinquish their "them versus us" philosophies, they begin to feel less angry and display an increased willingness to trust others with their deepest thoughts and feelings. Feeling more emotionally stable and more integrated in their identities, they now are able to explore other dimensions of their personalities. In other words, issues related to living as gay, lesbian, or bisexual in an oppressive society have become a backdrop for their lives, rather than the primary focus, thus freeing them to address other concerns. These clients have become ready for help with reintegration into the dominant culture and with the practical aspects of operationalizing and synthesizing their public and private identities.

Reframing the Past

Finally, Phase 5 clients may appreciate assistance with recasting past experiences and relationships in order to maintain a sense of life's continuity (Hanley-Hackenbruck, 1988, 1989). Relationships usually are outgrown and associations change as all individuals develop and mature, and there are times in life when people are "between friendships," with the old left behind and the new yet unformed. Few gay, lesbian, and bisexual individuals carry the same friendship networks throughout life because they have "shed their skin" so completely and some associations may have ended painfully upon coming out. Almost all sexual minorities, in addition, can recall at least some unpleasant experiences related to their "differentness," and some can remember a virtual lifetime of these distressing events.

Because clients often do not know where to file these kinds occurrences in their psychic scrapbooks, one of the major tasks of psychotherapy is to help them reframe their perspectives on the past. Some clients hope to rebuild bridges back into their families of origin, faith communities, and friendship networks; others desire to reformulate their personal histories in other ways. Because a sense of life's continuity is essential to all people, gay, lesbian, and bisexual clients often need to be reminded that their essential selves have remained intact and continue to evolve, even though they have formed and established new social and sexual identities.

Regressions naturally occur during the process of gay and lesbian identity synthesis and reintegration, and living with continued uncertainty is normative for most bisexual individuals. Contending with the stress of pervasive heterosexism, homophobia, and biphobia can erode defenses and allow critical and punitive conscience structures to be reactivated. At these times, clinicians provide perspective and objectivity, maximize evolving resources, and continue superego modification. For the most part, however, this stage of psychotherapy primarily addresses the normative developmental issues of adult life, including those of mentoring and generativity.

FACTORS AFFECTING MOVEMENT ALONG THE TRAJECTORY

Few individuals proceed through the identity development process in stepwise fashion and most, in fact, spiral back and forth through the stages, often over the course of a lifetime. Progression is rarely linear and the developmental tasks of several phases usually coexist and overlap (Berger, 1983). Hence, clients who are reluctant to "come out" or self-identify should not be seen as treatment-resistant or noncompliant. Rather, some clients are struggling with issues unique to bisexuality or to female gender role socialization, both of which affect the process and pacing of identity formation. Others are (appropriately) cautious and need additional time to integrate new experiences and emotional material, given the fluidity of their attractions, as well as the characteristics of their psychosocial adjustment and the social and relational dynamics that affect them. The following sections discuss these influences on the process of sexual minority identity formation.

Dynamics Unique to Bisexual Clients

Clinicians again are reminded of the complexity of helping bisexual men and women to achieve a positive sense of identity. The number of bisexual types, the varied patterns and histories of bisexually oriented individuals (discussed in Chapter 2), and the ongoing feelings of incertitude elucidate this intricacy (R. C. Fox, 1995; Klein, 1993; Paul, 1996; M. S. Weinberg et al., 1994; Zinik, 1985). Most of these clients face multiple relationship issues because frequently they eroticize the opposite sex before their own and have no homoerotic experiences until adulthood, and an estimated two-thirds of bisexual men are heterosexually married (R. C. Fox, 1993; Garnets & Kimmel, 1991; Toufexis, 1992; Zinik, 1985). The fluid patterns of attractions and relationships of those who are dually attracted obviously challenge the traditional emphasis on the role of biological sex in partner selection, and these assumptions and myths must be confronted (often repeatedly) as individuals proceed through the bisexual identity formation process (R. C. Fox, 1993; G. D. Morrow, 1989; Shuster, 1987).

Men and women who are bisexually oriented face another set of tortuous struggles in affirming their identities, in part because the legitimacy of bisexuality as a bona fide sexual orientation is denied by many members of the gay and lesbian community, the heterosexual majority, and the helping professions. As discussed in Chapter 5, many sexual minority individuals view bisexuality as cashing in on heterosexual privilege, as a failure to adjust to being gay or lesbian, or as a passing phase from heterosexuality to an authentic homosexual identity. Some people, though, are tentatively accepting, while others are prejudiced, resentful, or blatantly hostile (Klein, 1993; Matteson, 1996; Paul, 1996; Rust, 1993b; Shuster, 1987, 1992; Toufexis, 1992; M. S. Weinberg et al., 1994; Weise, 1992; Zinik, 1985). Given this widespread lack of support and validation, as well as the dearth of established communities to depend on for comfort and understanding, identity formation is virtually always a lonely passage for individuals attracted to both biological sexes (R. C. Fox, 1995; Toufexis, 1992).

Lesbian Perspectives on Identity Formation

Chapter 5 referred to sex differences in the process of identity development (Grace, 1992). These variations, including those related to stage sequencing, are thought to be based on differences in gender role socialization. Because men are conditioned to value instrumentality and autonomy, they frequently form their identities through sexual experimentation and thus are more likely than women to become sexually active before suspecting their gay identity (Groves & Ventura, 1983; T. Weinberg, 1978). Conversely, women are more relationally socialized and often construct their lesbian identities within emotional or romantic partnerships. Thus, they are more likely than men to become involved in a committed relationship before accepting their lesbianism (Cronin, 1974; Grace, 1992; Groves & Ventura, 1983; Troiden, 1979).

Relationality

The centrality of relationships in women's development has received increasing attention in recent years, and this perspective has come to be known as *self-in-relation theory* (Jordan, Kaplan, Miller, Stiver, & Surrey, 1991). Numerous writers, in addition to those cited previously, have expanded on the relational nature of women and their socialization to care for others and to be connected in intimate interpersonal relationships (Chodorow, 1978; Gilligan, 1982; G. D. Green, 1990; Kirkpatrick, 1991; Miller, 1976; Surrey, 1991). Accordingly, the female self develops and is maintained through connection and within the context of relationships.

Some feminist theorists (Bem, 1993; Unger, 1989) believe that those interpersonal strategies defined as *female* by the self-in-relation perspective "actually reflect positions in a social role hierarchy that have been incorrectly ascribed to gender" (L. S. Brown, 1994, p. 3). Accordingly, gender is seen as an artifact of sex and power relationships, and not a core feature of individual identity. For feminists of lesbian orientation who identify with this social constructionist position, the sociopolitical arena is central to the definition and construction of lesbian self-identification. To these women, becoming lesbian is a relational as well as political passage, which involves the unfolding of an identity within a matrix of current, historical, and community definitions. It also is a process whereby women form connections which define themselves within the context of relationships to one another rather than through definitions of female sexuality constructed by sexist or patriarchal distortions (Faderman, 1984; Phelan, 1993; Stephenson & Palladino, 1990).

Redefining Power

Feminist theologian Carter Heyward (1989a) illustrates this perspective when she describes "coming out" as an act of resistance to unjust power relations, in general, and to unjust gender relations in particular. This process, according to Heyward, is a public step of further opposition to male dominance and an opportunity for redefining power relations on the basis of women's sexuality. In this regard, a lesbian's experience of erotic power when joined with another woman empowers the empathy and mutuality of their same-sex relationships.

As discussed previously, many women enter the identity formation trajectory first within mutually intimate relationships and later through the lesbian community. From their association with other women, often they realize that they are second-class citizens, not only on the basis of sexual orientation but also because of their biological sex. They learn, further, that the heterosexism and male dominance of the majority culture largely is responsible for devaluing and oppressing both sexual minorities and women. These lesbians then transform this recognition of the relationship between the personal and the political into overarching explanations for most aspects of their lives. The awareness of a personal–political connection results for some in the creation of lesbian communities, some of which are known as "separatist" in that they do not form alliances with nonlesbians. The struggles of both separatist and nonseparatist lesbians with heterosexist power and patriarchy sometimes influences the course of their psychotherapy, as well as their choice of providers. Clinicians, therefore, must be especially sensitive to these issues when working with many lesbian clients (L. A. Lewis, 1984; Phelan, 1993).

Lesbian-Specific Models

Several lesbian-specific identity formation models have been developed to account for the relational nature of women's socialization and the need of some women to redefine themselves in relationship to power (Chapman & Brannock, 1987; L. A. Lewis, 1984; Sophie, 1982, 1986). Table 9.6 outlines three of these.

To avoid redundancy, the particular developmental stages delineated in Table 9.6 are not elaborated on further at this point because the processes are quite similar to those of the four models of lesbian and gay identity formation described in detail in Chapter 5. Readers are referred, though, to Chapman and Brannock (1987), L. A. Lewis (1984), and Sophie (1982, 1986) for the explicit ways in which these theorists conceptualize women's gender role socialization as influencing the sequencing of the developmental stages. The central focus of these contentions, however, is that lesbian identity is stabilized and integrated within the context of intimate and communal relationships rather than prior to, or apart from, these associations.

Traditional gender conditioning also is reflected during the identity formation process in the tendency of men to sexualize distress and in the inclination of women to reflect and become self-absorbed. Because men are taught to conquer their fear with action, they tend to "come out" more abruptly than women. They further may act more impulsively and less mindfully because they often feel a greater sense of urgency to tackle the problem. Consequently, many feel overwhelmed during the earlier stages of identity formation. Whereas greater ambiguity and fluidity appear to characterize this same process for women, the identity confusion and conflict in both sexes can resemble pathological processes (Gonsiorek & Rudolph, 1991; Schuker, 1996). Distinctions between typical "coming out" symptomology and diagnosable mental disorders were outlined in the previous chapter in order to help clinicians depathologize these predictable responses and thus avoid mislabeling gay, lesbian, and bisexual clients.

Fixed and Fluid Attractions

As was mentioned earlier, fluid patterns of sexual attraction are not uncommon in both lesbians and bisexual individuals, and these uncongealed configurations are among the primary factors influencing movement along the developmental trajectory for both populations. Though Sophie (1986) believes that linear models of identity formation have some validity, especially in the early phases, she believes that many directions for change are possible in later stages. She further contends that the notion of a *fixed* or rigid self-definition as a developmental endpoint for psychotherapy must be abandoned in favor of "flexibility in sexual identity" (p. 50). Others (discussed previously) also have argued for this concept of a *fluid* or flexible self-image (E. Coleman, 1988; Fox, 1995, 1996a,

TABLE 9.6. Lesbian Identity Formation Models

Chapman & Brannock (1987)	Lewis (1984)	Sophie (1982, 1986)
Same-Sex Orientation	Being Different	Lesbian Feelings
Incongruence	Dissonance	Coming Out to Self
Self-Questioning/Exploration	Relationships	
Self-Identification	Stable Identity	Coming Out to Others
Choice of Lifestyle	Integration	

1996b; Gonsiorek & Weinrich, 1991; Weise, 1992). Clinicians, thus, who allow for fluidity in sexual identity free their clients to explore the full range of their sexuality, including bisexuality.

Cass (1990), presents a somewhat more detailed conceptualization of these fluctuating amorous and sexual interests. Accordingly, she believes that erotic and emotional attractions or "preferences" themselves are, more or less, *fixed* (or immutable) for some individuals and *fluid* (or variable) for others. Further, she contends that the process of identity formation can influence not only the strength of the *fixed* attractions but the directionality as well as the intensity of the *fluid* preferences. In others words, the course of identity development may activate and drive the more variable inclinations, as well as reinforce the more immutable predispositions. Some of the ways in which the process of forming a sexual minority identity could influence the strength, directionality, and intensity of these attractions or preferences include the following:

- narrowing opportunities for sexual/social/emotional expression.
- building attitudes that attach a fixed quality to identity and preference.
- reinforcing behaviors that are consistent with that identity.
- providing a system of rewards that encourages commitment to a particular mode of behavior (Cass, 1990, pp. 252–253).

Few would disagree that contemporary concepts of gay, lesbian, or bisexual identity have been socially constructed primarily during the 20th century. Clients often need to be reminded of this fact as they confine their conceptualizations exclusively to the popular formulations of the present day. The development of identity is extremely sensitive to historical changes and social conditions, as well as to the influence of affirming and supportive communities (Faderman, 1984; Sophie, 1986). Further, the belief that the essential erotic and emotional attractions that largely define sexual orientation are themselves fluid is controversial (see Chapter 2 for a discussion of social constructionism and essentialism). Cass's four-point schema described previously allows psychotherapists to help their clients narrow opportunities, build attitudes, reinforce behaviors, and reward themselves for directing or strengthening their sexual and affectional preferences toward a heterosexual, homosexual, or bisexual orientation. Assuming that these core attractions are more fluid than fixed, clinicians may attempt to guide their clients in either direction. Chapter 13, however, discusses the limitations and adverse effects of religion-based psychotherapy that tries to "convert" or redirect the sexual orientation of those whose same-sex preferences are more fixed than fluid.

Psychosocial Adjustment

Personality variables, including psychosocial adaptation, are related to the developmental maturity of a sexual minority self. In an effort to describe individuals according to one of the six stages of the Cass model, Brady and Busse (1994) constructed a Gay Identity Questionnaire (GIQ), which they administered to 225 gay male subjects. The results indicated a significant positive relationship between stage of identity formation and a composite indicator of psychological well-being that assessed subjects' perceived happiness, loneliness, anxiety, sexual satisfaction, suicidal ideation, mental hygiene, and physical health. These findings underscored for the investigators the importance of psychological factors in the evolution of a gay identity and supported Cass's prediction that, as people move through the stages of her model, "self-perception changes from negative and ambivalent to a more positive and accepting view of self" (p. 10). Conversely, among the factors found by Brady and Busse to correlate inversely with the psychological adjustment of their subjects were loneliness, anxiety, suicidal ideation, and physical health. When facilitating identity formation in clients, then, psychotherapists can target these specific variables for clinical intervention.

Others also have noted the association between psychological adjustment, including self-esteem, and positive sexual minority identification (Miranda & Storms, 1989; Zinik, 1985). In one study, for example, 51 gay males who felt comfortable with their sexual identity were found to score low on anxiety, sensitization, and depression and high on self-concept (Schmitt & Kurdek, 1987). Conversely, Berger (1983) noted that gay and lesbian individuals who passed as heterosexual scored higher on measures of depression, awkwardness, and anxiety than did those who were able to share their sexual status. Further, informing others of a sexual minority orientation has psychological benefits, including greater satisfaction with the social support available from those who know (Berger, 1992a; Schmitt & Kurdek, 1987). Given that psychosocial elements are integrally related to identity development, studies such as those described previously can assist clinicians in targeting specific personality variables for treatment as they assist clients in the formation of their sexual minority identities.

Social and Relational Influences

Along the lines of the studies discussed in the previous section, Miranda and Storms (1989) discovered that self-labeling and self-disclosure are two coping strategies associated with positive gay and lesbian identification. Yet, as intrinsic as self-disclosure is to the phases of identity formation, most clients experience considerable difficulty with "coming out" to themselves and to others (Wells & Kline, 1987). D'Augelli (1991), for example, reported that the willingness of gay men in college to self-disclose was influenced strongly by their concerns with the opinions of others, and that the foremost challenge to their newly formed identities was the task of telling their families. Franke and Leary (1991) studied 184 subjects of both sexes who identified as gay, lesbian, or bisexual and likewise found that apprehension about the appraisals of others predicted substantially more of the variance in their openness than in the degree to which they accepted their own sexuality. In other words, individuals could be fairly comfortable with their own sexual orientation and yet apprehensive about self-disclosing to others.

Helping clients translate self-acceptance into self-revelation is a complex process, and, hence, many unspoken rules and obligations that structure social relationships shape decisions regarding how to manage information related to sexual orientation. Cain (1991a, 1991b), accordingly, found that choices both to disclose and to maintain secrecy were associated with a variety of relational, situational, and social factors unrelated to integration or synthesis of sexual identity. Harry (1993) identified some of these variables that related to being open with heterosexuals as income, sexual orientation of friends, type of occupation, and age. G. J. McDonald (1982) similarly noted several circumstances which significantly influenced the identity development process, namely gender, ethnicity, area of residence, and societal values. A person's stage of identity formation, then, is not necessarily predictive of where or to whom that individual "comes out" as gay, lesbian, or bisexual; therefore, clinicians must consider other factors, as well. Two important variables, traditional family values and family processes, are the focus of the following discussions.

Traditional Family Values

Traditional family values often influence the process of forming and disclosing a positive bisexual, gay, or lesbian self-image to significant others. B. S. Newman and Muzzonigro (1993) based their definition of these values on "(1) the importance of religion, (2) emphasis on marriage, (3) emphasis on having children, (4) and whether a non-English language was spoken in the home" (p. 213). They studied 27 gay male adolescents from African American, Hispanic/Latino, Eurasian, and Caucasian backgrounds to determine the effects of traditional family values on the course of identity development. Independent of other variables, "race alone had no systematic effect on how coming out was experienced. The presence of traditional family values, however, was related to the process of accepting a gay identity" (B. S. Newman & Muzzonigro, 1993, p. 224). Further, perceived rejection and disapproval were the biggest barriers to "coming out" for gay adolescents from highly traditional homes (see Chapter 10 for further discussion of sexual minorities of color).

Psychotherapists frequently must assist clients with recognizing the traditional family values of their childhood homes and with understanding how these standards, often with stringent rules around loyalty, frequently hinder not only the process of developing a positive gay, lesbian, or bisexual identity but also the disclosure of that status to significant others. In this regard, the psychotherapeutic task often becomes the examination of the values held by the family (religion, marriage, children, etc.) and the heterosexism through which they are transmitted. The specific makeup of these values and their methods of transmittal must be separated further from the *rigidity* with which they are held because, in many traditional families, most expectations, beliefs, rules, and directives are immovable and there is little room for deviation around many topics. From this vantage point, then, clients might be helped to see that the tight structure of the familial system undoubtedly is a source of numerous difficulties for other members, as well, and that their homosexuality is only one of several issues that trouble the family.

Family Processes

In addition to traditional values, other familial factors can influence the trajectory of gay, lesbian, and bisexual identity formation. M. J. Kahn and Nutt (1991) studied patterns of communication and relationships in the families of 290 lesbians and found that higher levels of intergenerational intimidation and intergenerational triangulation were significantly related to slower lesbian identity development and decreased disclosure. (*Intergenerational intimidation* refers to feeling pressured to conform to extended family values; *intergenerational triangulation* refers to feeling entangled in an unstable extended family relationship.) In other words, women who reported feeling intimidated or triangulated by their families of origin tended not to disclose their sexual orientation and thus formed their lesbian identities slower than did those who felt less threatened by familial rejection. Intergenerational intimacy, similarly, also decreased the likelihood of disclosure and women who reported feeling intimate with extended families remained heterosexually identified longer and developed their lesbian identities slower than those who felt less familial closeness.

M. J. Kahn (1991) also studied the differentiation of 81 lesbians from their families and found that intergenerational intimidation was significantly related to stage of identity development. Berg-Cross (1988) observed essentially this same pattern of fear and fusion when she reported on the individuation of young lesbians from their families of origin. Along similar lines, she also noted another factor that seemed to inhibit the process of lesbian identity development, namely, the tendency of many newly "out" women to escape into the "suffocating fusion" of early lesbian relationships.

As is true with individuals from traditional families (discussed earlier), clinicians may need to help clients identify and articulate the unspoken rules that structure their families of origin, as well as impose obligations and penalties on members. These rules often define behaviors indicative of loyalty to the clan, and defined as such, "coming out" as gay, lesbian, or bisexual may be considered the ultimate breach of fidelity to the family name. Clients also may need assistance with evaluating the extent to which intergenerational intimidation functions in their families of origin. By learning to consider family processes from an objective perspective, they can come to understand their fear of detriangulating, or of extracting themselves emotionally from enmeshed family systems, as a natural consequence of the anxiety and fusion operating within their kinship networks. This perspective often reduces self-criticism and unburdens clients to proceed with identity development. These clients, further, can be taught to monitor their tendency as members of enmeshed families to recreate similar dynamics in intimate relationships during the early stages of identity formation.

CONCLUSION

Psychotherapists again are reminded that few clients will proceed sequentially or smoothly through the phases of identity formation described previously. Most, in fact, will proceed and progress until some internal or external obstacle causes them to plateau or regress. These perspectives, as well as insight into the potential fluidity or variability of their attractions, should be presented to clients as natural and nonpathological variations on the identity development trajectory.

Bisexual and gender differences also influence "coming out" for many sexual minority clients. These variances, as well as fluctuating erotic inclinations, were described so that clinicians can adapt developmental models to the experiences of women and bisexually oriented individuals. Family-of-origin factors, such as fusion and rules or penalties around loyalty, likewise were addressed because they also affect the process and pacing of identity formation.

Although the basic approaches to psychotherapy, including empathic understanding and crisis management, obviously apply when working with sexual minority clients, certain therapeutic interventions are particularly significant and merit reiteration. Clinicians, for example, must address the isolation and depression of most gay, lesbian, and bisexual clients. The loss of a heterosexual life image must be grieved on some level and reformulated. Superego modification and the challenging of inhibition strategies also are necessary. Other important considerations include presenting the concept of "developmental lag" in a normative and affirming manner, assisting with the completion of adolescent tasks, and validating legitimate anger at oppression. Confronting dichotomous thinking and reintegrating and recasting the past, as well as addressing the normal developmental tasks of adult life, are essential to the psychotherapeutic process.

10

Sexual Minorities within Other Minority Populations

Sensitivity to the cultural context of their lives is essential to clinical work with sexual minorities of color. These clients often encounter more obstacles than mainstream individuals when attempting to form positive gay, lesbian, or bisexual identities because many encounter heterosexist stigmatization in addition to ethnic (or racial) intolerance on "coming out." After declaring their newly formed identities, these individuals become members of at least two marginalized groups, namely, the broader sexual minority community along with their own ethnic subculture. Although nonmajority culture gay and bisexual men can be conceptualized as holding dual membership, lesbians of color conceivably belong to three subcultural populations: one related to their ethnicity, another to their sexual orientation, and the third to their biological sex.

B. Greene (1994b), accordingly, describes a principle of "triple discrimination" (p. 391) as a situation in which androcentric, heterocentric, and ethnocentric biases have an impact on racial/ethnic minority lesbians. Hence, a complicated picture of oppression emerges as these individuals struggle to form multiple and overlapping identities that integrate gender, race, and sexual orientation (Reynolds & Pope, 1991). A Latina lesbian, for example, is first faced with understanding herself as a woman, as a Hispanic, and as a sexual minority and then is challenged to integrate these three cultural identities into a single "self" that is hardy enough to weather repeated encounters with sexist, racist, and heterosexist injustice. B. Greene (1997b) notes that this merger of identities is an extremely challenging process that often provokes "feelings of anger, sadness, or of being overwhelmed," and "for many, these issues represent a painful and challenging aspect of their everyday lives" (p. xiv).

H. B. McDonald and Steinhorn (1993) expand the concept of multiple minority group membership to include socioeconomic status. Many Mexican American gay men, for instance, have to grapple with belonging to a low socioeconomic group as well as to a community of color before contending with a same-sex orientation. Poverty, in addition to Afrocentric values, also reinforces the ties that many African American lesbians have to their ethnic communities. The financial assistance these women frequently contribute to their families of origin in many cases is essential for helping them maintain a reasonable standard of living (Mays & Cochran, 1988). Dworkin (1997) addresses the difficulties of being Jewish in a dominant Christian and anti-Semitic society and a sexual minority in a heterosexually oriented culture. The discussion in Chapter 13 expands further on the cultural clash involved in the integration of two marginalized identities: religious and sexual. The interactions of competing racial, sexual, religious and class identities, then, are extremely complex and seriously complicate identity formation and the "coming-out" process for numerous individuals (DiPlacido, 1998; B. Greene, 1994b, 1997a; Manalansan, 1996; E. S. Nelson, 1993; A. Smith, 1997).

IDENTITY FORMATION

Just as lesbians, bisexuals, and gay men form affirming identities in incremental phases (see Table 5.1), so do ethnic/cultural minorities. Sexual minorities of color, consequently, face the challenge of navigating two extremely difficult developmental processes simultaneously. Before its interaction with the gay, lesbian, and bisexual identity formation trajectory is discussed, however this chapter presents a model of ethnic minority identity development.

Minority Identity Development

The Minority Identity Development (MID) model of D. R. Atkinson, Morten, and Sue (1993) outlines a five-stage schema designed to assist psychotherapists in understanding the behaviors and attitudes of clients of color living in a White majority society, as those individuals "struggle to understand themselves in terms of their own minority culture, and the oppressive relationship between the two cultures" (p. 28). Like the sexual minority identity formation models presented earlier (see Table 5.1), the phases are not to be considered mutually exclusive but, rather, are meant to be experienced "as a continuous process in which one stage blends with another and boundaries between the stages are not clear" (p. 28). The model shown below describes client characteristics at each phase.

Conformity

Individuals at this stage:

- Admire, respect, and idealize members of the dominant group
- Unquestioningly accept the dominant group's cultural values
- Unconsciously depreciate themselves

or

- Consciously view their distinguishing characteristics as sources of shame
- View other members of their minority group according to the dominant group's beliefs about minority strengths and weaknesses
- View members of other minority groups according to the dominant group's system of minority stratification

Dissonance

Individuals at this stage:

- Become more aware that not all of the dominant group's cultural values are beneficial to them
- Grow in awareness of their minority group's cultural strengths

and

- Alternate between feeling ashamed and proud of themselves and their distinguishing characteristics
- Begin to question the dominant group's views of minority strengths and weaknesses
- Devote most of their psychic energy to resolving conflicting attitudes toward themselves, other members of their minority group, and the dominant group
- Start to feel the appeal of their minority group's cultural values
- Begin to question the dominant group's minority hierarchy

and

- Experience a growing sense of solidarity with other oppressed people
- View members of the dominant group with growing suspicion

Resistance and Immersion

Individuals at this stage:

- Explore and discover their history and culture, seeking information and artifacts that enhance their sense of identity and worth
- Honor and feel proud of their distinguishing characteristics
- Strongly identify with, and commit themselves to, their minority group
- Admire, respect, and idealize members of their minority group
- Unquestioningly accept their minority group's cultural values
- Experience a growing sense of solidarity with members of other minority groups, to the extent that they are seen as sharing similar forms of oppression
- Replace the dominant group's minority hierarchy with an ethnocentric stratification that values cultural similarity
- Totally reject the dominant society and culture
- Distrust and dislike all members of the dominant group

Introspection

Individuals at this stage:

- Experience dissonance between feelings of responsibility and loyalty to their minority group and ideas of personal autonomy
- Begin to concern themselves with group appropriation of individuality
- Grow uneasy with ethnocentric minority stratification

- Experience conflict between completely distrusting the dominant society and culture and selectively trusting members of the dominant group based on demonstrated attitudes and behaviors
- Acknowledge the usefulness of many dominant cultural values yet remain uncertain about integrating these elements into their minority culture

Synergetic Articulation and Awareness

Individuals at this stage:

- Experience a strong sense of self-esteem, self-confidence, and self-reliance as consequences of having developed their identities as individuals, members of a minority group, and members of a dominant society or culture
- Have a strong feeling of pride as members of their minority group without unequivocally accepting its values
- Couple strong feelings of empathy with their group experience with an awareness that each group member is an individual
- Join a strong sense of respect for the cultural values of other minority groups with an awareness that each group member is an individual
- Experience an increased understanding and support for all oppressed people, regardless of cultural similarity or dissimilarity to their minority group
- Selectively trust and appreciate members of the dominant group who seek to eliminate its oppressive attitudes and behaviors
- Open themselves to constructive elements of the dominant society and culture

Identity Development for Sexual Minorities of Color

Because lesbians, bisexuals, and gay men of color are faced with forming identities as members of (at least) two minority groups, the interactive nature of these development processes is discussed herein. Table 10.1 presents a schema that roughly approximates the parallel properties of the two trajectories.

During the first phases of both identity formation processes, individuals assume that they are still members of the dominant group and, thus, overvalue the norms of the majority culture as they unconsciously devalue themselves. Nevertheless, they feel *socially* different and try hard to be included, often fearful of behaving in ways that are contrary to White, heterosexual expectations.

Because most people of color are members of *visible* minority groups, their distinguishing characteristics usually are apparent to themselves and to others. Lesbians, bisexuals, and gay men, however, must struggle to develop an internal awareness of their differentness amid families and communities that often automatically assume their heterosexuality. At the beginning of Phase 2 of sexual minority identity formation, when these individuals begin to feel *sexually* different and privately label themselves as *possibly* gay, lesbian, or bisexual, their internal conflicts emerge and they frequently feel ashamed of the possibility. Similarly, in the *Conformity* stage of MID, feelings of shame about distinguishing racial/ethnic traits are common. Both populations often view members of nondominant groups (both others and their own) according to prevailing stigmas and stereotypes as they continue to overvalue the majority society and devalue minority cultures.

TABLE 10.1. A Comparison of Minority Identity Development and Sexual Minority Identity Formation

Minority Identity Development (ethnic/cultural) (Atkinson, Morten, & Sue, 1993)	Sexual Minority Identity Formation
	Phase 1
Conformity	Sensitization (Troiden) Pre-Coming Out (Coleman) Emergence (Grace)
	Phase 2
Dissonance	Identity Confusion (Cass, Troiden) Identity Comparison (Cass) Coming Out (Coleman) Acknowledgment (Grace)
	Phase 3
	Identity Tolerance (Cass) Identity Assumption (Troiden) Exploration (Coleman) Finding Community (Grace)
	Phase 4
	Identity Acceptance (Cass) Commitment (Troiden) First Relationships (Coleman, Grace)
	Phase 5
Resistance and Immersion	Identity Pride (Cass)
Introspection	
Synergetic Articulation and Awareness	Identity Synthesis (Cass) Integration (Coleman) Self-Definition and Reintegration (Grace)

The *Dissonance* stage of MID roughly parallels the third and fourth phases of gay, lesbian, and bisexual identity formation. Sexual minorities of color at Phase 3 begin to acknowledge their social, emotional, and sexual needs and to realize that the majority culture is less than affirming and supportive of their ethnic and sexual differences. As gay, lesbian, and bisexual people, they explore and experiment within their new subculture while, as ethnic minorities, they grow in awareness of their cultural heritage. New feelings of pride also are emerging even though members of both populations continue to experience occasional episodes of shame regarding their core identities. Sexual minorities of color, nevertheless, devote most of their energy during this phase to reconciling conflicts within themselves and with their majority and minority cultures. By Phase 4, ethnic minority lesbians, bisexuals, and gay men are beginning to resolve some of the dissonance they experienced earlier, and, in general, they are feeling more accepting of themselves both as sexual minorities and as people of color. As their identifications with both nondominant groups intensify, they become more aware of the majority culture's oppressive elements (i.e., racism and heterosexism).

The beginning of Phase 5 [*Identity Pride* (Cass, 1979)] and *Resistance and Immersion*

(MID) are virtually parallel processes. Individuals in this stage are learning as much as possible about their new subculture, experiencing a growing sense of pride and solidarity and strongly identifying with others like themselves. Consequently, they distance themselves from the racism and heterosexism of the majority culture and immerse themselves in their ethnic and sexual minority communities. Toward the middle of the fifth phase, however, people tend to grow uneasy with discriminating polarities based on ethnicity and sexual orientation. They come to see similarities as much as differences between themselves and members of the White, heterosexual majority culture. In addition, they grow to realize that there also are differences between and among members of their own minority groups. This *Introspection* (MID) often propels them to begin integrating their multiple identities.

The end of Phase 5 of sexual minority identity formation overlaps with *Synergistic Articulation and Awareness* (MID). As gay, lesbian, and bisexual people of color continue to integrate their ethnicity and sexual orientation with other personality traits into a singular, multifaceted self-concept, they begin to abandon dichotomies between their sexual and ethnic minority groups (i.e., gay vs. Asian American; lesbian vs. Latina) and between their minority group and the majority culture (i.e., African American and bisexual vs. White and heterosexual). Regardless of similarities and differences, their understanding and appreciation of other oppressed people increases and they now differentiate on the basis of perceived support rather than on ethnicity or sexual orientation. Their selective trust of dominant group members who seek to eliminate oppressive elements in the majority culture exposes them to its constructive components and allows them to proceed with normative tasks of adult development.

Ideally, the interaction between models of sexual and ethnic minority identity formation (discussed earlier) ultimately facilitates the development of a multicultural identity for gay, lesbian, and bisexual people of color living in a White, heterosexual majority culture. A Native American gay man, for example, will be able to appreciate the valuable elements in the dominant society, integrate his tribal culture into his overall identity, and incorporate his gay identity into his image of himself. In other words, his identity will have become integrated. The foregoing discussion also implies that individuals begin both models monoculturally identified with the dominant society and suggests that their ethnic and sexual minority identities are integrated simultaneously into the preexisting monocultural identity. This is seldom the case, however, because most people usually can undertake only one major developmental task at a time. Given the time and psychic energy required for identity formation, complete and concurrent immersion of self in two subcultures is virtually impossible. The models are presented together to highlight their interactive nature, but all phases and stages rarely happen contemporaneously. In other words, these processes are independent and parallel but rarely synchronized.

CULTURAL FACTORS

In addition to influencing ethnic minority identity development, numerous cultural factors have an impact on gay, lesbian, and bisexual identity formation for people of color. In other words, a number of variables affect how individuals proceed through these developmental models. B. Greene (1994b), for example, offers a range of factors for psychotherapists to consider when assessing the progress of clients in regard to developing positive ethnic and sexual minority identities (pp. 392–393):

- the function and significance of family and community
- the significance of bonds to the ethnic community
- the significance of procreation and perpetuating family lineage
- the function and expectancies of parents in the lives of their children
- the significance of the family as a source of economic and emotional assistance
- the function of religion/spirituality in the culture
- the degree to which individual clients are acculturated or assimilated
- important differences between the degrees to which individual clients and their families are acculturated
- the historical record of opposition or oppression that the specific group has experienced from dominant culture individuals and institutions
- the character and significance of the culture's traditional gender role stereotypes and their relative flexibility or rigidity
- the meaning attributed to gender and sexuality in the individual's culture

For the purpose of discussion, these factors have been grouped and are presented under three broad categories: family and community, acculturation, and gender and sexuality. Literature common to all sexual minority people of color, regardless of their particular cultural group, is summarized according to these classifications. Following this discussion, ethnic-specific considerations are addressed separately.

Family and Community

Garnets and Kimmel (1991) reviewed the literature on cultural diversity in identity formation and found that sexual minority identity development generally occurs within a context of family traditions and community values. Reconciling competing loyalties among different minority group subcultures, then, often becomes the major struggle for lesbians and gay men of color. In this regard, "they must participate in divergent social worlds, balancing demands and crossing boundaries of the different groups, including the gay male and lesbian community, one's ethnic culture, the majority culture, and for women, the women's or feminist community" (p. 156). These individuals, unfortunately, often experience discrimination and prejudice as "outsiders" in each community; nonetheless, they typically feel more comfortable in the sexual minority community but more strongly identified with their racial or cultural group.

In most ethnic groups, both family and community function as a refuge and buffer against racism in the dominant culture (B. Greene, 1994b). The boundaries of kinship in many ethnic cultures go beyond the nuclear family and extend to include members not related by blood. Because these affiliations often have served as safe havens in an oppressive society, sexual minorities frequently fear separation from their cultural group and rejection by it or by their families. Many thus will not risk jeopardizing their connections to their ethnic/cultural heritage by aligning themselves with the broader lesbian or gay community or even by divulging their same-sex orientation.

Caught between Cultures

In their literature review, Garnets and Kimmel (1991) discuss the high value placed on cooperation, interdependence, and commitment in many ethnic minority cultures. Like B. Greene (1994b, 1997a), they conclude that these norms often result in many lesbians and gay men of color not disclosing their sexual orientation to their families and, thus, remaining closeted and feeling like "outcasts" in their communities. Further, many ethnic groups view homosexuality as a "White Western" phenomenon and liken the acceptance of sexual minority identification to violating the social expectations of the culture by placing personal or individual desires above the needs of the group (p. 157). B. Greene (1994b), in fact, contends that these populations often are perceived by sexual minority members to be "more tenaciously antagonistic than the dominant culture" (p. 396). On the other hand, visible gay, lesbian, and bisexual communities consist primarily of majority-culture individuals who bring their values and norms into these groups. Identification with a predominantly White gay, lesbian, and bisexual community, therefore, may not have the same benefits for ethnic minorities that it does for Caucasian Americans. The result is that many gay, lesbian, and bisexual people of color feel torn between loyalty to (what often they perceive as) ethnocentric heterosexism and identification with Eurocentric sexual minorities (B. E. Jones & Hill, 1996; Loiacano, 1989; Nakajima, Chan, & Lee, 1996; Tafoya, 1996). B. Greene (1997a) notes that these individuals frequently experience "never being part of any group completely, leaving them at risk for feelings of isolation and estrangement and thus increased psychological vulnerability" (p. 235).

Lesbian, gay, and bisexual individuals from countries such as India, where British colonialism was particularly influential in shaping the norms and expectations of the culture, may experience another dimension to their cultural conflict. Many Indians, for example, view Great Britain as their "mother country" and thus may closely identify with Caucasians. Further, they often are from economically or educationally privileged backgrounds and, hence, may not relate to the disadvantaged conditions of many American ethnic/cultural minorities. Although these individuals may be seen as people of color because of their skin complexion, they do not experience themselves as ethnic minorities as may people of color who have been raised in the United States (B. Greene, 1994b). In understanding the cultural conflicts of not only these but all ethnic/cultural minority clients, clinicians must consider the diverse identifications and varied alliances of individuals "based on assumptions about the meaning of skin color as well as sexual orientation in different parts of the world" (p. 407).

Manalansan (1993) underscores this point in his review of the works of two Filipino gay immigrant writers (Silva and Pena) and addresses the complexity of problems faced by sexual minority individuals who have been raised in post-colonial cultures. He contends that the current emphasis on duality of experience (i.e., non-Caucasian and gay) is insufficiently multidimensional to describe the contradictory, often opposing, and sometimes even complementary transnational forces impinging upon these people; amid the controversy on multiculturalism, there have been few attempts to comprehend how transnational processes influence racial, national, ethnic, and sexual identities and accompanying world views. Manalansan (1996), nevertheless maintains that there is no universal "gay identity," contrary to the views perpetuated by both mainstream and sexual minority individuals and groups.

Resolving Cultural Conflict

Morales (1989, 1992, 1996) examined the interactive processes between ethnic minority communities and their sexual minority family members and presented a framework for understanding the course of change for lesbian, bisexual, and gay men of color as they try to reconcile dilemmas of dual or multiple minority group membership. He proposed a model in which he refers to the cognitive and lifestyle changes as *states* rather than *stages* because "it is possible that persons may experience several states or parts of states at the same time, unlike a stage model in which resolution of one stage leads to another" (Morales, 1992, p. 131). The Morales model includes many of the same concepts as those identified in Table 10.1 and discussed earlier in terms of the interaction between minority identification and sexual minority identity formation. Nevertheless, his five states are outlined separately in this section because the focus of the model directly relates to the discord felt by many bisexual, gay, and lesbian people of color as they attempt to address and integrate at least two conflicting cultural realities. The following outline has been adapted from his 1992 chapter (pp. 131–134) which includes suggestions for psychotherapists.

STATE 1: DENIAL OF CONFLICTS

Individuals in this state:

- Minimize the reality of racial discrimination
- Believe that their sexual orientation has limited consequences in their life
- Have an idealistic and utopian outlook that tends to dominate their perception of reality
- Need assistance from their therapists in developing a more accurate picture of how societal conditions affect their functioning

STATE 2: BISEXUAL VERSUS GAY OR LESBIAN

Individuals in this state:

- See the sexual minority community as an extension of White racist society
- Conceive of sexuality as sexual feelings for someone regardless of biological sex
- Assume a bisexual identity as a way to avoid being labeled and categorized by their own ethnic/cultural community
- Need assistance from their therapists in exploring feelings of hopelessness and depression resulting from the continual feeling of cultural conflict; and in imagining a sexual minority ethnic/cultural community

STATE 3: CONFLICTS IN ALLEGIANCES

Individuals in this state:

- Experience intense concern and anxiety about "taking sides" and betraying either their ethnic/cultural groups or other sexual minorities
- Feel torn between the emphasis in their minority culture on "sticking together" as a way of dealing with the oppression of mainstream society, and the gay, bisexual, and lesbian community's focus on the common struggles of all stigmatized groups
- Need assistance from their therapists in prioritizing allegiances rather than in

choosing sides so that their identities can shift from a monocultural perspective to one containing multiple dimensions

STATE 4: ESTABLISHING PRIORITIES IN ALLEGIANCE

Individuals in this state:

- Feel resentful and frustrated regarding the lack of integration among the communities of which they are members
- Experience anger and rage stemming from experiences of racism and subsequent rejection by members of the sexual minority community
- Separate Caucasian gay, bisexual, and lesbian friends from ethnic minority companions and continue to be identified primarily with their cultural communities
- Need assistance from their therapists in examining their rage and anger so that they may develop more proactive, rather than victimized, perspectives; this might include forming alliances with other sexual minority people of color

STATE 5: INTEGRATING THE VARIOUS COMMUNITIES

Individuals in this state:

- Feel a need to integrate their seemingly dualistic cultures into a single multicultural identity
- Experience anxiety, alienation, and frustration over the reality of limited options for integration
- Encounter pressure to be the "bridge" or "go between" for their ethnic/cultural groups and the sexual minority communities
- Face the constant challenge of conflicting allegiances and resulting feelings of being misunderstood by both populations
- Need assistance from their therapists in supporting their judgment and problem solving skills, and in encouraging them to expand their support systems to include people with similar multicultural perspectives

Acculturation

Given that a large number of ethnic/cultural minority individuals in the United States were born in their countries of origin, issues such as recency of immigration and degree of acculturation into U.S. society become psychotherapeutic concerns. Some new immigrants speak little or no English, whereas others learned and spoke fluent English in their native lands. Further, some have come from countries with a heavy U.S. influence and can be considered bicultural, as well as bilingual. For others still, not only is the language of the United States completely foreign, but so also is the culture.

Kitano (1989) provides a model for assessing the degree of acculturation of Asian Americans, the conceptualizations of which also can be applied to other ethnic/cultural populations. In this regard, Kitano believes that individuals be can classified along four dimensions:

- *High assimilation/low ethnic identity.* Individuals in this group identify primarily with Western values and have little identification with their ethnic culture.
- *Low assimilation/low ethnic identity.* Individuals in this group do not identify with either culture and tend to be marginal and sometimes dysfunctional.
- *High assimilation/high ethnic identity.* Individuals in this group are bicultural and have the ability to accept both cultural systems.
- *Low assimilation/high ethnic identity.* Individuals in this group tend to be recent immigrants and refugees.

Immigration

Culture provides specific plots or themes for who people are and what they might become, and immigration disrupts the life course and alters those narratives (Espin, 1994, 1997). Leaving a country of origin and migrating to another changes the scenario and requires individuals to rewrite their life stories. Because geographical as well as psychological, emotional, and behavioral boundaries are crossed in immigration, a new identity must be created. For sexual minorities coming to the United States, this entails the development of a lesbian, bisexual, or gay identity as socially constructed in this country rather than as defined in their native lands. In other words, people must learn not only how to be American but also how to be a sexual minority in the United States, particularly within the geographical region in which they settle. Hence, the processes of acculturation and identity formation may occur simultaneously.

Because they usually are not acculturated, new lesbian, gay, and bisexual immigrants rarely have contact with a sexual minority community, or even with individuals of same-sex orientation in their own ethnic group. Because of the previously discussed heterosexism of most cultures worldwide, the latter tend to be invisible and extremely closeted (B. Greene, 1994b). Most homosexually oriented clients, hence, describe extreme loneliness and alienation and often "agree that they feel like a minority within a minority in the United States" (Morales, 1992, p, 134).

Given the magnitude of the loss, mourning the separation from all that is familiar in their homelands is virtually universal among immigrants of all sexual orientations. This "culture shock" can be intensified depending on "perceived or real freedom to migrate, relative ease or difficulty of this process, sense of responsibility for those left behind, and conditions in both the home and host countries" (Espin, 1987b, p. 279). Espin (1987b, 1997) also discusses other factors that influence the nature of the adaptation. Her list includes such variables as language proficiency, ability to find a job, losses or gains in status or social class, educational level, degree of similarity between the two cultures, and reception by citizens of the host country. Intrapsychic factors such as ego strength, decision-making skills, and the ability to tolerate both uncertainty and gender role ambiguities are also indicated as variables correlated with adjustment to migration.

Espin (1987b, 1997) contends that these factors differ significantly, depending on biological sex. Women, for example, most likely played a traditional or subordinate role in their culture and, thus, may not have been consulted about the decision to emigrate. After arriving in the United States, usually they find a vast difference between their concept of appropriate gender roles (especially for women) and what they observe in the United States. They also may discover the possibilities for a different way of living given women's greater access to paid employment (Espin, 1994). When acculturation and adaptation are taking place, "modifications of women's gender roles may be more dramatic than those experienced by men" (Espin, 1987b, p. 281). For immigrant lesbians, this situation may be intensified further because of the newly found permission to "cross boundaries and transform their sexuality and sex roles" (Espin, 1997, p. 192). Some also experience prejudice based on their ethnicity in combination with bias due to their sexual orientation, whereas before migration they experienced discrimination solely because of their biological sex, sometimes on account of their lesbian status but rarely on the basis of their ethnicity.

Because women have been conditioned not to verbalize their distress, these clients often present with a high incidence of somatic complaints that may be symptoms of a masked depression. Their physical difficulties, in fact, may have prompted them to seek the services of a health care provider in the first place. Regardless of biological sex, however, most sexual minority immigrant clients usually have a number of serious concerns apart from difficulties related to their sexual orientation and sadness and depression may be present for years after the migration. Their loss is pervasive in that they have lost all that is predictable, such as friends, networks, routines, familiar foods, and their places in society. Posttraumatic stress reactions are not uncommon and may be manifested through nightmares, numbing of feelings, and overwhelming feelings of guilt.

Language

Language patterns, particularly comfort with the English language, can assist clinicians in classifying clients according to Kitano's (1989) acculturation continuum. In this regard, Morales (1992) believes that determining the frequency with which individuals speak their native language, and identifying those with whom they speak their primary versus secondary languages, can be invaluable in the appraisal of assimilation and acculturation. Individuals born and raised abroad tend to express a strong sense of identification with their country of origin and, subsequently, carry their native language with them throughout life. Further, under stressful conditions, people often revert to their original language as traumatic events are recorded in memory in the "mother tongue." Sexual minority immigrants who were persecuted before leaving their countries of origin may display this pattern in psychotherapy. These clients may have difficulty discussing their trauma in English and may find the services of a bilingual clinician helpful (Carballo-Dieguez, 1989).

Similarly, individuals who have learned English as a second language, whether in their native lands or in the United States, may have acquired a vocabulary in English for the practical matters of living and working. Often, however, they have retained the words of their native tongue to describe profound feelings, and their need to use this language to discuss either trauma or emotion complicates psychotherapy with these clients. The assistance of a native-speaking adjunct or a bilingual translator, hence, might be necessary to enhance treatment outcomes. In many instances, however, actually relating the painful event(s) in English may not be necessary if clients can describe the emotional aspects of the trauma in the (first) language of their "hearts." Although clinicians may not understand all that clients are communicating, their tone of voice, emotional intensity, and body language can provide the therapist with information sufficient to proceed with the resolution and integration of the negative experience(s) in whatever language can be understood by both parties.

On the other hand, bilingual clients may use a second language, such as English, to articulate certain words (especially sexual ones) that they are forbidden to verbalize in their native tongue (Espin, 1987b, 1994, 2000; B. Greene, 1994b). Because language reflects a culture's values, a client's first language may contain few words for *lesbian* or *gay* that are not derogatory, particularly if the culture views a minority sexual orientation negatively. This situation, unfortunately, is common, not only for most foreign-born sexual minority clients but also for those native to the United States who have internalized the heterosexism and homophobia of the dominant society.

In the case of foreign-born clients, however, a splitting of affect and behavior can occur when the *intimacy* and *emotions* related to sexuality (which are experienced in a native language) and sexual *behavior* (which can only be discussed in English) are not brought together or integrated within the context of psychotherapy. Espin (1987b) contends that this compartmentalization "may render unavailable certain areas of the bilingual's intrapsychic world" (p. 287). Further, De la Cancela (1985) believes that verbalizing feelings without describing the related sexual activities may be a burdensome challenge which offers minimal relief to the client. To avoid difficulties with splitting of emotion and conduct, referrals, adjuncts, or translators might be used to enhance psychotherapeutic integration.

Gender Roles and Sexuality

Comparative studies of same-sex practices provide new insights into sexual development because they have raised awareness of cultural influences on sexual expression in radically diverse societies. In many parts of the world, for example, popular terms for males who engage in same-sex behavior, such as *gay, homosexual,* and *bisexual*, have no context. Manalansan (1996) contends that even if the concept were operationalized in a phrase such as *men who have sex with men*, it still "is unable to capture the complex ways in which different cultures provide meanings and structures for such phenomena" (p. 393). He believes that sociocultural and phenomenological perceptions of sexual practices influence definition such that a first-generation Latino man from Venezuela who has sex with other men may be viewed by himself and others as heterosexual if he is married and maintains the active (or inserter) position in same-sex anal intercourse. Manalansan argues further that in the Harlem Black community, roles or types, such as the Latino categories of *pasivo* and *activo*, are not based on sexual activities but, rather, on the ability of the man to reverse roles in sexual situations. The gay orientation of an effeminate man, therefore, can still be overlooked if he is able to be flexible sexually and if he makes significant contributions to the Black community.

G. Herdt (1988) illustrates the variability of same-sex contacts globally and describes four forms found cross-culturally: age-structured homosexual behavior, gender-transformed homosexual practice, role-specialized homosexuality, and the modern gay movement. He also notes that bisexuality has different meanings in Western and non-Western settings and provides a linking framework for understanding classificatory schemes of homosexuality around the world (G. Herdt, 1990). In addition, in certain far-flung societies of Melanesia, Amazonia, central Africa, and western Egypt, sexual relations between adult and adolescent males are considered part of parenting and the maturation process (Adam, 1985). Finally, as discussed later in this chapter, the gender-transforming *berdaches* in North American tribal cultures were assigned specialized roles of mediation between the sexes as well as between the material and spiritual worlds. Given the variability of definitions, then, clinicians must take care to inquire about the meanings attached to sexuality, as well as same-sex orientation and behavior, in their clients' native culture(s). The dynamics presented could be viewed unknowingly from a biased, distorted, or uninformed perspective without this information.

Sexuality, for example, is a taboo topic that is rarely discussed in Asian cultures (C. S. Chan, 1992). Disclosure of a gay, lesbian, or bisexual identity, therefore, brings to the surface the subjects of sex, sexuality, and sexual orientation and usually implies that the person disclosing is sexually active. Parents and family members of Asian American sexual minorities often have as much difficulty acknowledging the sexual activity as the sexual orientation of their loved one. Focusing on the more overt sexuality, however, facilitates the avoidance or ignorance of the even more forbidden topic of being bisexual, gay, or lesbian.

Similarly, heterosexist masculine and feminine gender roles are assigned rigidly in most Hispanic cultures (Morales, 1992). As in Asian societies, open discussion of sex and sexuality between women is prohibited and women are expected to be sexually naive (Espin, 1984). Adolescent females, in particular, are encouraged to have *amigas intimas* (intimate female friends), as these relationships can serve to protect their virginity by diminishing their contact with males (Espin, 1984; Hidalgo & Hidalgo-Christensen, 1976; Ramos, 1994). Women perform sexual relations out of duty to their husbands; thus a lesbian orientation forces a culture that generally denies the sexuality of women to confront forbidden behavior directly.

Conversely, there is a known tolerance for same-sex relations among Hispanic males as long as it is not overtly labeled "homosexual" (B. Greene, 1994b). Just as women are expected to be pure, men must be macho and are "expected to have a sexual debut at a young age and to maintain a fairly promiscuous sexual behavior through life" (Carballo-Dieguez, 1989, p. 29). The sexual urges of Latino men supposedly are difficult to control and require frequent discharge. A macho man with a reputation for heterosexuality can be "forgiven" if he uses a *maricon* (faggot) to satisfy his sexual needs because, as discussed previously, sexual conduct is determined by the "masculinity" of the performance; for example, "Men who insert their penises are regarded as masculine; those who receive them are viewed as feminine and degraded" (Garnets & Kimmel, 1991, p. 158). Male-with-male sexual behavior, therefore, is tolerated if it is seen as manly but shamed and stigmatized if it is womanly in nature. Similarly, masculinized or "butch" lesbians who defy gender roles are subject to prejudice.

SPECIFIC POPULATIONS

Although members of all minority racial/cultural groups share numerous similarities of experience, such factors as ancestral heritage, country of origin, and cultural norms create differences between them (Garnets & Kimmel, 1991). This section highlights some of these elements that psychotherapists might observe in bisexual, lesbian, or gay clients from four major populations. In addition, consideration is given to the role of gender in each separate culture and its influence on the socialization of sexual minority men and women within that population.

African Americans

The African American community, in general, places a high value on the extended family, interrelatedness, religion, and parenthood (A. Smith, 1997), and gender roles are somewhat more flexible than in the majority culture and in many other ethnic minority groups. B. Greene (1994b, 1997) believes this partially is a derivative of the more egalitarian nature of many precolonial African tribes, as well as the high value placed on interdependence. While the need to adapt to slavery and racism made cooperation essential for those brought to the Western hemisphere as slaves, not all clients of African descent were born in the United States. Some, for example, were raised in Jamaica, Haiti, Trinidad, Puerto Rico, or other Caribbean countries and may be quite different culturally from each other, as well as from those with origins in the United States. Further, although the majority of Black Americans are from Baptist or Pentecostal religious traditions, some of them are Episcopalian or Catholic, much like a considerable number of those from West Indian nations. Interpretation of Christian scripture regarding homosexuality sometimes differs according to membership in one of these groups. Some believers, for example, select a certain set of biblical passages to castigate a gay or lesbian family member, whereas others cite different texts to justify his or her continuing acceptance (A. Smith, 1997).

Heterosexual relationships begin relatively early for many African Americans whereas other forms of sexual expression, such as masturbation, oral sex, and homosexuality, are less accepted, often for both religious and familial reasons (Wilson, 1986). Numerous authors have written about this intolerance of gay and lesbian sexuality, as well as about homophobic attitudes in the African American subculture (Adams & Kimmel, 1997; Capitanio, 1995; B. Greene, 1994b; Gutierrez & Dworkin, 1992; Icard, 1985/1986; B. E. Jones & Hill, 1996; Loiacano, 1989; Manalansan, 1996; Mays, Cochran, & Rhue, 1993; Peplau, Cochran, & Mays, 1997; J. L. Peterson, 1992).

B. E. Jones and Hill (1996) believe that attitudes of Black citizens about homosexuality gradually are changing in a positive direction, as indicated by discussion of the previously unmentionable topic in the African American media, by inclusion of gay, lesbian, and bisexual individuals in ethnically oriented political coalitions and in a few Black churches, and by antidiscrimination clauses in most African American civil rights organizations. They contend, further, that these more favorable perceptions reflect attitudes toward homosexuality in the broader society but also have developed because the increased incidence of HIV infection in Black men and women has forced many in the African American community to face the existence of homosexuality and bisexuality among its members. Negative feelings toward homosexuality continue to be prevalent, however, and the following three studies illustrate attempts to document the extent of prejudice empirically.

Accordingly, Bonilla and Porter (1990) surveyed 216 Hispanic, 1,005 Black, and 3,760 White adults and found that Blacks were less tolerant than the other ethnic/cultural groups regarding the morality of homosexuality. On the other hand, negative attitudes toward homosexuality were detected to be widespread among 391 Black heterosexual adults but were not more prevalent than among a comparison sample of Whites (Capitanio, 1995). Predictably (see Chapter 1), men's attitudes toward gay men were more negative than their feelings about lesbians or women's sentiments about gay men.

A final study compared the degree of disapproval of Blacks and Whites toward homosexuality in 2,006 employees of eight mental health facilities (Ernst, Francis, Nevels, & Lemeh, 1991). Data revealed less social tolerance of sexual minorities in the African American community than among Whites. This was particularly true among Black females, a finding that was contradicted by Capitanio's (1995) survey. Ernst et al. (1991), nevertheless, speculated that the attitudes of these women might have been shaped by the perception of a shortage of available Black men created partially by racially disproportionate incarceration rates and relatively high rates of premature death. To them, homosexuality seemed to be conceptualized as a "non-Afrocentric lifestyle originating in slavery and penal rape and contributing to a shortage of marriageable men" (Franklin, 1998, p. 18).

Many other African Americans also perceive homosexuality as a threat to their survival but for different reasons (Adams & Kimmel, 1997; Garnets & Kimmel, 1991). After having lived through generations of slavery, persecution, oppression, and numerous attempts to destroy them as individuals and as a culture, they place a strong value on the continuity of the heritage. Sexuality is viewed as a natural part of life that leads to childbearing, and individuals who do not engage in procreative sex are seen as contributing to racial genocide by not participating in the propagation of the race. According to some African Americans, childless gay Black men "are race traitors who can be symbolically absorbed into the social category of the privileged White homosexual" (Franklin, 1998, p. 19). African American lesbians, on the other hand, "are more likely to have had extensive heterosexual experience . . . and to have had prior heterosexual marriages and children" than are Anglo lesbians (Mays et al., 1993, p. 12).

Racism and Heterosexism

Internalized racism, separately or in combination with some of the factors discussed previously, also contributes to the devaluing of same-sex orientations in the African American culture. Historically in the United States, vast biological, moral, and intellectual differences were thought to exist between Caucasians and people of color, primarily Africans, and any genetic mixing of these supposedly different races was thought to create biological aberrations (Diggs, 1993). Mulattos, accordingly, were characterized as weak and degenerate intermediates between races whose infusion of Caucasian blood saved them from savagery. As Diggs (1993) reports, they "became the symbol of the consequence of transgressing the boundaries of species, either socially or sexually" (p. 7).

Diggs (1993) further hypothesizes that, in this transgression of normality, the pathologies of the mulatto and the homosexual intersected in that each had "confused the boundaries of the two-color or two-gender concept of the human species" (p. 8). Light-skinned African Americans and sexual minorities both shared undetectable, hidden taints which, if discovered, could have extremely negative repercussions not only in the dominant culture but also in the Black community which had internalized many of its views. Because of this potential oppression, both mulattos and sexual minorities lived in constant fear of being exposed or "outed" and employed constant surveillance to protect their shameful secrets. Although many in both populations established oral traditions about "coming out," few did so voluntarily given the consequences. As such, racism and heterosexism existed conjointly in the views of both the dominant culture and in the African American community.

Cultural Conflict

As mentioned previously, the sexual minority community is seen by many gay, lesbian, and bisexual African Americans as a White Eurocentric establishment with little interest in their concerns (Adams & Kimmel, 1997; B. E. Jones & Hill, 1996). Black lesbians, moreover, have been referred to as a "minority within a minority" (B. Greene, 1986) because they are not only members of an ethnic/cultural minority in the dominant culture but often experience themselves as unseen minority members in the primarily White lesbian community. Likewise, many Black men believe they must live a "double identity" and be relatively invisible in the gay community in order to avoid discrimination and rejection (e.g., Manalansan, 1996). African American sexual minorities, hence, often minimize their ethnicity in their associations with other gay, bisexual, and lesbian individuals and their sexual orientation when interacting with their own ethnic minority group. These people, as a result, often experience immense stress and anxiety as they "stand painfully juxtaposed between the fear of cultural estrangement from the African American community and the fear of racial and ethnic alienation from the gay and lesbian community" (B. E. Jones & Hill, 1996, p. 549).

African American sexual minorities, on the other hand, generally are accepted by others of their ethnicity if they lead socially constructive lives and make contributions to their families and to the Black community. This tolerance, however, is granted only if they remain silent about their homosexuality (B. E. Jones & Hill, 1996; Manalansan, 1996). Because "the strength of African American family ties often mitigate against outright rejection of gay and lesbian family members despite clear rejection of gay and lesbian sexual orientations" (B. Greene, 1997a, p. 224), most follow the norms of their subculture by not speaking of their homosexuality with their families who may be quite aware that members are lesbian or gay (Peplau et al., 1997). Maintaining this silence (and living with the often-accompanying feelings of separateness) allows them to take advantage of the powerful ties that connect both nuclear and extended family members in multiple networks of commitment and support (Boykin, 1998; B. Greene 1996; B. Greene & Boyd-Franklin, 1996a, 1996b).

On the other hand, a survey of 506 African American lesbians and 673 gay men revealed that most of these individuals had disclosed their sexual orientation to immediate family members, including mothers, fathers, and siblings (Mays, Chatters, Cochran, & Mackness, 1998). They had disclosed to fewer other relatives, and there was a clear preference to coming out first to females in the immediate family. Those who were older and reported initiating homosexual activity at a younger age were more likely to have disclosed to both immediate and distant family members.

Lesbians

Black lesbians frequently encounter racism, sexism, and homophobia in their experiences with others (B. Greene & Boyd-Franklin, 1996a, 1996b; Mays et al., 1993). B. Greene (1994b) discusses the fact that African American women do not fit the traditional stereotypes of the fragile, weak, and dependent female because slavery and racism have forced them to be stronger as well as more independent and assertive than their White counterparts. Hence, "they came to be defined as all of the things that normal women were not supposed to be" (p. 398). She further contends that prototypes depicting lesbians as masculinized women intersect with stereotypes of African American women in this regard, as both are viewed as "defective females who want to be or act like men" (p. 398). Due to sexism in both the Black and dominant cultures, and racism in the broader society, African American women often find themselves at the bottom of the racial and gender power structures. Heterosexual privilege, hence, may be the only social advantage available to them.

Being lesbian, further, is regarded as generally inconsistent with the role expectations of women in the Black community, given their lack of submissiveness to males (Loiacano, 1989). Because of their gender role discordance, they frequently are considered "not sufficiently subordinate to African American men," who, in turn, believe that strong women, not racist institutions, are responsible for their oppression (B. Greene, 1994b, p. 398). Even if lesbians often feel like outsiders within their own Black culture, most are attached firmly to their heritage. In fact, when both lesbians and gay men are asked about the relative potency of their identities, they frequently cite their African American lineage as primary and their sexual orientation as secondary (B. Greene, 1994b, 1997a).

Further, when they need help or support, African American lesbians usually turn to heterosexuals in the Black community rather than to members of the White lesbian population. Cochran and Mays (1986), accordingly, surveyed 450 Black lesbians and found that the women generally relied first on other African Americans rather than on White lesbians for such matters as driving them to the train station or airport, helping with running errands, loaning small and large amounts of money, waiting for a repair person, or asking to live with them if they were too sick or injured to care for themselves. When they truly needed assistance or support, in other words, these Black lesbians initially would turn to members of their own ethnic group.

Asian Americans

Asians are among the fastest growing ethnic/cultural groups in the United States, and as a result of large immigrations, the characteristics of Asian Americans have changed radically in recent years. With the exception of the Japanese, all other Asian groups consist primarily of foreign-born individuals. Indochinese have entered in record numbers, and thousands of Filipinos and Chinese likewise have immigrated. A large number of these immigrants left their countries of origin because of extremely harsh, dangerous, and oppressive conditions, and many continue to be victims of prejudice and discrimination in America. Among all major ethnic designations, Asian Americans are the most heterogeneous population. In fact, "some twenty-nine distinct subgroups that differ in language, religion, and values have been officially identified in the United States" (D. R. Atkinson et al., 1993, p. 195). In spite of these vast subgroup differences, however, many similarities exist between the various Asian populations. Several of these are discussed next and those characteristics that strongly affect the lives of individuals with same-sex orientations are highlighted.

Many aspects of Asian American and African American cultures are similar, specifically, the primacy of the family and community, cultural assumptions regarding definite roles for men and women, proscriptions against differences in behavior and identity, widespread homophobia, and pervasive heterosexism (C. S. Chan, 1989, 1992; B. Greene, 1997a; Liu & Chan, 1996; Nakajima et al., 1996). Shame, however, plays a bigger part in Asian cultures and dishonoring the family is to be avoided at all costs, especially in Confucian-oriented cultures. Even as adults with spouses and children of their own, individuals are expected to place their parents and families of origin above all other loyalties.

The primary purpose of marriage is to continue the family line, and, historically, in most Asian countries, it has not been considered a romantic affair. Unions often have been prearranged by family members to increase family kinship linkages, although these transactions are rare for assimilated Asian Americans. Men, but not women, theoretically are free to find romantic love or to have affairs with either men or women outside the marriage (Nakajima et al., 1996). Many sexual minorities, however, continue to accommodate their families by entering into a heterosexual marriage because "if a daughter or son is lesbian or gay, the child is seen as not only rejecting the traditional social role as a wife-mother or husband-father, but even worse, as also rejecting the importance of family and Asian cultural values" (Chan, 1992, p. 117). Because discussions of sex are taboo, open acknowledgment of a minority sexual orientation is seen as an act of overt rebellion which brings great shame on the family. In addition, disclosure is not only viewed as a rejection of the lineage but also as a failure on the part of one's parents. The mother is to be particularly blamed because she is considered responsible by family and peers for the appropriate socialization of the children (B. Greene, 1994b, 1997a).

C. S. Chan (1992) contends that sexual minority Asian American clients describe to psychotherapists issues with two common themes: the fear of family rejection for being gay or lesbian and the anticipation of complete parental misunderstanding. Clients further report feeling selfish or guilty for choosing a personal life instead of one that would please their elders. Gay men may feel this guilt or "loss of face" especially keenly since, in Confucian tradition, "men are the carriers of the family name, kinship linkage, and family heritage" (Garnets & Kimmel, 1991, p. 159). In this regard, Wooden, Kawasaki, and Mayeda (1983) studied 13 Japanese American gay men and found that only half of them had disclosed their sexual orientation to their families, and their gay identity development on the Cass (1979) model reflected reservations about synthesizing all aspects of their identity. The authors suggest that the men's reluctance to be more visibly and actively gay could be explained partially by their fears of rejection by family and community.

Similarly, C. S. Chan (1989) surveyed 35 highly educated lesbian and gay Asian Americans (ages 21 to 36) who reported that disclosing their sexual orientation to their parents was the most difficult task of their "coming-out" process. In fact, 26 (74%) had not yet done so at the time the study questionnaire was distributed, and 77% felt it was harder to "come out" to other Asian Americans than to lesbians or gay men because of the high risk of rejection and stigmatization. More than half of Chan's subjects said that even the existence of sexual minorities among Asians was denied when asked to describe their ethnic group's perception of gay and lesbian Asian Americans. One person commented that there was no frame of reference to understand homosexuality in his or her culture. C. S. Chan (1997) notes, accordingly, that modern homosexual identities are Western constructs and that there are no comparable sexual identities in Asian cultures. The entire concept, in fact, "may be literally inconceivable except to those who are relatively highly acculturated into a Western identity" (p. 246).

Cultural Clash

Just as C. S. Chan's (1989) 35 respondents felt fairly invisible within their Asian American communities, they also seemed to share a perception that the gay and lesbian population did not acknowledge their existence either. When asked in which community they participated in social or political events, 26 individuals (74%) said they engaged in these kinds of activities only with other lesbians or gay men, 9 (26%) participated with both groups, and no subject reported that he or she shared in these activities only with other (presumably heterosexual) Asian Americans; 20 (57%) described feeling more comfortable in the gay and lesbian community than in their ethnic minority group. Surprisingly, however, given the high rates of participation and comfort reported, 30 (86%) said that they did not feel acknowledged and accepted in the gay and lesbian community. Apparently, like a considerable number of other sexual minority people of color, many did not feel totally comfortable in either group. Unlike African Americans, however, "when a choice of identification is required, more respondents identified themselves as lesbian or gay than as Asian American" (p. 128). Seven (20%) refused to choose because it would mean denying an important part of their identity.

Like members of other ethnic minorities, many Asians see homosexuality as a White Western phenomenon, or as an outcome of too much assimilation and a consequence of losing touch with Asian tradition (B. Greene, 1994b, 1997a). This Eurocentric focus of the gay and lesbian community, as well as the pervasive heterosexism in their own ethnic group, leaves many sexual minority Asian Americans feeling marginalized and caught between two conflicting cultures (Nakajima et al., 1996). "Similar intricate and complex conflicts of loyalty are also observed in lesbians [and presumably gay men] of color from other ethnic groups" (B. Greene, 1994b, p. 406). Because gay and lesbian Asian Americans challenge deeply embedded cultural assumptions about gender roles, they have difficulty conforming to the traditional expectations of family and community. They likewise hold different world views than those of European origin who tend to predominate in the lesbian, gay, and bisexual communities.

Further, individuals designated "Asian" are from many ethnic or cultural groups, such as Filipino, Chinese, Japanese, Korean, Vietnamese, Indian, and numerous other Southeast Asian heritages, as well as from various linguistic backgrounds, socioeconomic classes, and religions (e.g., Confucianism, Buddhism, Taoism, Hinduism, and Islam) within these populations (Manalansan, 1996; Nakajima et al., 1996; Ratti, 1993). There may be very few commonalities, hence, between "a bisexual fourth-generation Japanese American woman and a recently emigrated gay man from Pakistan" (Nakajima et al., 1996, p. 564). Because they have been socialized in dissimilar cultures and even subcultures, sexual minority "Asian" Americans may even be somewhat alienated from each other; or, rather than feeling torn between two cultures, they may experience cultural clash or dissimilarity with several of them.

Lesbians

C. S. Chan (1989) argues that the "passive but exotic" sexual stereotype of Asian women may be so strong that the possibility that they "could be lesbian may not even enter into the picture" (p. 19). Garnets and Kimmel's (1991) summary of the literature supports this denial of the existence of lesbianism in Asian communities. In fact, these writers conclude that if women do acknowledge their same-sex orientation, they are "perceived as tarnishing the family honor by not being dutiful daughters, by rejecting the role of wife and mother, and by rejecting the role of passive reliance and deference to men and the submersion of identity within the family structure" (p. 159). Due to this expectation for passivity and submissiveness, C. S. Chan (1989) contends that many Asian American women, regardless of their sexual orientation, feel discriminated against based on their ethnicity and gender. In this regard, the 19 lesbians in C. S. Chan's (1989) aforementioned study of 35 sexual minority Asians reported that they experienced more discrimination because they were of Asian descent than because they were lesbians.

An unmarried Asian woman, regardless of her age, is considered part of her family of origin, with her father often feeling responsible for her welfare. She also has no identity of her own (let alone a *sexual* identity) until she is married. "Asian American lesbians, because they are not married in the traditional sense, are rarely considered to have separated from their families, regardless of financial or professional status" (C. S. Chan, 1992, p. 120). Further, having an unmarried daughter often brings shame to a family, as well as blame to the mother for not raising her daughter appropriately (B. Greene, 1994b). Rejection of a lesbian child is not uncommon because Asian parents frequently refuse to acknowledge that their daughter is "anything but a sexually active unmarried woman" who is no longer "fit to become married or to be a real part of the family again" (p. 122). Those who openly identify as lesbian, thus, are likely to be those who are relatively assimilated into Western culture and ideas and feel safe in non-Asian environments (C. S. Chan, 1997).

Hispanics/Latinos and Latinas

There is no single label that describes adequately this ethnically, racially, and linguistically diverse group that includes individuals of Mexican, Spanish, Puerto Rican, Cuban, and Central and South American descent. The lack of more explicit terminology necessitates the interchangeable use in this section of the *Hispanic* and *Latino/Latina* designations when speaking of people linked by a somewhat common cultural heritage that espouses *la familia* as its core central value (Gonzalez & Espin, 1996). Reference is made to specific countries of origin, though, when it is appropriate to do so.

Hispanics, as a combined population, "are the fastest growing ethnic minority in America" (D. R. Atkinson et al., 1993, p. 241). These individuals tend to cluster together in the United States (90% live in nine states), generally reside in densely populated urban areas, have comparatively elevated birth rates, and suffer from the same problems of poverty and high unemployment that confront other ethnic/cultural minorities living in inner cities. Because the ancestral immigrants of many Latinos/Latinas originated in nonindustrial and agrarian-based countries, they often lack the vocational and linguistic skills needed in a technological society. The major exception to this commonality was the first wave of Cuban immigrants who were middle class and educationally specialized when they migrated. Some other foreign-born Latinos/Latinas also were raised in middle- and upper-middle-class families in their own countries; nonetheless, their lack of English and stalemates with professional licensing boards, in addition to societal and workplace discrimination, have resulted in low socioeconomic circumstances for many of them (Morales, 1992).

The heterogeneity of Hispanics is mediated further by their generational standing in the United States, degree of assimilation, biculturalism, language preference (e.g., English, Spanish, Portuguese, indigenous languages, or mixtures and variations of these), gender, racial mix, and political status as native or documented/undocumented immigrant (Comas-Diaz, 1990; Espin, 1997, Gonzalez & Espin, 1996). Refugees comprise a large number of those arriving from Central America, particularly El Salvador, Honduras, and

Nicaragua, and their profiles tend to differ from other Latino/Latina groups. Due to civil wars in their countries, they have come to the United States following a history of oppression and exploitation, often without preparation or support from abroad. Many have severe emotional problems resulting from the traumas of war and torture, such as suspiciousness, paranoia, depression, hopelessness, and helplessness (Comas-Diaz, 1990). In these ways, they may resemble refugees from the conflicts in Indochinese countries and other parts of the world. Homosexuality in Latin cultures exists against this vast backdrop of situational variance and emotional complexity and, to Gonzalez and Espin (1996), invokes "a fictional category that cannot possibly contain the diversity of motivations, behaviors, identities, and institutions that it purports to name" (p. 583).

As with Asians, the boundaries of kinship extend beyond the nuclear family in Hispanic cultures (B. Greene, 1997a). This *familismo* (familism) emphasizes interdependence, affiliation, and cooperation and usually includes numerous individuals in the extended family. Grandparents are honored as especially integral, and godparents (who function as coparents) are regarded as *compadre* or *comadre*, or part of the family. Other people close to the family might include aunts, uncles, cousins, people from the same hometown, or even good old friends (Carballo-Dieguez, 1989). *Simpatia* requires social politeness and smooth relations and considers confrontation as offensive and improper. Somewhat similarly, *respeto* refers to the need to treat others, especially the elderly, with dignity and respect. Gender roles are rigid and clearly defined. Men's behavior, in this regard, is governed by *machismo*, which pertains to a code of virility and masculine conduct that prizes aggressiveness, invulnerability, and sexual prowess, as well as to the responsibility of a man to protect, defend, and provide for his family (Gonzalez & Espin, 1996; Morales, 1996). According to this standard, bisexuality does not make a man homosexual as long as he plays the appropriate masculine penetrative sex role. *Marianismo* (referring to the Virgin Mary) is the female counterpart of *machismo* and defines conduct for pure and good women, who are supposed to be self-sacrificing mothers and subservient to men. This rigid dichotomy of gender "operates not only between heterosexual partners but also informs how homoerotic desire plays out in Latino cultures" (Gonzalez & Espin, 1996, p. 587). Morales (1992) contends further that all Hispanic cultural values that define the nature of relationships with family, friends, and community affect the socialization of Latina lesbians and Latino gay men.

Cultural Conflict

Several writers (Espin, 1984, 1987a; B. Greene, 1997a; Hidalgo & Hidalgo-Christensen, 1976; Morales, 1992) claim that the Latino/Latina community has more negative attitudes toward sexual minorities than does the dominant culture. They also suggest that this pervasive heterosexist influence and oppression within Hispanic cultures leaves many lesbians and gay men feeling an intense need to remain closeted because "coming out" frequently is perceived as analogous to an act of treason against family and culture. Although leading a double life carries a heavy psychological burden, most choose this option rather than risk the loss of contact with their ethnic community and lack of support for their Hispanic identity (Espin, 1987a, 1997).

Like other sexual minority people of color, gay Latinos and Latina lesbians often feel caught between the strong rejection of same-sex orientations in their ethnic group and the racism of the predominately Caucasian lesbian and gay community. The strongly interdependent Hispanic culture exerts a powerful influence in the lives of many, and these individuals often fear stigmatization by fellow Latinos and Latinas far more than they fear rejection by mainstream society. In describing this difficult situation, Espin (1987a) contends that "coming out to self and others in the context of a sexist and heterosexist American society is compounded by coming out in the context of a heterosexist and sexist Latin culture immersed in racist society" (p. 35).

Regarding the "polycultural" integration of their cultural, racial, and religious identities with their self-concepts as lesbians and women, Espin (1987a) questioned 16 highly educated lesbians of Cuban descent. Fifteen of the women had been born in Cuba and most had immigrated to the United States during their childhood years. All had come to the United States prior to age 22 and were from various socioeconomic backgrounds. Although 14 had been raised Catholic, only 3 of the 16 subjects were practicing their religion at the time of the survey. (They were members of Dignity, a national organization of gay and lesbian Catholics.) When asked if being lesbian or being Cuban was more important to them, 12 responded that both were equally important. Most of the women, however, reluctantly chose to be among Anglo lesbians rather than among heterosexual Latinas and Latinos. According to Espin (1987a), "even when they believe that it is easier to be Cuban among lesbians than it is to be lesbian among Cubans, they do not feel fully comfortable not being both. In fact, what most of them say is that they feel more whole when they can be out both as Cubans and as lesbians" (p. 48). Thus, rather than having to choose between their two cultures, they would prefer a single identity that includes all facets of themselves.

Various Hispanic gay and lesbian community organizations designed to help individuals integrate their identities exist in cities around the country (see Resources section). For example, LLEGO (the National Latino/Latina Lesbian and Gay Organization) is headquartered in Washington, DC. La Red (the network) or the Lesbica y Homosexual del Continente Americano (a Latin American lesbian and gay human rights association) is situated in Los Angeles and not only provides support but also serves political and human rights functions. La Red specifically was founded in 1991 to address the problems of sexual minorities in light of the abuse and repression committed against them by governments and religious institutions throughout the Western hemisphere. As such, it exposes specific incidents of violence and oppression against lesbians and gay men anywhere in the Americas.

Lesbians

As discussed previously, gender roles are applied rigidly in Latin cultures, and women are expected to be submissive to their male superiors, respectful, and sexually virtuous (Greene, 1997a). Making a lesbian orientation public not only disregards these cultural prescriptions but others as well. For example, the value of *simpatia* (smooth relations and avoidance of conflict) is violated because the disclosure is seen as a form of direct and willful confrontation. Further, the family has lost face and parents, grandparents, and other *compadres* and *comadres* have not been granted proper respect (*respeto)*.

Espin (1987a) notes that Hispanic families tend to treat their lesbian members with silent tolerance and rarely with overt rejection. Although these women are not denied a place in the family, neither is there open acknowledgment of a lesbian sexual orientation. Both sides seem to consent to an informal pact not to discuss the issue with each other.

Because Latina lesbians are generally "single" and self-supporting, their families (like those of African American lesbians) tend to rely on them for assistance and advocacy for themselves or for the group. For both them and their families, then, disclosure that their *amistad intima*, or close friendship, includes erotic attraction could jeopardize not only family relationships but also the possibility of providing service to the Hispanic community (Espin, 1987a; Gonzalez & Espin, 1996).

Lesbian writer Cherrie Moraga (1983) contends that it was due to her sexual orientation that she learned about silence and oppression. It was also through her lesbianism that she was able to identify and empathize with her mother's oppression as a poor and uneducated Chicana. Given the fixed hierarchy in Latin cultures of male dominance and female subordination, Hispanics generally view both outspoken women and Latina lesbians (who are recognized as such only if they are masculinized to some degree) as a threat to the established order of their culture (Gonzalez & Espin, 1996). In this regard, Trujillo (1991) asserts that the open acknowledgment of lesbians has the potential to raise the consciousness of all Latina women and cause them to question the assumptions of female inferiority and male supremacy. If this is a possibility, those who shape the norms of the culture have every reason to keep women who love women silent and invisible.

Native Americans

Native American populations are as diverse as Asian American and Hispanic communities in the United States. The federal government recognizes some 505–511 American Indian tribes, and states identify an additional 365 native bands and clans. Between 150 and 200 tribal languages are still spoken today. Individuals of Native American ancestry are dispersed throughout the country with approximately half residing in urban areas and one-quarter living on reservations. People from different tribes may be quite dissimilar from each other, just as those raised in cities may differ from those living or raised on reservations.

Whom is considered to be a Native American varies according to whether the Bureau of Indian Affairs, the United States Bureau of the Census, or the particular tribe assigns the classification. Some who designate themselves as American Indian live in cities, speak only English, and feel minimal identification with their culture or tribe. Others are quite traditional, speak and think in their native language, and comprehend little English. In between these two polarities are individuals who primarily are acculturated in their Native traditions but function adequately in the dominant culture, as well as people who marginally are assimilated into mainstream society while only tangentially identify with their tribe. Although this latter group often has considerable difficulty coping with both worlds, other Native Americans are truly bicultural and move between their tribal heritage and the dominant culture with relative ease (LaFromboise, Trimble, & Mohatt, 1993).

Regardless of locale of residence or tribal background, however, unemployment is extremely high, with the mean hovering at around 30% for reservation Indians. In addition, the average educational level of Native Americans is the lowest of any major ethnic group, school dropout rates are high, and nearly one-third of all adults are classified as illiterate (LaFromboise, 1988; Thomason, 1991). Native children were forbidden to attend public schools prior to the 1930s and were required to attend federal boarding schools. This resulted in young people often being removed from their families and tribes at 6 years of age. As of 1994, fully 25% of these children were still attending these boarding schools and they continue to have "a devastating impact on Native American lives, deliberately interfering with language, culture, spirituality, and sexuality" (Tafoya, 1996, p. 610).

The radical disruption of American Indian tribal culture and heritage has made Native people "aliens in their own land" (LaFromboise, 1988, p. 124) for more than 100 years. The result of being constrained on reservations, compelled to leave the tribe and attend boarding school, or forced to acculturate to urban living has had not only educational consequences but also various psychosocial effects. Many individuals, for example, are confronted with an extremely large number of stressors which include prolonged unemployment and subsequent poverty, substandard housing, malnutrition, and inadequate health care. Preliminary research, basically anecdotal at this point, further indicates that sexual abuse, including intergenerational incestual abuse, is high (Tafoya, 1996). The results of living with these kinds of antagonistic conditions often are shortened life expectancies, depression, alcoholism, drug abuse, and elevated suicide rates. Incidences of delinquency and arrest are here among the highest of any ethnic group.

In spite of the destruction of their societies and the adverse social, physical, and emotional aftereffects, the majority of Native people are bound tightly to their tribes and families and the primary basis for identity remains their ethnicity (Tafoya, 1996). This cohesion is particularly strong during times of crisis. When problems arise for individuals, the family, kin, and friends come together to draw those who are suffering out of isolation and back into the social life of the clan. Thus, "the collective treatment of psychologically troubled individuals in tribal groups not only serves to heal the individual but also reaffirm the norms of the entire group" (LaFromboise, 1988, p. 133). Often, traditional healers, who are viewed as safekeepers of ancient legends, are called on to assist the tribe in restoring well-being to people with "excessively individualistic behavior" so that they can live harmoniously with nature by following the traditions of the clan. Those in such disharmony are thus helped to develop "the discipline necessary for the maintenance of cultural values and community respect" (p. 132).

Healers

These healers, medicine men and women, or value keepers of the tribe, have been viewed as doctors, historians, counselors, and spiritual leaders. In the past, they usually were held in high esteem; served as couriers, guides, priests and priestesses, prophets, warriors, peace mediators, and communicators with the spirit world; and performed complex rituals that invoked the spirit world in restoring health and unifying the physical, social, psychological, and spiritual aspects of the afflicted person's being (Grahn, 1986). Accordingly, "prevention and intervention always have a religious and cosmological framework; the medicine man [or woman] both prays and doctors. Religion and psychology intertwine" (LaFromboise et al., 1993, p. 148).

These healers were thought of as "two-spirited people," which is "a term that can encompass alternative sexuality, alternative gender, and an integration of Native spirituality" (Tafoya, 1996, p. 603). These individuals, regardless of biological sex, possessed the female and male spirit. Before European colonialism, "physical anatomy was not inextricably linked to gender roles and that mixed, third gender, or alternative gender roles were at one time accepted and integrated into tribal life" (B. Greene, 1994b, p. 401). Estimates are that well over half of the surviving North American Native languages, for example, have terms for tribal members who were not completely male or female. The concept of sexuality and gender, hence, did not include such mutually exclusive polarities as female and male or homosexual and heterosexual. An individual's sexuality, rather, was viewed along a continuum and a wide range of sexual and gender behaviors was acceptable (Tafoya, 1992, 1996). Edward Carpenter (1987), a 19th and early 20th century British writer, referred to these individuals as *intermediate types* who "became students of life and nature, inventors and teachers of arts and crafts, or wizards . . . and sorcerers; they became diviners and seers or revealers of the gods and religion; and they became medicine-men and healers, prophets and prophetesses" (p. 160).

Jacobs (1968) studied the 99 tribes that kept written records before the European colonists arrived on American soil. Of these 99 clans, 88 made specific reference to same-sex behavior, and 21 described the functions of two-spirit, cross-dressing people who assumed the labor, clothing, and social rank of the other sex while establishing sexual and even marital relationships with their own sex (Grahn, 1986). In 12 of the 21 tribes, these individuals were the medicine people or shamans of the group, and the Crow, Cheyenne, Dakota, and Illinois tribes used them for high spiritual ceremonies. They were referred to by close to 150 different names, some of which translate to mean hermaphrodites, lesbians, priests, magicians, men-witch-women, not-men/not-women, and manly hearted women. Families often felt honored by having such a sacred person among their members because that individual brought wealth and success to the entire kinship (Grahn, 1986; Roscoe, 1987a).

Jacobs examined only the tribes of the United States. The Gay American Indian (GAI) history project investigated the existence of the *berdache*, cross-dressing individuals, from the Arctic Circle to Central America and found references to these people in more than 130 North American societies (Roscoe, 1987b). W. L. Williams (1996), on the other hand, located and studied androgynous or *two-spirit people* in the continental United States, Alaska, Canada, Mexico, Indonesia, Thailand, Polynesia, the Philippines, and on three of Hawaii's islands. Tafoya (1996) and W. L. Williams (1996) argue against the term *berdache* to describe any of these Native people because it was imported into various lands by Europeans and has the implication of an effeminate male who was the recipient of anal intercourse. They contend that this concept is misleading because it excludes individuals who were biologically female, is a term not present in the languages of Native people, and confounds differences in sexual and gender-related activities and roles. They suggest that the designation *two-spirit people* is more accurate because it "prompts a different way of thinking about the association between homoeroticism and the sacred" (W. L. Williams, 1996, p. 417)].

The tribes (11 of the 99 who kept written records) which Jacobs (1968) reported having denied the presence of any form of homosexuality all lived along the East Coast, which was the area of the country with the longest contact with White settlers and Christianity. Grahn (1986) and Tafoya (1996) contend that the heaviest persecution of homosexuals in Spain and other European countries coincided with the most intense period of colonization of Native Americans. The European missionary attitude toward sexual variance was one of intolerance and condemnation (W. L. Williams, 1996), and when settlers entered Indian villages, they often first killed the cross-dressing people before annihilating the others. The Spanish explorer Balboa, in fact, took the lives of biologically male two-spirit people of California tribes by unleashing wild dogs to attack what he referred to as "sodomites." Even when they were not murdered outright, these gender nonconforming individuals often were scorned, insulted, belittled, mocked, ridiculed, shamed, and persecuted. They, in turn, sometimes disguised their identities or "changed their behavior for the sake of their people's safety" (Grahn, 1986, p. 45).

Cultural Clash

A considerable number of Native Americans lack trust in the government and the majority culture. Broken treaties, the confiscation of their lands, violence, and attempted genocide have produced in many an extreme wariness of "outsiders" or non-Indians. Without committing overt atrocity, representatives of the church and government have tried nonetheless to separate them from the ways of their tribes and to alienate them from their own people and traditions. The "patronizing attitudes and missionary zeal" of those who came to save "savages" from ignorance and eternal damnation also have contributed to the intense mistrust with which many Native Americans regard White society (LaFromboise et al., 1993, p. 149).

Most sexual minority Native people have observed or experienced the unqualified heterosexism adopted by their own communities from missionaries, government workers, and Bureau of Indian Affairs agents and Christian American Indian converts themselves (Roscoe, 1987b). Homophobia, in fact, is so intense in some tribes that many reservation Indians assume they must move to cities to find acceptance from other sexual minorities (Tafoya, 1992). Openly gay, lesbian, and bisexual individuals are ridiculed, "considered queer," and mocked by both White and Indian society (Grahn, 1986, p. 55). Intense hostility and "vehemence among nongay Indians" is reflected in reported incidents of homicides on reservations, some of which were committed by means of cruel and sadistic methods (Roscoe, 1987b, p. 71). Most sexual minorities, not surprisingly, remain closeted in order to secure a favorable position with the dominant White society, as well as within their own tribe. Few, in fact, speak of their sexuality with their families but, rather, contend that they have "just always known" (Tafoya, 1996, p. 612). Further, many have internalized the majority culture's negative stereotypes of Native Americans, their "savagery," poverty, drinking, and drugs (Lone Dog, 1991).

For these reasons, gay, lesbian, and bisexual Native people often have difficulty identifying exclusively with their cultural heritage, even though "one's membership in the clan, family, tribe, or nation never changes, regardless of one's sexual orientation" (Tafoya, 1996, p. 612). They thus experience being a minority in the majority culture as well as a subculture within the Native American community. Most also feel pulled between the traditional tribal and mainstream cultures of the United States (L. B. Brown, 1997; Thomason, 1991); nevertheless, the GAI, founded in 1975, has helped a number of individuals reconcile this discord by integrating their identities in positive ways. GAI also has served valuable political and educational functions. Like similar groups organized by and for sexual minorities of color, however, most of the services provided by GAI and similar organizations are unavailable to Native people living outside large cities or to those in the early phases of identity development. Fewer publications are available to them than to sexual minority members of other ethnic/cultural groups (Gock, 1996). Most people, consequently, struggle with cultural conflict alone.

Lesbians

With the colonization of Native Americans and the establishment of a social order resembling European patriarchy, those who most closely observed tribal rituals and customs suffered the most severe losses of status, power, and leadership. The respected and two-spirit cross-dressing men and women were the most obvious individuals in this group. Lesbians, particularly those on reservations, not only lost status and respectability but also became targets for oppression for another reason. Motherhood is an important role for Native women because children are seen as the future of tribes which may have lost many members in 19th-century battles with settlers for their lands. Because lesbians are assumed to be childless, they are devalued for not doing their part to ensure the continuity of the culture. Therefore, out of respect to family, tribe, and tradition, many lesbians have children (B. Greene, 1994b).

Native American lesbians and feminists may have a special interest in the revitalization of the culture, language, and religion of their ancestors. To many, this "retraditionalization" entails the restoration of women's precolonial roles as caretakers and transmitters of cultural knowledge, and as healers, legal specialists, and tribal governors (LaFromboise et al., 1993). These former functions, which included the authority to make decisions on all tribal levels, have faded with the visibility of Native American lesbians in contemporary society. Women who once assumed roles designated masculine and were especially honored and respected by the tribe are today forced into closets of secrecy in order to serve patriarchal interests (P. G. Allen, 1986).

PSYCHOTHERAPEUTIC CONSIDERATIONS

When treating sexual minority clients of color, clinicians are challenged to unravel the complex interplay of dynamics related to ethnicity, gender, and sexual orientation (B. Greene, 1997a). Although there are an increasing number of publications that address these issues in assessment and treatment, there are few empirical studies available to guide clinicians (Gock, 1996), although more are beginning to appear in the literature (e.g., Adams & Kimmel, 1997; Peplau et al., 1997). Psychotherapists, thus, currently have to rely on what little specific information is attainable, as well as their clinical experience and observational abilities, when working with these individuals.

Specifically in reference to gender, psychotherapists are reminded that "lesbian women of color exist within a tangle of multiply devalued identities surrounded by the oppression and discrimination that accompany institutionalized racism, sexism, and heterosexism. . . . Unlike their ethnic identities, their sexual orientation and sometimes their gender may be devalued by those closest to them in their families" (B. Greene, 1994b, p. 412). On the other hand, gay and bisexual men have lived from childhood as members of the more privileged sex in their cultures and, hence, do not reach adulthood having their gender itself devalued. These individuals may have been denigrated because their appearance and behaviors were considered inappropriate for little boys, but they probably were not devalued because they were male.

As discussed earlier in this chapter, clinicians also must consider the influence on their clients of social class, religion, geographic region of residence or origin, traditionalism, and family cultural values regarding privacy, sexuality, and relationships, in addition to their gender, ethnicity, and sexual orientation (A. Smith, 1997). Not only are there between-group differences within ethnic and sexual minorities as well as across genders but there are also within-group differences among these populations. In others words, psychotherapists can deprive themselves of much clinically rich material if they single out any one of these personal or demographic factors for attention in either assessing or treating their clients. On the other hand, however, they can focus so holistically that they miss the critical significance of a particular element (or combination thereof). Examples of these composite variables might include a Native American lesbian, a member of a small tribe that lost most of its members in the Indian massacres of the last century, who feels intense tribal pressure to marry and reproduce, or an African American gay man, the only child of a mother who was widowed during his preschool years, who feels responsible for sparing her the shame she might experience from her family, church, and community, if he discloses his sexual orientation.

In counseling any sexual minority of color, C. S. Chan (1992) advises clinicians not only to be familiar with cultural issues in a general sense but also to be attuned to specific factors within the context of each client's situation. For the purposes of guiding psychotherapists through this kind of individualized assessment, she suggests the following questions:

- Is the client an immigrant, or born in the United States?
- To which ethnic group does the client belong?
- What are the specific cultural values of the client, the client's family, the client's ethnic group?
- How closely does the client observe traditional customs?
- What is the client's socioeconomic level?
- What is the client's degree of bilingualism?

The issues inherent in these questions have been discussed earlier in this chapter. Once specific factors of this nature have been given appropriate consideration, the manner in which they converge and operate dynamically within a specific client should be determined.

Assessment of Multicultural Integration

L. S. Brown (1989b), as well as Lukes and Land (1990), discuss the application of established theories of ethnic identity and bicultural socialization to the lives of lesbians, bisexuals, and gay men. The latter writers offer a conceptual framework for assessing the experience of these clients, which includes at least four variables that influence the extent to which sexual minorities of color become multicultural. These factors also can serve as indicators to psychotherapists that two or more cultural identities have become integrated. The following questions have been developed from Lukes and Land's variables and can be used as models of inquiry in assessing degrees of multicultural socialization and resources for navigating within and between various cultural communities.

Cultural overlap

- "How are your ethnic and sexual minority groups like the majority culture?"
- "What do all of your cultural groups have in common?"

Existence of cultural translators, mediators, and models

- "Who taught you how to function in your three (ethnic, sexual, majority) cultures?"
- "Who did you watch in order to learn how to move back and forth between the cultures?"

Problem-solving skills

- "What skills do you use to operate successfully within each of your three cultures?"
- "What skills do you use to succeed in navigating between and among all three of your cultures?"

Degree of bilingualism

- "What language patterns do you use with members of each of your minority cultures as well as with those from the dominant society?"
- "How do you translate communication across all three of your cultural groups?"

Resource Identification

As discussed previously, the more clients are able to see common elements in their various communities, the more integrated will be their overall identities. This "whole-seeing" perspective provides them the means to function adequately in more than one cultural milieu. Obviously, having mentors or models after which to pattern their behaviors can also facilitate this ability. If clients do not have cultural mediators in their lives, clinicians can help them identify such individuals. In addition, people who are multiculturally socialized have developed skills and linguistic abilities for navigating within and between the various cultures. Often they are unaware of these abilities and psychotherapists can provide assistance in identifying and strengthening them.

Sexual minority clients of color also have developed resources that enable them continually to combat racism and discrimination. These individuals have been forced to learn useful coping mechanisms to confront pervasive homophobia and heterosexism, and clinicians may need to remind them that they use all these skills and aptitudes on an ongoing basis (B. Greene, 1994b, 1997a). The psychotherapist's task, then, is to help ethnic minority bisexual, gay, and lesbian clients develop an awareness of these struggles, identify their coping resources, and reassure them of their ability to manage these conflicts (Morales, 1989).

Appropriate Support

It is imperative that clinicians understand each client's perception of his or her personal oppression and that individual's idiosyncratic strategies for coping with discrimination. Otherwise, if psychotherapists see only the dominant culture's perspectives on race, sexual orientation, or gender, they could be in "danger of perpetuating ethnocentric, heterocentric, and androcentric biases" (B. Greene, 1994b, p. 393). Like all conditions that bring people to psychotherapy, that which clinicians may consider a problem or source of difficulty may not be viewed as such by a particular client. Thus, psychotherapists must avoid seeing clients through their own eyes but rather must view them through the perspectives of the individuals seated before them. In this regard, Nakajima et al. (1996) suggest that therapists of Asian clients emphasize that it is not always essential for healthy development to come out to family members, regardless of how much pressure the counselee may feel from non-Asian American friends or how important the clinician might see this action for his or her growth. Similarly, in a survey of 2,393 lesbians, Morris and Rothblum (1999) found only moderate correlations between ethnicity and five aspects of lesbian sexuality and the coming-out process: Sexual Orientation, Years Out, Outness/Disclosure, Sexual Experience, and Lesbian Activities. In other words, those variables that typically are associated with an integrated identity do not hold true for all lesbians. Aspects of the lesbian experience were most intercorrelated for African American women in the Morris and Rothblum study, followed next by Native American subjects. Unlike these two groups, however, Latinas had nonsignificant correlations between Years Out and Outness/Disclosure. Caucasian and Asian American lesbians had the fewest intercorrelations, most of those for the Asian women were insignificant.

Along the lines of the study described previously, B. Greene (1994b) provides another example of cultural objectivity when she discusses the common instance of a sexual minority client of color who may be unwilling to identify as bisexual, lesbian, or gay when all available information would indicate to the clinician that one of these labels is appropriate. Rather than assuming that the client's reluctance is a reflection of internalized homophobia, she asks psychotherapists to consider whether his or her "avoidance of the [homosexual] label has its origins in culturally prescribed methods of managing potential conflicts" (p. 396). Moreover, she indicates that there are "culturally distinct or different concepts of what constitutes a lesbian [or gay] identity" (p. 396), as well as taboos in many cultures against discussing sexuality or sexual behavior. Clinicians should avoid assuming that a client is in the early phases of gay or lesbian identity development without first considering the client's presentation of self within the context of potentially relevant cultural variables and identities (Gock, 1996; Tafoya, 1996).

In further regard to psychotherapeutic blind spots, B. Greene (1994b, 1997a) discusses possible countertransference issues that may arise with sexual minority clients of color. Because of the various forces of oppressions that a particular client or population may have endured or may be currently experiencing, clinicians can become overly involved in the individual's pain and lose objectivity. A loss of focus also may occur because the client's description of events has offended the psychotherapist's social conscience or elicited guilt for not having personally done enough to remedy society's injustices. Clinicians, in these cases, may feel sorry for the person and fail to set limits, or bend over backward to accept and accommodate the client, and, thus, fail to maintain appropriate psychotherapeutic boundaries. Sexual minority clinicians, particularly those of color, could possibly overidentify and similarly weaken the psychotherapeutic alliance.

To summarize, then, clinicians must affirm and encourage gay, lesbian, and bisexual clients of color without losing the perspective necessary for effective psychotherapy. Many of these individuals are emotionally vulnerable and feel isolated and estranged from at least three cultures—their own ethnic/cultural group, the sexual minority community, and the dominant society. They often need assistance in understanding their conflicting emotions, as well as help in managing the justifiable anger produced by having to make primary and secondary identity choices (B. E. Jones & Hill, 1996; Nakajima et al., 1996).

In addition to receiving knowledgeable and appropriate support within the clinical setting, however, these clients need affirming and mirroring communities in which to live, love, and work. The *Gayellow Pages* and other national or regional directories (see Resources section) list the names and addresses of numerous support and advocacy groups for sexual minority clients of color. As mentioned previously, most of these are headquartered in large urban centers, but clients in rural or small communities can communicate with others like themselves by telephone, letter, e-mail, or on the Internet when they are unable to visit cities. Ethical practice assumes that psychotherapists will identify and share these resources with their clients.

CONCLUSION

As discussed in this chapter, racism and ethnocentrism, as well as heterosexism complicate the parallel processes of minority identity development and sexual identity formation for gay, lesbian, and bisexual people of color. Levels of acculturation and culture-bound gender role expectations further influence their psychological adjustment and social functioning. Sexual minority African, Asian, Latino, and Native Americans often experience cultural conflict between the lesbian, gay, and bisexual community and their specific racial/ethnic groups. These discussions are offered to orient clinicians to multicultural dynamics and considerations for affirmative psychotherapy.

11

Career Choice and Development with Sexual Minority Clients

At the turn of the 21st century, the U.S. Congress had yet to legislate the Employment Non-Discrimination Act (see Chapter 4), which would explicitly prohibit job discrimination on the basis of sexual orientation. Chapter 4 addresses current legal issues facing sexual minority employees. This chapter adapts and applies theories of career choice and development to sexual minority clients to further and more fully explain the vocational selection and maturation of gay, lesbian, and bisexual workers. In addition, this chapter addresses lesbian-specific employment issues before suggesting career assessment, intervention, and resource recommendations.

THEORETICAL ADAPTATIONS TO SEXUAL MINORITY CLIENTS

Although many career counseling textbooks now contain excellent sections on racial and cultural minorities, most fail to mention the career choice and development of lesbians and gay men (Elliot, 1993). In terms of research and practice, the most influential theories of vocational selection and maturation for the general population include Holland's theory; the theory of work adjustment; the lifespan, lifespace approach to careers; Gottfredson's theory of circumscription and compromise; Krumboltz's learning theory of career choice and counseling; and a sociological perspective on work and career development (D. Brown & Brooks, 1996). Three of these six theories of career choice and development have been examined specifically concerning their relevance to lesbians and gay men. These analyses investigate the appropriateness of Holland's theory (Mobley & Slaney, 1996), the lifespan, lifespace approach to careers (Dunkle, 1996), and Gottfredson's theory of circumscription and compromise (Morgan & Brown, 1991). Although the other three approaches have not been explored explicitly regarding their applicability to sexual minority persons, some of their theoretical constructs (i.e., work adjustment, social learning, status attainment, and labor markets) are addressed in the professional literature on gay, lesbian, and bisexual career development. These theories and their conceptual components provide the framework for the following discussions. Accordingly, psychotherapists may inform their clinical interventions with these theoretical adaptations in order to more accurately assess and address the vocational concerns of their sexual minority clients.

Holland's Theory

Holland (1992) assumed that most personality styles and occupational environments can be classified according to one of six types: *Realistic, Investigative, Artistic, Social, Enterprising*, or *Conventional*. These personality styles and occupational environments interact to determine vocational behavior. Individuals seek vocational surroundings that allow them to exercise their abilities and aptitudes, express their values and viewpoints, and assume appropriate roles and responsibilities. Workers find these surroundings reinforcing and satisfying when environmental patterns reflect their personality patterns. In regard to interactions between the worker and the workplace, incongruence facilitates change and congruence fosters stability in vocational behavior. Individuals resolve incongruence by seeking new and congruent environments or by changing personal attitudes or habits. The reciprocal interactions of these individuals and their serial employment generally leads to a cyclical sequence of success and satisfaction.

Mobley and Slaney (1996) examined the relevance of Holland's theory for lesbian women and gay men. Their analysis is organized around three central concepts: (1) personality styles, (2) occupational environments, and (3) congruence. Accordingly, they compare perspectives on career development provided by Holland's (1992) theory and by Cass's (1979, 1983/1984, 1984) model of gay and lesbian identity formation. The following discussions briefly summarize these comparisons.

Personality Styles

Mobley and Slaney (1996) challenged the theoretical assumption that personality styles measured by the six Holland types (i.e., *Realistic, Investigative, Artistic, Social, Enterprising*, or *Conventional*) "are maximally relevant to career choice and development" for lesbian women and gay men (p. 127). They further hypothesized that Cass's model of gay and lesbian identity formation may have descriptive significance for understanding the vocational development of sexual minority persons in ways that qualify or complement Holland's theory. Accordingly, the development of personality style and Holland type might be qualified by the stage of gay or lesbian identity formation into which a sexual minority person might be classified. Cass (1979, 1983/1984, 1984) observed, for example, that people attracted to persons of their own sex lack a clear sense of themselves during the early stages of *Identity Confusion* and *Identity Comparison*. Further, a hypothetical relationship between identity development and career indecision has been delineated (Newman, Fuqua, & Seaworth, 1989) and investigated (Weyhing, Bartlett, & Howard, 1984) in the professional literature. For instance, Newman et al. (1989) outlined an extended reciprocal model that best reflects current thinking about the association between anxiety and career indecision. This pattern represents a reciprocal interaction between anxiousness and vocational undecidedness, as well as between both of these variables and inadequate identity formation. In other words:

The inhibitory effects of poor identity formation on career development may prevent the client from establishing a professional identity, which comprises a major component of identity formation in our culture. The anxiety, which may initially have resulted from identity confusion, would likely serve to further inhibit effective situational responses to the client's environment, thus further exacerbating the identity issues. (p. 227)

Based on the emotional variance that sexual minority persons experience during the course of gay and lesbian identity development, Mobley and Slaney (1996) concluded that "it is important [for clinicians and their clients] to understand how the career assessment process might be affected" (p. 128).

Occupational Environments

Holland (1992) assumed that most occupational environments can be classified according to same six types used to categorize personality styles (i.e., *Realistic*, *Investigative*, *Artistic*, *Social*, *Enterprising*, or *Conventional*). Mobley and Slaney (1996), however, proposed that Cass's model of gay and lesbian identity formation may recommend a completely different context for appraising vocational settings. From this perspective, "the emphasis [for counselors and their counselees] may be on assessing the receptivity of the environment to lesbian and gay concerns and issues" (p. 128). Accordingly, Cass's theory indicates that the preferred type of occupational environment may vary depending on an individual's stage of sexual minority identity development.

Congruence

Holland (1992) hypothesized "vocational satisfaction, stability, and achievement depend on the congruence between one's personality and the environment in which one works" (pp. 10–11). Similarly, Cass (1979) speculated that "stability and change in human behavior are dependent on the congruency or incongruency that exists within an individual's interpersonal environment" (p. 220). Whereas Holland recommended that individuals search for congruence between their personality types and those of other workers in the workplace, Cass suggested that sexual minority persons seek congruency between their attitudes and those of other colleagues toward lesbian women and gay men.

The Theory of Work Adjustment

The theory of work adjustment (Dawis & Lofquist, 1984) assumes that the worker has needs that can be satisfied by the workplace and that the employer has requirements that can be satisfied by the employee. When the needs of the worker and the requirements of the workplace correspond, both employee and employers experience and express satisfaction. When change inevitably disrupts the correspondence between worker needs and workplace requirements, attempts to recover this ideal state are called adjustment (Dawis, 1996) and may require vocational guidance or psychotherapeutic intervention.

In specific reference to lesbian women, Fassinger (1995, 1996) discussed the process by which sexual minority workers adjust to the workplace. According to her, "the most salient barrier to the vocational . . . adjustment of lesbians [and gays] is the cluster of environmental variables related to occupational stereotyping, discrimination, and harassment" (p. 166). Similarly, the professional literature on gay, lesbian, and bisexual career development often has considered how negative stereotypes, employment discrimination, and sexual harassment obstruct the work adjustment of sexual minority employees (Badgett, 1996; Chojnacki & Gelberg, 1994; Elliott, 1993; A. L. Ellis, 1996; Hetherington, Hillerbrand, & Etringer, 1989; Hetherington & Orzek, 1989; Kitzinger, 1991; Pope, 1995, 1996; Schmitz; 1988).

The theory of work adjustment further assumes that employers possess capacities than can be used to satisfy employee needs (e.g., equitable earnings, favorable conditions, amiable coworkers, and impartial managers). In a homophobic or heterosexist workplace, however, these work reinforcers may be inadequate to meet the demands of gay, lesbian, and bisexual workers who place high value on being able to express their sexual orientation through, at, and outside work (Chung, 1995). Not surprisingly, the professional literature on sexual minority career development also has discussed frequently the importance of identity self-disclosure and coming out on the job (Badgett, 1996; Elliott, 1993; A. L. Ellis, 1996; Fassinger, 1995, 1996; Morgan & Brown, 1991; Kitzinger, 1991; Pope, 1995, 1996).

Finally, the theory of work adjustment defines flexibility as the degree to which the worker or the workplace can tolerate disagreement prior to the initiation of adjustment behavior. During the developmental stage of *Identity Pride* (Cass, 1979, 1983/1984, 1984), gay and lesbian individuals tend to discriminate between people based on sexual orientation or identification and adopt a "them versus us" philosophy. At this phase of identity formation, worker flexibility is inclined to be low as gay and lesbian employees apply a "heterosexual versus homosexual" dichotomy to adversarial relationships with colleagues and supervisors. Nonetheless, worker flexibility is likely to increase during the developmental stage of *Identity Synthesis* (Cass, 1979, 1983/1984, 1984), when gay and lesbian employees integrate their sexual identities with their occupational self-concepts.

The Lifespan, Lifespace Approach to Careers

As Mobley and Slaney (1996) did with Holland's theory, Dunkle (1996) considered how the identity formation of lesbian women and gay men, as delineated by Cass (1979, 1983/1984, 1984), influences their vocational development, as outlined in the lifespan, lifespace approach to careers (Super, Savickas, & Super, 1996). Dunkle (1996) identified common theoretical assumptions between these two processes:

> Both are developmental and involve the progression through a series of life stages. Both . . . also emphasize that career identities and gay and lesbian identities are multidetermined. Finally, both . . . maintain that, for many reasons, individuals can recycle through stages or become foreclosed at any stage. (p. 151)

Further, he organized his considerations according to five stages of career development, as proposed by Super et al. (1996): *Growth*, *Exploration*, *Establishment*, *Maintenance*, and *Disengagement*. The following discussions supplement as well as summarize his conclusions. These summaries illustrate for psychotherapists the reticulating effects of these parallel trajectories.

Growth

The *Growth* stage of the lifespan, lifespace approach (ages 4 to 13) involves four major tasks of career development (Super et al., 1996): "becoming concerned about the future, increasing personal control over one's own life, convincing oneself to achieve in school and at work, and acquiring competent work habits and attitudes" (p. 131). Whereas Cass (1979, 1983/1984, 1984) assumed that gay and lesbian identity formation begins with conscious awareness that information regarding homosexuality has personal relevance, Troiden (1979, 1989) believed that the first stage of the process (i.e., *Sensitization*) occurs before puberty and is characterized by childhood feelings of social difference and gender nonconformity. Prior to lesbian self-identification, for example, young girls frequently describe themselves as (1) not being interested in boys; (2) feeling unfeminine, ungraceful, and not very pretty; and (3) considering themselves more masculine, independent, and aggressive than other female children. Before gay self-labeling, conversely, young boys often describe themselves as being more interested in the arts and less interested in sports than other pre-adolescent males. In regard to the lifespan, lifespace approach, Dunkle (1996) suggested that these early experiences of social discordance and gender discrepancy may affect career-specific developmental task performance and mastery during childhood.

Exploration

Between the ages of 14 and 24, individuals face the developmental tasks of crystallizing, specifying, and implementing a vocational choice (Super et al., 1996). According to Dunkle (1996), however, "the process of gay and lesbian identity formation may pose several challenges at the exploration stage of career development" (p. 152). During the early phases of *Identity Confusion* and *Identity Comparison* (Cass, 1979, 1983/1984, 1984), for example, various psychosocial stressors (e.g., internalized homophobia, and employment discrimination) are likely to impair vocational maturity. In other words, the coming-out process often competes with an individual's concentration on occupational challenges.

Establishment

The *Establishment* stage of the lifespan, lifespace approach (ages 25 to 44) involves the developmental tasks of stabilizing, consolidating, and advancing in an occupation (Super et al., 1996). When new gay or lesbian identities emerge at this phase of vocational development, sexual minority employees may change careers nonetheless and recycle through a minisequence of *Growth*, *Exploration*, and *Establishment*. During this recycling process, these workers may reexamine themselves and their environments to initiate appropriate employment in which to implement their newly emerging self-concepts (Dunkle, 1996).

Maintenance

Between the ages of 45 and 65, individuals face the developmental tasks of holding on, keeping up, and innovating their vocational choices (Super et al., 1996). According to Dunkle (1996), however, a substantial number of adults who begin to self-identify as gay or lesbian between midlife and retirement may have to cope with the stage-specific stressors of early identity formation during the *Maintenance* stage of career development. In addition, lesbian women and gay men in the later phases of *Identity Acceptance*, *Identity Pride*, and *Identity Synthesis* (Cass, 1979, 1983/1984, 1984) may have to contend with workplace self-disclosure and employment discrimination.

Disengagement

The *Disengagement* stage of the lifespan, lifespace approach (over age 65) involves the developmental tasks of career deceleration, retirement planning, and retirement living (Super et al., 1996). In his reflection on this final phase of vocational development, Dunkle (1996) summarized Berger's (1982b) discussion of older lesbian women and gay men. According to Dunkle (1996), Berger asserted that older gay and lesbian adults may experience less stress during the coming-out process because they (1) may be less dependent on family members for emotional and financial support; (2) "may be more accustomed to stigmatization," having grown up in an era "when attitudes toward homosexuality in the United States were more negative than today"; (3) "may have passed for many years as heterosexual"; and (4) may "have developed a lifetime's worth of social networks" (p. 156). Berger (1982b) also suggested that compared to older heterosexual adults, gay men and lesbian women may be better able to contend with negative stereotypes about aging based on their experience of contending with homophobia and heterosexism. If so, then gay and lesbian retirees may feel less stressed during this culminating stage of their careers.

Gottfredson's Theory of Circumscription and Compromise

Morgan and Brown (1991) explored the applicability of Gottfredson's (1981) theory in relation to increasing counselor awareness of lesbian career experience. Although their exploration was limited to women, their analysis may be applied further to improve clinical understanding of gay male career development. Gottfredson (1996) delineated four developmental stages during which individuals circumscribe vocational alternatives based on internal factors (i.e., self-concept and personal preferences) and external variables (i.e., perceptions of job accessibility and occupational images, such as sex type and prestige level). She also hypothesized that, when forced to compromise their career choices, individuals will abandon their vocational interests before relinquishing their preferred job status. Consequently, sex type is surrendered only after all other options are exhausted. Based on speculations that gay men (Chung, 1995) as well as lesbian women (Fassinger, 1995, 1996) adopt broader definitions of gender-appropriate work, however, Gottfredson's theory would predict that sexual minority persons might demonstrate different career decision-making patterns than their heterosexual peers (Morgan & Brown, 1991). Psychotherapists first can help gay, lesbian, and bisexual clients increase self-awareness of these specific patterns which then can be reinforced or modified, if necessary, to facilitate vocational selection and maturation.

Krumboltz's Theory of Career Choice and Counseling

Krumboltz (1979, 1996) established his theories of vocational guidance on principles of social learning. S. L. Morrow, Gore, and Campbell (1996) discussed similar concepts in their application of a social cognitive framework to the career development of lesbian women and gay men. Specifically, these constructs included vicarious learning and social persuasion. According to S. L. Morrow et al. (1996), these "important determinants of self-efficacy beliefs" (p. 140) interact over time with outcome expectations to influence educational and vocational interests.

Although media depictions increasingly represent women and men in nontraditional vocations, S. L. Morrow et al. (1996) acknowledged that the preponderance of occupational role models are still gender stereotypical; thus, "social persuasion operates in the direction of encouraging young children to engage and achieve in gender-congruent activities" (p. 140). Further, S. L. Murrow et al. (1996) affirmed that a lack of appropriate role models or negative social persuasion may undermine self-efficacy beliefs, thereby hindering or restricting the development of career interests. Conversely, they asserted nonetheless that vicarious learning may provide adequate reinforcement to fortify self-efficacy beliefs in the absence of immediate experience, positive social persuasion, or same-gender imitation. Under these circumstances, "even faced with a nonsupportive environment, lesbian or gay children might continue to develop interests based on exposure to gender-nonstereotypic models" (p. 140).

Other contributors to the body of professional literature on sexual minority career development discuss the importance of using gay and lesbian role models in the process of vocational guidance (Hetherington, et al., 1989; Pope, 1995). Based on a review of 15 articles and a frequency count of population-specific career counseling techniques, for example, Pope (1995) concluded that "supporting and encouraging gay and lesbian professionals as role models" (p. 194) is one of the interventions most widely recommended for sexual minority clients. Similarly, Hetherington et al. (1989) suggested tapping into the gay and lesbian community for role models to increase client awareness of occupational alternatives.

A Sociological Perspective on Career Development

A sociological perspective on work and career development (Hotchkiss & Borow, 1996) assumes that status attainment and labor markets are among the influences that interact to affect the vocational behavior and occupational achievement of contemporary workers. The following discussions are organized around these concepts.

Status Attainment

The basic theory of status attainment assumes that the attitudes of significant others about appropriate educational and occupational levels affect the vocational status of workers (Hotchkiss & Borow, 1996). Included among these attitudes are negative occupational stereotypes of sexual minority persons. In their discussions of career counseling with gay men and lesbian women, for example, Hetherington and her colleagues (Hetherington et al., 1989; Hetherington & Orzek, 1989) cited a survey of 120 college students (Botkin & Daly, 1987) which demonstrated stereotypical attitudes based on gender as well as sexual orientation. According to this sample of the general population, the top three professions presumed (1) for heterosexual men were doctor, photographer, and engineer; (2) for gay men were photographer, interior decorator, and nurse; (3) for heterosexual women were interior decorator, nurse, and dietitian; and (4) for lesbian women were auto mechanic, plumber, and truck driver. Whereas heterosexual and gay men were assumed to share one common professional interest (i.e., photography), gay men and heterosexual women were assumed to share two common vocational ambitions (i.e., interior design and nursing). In other words, gay men were presumed to be more similar vocationally to heterosexual women than to men. In addition, Hetherington and Orzek (1989) observed that "the occupations listed for lesbian women do not require a college degree" and concluded that "lesbian women may therefore experience deep negative stereotypes because of their sex" (p. 68) along with their lesbianism. To the extent that their significant others internalize and express these stereotypical attitudes, gay and lesbian students and workers are inclined to experience or self-impose restrictions on their attainment of academic and career status. While systemic strategies can be designed to modify or eliminate external barriers to occupational achievement, psychotherapeutic interventions can be developed to explore and resolve internal impediments to vocational fulfillment.

Labor Markets

The sociology of labor markets suggests that socioeconomic conditions influence vocational growth (Hotchkiss & Borow, 1996). In addition to Gottfredson's (1981) theory of circumscription and compromise, Morgan and Brown (1991) explored the applicability of Astin's (1985) model of career choice and work behavior with specific regard to lesbian women. Comparable to their discussion of Gottfredson's approach, their analysis of Astin's paradigm may be applied further toward understanding the occupational development of gay men.

According to Morgan and Brown (1991), "Astin's model explores the interactions between personal characteristics and social forces and describes how socialization influences each person's view of the [employment] opportunity structure" (p. 285). An especially interesting aspect of this paradigm for application to gay and lesbian career issues is its perspective on how the opportunity structure shifts over time as a result of sociological patterns and trends. "This ability to account for changes in the perceived structure of [employment] opportunity has relevance to the vocational concerns of women [and men] in the process of coming out as lesbians [and gays]" (p. 285). To the degree that economic conditions affect social tolerance toward sexual minority workers (Boswell, 1980, 1994), the sociology of labor markets is pertinent to a clinician's accurate appraisal of gay, lesbian, and bisexual career experience.

LESBIANS AND WORK

Along with employment discrimination, many lesbians encounter sexism in the workplace. Twice oppressed, sexual minority women often experience a higher risk for occupational stress and impairment than do their gay male and heterosexual coworkers. The following discussions thus address lesbian-specific vocational issues. Morgan and Brown (1991) base their observations regarding lesbian career development on data from two large samples, namely The National Lesbian Health Care Survey data ($n = 1,925$) of Bradford and Ryan (1988) and the research findings of Blumstein and Schwartz (1983). In the latter investigation, heterosexual and same-sex couples ($n = 1,455$ lesbians) were studied to determine how they handle issues of money, work, power, and relationship maintenance. After reviewing the surveys, Morgan and Brown (1991) note that 85% to 91% of all lesbians work for pay outside the home. Although her data are not precisely comparable, Hall (1986) contends that between 70% and 85% of this work is full-time employment.

Vocational Identification

In contrast to heterosexual women, lesbians grow up assuming that their own incomes will be their primary means of financial support. Most do not assume that they will be financially supported by anyone else and anticipate that their economic security will depend on their ability to provide for themselves (Browning, 1987, 1988; Clunis & Green, 1988; Elliott, 1993). Of the 18 lesbians interviewed by Hall and Gregory (1991), most had high expectations about vocational fulfillment and were strongly identified with, and stimulated by, their work. Most contended that they "had been groomed for such career focus from childhood" (p. 126). They felt a commitment to their financial independence and said they would be willing to provide for their partners but could never let themselves similarly be supported.

The egalitarian values of many lesbians encourage financial independence. Based on their ideas of equity, they do not subscribe to the subordinate–dominant role dichotomy implied by unequal financial arrangements. Thus, there are few lesbian equivalents of the heterosexual concept of "housewife." Because women cannot marry legally and share each other's benefits, few lesbians are able to support their partners financially. Nonetheless, many choose jobs considered nontraditional or gender discordant and thus higher paying than those regarded "women's work" (Hall, 1986).

Lesbians tend to be underemployed and underpaid, even when their incomes are compared generally to women's wages in the United States (which are currently 74% of men's earnings in comparable occupations). On average, economic discrimination prevents two women who form a same-sex couple from earning as much as the average gay male or heterosexual pair (Browning, 1987, 1988). According to Morgan and Brown (1991), this "economic reality may also influence lesbians to consider nontraditional fields from very early in their vocational development" (p. 278) because men's work pays more than women's. Thus, choosing work in unconventional occupations may be "one way for lesbians to bridge gender-related wage gaps and mitigate the effect of living without a man's higher wages and better economic opportunity" (p. 278). Because lesbians frequently do not adhere to conventional gender roles, they are more able to choose careers not considered traditional for women, and thus raise their standards of living.

Lesbian Couples and Employment

Eldridge and Gilbert (1990) studied 275 dual-career lesbian couples (ages 20 to 59) and found that career commitment was not associated with relationship satisfaction in individual women but that being "out" on the job was (65% of the 550 women surveyed had not disclosed their sexual orientation to their employers, and 37% had not told anyone in their work setting). A unique finding of their study, however, was the discovery that different levels of career commitment between partners correlated negatively with relationship satisfaction. In other words, if two people differed significantly in their career commitments, the likelihood of dissatisfaction within their relationship increased.

Along this same line, Hall and Gregory (1991) interviewed nine couples of lesbian women (ages 32 to 50), the majority of whom had postgraduate degrees, and found that the less occupied partner was more likely to complain about the lack of shared time and to feel stress more within the relationship than her busy counterpart. Further, when the discrepancies between each partner's work commitment became too intense, one tended to concentrate on the couplehood while the other focused on her job. The partner oriented toward work was inclined to see the relationship "in terms of renewal—a resting place on the way to career goals" (p. 128). The other was more likely to see the partnership as an end in itself.

Frequently in same-sex relationships, when one partner moves to another city or state, there often are few resources to help the other find a job. Thus, some sexual minority couples must live apart to advance in their careers. In one study of lesbian pairs (Peplau, Padesky, & Hamilton, 1982), extreme geographic separation was a major factor in 19% and a minor factor in 16.7% of the terminated relationships.

CAREER COUNSELING WITH SEXUAL MINORITY CLIENTS

Along with those of sexual minority women, the occupational experiences of gay and bisexual men often differ from those of heterosexual workers. Comparable to vocational guidance with their sexual majority counterparts, however, career counseling with gay, lesbian, and bisexual clients includes assessment and intervention, as well as information and referral. These specific procedures of the generic process provide a framework for addressing the special needs of sexual minority populations.

Assessment

As reflected earlier in this chapter among the theoretical reviews, sexual identity development and environmental factors are central variables in career assessment with gay, lesbian, and bisexual workers (Gelberg & Chojnacki, 1996; Prince, 1997). After summarizing these critical factors, this section suggests recommendations for vocational appraisal with sexual minority clients.

Sexual Identity Development

At least two of the theoretical adaptations and applications discussed toward the beginning of this chapter consider the reciprocal relationship between gay, lesbian, or bisexual identity formation and sexual minority career development (Dunkle, 1996; Mobley & Slaney, 1996). Gelberg and Chojnacki, (1996) also developed a comprehensive model that integrates a number of principles of lesbian and gay identity and career development, as well as information from adult lifespan and career evolution. These authors note "that to omit consideration of any of the factors of adult development, career development, gay/lesbian/bisexual development, and person-environment match results in career and life counseling that lacks both depth and scope" (p. 121). Accordingly, as outlined in Chapters 5 (Table 5.1) and 9 (Table 9.6), individuals progress through at least five developmental phases in the process of forming a positive gay, lesbian, or bisexual identity. The following discussion describes some conceivable effects of identity acquisition on vocational maturation.

PHASE-SPECIFIC ISSUES

People at the first phase of identity development usually feel socially different from their peers and very much alone. Frequently, these individuals are quite depressed, and if they are doing much of anything concerning their careers, it is at great personal expense. If they can mobilize the energy, they often diligently try to be successful in order to gain approval for their efforts. Some become overachievers as a way of compensating for their feelings of differentness (Terry, 1992; J. D. Woods, 1993), and they assume that if they do well vocationally, they will be noticed for their accomplishments and not for their idiosyncrasies. This ability to sublimate emotions and channel effort into work and achievement often facilitates passage through these initial painful stages of development. Further, individuals with this capacity are often those who establish their careers first and then self-identify later in life.

The second phase of development involves intense confusion about feelings of sexual differentness, and due to the intensity of this emotional distress, most individuals experience some degree of vocational disruption. Denial, efforts to change an undesired sexual orientation, hyperheterosexuality, or even substance abuse are common. Those who are preparing for a particular line of work or otherwise trying to get started professionally are most at risk. Frequently, vocational choices result from efforts to keep a possible minority sexual orientation concealed or denied (Elliott, 1993). Whatever the strategy employed to handle their unwanted attractions, the career development of these persons is truncated to some extent. Only a few people, primarily those with either a strong ability to sublimate desire or those with a well-established career, likely are able to continue along their vocational paths without being detoured by fear, anxiety, or other upsetting emotions.

Once people are able to tolerate the probability of being lesbian, bisexual, or gay, they experience a natural need to explore and find a community of like-minded individuals. This process of seeking, experimenting, and otherwise coming out at Phase 3 usually is all-consuming, both in terms of time and energy. Consequently, few are able to undertake this life-altering challenge while focusing on setting themselves up in a job or a career. Because of the developmental lag (Grace, 1992) between chronological and psychological maturity, the adolescent and young adult tasks of forming identity and establishing intimacy in relationships take precedent over adult and later life responsibilities of career development and generativity.

Because individuals at the fourth phase of identity formation have come to accept their minority sexual orientations, they are more settled than they were at previous times in their lives. Most are relatively at peace with themselves, in spite of the new insecurities and difficulties involved in integrating into the gay, lesbian, or bisexual community and possibly in establishing their first intimate relationships. Many are now ready to turn toward their careers. For some, this involves a reevaluation of choices, such as using "counterfeit" strategies designed to lead coworkers to assume heterosexuality or avoidance of sexual orientation altogether, made earlier when their world views and self-concepts were very different (J. D. Woods, 1993). Others focus on career development for the first time and still others reinvest in work that had been either physically or emotionally postponed while they were involved with activities related to developing their sexual minority identities.

Often the legitimate rage that individuals feel at the beginning of Phase 5 diverts them from their career paths once again. Confronting heterosexist oppression sometimes engages their attention and becomes a job in and of itself. Further, their "them versus us" dichotomies can alienate the heterosexual majority and thus generate negative consequences vocationally, particularly if a supervisor or employer is one of those who feels antagonized. Most, fortunately, have the ability to modulate their anger and, therefore, rarely suffer complete vocational disruption at this point in their identity formation. (Those who do experience an extensive amount of compromise usually find it occurring earlier in the developmental process.) Sexual minorities at all phases, nonetheless, continue to experience some degree of adversity in the workplace (J. D. Woods, 1993). As people mature into their gay, lesbian, and bisexual identities, however, most fortunately acquire the internal resources to cope with the on-going oppression. When they progress toward the end of Phase 5, an integration of identity occurs and concerns regarding sexual orientation recede into the background. Most of their resources now can be spent addressing the normative developmental issues of adult life, with work and its meaning and place in their lives being one significant area of attention.

CAREER CHOICE AND COMING OUT

Career choice is influenced strongly by the age at which people self-identify as members of a sexual minority. For example, the career development of lesbians who acknowledge their sexual orientation before leaving high school is more likely to be affected directly by their lesbian identity than that of those who come out later in life. Because of their early exposure to the lesbian community and possible encounters with lesbian role models, they may have more opportunities to make informed career decisions. The amount of homophobia in their social environment, however, and the qualitative nature of this early exposure are key variables regarding whether doors to the future are opened or closed (Morgan & Brown, 1991). Conversely, when people self-identify as lesbian, gay, or bisexual later in life, a crisis often ensues and choices become very difficult. Individuals struggle over whether to change occupations entirely or to work at integrating their newly identified sexual orientations into their existing vocations. Regardless of the actual choices, both career development and the coming-out process are delayed.

As mentioned previously, identity formation and career development are interactive rather than parallel processes; thus, sexual orientation and occupational choice must be blended on some level in order for sexual minorities to achieve career satisfaction (Orzek, 1992). As people move through phases of identity development, issues of vocational choice will resurface and must be reevaluated. Decisions made in earlier stages may no longer fit as more comfort is established with a gay, lesbian, or bisexual identity. In these cases, closets get suffocating and individuals become unwilling to live with dual identities or to live in one town and work in another (J. D. Woods, 1993).

DEVELOPMENTAL DELAYS

Few individuals are able to navigate the identity formation process without some delay in their vocational development. Although most people are resilient enough to eventually create a reasonably viable career path, far too many feel the negative effects for the remainder of their work lives. In this regard, O'Neill and Ritter (1992) describe five nonviable employment patterns among lesbians and gay men, regardless of their educational levels (pp. 16–17):

- *The Brokenhearted*: "those who feel so broken early on in life that they are no longer able to hope or to imagine that anything they plan will materialize."
- *The Underachievers*: "those who can still dream but fail to realize their potential due [either] to prejudicial treatment in their work environment **or** to a realistic appraisal of their work situation and the futility of achieving upward mobility as a lesbian or gay individual."
- *The Underemployed*: "those who may have wanted to 'be something' when they grew up but whose fear of exposure keeps them hidden and thus underemployed relative to their talents and skills."
- *The Shifters*: "those whose vocational plans are interrupted by their inability to focus energy away from issues related to their sexual orientation."
- *The Pretenders*: "those who truly achieve the substance and trappings of their life images but at the price of pretense and incongruity."

When clinicians detect patterns such as those described previously, they are able to forestall processes of this nature before they become so pervasive that a person's vocational path is severely and permanently hindered. Gonsiorek (1993) contended, nonetheless, that "some degree of career restriction and diminishment of choice is likely for most gay and lesbian people in the current socio-political climate" (p. 256). Ideally, however, the constraints can be decreased by affirmative and supportive psychotherapy so that truly nonviable career patterns can be avoided or adjusted.

Environmental Factors

The effects of environmental influences on gay, lesbian, and bisexual development are discussed throughout this specific chapter and entire book. According to Prince (1997), Betz and Fitzgerald (1995) offer a useful model for understanding these factors and classify them as either structural or cultural. Structural influences refer to societal and organizational characteristics (i.e., heterosexism) that restrict access to vocational opportunities; cultural variables involve attitudes and beliefs, including occupational stereotypes, that result from socialization. These structural and cultural factors, thus, are addressed in the following discussions.

ORGANIZATIONAL HETEROSEXISM

Most mainstream organizations want "majority culture" employees and do not want to hire, retain, or promote sexual minorities (Levine, 1989; Terry, 1992). For lesbian, gay, and bisexual workers, *majority culture* translates to mean *heterosexual,* or *heterosexual appearing,* even at social functions such as the annual company dinner or picnic. According to Hall (1986), "any deviation from this norm, if not compensated for by extraordinary achievement or Affirmative Action laws, results in everything from less status, less opportunity, and loss of co-workers' esteem, to ostracism, harassment, and firing" (p. 72).

In regard to the climate of heterosexism in the workplace, Hall and Gregory (1991) interviewed nine couples of lesbian women (ages 32 to 50), the majority of whom had postgraduate degrees, and found that the women employed in large corporations commonly had joined an underground network of other sexual minority employees with whom they could be genuine. None felt as if they would be fired if their sexual orientation came to light, but they all believed that such a disclosure would interfere with their chances for promotion. In other words, their lesbianism was a "strike" against them. B. E. Schneider (1986) found that lesbian self-disclosure at work decreases as income increases and speculated either that higher-paying work environments are more homophobic or that better-paid workers have more to lose if they are terminated. Similarly, J. A. Lee (1977) studied 24 gay men and observed that those whose social status was built around the assumption they were heterosexual experienced the most fear, guilt, and anxiety.

OCCUPATIONAL STEREOTYPES

In addition to basing career choice on the presence or absence of role models, individuals frequently make career plans or restrict their decisions around stereotypes (Hetherington & Orzek, 1989). Lesbians and gay men may be drawn to certain professions because they perceive tolerance for their sexual orientation or because they see others like themselves occupying those jobs (Murray, 1991). Some, however, may be discouraged "from entering these professions because of their fear of being stereotyped or because of their own homophobia" (p. 53). For example, the popular belief that a high percentage of male actors are gay may frighten young thespians from entering a career in the theater. Neuringer (1989) challenged this stereotype, however, when he analyzed empirical literature and concluded that the percentage of gay men in the acting profession is no higher than in the general population.

Some occupations (i.e., interior decorating or floral design for men; physical education or mechanics for women), nonetheless, become associated with minority sexual orientations. Levine (1989) and Harry (1982b) contend that societal homophobia not only prevents sexual minorities from obtaining good jobs but also drives many gay men into nonprestigious, low-paying, white-collar or service jobs generally considered inappropriate for the truly "masculine" members of their sex. Public opinion polls support the notion of gay men doing supportive, decorative, or expressive forms of "women's work" but oppose them working in occupations considered maternal or feminine (Elliott, 1993; Levitt & Klassen, 1974; W. Schneider & Lewis, 1984). Similarly, the public disapproves of sexual minority males doing "men's work" that expresses stereotypically masculine traits such as rationality, toughness, and aggressiveness. Thus, gay men are permitted by society to be artists, beauticians, florists, interior decorators, musicians, photographers, and retail clerks but not judges, doctors, policemen, government officials, clergy, teachers, principals, or camp counselors. Levine (1989) contends that "these attitudes prompt job discrimination against gay men" (p. 263), isolate them in certain lines of work, and result in problems with hiring, retention, and advancement. Also, fear of these outcomes drives many sexual minority males into "sissy" lines of work.

Similarly, stereotypes about women who affirm and disclose their lesbianism prohibit them from working with youth or engaging in occupations in which they might influence the attitudes of others. B. E. Schneider (1986) found that the nature of the employment setting thus affects the degree to which women are out at work. For example, lesbians are more likely to be open about their sexual orientation when they work in small, nonbureaucratic settings, in female-dominated organizations, with adults rather than children, and in human service professions. In most other kinds of settings, women tend to remain closeted in order to avoid being stigmatized and to keep their jobs.

Appraisal

As described in the preceding pages, sexual identity development and environmental factors influence career assessment with gay, lesbian, and bisexual workers. After discussing vocational appraisal with sexual minority populations, Prince (1997) concluded that "ethical career assessment requires the elimination of oppressive assessment practices and the creation of affirmative tools and methods" (p. 235). Accordingly, clinicians can seek first to understand the range of developmental, social, and cultural variables that can influence both the responses of gay, lesbian, and bisexual clients and the interpretations of career professionals. In addition, counselors can reduce the invisibility of sexual orientation in assessment tools and practices. Affirmative appraisal can begin with "routine questions or statements that acknowledge sexual orientation as openly and positively as other demographic variables such as race, ethnicity, gender, or religion" (Prince, 1997, p. 235). Supplementary assessments can be used to gather information about sexual identity development and environmental factors that influence sexual minority career choice and development. For example, clinicians can gather important historical and circumstantial data concerning sexual identity formation through questionnaires, interviews, or homework assignments that request the following information:

- Age at initial awareness of sexual orientation
- Number of family members, friends, employers, and associates to whom sexual orientation has been disclosed
- Level of social isolation
- Quality of gay, lesbian, and bisexual community attachments
- Experience of discrimination in academic and occupational environments

Finally, counselors can adapt strategies for intercultural assessment (Jones & Thorne, 1987) to career appraisal with gay, lesbian, and bisexual workers. Before evaluations are administered, for example, sexual minority clients can be assigned to write about their experiences of the "coming-out" process. After outcomes are interpreted, they can be instructed to describe the relationship between their sexual orientation and test results (Prince, 1997).

Intervention

A comprehensive review of the relevant literature widely recommends nine interventions for career counseling with gay, lesbian, and bisexual clients (Pope, 1995). One-third of these approaches involve professional development and require clinicians to:

- Learn the model of sexual identity development (see Chapters 5 and 9)
- Examine their own biases
- Be gay, lesbian, and bisexual affirmative

The other two-thirds encourage counselors to:

- Use special assessment procedures
- Openly discuss employment discrimination
- Openly discuss coming out in the workplace
- Help clients overcome internalized negative stereotypes
- Support and encourage gay and lesbian professionals as role models
- Work with both partners in a same-sex relationship on dual-career couple issues

The first of these latter six strategies is discussed under *Assessment* in the preceding section. The other five are described under separate subheadings in the following paragraphs.

Discuss Employment Discrimination

Anticipatory anxiety about workplace prejudice affects the career choice and development of gay, lesbian, and bisexual persons. Psychotherapy, however, frequently involves testing the reality of a client's fear. Although often prevalent, formal and informal employment discrimination are seldom universal. Accordingly, clinicians can help clients accurately assess and carefully distinguish between their negative expectations based on historical experiences of oppression and the actual threat present in the occupational environment.

Discuss Coming Out in the Workplace

An earlier discussion of theoretical adaptations and applications to sexual minority clients cites the importance of identity management for work adjustment. To facilitate the development and integration of sexual identity and occupational self-concept, psychotherapists can help sexual minority workers develop individualized plans for coming out in the workplace. These personal strategies should consider the risks and benefits of disclosure based on an accurate assessment of employment discrimination.

Challenge Negative Stereotypes

Some of the negative stereotypes that gay, lesbian, and bisexual clients internalize are discussed among the environmental factors to be appraised in the career assessment of sexual minority workers. These biased generalizations often needlessly restrict occupational selection and restrain vocational development. Accordingly, clinicians can help clients examine the adaptive and defensive functions of these overdetermined representations. Psychotherapists can facilitate self-analysis of homophobic and heterosexist introjects that accurately reflect and respect occupational environments as well as unnecessarily circumscribe and compromise career choices.

Support and Encourage Role Models

The absence of sexual minority role models discourages many gay, lesbian, and bisexual workers from entering certain professions based on the assumption that those occupations are not open to them (Elliott, 1993). For example, if sexual minority adolescents grow up without ever seeing an openly lesbian or gay school teacher, physician, minister, priest, or politician, they may conclude that such a career is closed to people like themselves. Accordingly, sexual minority clients in the early stages of sexual and vocational identity development can be referred to gay, lesbian, and bisexual business and professional organizations for mentoring relationships (see the Resources section, below).

Explore and Resolve Dual-Career Couple Issues

In regard to sexual minority women specifically, dual-career issues are addressed earlier in this chapter. These dyadic concerns, along with those of male couples, also include presenting gay or lesbian relationships and introducing same-sex partners to employers and coworkers. In others words, the discussion of coming out in the workplace often involves a conversation concerning whether and how to disclose relational status as well as sexual orientation. This process frequently is complicated by partner differences in identity development and occupational environment. Ideally, these dilemmas can be explored and resolved in individual as well as conjoint therapy.

Resources

Psychotherapists can help many gay, lesbian, and bisexual clients by becoming familiar with federal, state, and local employment practices regarding sexual minorities in the public and private sectors (Elliot, 1993; Gelberg & Chojnacki, 1996; Shannon & Woods, 1991). Accordingly, HRC WorkNet is "a national source of information on workplace policies and laws surrounding sexual orientation and gender identity" (Human Rights Campaign, 2001). Online information includes WorkAlert, a monthly update on workplace news and developments; "how to" tools for workplace advocates; the WorkNet employer database of companies with nondiscrimination policies, domestic partner benefits, and sexual minority employee groups; lists of states, counties, and cities that prohibit employment discrimination based on (1) sexual orientation and (2) gender identity; and an index of jurisdictions with domestic partner registries.

In addition, clinicians can refer gay, lesbian, and bisexual individuals to sexual minority business and professional groups. These alliances often provide clients with social networks which facilitate further development and integration of their vocational and sexual identities. Gayellow Pages (2000) is a directory of U.S. and Canadian associations, companies, supports, and supplies for the gay lesbian, bisexual and transgender community. Online information includes a catalog of business and professional organizations and resources for sexual minority workers.

CONCLUSION

Two years after homosexuality was officially classified as a mental illness in the American Psychiatric Association's (1952) first edition of the *Diagnostic and Statistical Manual of Mental Disorders* (DSM), Lambert (1954) asserted that vocational guidance was "the most constructive therapeutic approach that could be made in helping homosexual clients improve their social adjustment" (p. 254). Three years into the post-Stonewall gay liberation movement, Blair (1972) echoed Lambert's (1954) earlier assertion with a claim that "homosexuals in this society are more likely to need an employment counselor than a psychiatrist" (p. 7). In accord with these claims, this chapter helps therapists to adapt and apply theories of career choice and development to sexual minority clients in order to advance and more fully account for the vocational preferences and progressions of gay, lesbian, and bisexual workers. Additionally, the discussions of lesbian-specific employment issues address the oppressive conditions of sexism as well as heterosexism in the workplace that sexual minority women might encounter, internalize, and present to clinicians for psychotherapeutic and systemic intervention. Finally, the vocational appraisal, guidance, and resource recommendations offer career counselors strategies and techniques for affirmative practice.

12

Health and Medical Concerns

As discussed throughout this book, stigmatization results in high levels of stress among many sexual minority persons. This distress, in turn, can render lesbians, bisexuals, and gay men more vulnerable than heterosexuals to depression, suicide, alcoholism, drug use and dependency, human immunodeficiency virus (HIV) infection, certain cancers, and cardiovascular disease (Cochran, 1999; Harrison, 1996; Lehmann, Lehmann, & Kelly, 1998; Saunders, 1999). In addition, many lesbians and gay men encounter heterosexist bias from medical and critical care personnel, allied health professionals, and rehabilitation counselors, as well as prejudice directed toward them as parents and toward their children. Their problems often include medical screening of prospective birth parents, assistance with donor insemination procedures, prenatal care, preparation for birth, and routine and emergency pediatric care, along with problems related to gay men's sexual health (Albarran & Salmon, 2000; Carroll, 1999; Harley, Hall, & Savage, 2000; Kenney & Tash, 1992; Patterson, 1995a, 1996, 1998; Perrin & Kulkin, 1996; Rankow, 1995; Scarce, 1999). Because the unique healthcare needs of sexual minority populations often are ignored or misperceived, the most significant health risk for many lesbians and gay men is that they avoid routine healthcare (Harrison, 1996; Harrison & Silenzio, 1996).

BARRIERS TO SEEKING HEALTHCARE

In addition to negative attitudes or information deficits on the part of medical personnel, limited finances prevent sexual minorities from seeking screening for diseases and the relevant treatment (J. C. White & Dull, 1997). Lack of health insurance coverage is the primary obstacle for many (Burnett, Steakley, Slack, Roth, & Lerman, 1999). Bradford and Ryan (1988, 1991), for example, found that 32% of the respondents in their National Lesbian Health Care Survey (*n* = 1,925) were uninsured. Another survey, conducted in 1992, indicated that 42% of the gay men and lesbians surveyed also lacked health insur-

ance (Badgett, 1999). Although increasingly more companies are offering domestic partner and other benefits (see Chapter 4), there still are millions of sexual minorities who do
not have access to health coverage, either in their own names or through a significant
other. Those who do have domestic partner benefits appear to be concentrated in a few
fields of employment—higher education, nonprofit organizations, legal services, computer programming, newspapers and publishing, and hospitals (Badgett, 1999).

Provider Bias

Bias toward gay, lesbian, and bisexual patients also can influence the willingness of sexual minorities to seek care from the mainstream medical establishment (Carroll, 1999;
Scarce, 1999). For example, G. B. Smith (1993) measured attitudes toward gay men and
lesbians, as well as levels of homophobia, among 165 psychiatric nurses (ages 24 to 70).
Although most of these professionals demonstrated neutral or mildly positive attitudes,
57% indicated moderate and 20% indicated severe levels of homophobia. Smith thus
concluded that nurses express cognitive acceptance of lesbians and gay men, but also
hold negatively charged sentiments that potentially could affect the quality of healthcare
delivered to these patients.

Similarly, less than two-thirds (62.4%) of 117 family medicine residents surveyed indicated that they were comfortable with homosexuals, and a number of them retained the
notion that gay men deserved to get AIDS (acquired immune deficiency syndrome)
(Prichard, Dial, Holloway, & Mosley, 1988). Likewise, another group of family practice
residents and psychiatric residents and faculty (n = 72) were polled and generally scored
in the low range on a homophobia index; nonetheless, 4.2% felt gay men with AIDS "got
what they deserved" (Chaimowitz, 1991). Other surveys of 144 rural nursing personnel
(D'Augelli, 1989a), 161 students training for health professions (Royse & Birge, 1987),
and 200 undergraduate nursing education students (Eliason & Raheim, 2000) also indicated generally negative attitudes and high levels of discomfort that were inversely associated with empathy toward AIDS patients and sexual minorities and the quality of care
these patients might receive. In regard to women, 120 female undergraduate nursing students were administered questionnaires; 50% indicated that lesbians were not acceptable
in society, 15% felt there should be laws against lesbian sexual behavior, and only 24%
were willing to invite a lesbian to their home (Eliason & Randall, 1991).

Psychotherapeutic Issues

Among healthcare providers, negative attitudes toward gay, lesbian, and bisexual populations—as well as lack of information on their specific health concerns—create barriers for
sexual minority patients who seek healthcare services. While systemic change can help
them overcome or circumvent many of these external obstacles, psychotherapists also
may need to assist these clients in examining their internal impediments to healthcare
utilization. For example, overdetermined negative expectations of provider bias or
ignorance could reflect internalized homophobia and should be explored. In other words,
some sexual minority patients automatically and unconsciously might assume and anticipate provider prejudice and inexperience from affirming and informed professionals.
Clinicians, therefore, are encouraged to apply both intrapsychic and structural intervention to modify internal and external barriers to healthcare treatment.

CHEMICAL DEPENDENCY

Alcohol and other substances constitute a major problem for many lesbians, bisexuals, and gay men (Abbott, 1998; Bergmark, 1999; Cabaj, 1995, 1996c; Crosby, Stall, Paul, & Barrett, 1998; Israelstam & Lambert, 1986; T. S. Weinberg, 1995). In particular, a high use of methamphetamines, cocaine, and "psychedelic" drugs, such as MDMA ("Ecstasy"), has been reported (J. Beck & Rosenbaum, 1994; Gorman, 2000; Klitzman, Pope, & Hudson, 2000). Various authorities have estimated that between 28% and 35% of the sexual minority population has difficulty with the ingestion of substances, compared with 10% to 12% of the general population (Cabaj, 1995, 1996c; Finnegan & McNally, 1990; Glaus, 1988; Kominars, 1989; Kus, 1990; H. B. McDonald & Steinhorn, 1993; Schaefer, Evans, & Coleman, 1987; Ziebold & Mongeon, 1985). Consistent with these estimates are findings from a survey of 3,400 gay men and lesbians indicating that substantially more of them used alcohol, marijuana, or cocaine than did people in general (McKirnan & Peterson, 1989a). Although they did not necessarily use cocaine and marijuana with more frequency and intensity, these lesbians and gay men did reveal higher rates of alcohol problems. Although in the general population, substance use significantly declines with age and women ingest fewer drugs and less alcohol than do men, neither pattern holds in the experience of gay men and lesbians (Bergmark, 1999). In fact, older lesbians have more alcohol problems than do heterosexual women in a comparable age range (Abbott, 1998; Eliason & Hughes, 2000; Falco, 1996).

Similarly, Skinner (1994) compared prevalence rates for a sample of 190 lesbians and 265 gay men to those obtained for the general population from a National Household Survey on Drug Abuse (NHSDA). Among the "early" adults (ages 18 to 25), 37.5% of gay men and 23.5% of lesbians had used marijuana in the last month, compared to 16.5% of men and 9.1% of women in general. Among the "young" adults (ages 26 to 34), 81.3% of gay men and 66.7% of lesbians had used alcohol in the past month, compared to 73.7% of men and 55.2% of women in general. Skinner and Otis (1996) later compared self-report data from 1,067 lesbian and gay respondents to comprehensive societal information from the NHSDA. Their subjects were found to have higher prevalence rates for the use of marijuana, inhalants, and alcohol, but not for cocaine. On the basis of comparative data, Skinner (1994) concluded that alcohol and drug use in the United States gay and lesbian community comprises a public health concern that demands immediate attention.

As with other research that involves hidden sexual minorities, measuring the extent of substance-related disorders among bisexuals, lesbians, and gay men is bound to be inaccurate. Locating subjects in lesbian and gay bars has resulted in biased samples for some studies. Further, imprecise definitions and changing terminology (i.e., use, abuse, addiction, alcoholism, dependence, heavy drinking, problem drinking), as well as the use of self-report and non–control group designs, have created methodological concerns and have rendered certain findings highly questionable (Abbott, 1998; Bux, 1996; Cabaj, 1995, 1996c; Eliason & Hughes, 2000; Hughes & Wilsnack, 1997; Nardi, 1982; Razzano et al., 2000). The following discussions, therefore, proceed under the assumption that considerable substance use and dependence exists within the sexual minority population, but certainly future research will be necessary to determine the precise extent of the problem. Moreover, because the literature primarily addresses alcohol, a lower number of references to other psychoactive substances are cited here. Until more drug-specific studies of sexual minority addicts become available, therapists are left to rely on the mainstream drug research data and must adapt this information accordingly. Further, clinicians should consider similarities between alcoholism and other substance addictions and apply crossover treatment interventions to sexual minority clients, as deemed appropriate.

Lesbian Substance Use

Lesbian and bisexual women have been reported to use or abuse alcohol and other drugs at higher rates than do heterosexual women (Abbott, 1998; Cochran, 1999; Cochran & Mays, 2000b; Eliason & Hughes, 2000; Koh, 2000; Lehmann et al., 1998; Moran, 1996; Mosbacher, 1988; Roberts & Sorensen, 1999; J. C. White & Levinson, 1995). A research project in New Zealand involved a survey of 561 lesbians (Welch, Howden-Chapman, & Collings, 1998). Results revealed that 90.2% had consumed alcohol and 32.6% had used cannabis at least once in the past year; 75.8% had used cannabis and 30.8% had used other recreational drugs at some time in their lives. The alcohol consumption of 57 American lesbians and 43 heterosexual women was compared, first by Saghir, Robins, Walbran, and Gentry (1970) and later by C. E. Lewis, Saghir, and Robins (1982). Initially, a history of excessive or alcoholic drinking was found among 35% of the lesbians compared to 5% of the heterosexual women. Reanalysis of the data 12 years later revealed that 28% of the lesbians and 5% of the heterosexuals were rated as alcoholics, and 33% of the lesbians and 7% of the heterosexuals were rated as heavy drinkers. On a positive note, recent studies have indicated that more lesbians than heterosexual women are in recovery from substance abuse problems (Cochran, 1999; Eliason & Hughes, 2000; Razzano et al., 2000). One survey (Razzano et al., 2000), coincidentally, found approximately the same percentages of women had used alcohol or drug-related services within the past 5 years (23% of 63 lesbians, compared with 4% of 57 heterosexual women) as were found to drink inordinately in the Saghir et al. (1970) and C. E. Lewis et al. (1982) studies just cited.

Heterosexist Oppression and Other Contributing Factors

Heterosexist oppression, internalized homophobia, and ensuing conflicts about sexual orientation are thought to be major contributors to the high rates of chemical dependence and abuse among lesbians, bisexuals, and gay men (Beatty et al., 1999; Cabaj, 1995, 1996c; Finnegan & McNally, 1987, 1989, 1990; Glaus, 1988; Hughes et al., 2000; Israelstam & Lambert, 1989; Nicoloff & Stiglitz, 1987; Ratner, 1988; Shifrin & Solis, 1992; Sorensen & Roberts, 1997). As discussed throughout this book, stigmatization adversely affects mental health, psychic structures, and overall functioning, thus creating intense emotional distress, depression, anxiety, loneliness, and a range of other dysphoric emotions. Societal homophobia exacerbates feelings of fear, low self-worth, isolation, alienation, and shame for a considerable number of sexual minorities (Finnegan & McNally, 1987, 1990; Ghindia & Kola, 1996). Consequently, many "who are at risk for chemical dependency may drink or use other drugs to medicate their depression, to fill the void, to kill the pain, or to create the illusion of not being different" (Finnegan & McNally, 1987, p. 41). Since sexism combined with heterosexism creates a double form of oppression for lesbians, both sexism and homophobia must be taken into account when focusing on the etiology and treatment of substance dependence and abuse in lesbians (Underhill, 1991). Accordingly, McNally and Finnegan (1992) described a model by which women in recovery accept and integrate two subidentities of *lesbian* and *alcoholic* into a single distinct identity of *lesbian recovering alcoholic.*

Milliger and Young (1990) surveyed 126 homosexuals who were recovering from alcoholism using, among other measures, the Gay Perceived Acceptance Social Isolation Scale (PASI). Since struggles with sexuality were found to heavily influence high PASI ratings, the authors concluded that resolving these conflicts could increase acceptance, reduce isolation, and thus improve prognoses for long-term recovery from alcoholism. Along this same vein, Kus (1988) surveyed 20 recovering alcoholic gay men, none of whom reported seeing a positive aspect of being gay until after establishing their sobriety. Many, also, did not recognize the extent of their internalized homophobia before initiating recovery. In a later work, Kus (1990) concluded that "sobriety leads to acceptance, and not the other way around" (p. 69). In other words, struggles with sexual orientation contribute to substance dependence and abuse and cannot be resolved independent of the recovery process. Hence, without an acceptance of their homosexuality, sobriety is difficult for lesbians and gay men to maintain.

Tension Reduction

McKirnan and Peterson (1988) hypothesized a "stress–vulnerability" model of substance abuse, wherein individuals with culturally specific stressors would show elevated rates of alcohol and drug abuse. They tested their model among gay men and found that the tension-reduction expectancies of alcohol effects had a substantial influence on use, as did the frequenting of bars as a social resource to reduce loneliness. Two other variables, negative affectivity (presumably depression and other dysphoric emotions) and sexual orientation discrimination also affected chemical abuse. They tested their model on 3,400 gay men and lesbians (McKirnan & Peterson, 1989a, 1989b), and data supported their stress–vulnerability perspective. In other words, heterosexist oppression, combined with expectancies of relief through chemicals, renders many gay, lesbian, and bisexual individuals vulnerable to alcohol and drug problems.

STRESS

Several other writers also cite the relationship between culturally induced stress and substance use and abuse in adults (S. E. James & Murphy, 1998; Jordan, 2000; Prairielands, 2000; Safren, 1998), and Chapter 6 details the use of chemicals in sexual minority adolescents. One study (DeBord, Wood, Sher, & Good, 1998) followed 39 gay, lesbian, or bisexual and 156 heterosexual college students for 4 years after matriculation. As predicted, the relationship between psychological distress scores and alcohol dependence was stronger for gay, lesbian, and bisexual subjects. Parks (1999) likewise found that alcohol use served a social function for 31 lesbians as they began to struggle with their attractions to women and the subsequent conflict with heterosexist expectations and values. Alcohol was a far more available commodity than was adult or peer support for many of the subjects at this difficult time in their lives. Other women have been found to use food, sometimes in addition to alcohol, to regulate affect (Heffernan, 1998a, 1998b). Of 263 lesbians studied, those who were more angry and frustrated felt a stronger urge to eat in order to manage their dysphoric emotions and to feel comforted. While high rates of heavy drinking and drug use were not found in this sample, those women who drank excessively tended to have more avoidant coping styles and to rely on bars as their primary social setting.

Psychoactive substances, then, frequently are used to tranquilize the tension and mitigate the stress created by being gay, lesbian, or bisexual in a heterosexist society (Cabaj, 1995, 1996c; Gorman, 2000; H. B. McDonald & Steinhorn, 1993; Shifrin & Solis, 1992). Cabaj (1995) further notes that "substance abusing gays and lesbians . . . may be particularly vulnerable to the false promises of so-called conversion or reparative therapy" (p. 98) (see Chapter 13). He explains that the desire to change sexual orientation usually recedes after abstinence from substances, but that these individuals need treatment that is open, accepting, and affirming in order to explore and resolve their internalized homophobia and maintain their sobriety.

MIRRORING

As discussed throughout this book (Chapters 3, 8, 9, 14, and 16), sexual minorities often missed the parental mirroring that is provided to heterosexual children and adolescents. Accordingly, Cabaj (1995) contends that "substance use serves as an easy relief to the tensions created in gay men and lesbians in this developmental process, providing acceptance, and, more importantly, mirroring the 'comforting' dissociation developed in childhood" (p. 102). The dissociative state created by alcohol and other drugs provides relief from emotions and anxiety, "mimicking the emotional state many gay people had to develop in childhood to survive" (p. 102). This detached condition is comforting in that it helps many sexual minorities brace for rejection, engage in social and sexual encounters with others like themselves, or live in a closet where denial and dissociation are essential. Cabaj (1995) notes that many have their first homosexual erotic experiences while drinking and that this association between sexuality and chemicals is "a very powerful behavioral link," which is difficult to "unlink" later in life (p. 103). In his study of methamphetamine and other drug use in gay and bisexual men, Gorman (2000) acknowledges this association between the consumption of chemicals and the context and meaning of sexual experiences. A dissociative state usually is not clinically significant, however, if recovery from substances is sustained and individuals are able to resolve underlying homophobia and find sober methods of tension reduction. If the dissociation persists, or if there is a solid history of dissociation, therapists should consider the possibility of a dissociative identity disorder since there are cases in the literature of these conditions being associated with substance abuse in gay males (McDowell, Levin, & Nunes, 1999).

Childhood Sexual Abuse

Abusive home and childhood environments also have been shown to contribute to high rates of substance use and abuse among sexual minorities (J. M. Hall, 1998, 1999; Roberts, 1999). In this regard, Hall (1996) performed an in-depth study of alcohol recovery experiences of 35 lesbians (ages 24 to 54) and found that 35% of the women had survived childhood sexual abuse. This group reported multiple addictions, self-harm, isolation, sexual problems, depression, self-loathing, physical illness, and difficulties with work and employment. Those women who did not report childhood sexual abuse were more socially and occupationally stable, self-satisfied, and physically healthy. Hall concluded that the alcohol problems of this latter group were more circumscribed and responsive to conventional intervention. The histories of the women who had been sexually abused as children, however, appeared to intensify health risks that complicated alcohol recovery, thus necessitating more comprehensive clinical attention. S. T. Perry (1995) also sampled the relationship between coercive sexual activities and the use of substances, primarily alcohol and marijuana, in lesbian and bisexual women (n = 152). Findings revealed an association not only between past abusive events and chemical use but also between current high-risk sexual behaviors and the use of alcohol and marijuana.

Neisen and Sandall (1990) conducted a retrospective inpatient chart review at the Pride Institute, a treatment program for alcoholic and drug-dependent lesbians and gay men. Of the 201 patients whose files were surveyed, nearly 50% had reported being sexually abused in childhood. Other writers also have noted a high incidence of sexual abuse among gay and lesbian problem drinkers and drug addicts and speculated that the violations occur within the context of disinhibited, disorganized, and chemically dependent family systems (Bradford & Ryan, 1988, 1991; Glaus, 1988; J. M. Hall, 1998, 1999; Shernoff & Finnegan, 1991). Along these same lines, Loulan (1987) surveyed 1,566 lesbians and detected that 49% of those identified as current or recovering alcoholics or addicts, compared to 34% of those identified as nonalcoholics or addicts, had been sexually abused in childhood. She also found that 50% of the women raised in alcoholic homes had histories of childhood sexual abuse, contrasted with 32% of those raised in nonalcoholic households. In addition, Loulan discovered that 57% of the alcoholic, addicted, and recovering lesbians had been raised in alcoholic homes, thus suggesting a strong correlation between lesbian chemical dependency and family alcoholism. Data from a study of 341 gay men similarly revealed that a familial history of substance abuse accounted for half the variance of alcohol abuse and over one-third the variance in drug abuse among those who completed the survey (Ghindia & Kola, 1996). In other words, high levels of chemical dependency in family members were significantly associated with alcohol and drug abuse in the gay men questioned.

Power and Powerlessness

Some psychodynamically oriented theorists hypothesize that excessive drinking or drug use by some gay men has its origins partially in concerns related to dependency, power, and masculinity (Lemle & Mishkind, 1989; Siegel & Lowe, 1994). For gay men, who often have grown up feeling less manly and less influential than heterosexual males, drinking is "associated with increased power-related behaviors such as assertiveness, sexual advances, and verbal or physical aggression" (Nicoloff & Stiglitz, 1987, p. 285). These behaviors are seen as compensatory in men who were considered gender-discordant or feminine as boys, but who feel in control and hardy under the influence of drugs or alcohol. The HIV epidemic also has rendered numerous gay men feeling hopeless and vulnerable. The use of methamphetamines and other chemicals provide some with a sense of energy and the illusion of self-confidence (Marion, 1996). Many of these same dynamics also manifest themselves in lesbians, who often accept their dependency needs less readily than do heterosexual women (Nicoloff & Stiglitz, 1987). Since aggressive and assertive behavior changes point directionally toward masculinity, some women are thought to use chemicals as a means to reduce sex role conflict. Feeling powerless, both as women and

as lesbians, the confidence and positive self-esteem they experience when drinking reinforces their dependence on substances. Therapy with both gay men and lesbians, then,
must assist clients in feeling empowered and congruent in their sex role without the use of
drugs and alcohol.

Racism

Sexual minorities of color are confronted with an additional aspect of oppression in the
form of racism. As described in Chapter 10, they often feel trapped between the racism
and heterosexism of the broader culture and the homophobia of their ethnic communities, leaving them caught between cultures. To alleviate this strain and distress, many rely
on drugs and alcohol (Cabaj, 1996c; Gonzalez & Espin, 1996; Icard & Traunstein, 1987;
Sterk & Elifson, 2000; Tafoya, 1996). The incidence of substance abuse and dependence
among gay men, lesbians, and bisexuals of color, however, is somewhat speculative as researchers only recently have begun to investigate rates of occurrence among these populations. Further, many sexual minority members of ethnic groups conceal their sexual orientation in order to maintain a favorable status in their cultural communities (see
Chapter 10).

Assessment

As with all substance abuse evaluations, assessments of chemical dependency in bisexuals, lesbians, and gay men must be specific regarding the frequency, range, and quantity
of use, as well as the impact of the substance(s) on all areas of their lives. In light of the
contributing factors discussed previously in this chapter, these appraisals also must assess
for the following: childhood physical and sexual abuse; family alcohol and drug use; relationship with family of origin; history of depression, grief, and loss; suicide attempts; past
and present domestic violence; current relationship status; parenting history; previous or
current heterosexual marriage; career and economic status; and support network (Cabaj,
1996c; Glaus, 1988; Gorman, 2000; Kus, 1990; Prairielands, 2000; Shernoff & Finnegan, 1991). Specifically, "coming-out" histories must be taken with sensitivity and as
much specificity as clients will allow (Cabaj, 1996c; Finnegan & McNally, 1987). Therapists might need to remind themselves, however, that many sexual minority clients began
drinking to limit awareness of their same-sex erotic and emotional attractions. Thus, they
may deny adamantly their sexual behaviors, fantasies, and feelings due to internalized
heterosexism, homophobia, and shame. Nevertheless, asking questions related to choice
of sexual partner offers clients an opportunity to disclose, conveys a message that sexual
orientation is a legitimate concern, and addresses the issue of hidden anguish, which, if
not shared, may result in feelings of alienation or loneliness or in unsuccessful treatment
outcomes.

Treatment

When bisexuals, lesbians, and gay men actually enter treatment for chemical dependency,
they often do so with a measure of mistrust. Their fears and suspicions are not unfounded, however, since many alcohol treatment programs either avoid or only reluctantly address concerns relevant to their sexuality (Hellman, Stanton, Lee, Tytun, &

Vachon, 1989; Israelstam, 1986; Kus, 1990, 1995; Neisen & Sandall, 1990; Nicoloff & Stiglitz, 1987; Travers & Schneider, 1996; Weinstein, 1993). Additionally, sexual minority clients frequently anticipate that the staff will not protect them if they are harassed by other patients. While some patients may be required by therapists to reveal their sexual orientation in group counseling, others may be forbidden to self-disclose by staff who contend that a divulgence of homosexuality may disrupt the serenity of other patients or who consider disclosure an irrelevant distraction from the real issues of alcoholism. For these reasons, some authorities (e.g., MacEwan, 1994) suggest that group therapy may be undesirable for sexual minority clients, particularly gay men.

In any case, gay, lesbian, and bisexual clients face several dilemmas during treatment. If they reveal their sexual orientation, they face possible alienation from other patients or rejection by peers or staff. If they do not come out, they can be labeled as untruthful. If they point out their differences from heterosexual clients, they can be seen as asking for special privileges or jeopardizing the recovery of others. If they accept generic treatment, however, their own recovery may be endangered (Prairielands, 2000).

Thus, whether the therapeutic climate is permissive, prohibitive, or coercive, clients must decide whether or not to self-disclose. If they decide to remain closeted, however, they perpetuate the dishonest communication patterns that were originally established around sexual orientation and chemical dependency. In addition, maintaining secrecy may prevent them from exploring and resolving significant recovery issues (Nicoloff & Stiglitz, 1987). Cabaj (1995) strongly believes that sexual orientation needs to be addressed early in recovery since "relapse is almost certain if the gay [lesbian, or bisexual] person cannot acknowledge and accept his or her sexual orientation" (p. 106). Early recovery is a time when many may seek a change in sexual orientation, blaming homosexuality for their substance abuse. Thus, by engaging in denial and attempting to alter the unchangeable, anxiety and depression often lead to relapse. In other words, unless clients are helped to examine their internalized homophobia and are provided ways to live as sober lesbian, gay, or bisexual individuals, the prognosis for recovery is poor.

Internalized Homophobia

In addition to standard protocols for treating chemical dependency, most programs that specialize in the recovery of sexual minority clients (see Resources section for examples) directly address the homophobia and conflicts with sexual orientation that initially contributed to the drug or alcohol problems (Cabaj, 1995; Glaus, 1988; Kus, 1990, 1995; Ratner, 1988; Weinstein, 1993). In these curricula, clients are provided information and perspective on gay and lesbian identity formation, as well as the sociocultural roots of sexual minority oppression and their relationship to substance abuse. Since denial is common to struggles with both substance abuse and sexual orientation, clinicians can expect to encounter various degrees of resistance when openly addressing these issues. Treatment, however, must not collude with keeping the dual stigmas of alcoholism and homosexuality hidden and secret. In fact, if either stigma is rendered invisible in therapy, "then the treatment is incomplete and inadequate" (Finnegan & McNally, 1987, p. 77).

Since homophobia and substance abuse produce similar negative effects, clients can be taught to identify feelings common to the "dual oppressions." Possibilities include denial, anxiety, fear, suspicion, hostility, anger, rage, arrogance, guilt, shame, self-pity, depression, powerlessness, helplessness, hopelessness, fragmentation, isolation, alienation, confusion, self-deception, passivity, victimization, inferiority, self-loathing, and low self-esteem (Cabaj, 1995; Finnegan & McNally, 1987). Treatment must actively teach clients to integrate both stigmatized identities given that their dynamics are intrapsychically parallel (Cabaj, 1995; Diamond-Friedman, 1990). Since clients become stigmatized in two domains (alcoholism and homosexuality), they must recover along two trajectories following a similar common path—awareness, admission, acceptance (surrender), and reconstruction (Finnegan & McNally, 1987).

Sexism

Lesbians especially need therapists who are sensitive to the concerns and communication preferences of women. In this regard, 35 chemically dependent lesbians who were asked to describe barriers in their alcohol treatment identified the persuasive styles of staff as pivotal to recovery. A confrontational approach caused problems for some women, most of whom preferred an influential style that is characterized by flexibility, negotiation, support, and avoidance of ultimatums (Hall, 1994a). If the style of the staff is argumentative, a crisis can be precipitated in women with histories of physical and sexual trauma since activation of the original dynamics can be overly stimulating and counterproductive to recovery. Hall's findings also challenge the assumption that alcoholics are manipulative and, therefore, require coercion to establish and maintain recovery. Other lesbians have reported feeling threatened by masculine and heterosexist bias in a treatment center, and, in one New Zealand study, 50% of the lesbian participants in such a situation said they hid their sexuality throughout the regimen (MacEwan, 1994).

In addition to objecting to the patriarchal image of God and the antifeminist, nonrelational concept of a Higher Power as presented in Alcoholics Anonymous (AA) and other 12-Step groups, lesbians frequently are offended by the pervasive sexism, male domination, and emphasis on overcoming obstacles by surrendering personal power rather than by promoting a healthier sense of self-reliance (Glaus, 1988; MacEwan, 1994; Razzano et al., 2000). In this regard, 35 recovering lesbians were interviewed (Hall, 1994b), 74% of whom were involved in AA. Only a few of these 26 women attended lesbian AA meetings exclusively, and the majority acknowledged considerable tension when participating with the general AA population. They described their tension as a conflict between assimilation and differentiation, between authority and autonomy, and between philosophical ideologies and political realities.

Aftercare Preparation

Ziebold and Mongeon (1985) noted that the usual goal of alcohol treatment programs—to return clients to the "mainstream of life" (p. 6)—is questionable for recovering gay men, bisexuals, and lesbians whose marginalization from the broader culture has contributed to their problems with chemicals. Unlike heterosexual clients, their treatment must include preparation for returning to a sexist and heterosexist society without relapsing into using chemicals to deal with oppressive conditions (Cabaj, 1995; D. Crawford, 1990; Finnegan & McNally, 1987; Israelstam & Lambert, 1986; T. M. Smith, 1987; Underhill, 1991; T. S. Weinberg, 1995; S. Whitney, 1982). In this regard, sexual minority clients must be helped to establish social support from others like themselves before they go back to their own communities, which often include a gay or lesbian bar as the only gathering place for group socialization. Treatment, in other words, must assist them in living chemical-free in a gay and lesbian environment that values sober socializing and sober sex.

Environmental resources, such as gay and lesbian AA meetings, to support individuals in recovery are scarce in rural areas and often are available only in large cities (Kus, 1987). Therefore, many individuals need assistance in establishing alternative sources of support that they can access in their daily lives. Telephone and Internet contacts may prove helpful in this regard. Because, as already discussed, some recovering sexual minorities are distressed by the heterosexism and covert or overt homophobia at regular meetings of AA and other 12-Step groups, alternatives may need to be generated (Kus, 1990).

Engaging in sexual activities while sober also can be problematic for some recovering sexual minorities since, before recovery, they may have come to associate chemicals with same-sex intimate activity. If substance use was linked with sexual expression either to numb feelings of fear, denial, or anxiety or to intensify the experience, sober sex may be quite difficult to achieve (Cabaj, 1996c). Relationship problems also may be an issue in recovery since chemicals either may have been used to facilitate friendships and relationships or may have affected them negatively (Bryant & Demian, 1995; T. M. Smith, 1982). As evidenced throughout the previous discussions, many of these concerns are common to both the gay and lesbian experience of substance abuse and dependence. Each in some way may have contributed to the chemical abuse and, thus, has been affected by it. Therefore, all of these relevant treatment issues must be addressed clearly and specifically with each client (Cabaj, 1996c; Crawford, 1990).

Staff Awareness

Often, staff of drug treatment programs lack information about many of the important issues that affect sexual minority clients, and these clinicians may need population-specific inservice education related to both drug abuse and alcoholism. They also may require specific training regarding how oppression and discrimination contribute to struggles with sexual orientation and chemical dependency (Cabaj, 1996c; Eliason & Hughes, 2000; Kus, 1990, 1995; Nicoloff & Stiglitz, 1987; Prairielands, 2000; T. M. Smith, 1982; Travers & Schneider, 1996; Zigrang, 1982).

Clinicians also may need additional information about the concerns of lesbian and gay couple and family relationships (see Part IV, this volume). Because lesbians are more likely than gay men to be in committed relationships and to be parents, there may need to be an emphasis on family and parenting concerns, as well as on the unique dynamics of relationships between two women, when working with some lesbian substance abusers (Anderson, 1996; Cabaj, 1995). Gay male couples and their families will be affected similarly by chemical use, however, and both gay and lesbian couples may need assistance in overcoming the damaging effects that substances have had on their relationships and family life (Cabaj, 1996c).

Adjuncts to Therapy

Bibliotherapy can be useful in the recovery process, and clients can be referred to AA manuals and pamphlets, 12-step guides, and books on meditation, recovery, and spirituality, some of which have been written specifically for lesbians and gay men (Bittle, 1982; Kettelhack, 1999; Kus, 1989). Whether or not they have access to minority-specific AA meetings, individuals should be helped early in treatment to find a gay or lesbian (affirming) sponsor who can help them live without chemicals in their own communities. In addition, partners and other family members can be enlisted to participate in recovery and aftercare programs, as well as be invited to Al-Anon and other family support groups (Cabaj, 1996c; Glaus, 1988; Kus, 1990, 1991). Having both members of a couple involved throughout these processes is particularly important since the pair may need assistance in repairing a relationship that undoubtedly has been damaged by the effects of chemical use. Finally, the Resources section contains a list of treatment centers and other resources designed especially for chemically dependent clients, their families, and their therapists.

LESBIAN HEALTH CONCERNS

The Women's Health Initiative (WHI) is a collection of studies sponsored by the National Institutes of Health in which 164,500 women aged 50 to 79 are being followed for 15 years (K. A. Matthews et al., 1997). There are three components to the project: randomized controlled clinical trials, an observational study, and a community prevention study. Preliminary data (n = 93,311) from 40 WHI study centers representing geographic and ethnic diversity indicate several increased health risks among lesbians when compared with heterosexual women, including higher lifetime smoking habits, more depression, a higher prevalence of obesity, more alcohol consumption, and a lower frequency of Papanicolaou (Pap) tests (Bowen, 1999; Valanis et al., 2000). In addition to these health risks, other problems, such as higher caffeine use, less healthy diets, and heavier ideal body weights, have been identified (Herzog, Newman, Yeh, & Warshaw, 1992; Koh, 2000; N. Moran, 1996). While many lesbians have regular Pap smears (54% within the past year, and 71% in the last 2 years), and mammograms (70% within the past year, and 83% in the last 2 years), many others are not taking advantage of these important tests at the recommended rate (Diamant, Schuster, & Lever, 2000).

Lesbians and the Healthcare System

Data from a nationwide survey of 1,925 lesbians sponsored by the National Lesbian and Gay Health Foundation (Bradford & Ryan, 1988; Bradford et al., 1994) indicated that respondents generally lacked confidence in the healthcare system. Further, many of the midlife lesbians (ages 40 to 60) in the sample had fairly serious health needs that did not appear to be appropriately met, and they had not found providers who delivered services impartially to sexual minority women. Their most frequently cited problems were in the critical area of gynecological care, which included Pap smears and breast examinations. In this regard, 17% said that their primary providers provided care as if they were sexually active with men. One-quarter of the midlife lesbians who received gynecological treatment in the public healthcare system experienced similar heterosexist treatment from their physicians (Bradford & Ryan, 1991).

Unfavorable Reactions

Results of several studies have found that lesbians generally are reluctant to seek healthcare, and many have reported having experienced negative reactions from healthcare providers (Carroll, 1999; O'Hanlan, 1995, 2000; White & Dull, 1997). Further, findings from one study of 45 lesbians (Stevens, 1994) reflected that they experienced heightened vulnerability in healthcare settings and relied on a repertoire of protective strategies in these environments. These defensive approaches included screening providers, seeking those who reflect the lesbian experience, maintaining vigilance, controlling information, bringing a witness, and challenging mistreatment. Several other studies likewise discovered that lesbians often are uncomfortable in healthcare situations that feel more heterosexist than lesbian-affirming and supportive, as well as more intimidating than respectful, empowering, or negotiating (Buenting, 1992; Carroll, 1999; Mathieson, 1998; Rankow, 1995; Saulnier, 1999; Stevens, 1992, 1995, 1996; Stevens & Hall, 1990; Trippet & Bain, 1992, 1993). Because of such experiences, many of these women delay seeking healthcare as they anticipate and calculate the risks of self-disclosing their sexual orientation. When services are sought, scanning and monitoring strategies frequently are employed to reevaluate the presumed dangers in the environment.

Some 13% of the midlife lesbians in Bradford and Ryan's (1991) sample indicated that they felt they could not come out to their primary physician. These data reflect the views of primarily Caucasian women (90%) and can be contrasted with a multiethnic sample of lesbian and bisexual women, ages 20 to 75 (DiPlacido, 2000). Accordingly, the 403 subjects who responded to a survey included 49% women of color. Of this population, 25% of Latinas, 20% of White women, and 15% of Black women concealed their sexual orientations from their physicians. In contrast, only 31% of lesbians in another study (n = 53) had disclosed their sexual orientation to their healthcare provider (Lehmann et al., 1998). This low figure compares with 61% from a presumably more "out" sample of 6,935 self-identified lesbian readers of a national biweekly gay, lesbian, and bisexual new magazine (Diamant et al., 2000).

Affirmative Responses

Federal responses to the health status of lesbian and bisexual women was limited until 1993 when representatives of the Department of Health and Human Services met with members of lesbian and gay health organizations. Several initiatives emerged from a series of meetings, one of which was a lesbian health agenda that included lesbian and bisexual women in the large, longitudinal Women's Health Initiative (discussed previously in this chapter). Also, as a result of these meetings, a Committee on Lesbian Health Research Priorities, Institute of Medicine, was authorized to conduct a workshop to examine the need for future research on the health of lesbians, focusing on existing data and evaluating research methodologies. Authorities in various areas were invited to present and participate.

In her testimony on behalf of the American Psychological Association at the lesbian health committee workshop, Patterson (1997b) noted that little is known about the mental and physical health of lesbian and bisexual women due to the near absence of questions about sexual orientation in health research on the general population. "Opposition to including sexual orientation as a demographic or independent variable in research has been quite potent" (p. 2). Her testimony, therefore, advocated the modification of federal research policy to include sexual orientation in clinical, services, and prevention research. The workshop proceedings were translated into an extensive report (Solarz, 1999) that identified reasons for directing attention to the study of lesbian health issues, examined the complexity of looking at lesbian health and the numerous methodological difficulties involved, identified research gaps and priorities, and offered recommendations for improving the knowledge base on lesbian health. Implementation efforts were begun after the release of the report, but the process will be long and continuous, given the minimal efforts thus far by the federal government on behalf of lesbian and bisexual women's health. For example, the government's "blueprint" for health care in the next century, *Healthy People 2010*, contains virtually no references to the healthcare needs of sexual minorities ("Lesbian Health," 2000).

Breast Cancer

Due to different reproductive events, including having children later or not having them at all, as well as factors such as those discussed in the previous section, lesbians may be at a higher risk for breast cancer than are heterosexual women (Bowen, 1999; Burnett et al., 1999; Lauver et al., 1999; "National Focus for Lesbian Survivors," 2000). In spite of this possible increased susceptibility, many lesbians do not avail themselves of frequent mammography screening. Concern among researchers and practitioners has led to several studies that explore lesbian health risks for breast cancer and are being conducted at various centers across the United States (discussed throughout this section). In addition, women from the Mautner Project, an organization that serves lesbians with cancer (see Resources section), organized the first national symposium of lesbians and cancer in 2000. Designed to establish an agenda for lesbian cancer research and support services, the conference was attended by individuals from lesbian cancer-advocacy organizations and representatives from government agencies and the medical community.

Numerous issues arise for lesbians who have been diagnosed with breast cancer, many of which are quite similar to those that involve gay men with HIV infection. So much so, in fact, that some gay male writers have challenged other gay men to become involved in the struggles of lesbians with breast and other cancers, just as lesbians have assisted gay men in their fights against AIDS (Gallagher, 1997b; Phelps, 2000). In addition to increasing recognition given to the concerns of lesbians with breast cancer, women with the diagnosis are finding considerable support from current publications, an increasing number of which are giving recognition to their trials (Love, 2000).

Difficulties with Healthcare Providers

Even if the lesbians with a cancer diagnosis have established open communication with their primary care physicians about their sexual orientation, referrals to specialists for consultation and treatment may evoke new predicaments about disclosure and lifestyle (Haber et al., 1995; A. K. Matthews, 1998). Fear of stigmatization and of compromised care often intensify the anxiety related to the cancer itself. If lesbians have partners, issues about visitation, support during examinations, and authorization for emergency treatment may arise in medical facilities and hospitals. Family-of-origin members may ask questions about the presence of a significant other, feel uncomfortable with lesbian visitors, or want to take an ill woman "home" with them. In turn, the lesbian partner may feel unacknowledged and betrayed. Although the drafting of durable and medical powers of attorney can be used to reduce or eliminate some of these problems (see Chapter 4), le-

gal documents cannot replace or eliminate the need for personal disclosure of sexual orientation and relationship status to medical personnel or family members.

Social Support

Breast cancer support groups usually are geared toward the concerns of heterosexual
women, and lesbians in these groups have trouble relating to discussions about whether
husbands or boyfriends will still find them engaging or if they will be able to find a male
partner after surgery (Haber et al., 1995). While many lesbian survivors of breast cancer
are concerned with the same issues of femininity, or if present or future partners will find
them attractive, they nevertheless can feel alienated by the heterosexist nature of the support group conversations. Hence, they may receive little sustenance or comfort in these
groups (A. K. Matthews, 1998). Some lesbians feel they have little in common with a
group of heterosexual women, other than the fact that they all have breast cancer. This
lack of identification leads many to stop attending (Gallagher, 1997a).

   Because the lesbian cancer survivor's partner also is a woman, she may "experience
her own heightened sense of vulnerability to the disease" (Haber et al., 1995, p. 66). The
partner, therefore, may need therapeutic assistance in clarifying her own fears "so that
she does not distance herself from the patient" (p. 66). Also, as mentioned previously,
partners can feel excluded by family members and medical personnel as support during
treatment for breast cancer typically is provided by male spouses (A. K. Matthews,
1998). Moreover, lesbian patients and their partners may be uncomfortable with the aftercare services provided by cancer agencies since, as with support groups and healthcare
providers, issues of difference and heterosexism can be present (Gallagher, 1997a).

Gynecological Problems

Many lesbian and bisexual women have had intercourse with men at some time in their
lives, yet healthcare providers often fail to take a comprehensive sexual history from
these patients because of assumptions that they only have been sexually active with
women (Diamant, Schuster, McGuigan, & Lever, 1999; Patel, DeLong, Voigl, & Medina,
2000; J. C. White & Levinson, 1995). Data from numerous studies indicate that this presumption is inaccurate. For example, in a sample of 6,935 self-identified lesbians
(Diamant et al., 1999), 77.3% reported at least one or more male sexual partners in their
lifetime, 70.5% noted a history of vaginal intercourse, 17.2% had experienced anal intercourse, and 17.2% had acquired a sexually transmitted disease. Responses from a
subsample of 3,816 female teenagers similarly indicated that lesbian respondents (33%)
were about as likely as heterosexual teens (29%) to have been sexually intimate with
males, and 22% of the bisexual and lesbian young women reported frequent intercourse
(Saewyc, Bearinger, Blum, & Resnick, 1999). Along these same lines, data from the
Women's Health Initiative indicated that 35% of the lesbians and 81% of the bisexual
women surveyed had been pregnant (Valanis et al., 2000).

   In one survey of gynecological difficulties in 1,921 lesbian and 424 bisexual women
(S. R. Johnson, Smith, & Guenther, 1987), differences in abnormal Pap smears, cystitis,
genital herpes, gonorrhea, and vaginal infections were associated with differences in reported frequency of (prior) coitus with men (95% in bisexuals and 77% in lesbians). Bisexual women, therefore, were more likely to report these conditions than lesbians,

whose overall sexual behaviors are associated with a lower risk of most sexually transmitted diseases. Similarly, findings from a study of 186 Canadian lesbians (N. Moran, 1996) indicated that the women tended to get Pap smears and examine their breasts less frequently than other women, even if they were at high risk. They were less prone to gynecological complaints, however, especially infectious diseases. Cervical smear abnormalities have been found in women who have reported never being sexually active with men, nonetheless, and Pap tests are recommended for lesbians in accord with current health guidelines (J. V. Bailey, Kavanagh, Owen, McLean, & Skinner, 2000; Marrazzo, Stine, & Koutsky, 2000).

The effect of nonheterosexual factors on the vaginal flora has been studied (McCaffrey, Varney, Evans, & Taylor-Robinson, 1999). For example, in a study of 91 lesbians, bacterial vaginosis was diagnosed in 51% of them. Most of these women previously had a male sexual partner, but not in the previous 12 months. A detailed analysis of their sexual practices did not associate the presence of bacterial vaginosis with any same-sex activity that would have the propensity to pass vaginal secretions from one woman to another. Cervical, ovarian, and other cancers, as well as menstrual difficulties, pelvic inflammatory disease, human papillomavirus, trichomonas vaginalis, and other sexually transmitted diseases, also occur in lesbians. Clinicians, therefore, should be prepared to discuss these concerns with clients and to refer them for medical evaluation (Ferris, Batish, Wright, Cushing, & Scott, 1996; S. R. Johnson et al., 1987; Kellock & O'Mahony, 1996; Koh, 2000; Marrazzo et al., 1998; O'Hanlan, 2000; O'Hanlan & Crum, 1996; A. Patel et al., 2000).

Lesbians and HIV Infection

While far more gay and bisexual men are infected with HIV, lesbians remain vulnerable to this disease and should learn techniques to protect themselves (Munson, 1996). Lesbian and bisexual women, like many gay men, have a number of social factors that affect HIV risk—including social isolation, multiple stigma, drug use, and vulnerability to violence—and thousands of them are living with HIV infection (Case, 1999). Although the majority of these HIV-positive women have been infected through either intravenous drug use or sex with men, female-to-female transmission remains a possibility. While the virus is not easily transmitted between women, the Centers for Disease Control and Prevention nevertheless funded a research project on HIV-positive lesbians and other women who have sex with women (Rochman, 1999a).

Physical and Sexual Abuse

As discussed previously, the rate of physical and sexual abuse among sexual minorities with substance use and misuse problems is high (J. M. Hall, 1998, 1999). Bradford and Ryan (1988, 1991), more specifically, found that, among 1,925 lesbians who responded to the National Lesbian Health Care Survey, 49% had experienced physical or sexual abuse at some time in their lives. One-third (34%) had been abused either sexually or physically in childhood, and 8% had experienced both forms of abuse. Hyman (2000) designed a study to examine the long-term consequences of child sexual abuse in the population investigated by Bradford and Ryan. The four spheres considered include physical health, mental health, educational attainment, and economic welfare. Preliminary data suggested that the type of sexual abuse experienced in childhood was a significant predictor of level of education attained and annual earnings.

Bernhard (2000) compared lesbians (n = 136) to heterosexual women (n = 79) and found that significantly more lesbians (51%) than nonlesbian women (33%) reported having experienced nonsexual physical violence. The differences between the two populations that were experiencing sexual violence was not statistically significant (lesbians, 54%; heterosexuals, 44%), although lesbians described proportionately more occurrences. Finally, results from another study (Hughes et al., 2000) reflected that 41% of lesbians (n = 550), compared with 24% of heterosexual women (n = 279) had been forced to engage in nonconsensual sex before age 15. The rates of nonsexual violence were equally high for both groups (lesbians, 45%; heterosexual women, 41%).

Mental Health

Some studies have shown that lesbians have a higher incidence of mental health problems, particularly depression, than do heterosexual women (Bowen, 1999; N. Moran, 1996; Valanis et al., 2000), while other research has not found statistically significant differences between the groups (Hughes et al., 2000). Hughes et al., however, speculate that "lesbians' high rates of use of mental health services, especially therapy/counseling, may act to buffer stress and thus protect against depression" (p. 71). In their multisite mental health study of 829 women, sadness and depression were primary reasons for seeking counseling in both lesbian and heterosexual populations, however. Often healthcare providers fail to acknowledge this depression. In addition, many lesbians have reported difficulties in discussing the nature of their depression with medical personnel (Rankow, 1995; J. C. White & Dull, 1997; J. C. White & Levinson, 1995).

Hughes et al. (2000) also found that lesbians in their study (n = 829) were significantly more scared or anxious than were heterosexual women, and they had experienced more suicidal feelings. When asked if they had seriously considered committing suicide at some time in the past, 51% of lesbians, compared with 38% of heterosexual subjects, reported in the affirmative. Most of the actual reported suicide attempts (lesbians, 22%; heterosexuals, 13%) had occurred when the women were adolescents or young adults. Likewise, findings from the Boston Lesbian Health Project (n = 1,633) indicated that reported suicide attempts decreased considerably after adolescence and coming out (Sorensen & Roberts, 1997). Self-mutilation, particularly cutting on the skin, by young lesbians also has been described, but the extent is unknown (Rochman, 2000). Conflict about their sexual orientation often is cited as a primary reason, but the high rate of physical, sexual, and emotional abuse among sexual minorities must be factored into the equation. While cutting sometimes is equated with suicide attempts, motivations undoubtedly are complex and somewhat idiosyncratic.

In a study designed to identify health risks in lesbian and bisexual women (n = 1,124), struggles with depression, anxiety, and eating were reported (Markovic & Aaron, 2000). Lesbians have been shown to report moderate and severe levels of stress due to emotional difficulties, problems with sexual identity, and issues associated with being female (Bernhard & Applegate, 1999). They also have noted the same concerns about depression and relationships as have other women (Sorensen & Roberts, 1997), although one study (Hughes et al., 2000) found that lesbians were significantly more likely to describe problems with a partner or spouse as the reason for seeking therapy (see Chapter

15 for discussions about sex role socialization "doubled" in lesbian couples). Other research likewise found that relationship problems were more likely to lead lesbians than heterosexual women to seek therapy, as were concerns with depression and sexual orientation (Razzano et al., 2000).

Clinical Considerations

Like other sexual minority persons, lesbian and bisexual women often encounter negative attitudes and lack of information among healthcare providers as barriers to seeking diagnostic and treatment services (Ponticelli, 1998). In addition, they frequently experience high rates of physical and sexual abuse, as well as gender-specific health concerns, including breast cancer and gynecological ailments. Based on the research data summarized in the preceding discussions, psychotherapists are reminded to assess histories of physical conditions affecting these clients that may require medical evaluation and intervention and that might otherwise precipitate or exacerbate psychological distress and disturbance.

GAY MEN'S HEALTH CONCERNS

HIV infection and AIDS are the most deadly and publicized health issues of gay men. Accordingly, their communities have been altered dramatically in the face of this disaster (Paul, Hays, & Coates, 1995): "Urban gay male culture has shifted from one that exulted in youth, freedom, and pleasure to one in which illness, death, and loss are omnipresent" (p. 348). AIDS has impacted gay men on the individual level in terms of their behaviors, attitudes, and emotional well-being. It also has affected their interpersonal relations and social networks, as well as changed the gay community's structure, institutions, and directions. Finally, the disease has changed gay men's relationship with the larger society, having "been used as a symbol for expressing negative attitudes toward groups disproportionately affected by the epidemic" (Herek, 1999a, p. 1106). For these reasons, the focus here is primarily on the effect of HIV and AIDS on the lives of these individuals.

Sexually transmitted diseases (STDs) and other genital and rectal problems also are prevalent among gay men (Goldstone, 1999; Kauth, Hartwig, & Kalichman, 2000; Shalit, 1998). This portion of the chapter, for the most part, discusses these within the context of HIV infection because the avenue for their transmission (i.e., unprotected sex) is similar to that of HIV. Many gay men who have not been infected with HIV do incur these ailments, however, as the rates of STDs "skyrocketed" among gay men before the advent of AIDS and again are rising (Kirby, 1999a, p. 41; Paul et al., 1995, p. 349). A large percentage have contracted an STD, including body lice, hepatitis B, herpes simplex, genital warts, and rectal gonorrhea. In addition, an estimated 35 of every 100,000 gay and bisexual men each year contract the human papillomavirus that is thought to lead to cervical cancer in women and anal cancer in men who have sex with men. Further, syphilis, a disease thought to have been virtually eradicated, has risen among gay men in Los Angeles and three other urban centers (Condon, 2000). The high level of STDs suggest to public health officials an erosion of safer-sex practices among gay and bisexual men and foreshadow "what could be a new wave of HIV infections" (Kirby, 1999a, p. 40).

High-Risk Sexual Behaviors

The first of these conversations involves the relationship between sexual behaviors thought to put individuals at high risk for HIV transmission and the use of drugs and alcohol. Definitions of high-risk sexual behaviors, however, appear to differ across studies. For example, some investigators use an extremely broad term such as *unprotected receptive and insertive anal/oral sex* (Robins, 1998) as a definition. Others are quite specific—for example, *unprotected anal intercourse with a nonmonagamous partner* (Stall, Paul, Barrett, Crosby, & Bein, 1999)—while still others are somewhat narrow in their definitions, for example, *unprotected anal intercourse* (Klitzman et al., 2000; Seage et al., 1998) and *receptive anal intercourse* (Boles & Elifson, 1994). The following discussion, then, should be read with the notion in mind that, just as experts differ in their definitions of high-risk sexual behaviors, many gay and bisexual male clients likewise lack agreement as to what constitutes safe or safer sexual practices.

Reporting accuracy is another issue involved when surveying gay and bisexual men about their sexual behaviors. For example, a total of 1,063 gay and bisexual men at sexually transmitted disease clinics were screened and interviewed to evaluate their rate and accuracy of disclosing HIV risk behavior (Doll, Harrison, Frey, & McKirnan, 1994). Although 523 participants reported episodes of unprotected anal sex during the interview, 29% failed to report these incidents during the screening. Further, subjects who failed to report unprotected anal sex were less inclined to disclose unprotected oral sex as well. Men who disclosed no HIV risk behaviors reported greater participation in gay organizations, greater perceptions of peer support for condom use, fewer episodes of unprotected anal sex, and lower rates of substance abuse treatment. Because the participants in this investigation were asked about drug and alcohol use and treatment, as well as about unprotected oral and anal sex, the possibility exists that they also underreported their chemical use. This point also should be taken into consideration when reading the following set of studies.

Substance Use and High-Risk Sexual Behaviors

The use of alcohol and drugs, including marijuana, nitrite inhalants (poppers), amphetamines, MDMA (Ecstasy), cocaine, and injectable substances, has been associated with high-risk sexual behaviors and with HIV infection (Boles & Elifson, 1994; Craib et al., 2000; Crosby, Stall, Paul, & Barrett, 2000; Ekstrand, Stall, Paul, Osmond, & Coates, 1999; Halkitis, 2000; Jurek, 1999; Knox, Kippax, Crawford, Prestage, & Van de Ven, 1999; Midanik et al., 1998; Robins, 1998; Seage et al., 1998; Vanable, 1998; Winters et al., 1996). Seage et al. (1998), for example, found that the gay men ($n = 508$) in their study were significantly more likely to have unprotected anal intercourse with their nonsteady, as opposed to steady, sexual partners after drinking than when sober. Further, the men who combined high-risk sexual behaviors with substance use were more likely to have a drinking problem. Along these same lines, researchers with the San Francisco Men's Health Study followed 337 gay and bisexual men who were baseline HIV negative for 6 years (Chesney, Barrett, & Stall, 1998). Every 6 months blood was drawn for HIV testing, and the subjects were interviewed to assess risk behaviors and the use of alcohol and other substances. Results reflected that the 39 men who became infected more consistently used marijuana, nitrite inhalants, amphetamines, and cocaine than did those men who remained HIV negative. Similarly, Robins (1998) studied 166 gay men and found that binge drinking, popper use, and illicit drugs were each associated significantly with high-risk sexual practices. Klitzman et al. (2000) likewise questioned 169 gay and bisexual men and found that Ecstasy use was strongly and significantly correlated with a history of unprotected anal intercourse. This association remained equally strong even after controlling for age, ethnicity, and all other forms of drug use, including alcohol.

Psychosocial Factors

Personality and cognitive factors influence substance use and sexual risk for HIV infection among gay and bisexual men. Sensation-seeking personality characteristics, for example, have been found to vary along with both substance abuse and sexual risk behavior. In a study of 289 gay and bisexual men (Kalichman, Tannebaum, & Nachimson, 1998) alcohol and other drugs were associated with sexual risk behavior. Sensation-seeking participants, however, reported taking significantly more sexual risks than those who only used substances before sex. Additionally, sensation-seekers expected substance use to enhance their sexual pleasure and therefore expected themselves to use substances before sex. The researchers concluded that modifying expectations that substance use will increase sexual enjoyment may be an important strategy to reduce the risk of HIV infection among sensation-seeking gay and bisexual men. Another study of 297 HIV-negative gay and bisexual men similarly found only the pleasure of unprotected anal intercourse and substance use to be significant predictors of the frequency with which participants engaged in high-risk sex (Kelly & Kalichman, 1998).

Vanable (1998) also examined the expectancies of 1,183 gay and bisexual men and found expectations that alcohol enhances sexual responding and reduces tension. These expectations were related to the use of alcohol in sexual settings, particularly those in which concern about avoiding risky behavior is presumed to be the highest (e.g., sex with casual partners). High-risk sexual activities in these settings, when participants are sober, would tend to be inhibited or constrained in most individuals. In another study (Crosby et al., 2000), gay and bisexual men who dropped out of substance abuse treatment, compared with treatment "graduates," were more likely to report injection drug use and recent substance use. Further, they tended to have social problems related to substance use and self-blaming coping strategies, as well as to have used sex for tension relief.

Mood, HIV, and Chemical Dependency

Relationships between affective disorders, HIV-related events, and chemical dependency have been found (D. Greene & Faltz, 1991; Rosenberger, Bornstein, Nasrallah, & Para, 1993; Rotheram-Borus, Murphy, et al., 1999). Rosenberger et al. (1993) assessed 166 HIV-positive and 31 HIV-negative gay and bisexual men and found a high lifetime prevalence of affective and substance use disorders; almost half of the participants met the criteria for both conditions. HIV-related events were associated most closely with onset or recurrence of an affective disorder. Many of these men apparently were predisposed to depression, given that an association was discovered between a positive family history of mood disturbance and a diagnosis of lifetime affective disorder. Even for individuals without these familial or personal patterns, the hopelessless of recovering gay men who are diagnosed with HIV infection may develop into rationalizations for relapse into chemical dependency (D. Greene & Faltz, 1991). Multiple AIDS-related losses also have been found to be associated with substance use in HIV-negative gay men (n = 87; Jurek, 1999). Jurek (1999) for example, found that the repeated, uncontrollable losses that many gay men experience due to AIDS lead to other maladaptive attitudes and behaviors, namely internalized homophobia and substance use.

A preponderance of HIV-positive men with substance abuse problems discontinue or reduce their chemical intake before or upon knowledge of their infection (Rotheram-Borus, Murphy, et al., 1999; Sullivan et al., 1993). Those men who continue to drink or use drugs experience higher levels of depression, distress, and diminished quality of life (Ferrando et al., 1998). In addition, Ferrando et al. found that 42% of their HIV-positive gay and bisexual subjects (n = 183) had lifetime substance use disorders, compared with 27% of their HIV-negative participants (n = 849). Similarly, 337 youth who had HIV were questioned, and one-third indicated amphetamine use in their lifetime, with 21% reporting current use (Rotheram-Borus, Mann, & Chabon, 1999). Users also initiated drug use at younger ages, used more types of drugs, had more sexual partners and more sexual encounters, reported more emotional distress, and employed escape coping behaviors significantly more.

Substance Use Treatment

Reductions in unprotected anal intercourse (UAI) often occur when individuals are treated for their chemical use. Accordingly, 456 gay men were followed for a year after treatment, and significant reductions in UAI were detected (Stall et al., 1999). While lapses to unsafe sex were common during treatment, those men who continued UAI were those who were considered a higher risk at intake, given that they were younger and had heavier concurrent use of alcohol or amphetamines, as well as a greater number of sexual partners. These individuals continued to be more sexually active after treatment and were more likely to combine substance use with sexual behavior.

Factors That Influence Infection

In the early part of the 1990s, HIV prevention efforts appeared to be effective in some segments of the gay male population (Vincke, Bolton, & Miller, 1997), but numerous adolescents and adults continue to practice high-risk behaviors (Botnick, 2000; Coxon & McManus, 2000; Maguen, Armistead, & Kalichman, 2000; Rosario, Meyer-Bahlburg, Hunter, & Gwadz, 1999). African American gay men are five times more likely to contract HIV infection than are other gay men, and their AIDS death rates are nearly 10 times higher than for Caucasians (Kilbourn, 1999). HIV infections among gay men in San Francisco tested at anonymous testing sites tripled, from about 1.3% a year in 1997 to 3.7% per year in 1999. If these percentages were extrapolated for another decade, this "would lead to a 37% level of infection in ten years" (Rotello, 2000, p. 88). Rotello noted that this rate of infection is higher than in almost every country in sub-Saharan Africa. During the years for the data he provided, gay men began taking protease inhibitors (that block HIV replication once it infects a cell) and combination drug therapies that drove down their viral loads and made them seem far less infectious. Recent treatments also have allowed many of the estimated 800,000 to 900,000 people in the United States who live with HIV infection to return to work, instead of going home to die (Temple-

Raston, 2000). Rather than new infections dropping, however, they have risen dramatically to about 40,000 a year. In part, this is due to the rise in the practice of unsafe sex (or "barebacking" as some call it) among gay and bisexual men, many of whom may believe that new drugs, some of which may stop the virus from penetrating cells, have quashed the epidemic (Kirby, 1999a).

Underestimation of Risks

In one study (Vanable, Ostrow, McKirnan, Taywaditep, & Hope, 2000), 17% of 554 gay and bisexual men surveyed were HIV positive. A substantial minority reported a lower concern for HIV because of recent treatment advances. In response to hypothetical scenarios describing sex with an HIV-positive partner, participants rated the risk of unprotected sex to be lower if the other person was taking a combination of treatments and his viral load was not detectable. The investigators noted that an undetectable viral load does not eliminate infection risks, however.

There is some evidence that repeated testing for HIV infection is being used as a personal strategy to reduce risk for acquiring the disease (Leaity et al., 2000). In a study of 1,446 individuals at a testing clinic, gay men who had three or more previous tests were more likely than other gay men to report unprotected anal intercourse. Repeat test takers further reported more sexually transmitted diseases than did the other individuals in the survey. Although testing rates may be lower in small cities than in urban areas, little information is available on comparisons between rural and urban areas (Heckman et al., 1995). Risk behaviors also may be lower among individuals who live in rural parts of the United States, however, given the differences in drug availability and sexual practices there (Brunette et al., 1999).

Illusion of Safety

Many gay and bisexual men appear to reassure themselves with a belief that being in a relationship with a primary partner protects against HIV infection. A review of research on AIDS prevention, for example, indicated that minority and nonminority heterosexual adolescents and adults, gay men, injection drug users, and commercial sex workers are less likely to practice safer sex with close relationship partners than with "casual" sexual partners (Misovich, Fisher, & Fisher, 1997). The authors noted in their summary that practicing unprotected intercourse with a committed partner who has not been tested for HIV infection is a major and unrecognized source of risk. Wagner, Remien, and Carballo-Dieguez (1998) documented this risk in their study of 75 couples with opposite HIV status (i.e., only one member was HIV positive), 67% of whom reported sex outside of the primary relationship by one or more members of the couple. Rates of unprotected anal intercourse were 25% with "one-night stands" and 33% with "other" partners. Moreover, 54% of the men who engaged in anal sex with their partners did not always use condoms.

Bosga, de Wit, de Vroome, Ernest, and Houweling (1995) investigated 164 gay men who engaged in unprotected anal sex with primary and casual partners in order to determine their subjective perceptions of the risks associated with their sexual behavior. The majority of participants who engaged in unprotected anal sex with their primary partners did not subjectively perceive their behavior as risky. For partners from couples of unknown HIV status, this discrepancy between perception and risk was explained by their not having had sex with others known to be HIV infected or to have AIDS. For those from HIV-negative couples, the variance was explained by their not having had friends or relatives who were ill or had died. Nonetheless, men who engaged in unprotected anal sex with casual partners generally recognized the risk involved in their sexual behavior.

Childhood Sexual Abuse

A history of childhood sexual abuse has been discussed previously in this chapter as being related to substance abuse and dependency in many sexual minority individuals. Likewise, sexual trauma early in the lives of lesbians was found to be associated with later mental health and physical problems. Similarly, studies have shown that childhood sexual abuse is correlated with numerous difficulties in gay and bisexual men, including a high risk for HIV infection. For example, findings from one study ($n = 1,001$) reflected significant associations between childhood sexual abuse and mental health counseling and hospitalization, psychoactive substance use, depression, suicidal ideations and actions, sexual identity development, and high-risk HIV behaviors, including unprotected anal intercourse and injection drug use (Bartholow et al., 1994).

Of 327 gay and bisexual men in another study (Lenderking et al., 1997), 35.5% reported having been sexually abused as a child. Those who were abused tended to have more lifetime male sexual partners, childhood stress, and unprotected receptive anal intercourse in the past 6 months. Finally, 182 Puerto Rican men who had sex with men were divided into three groups, depending on the nature of childhood trauma and their perceptions of the events (Carballo-Dieguez & Dolezal, 1995). Those who reported experiencing the most distress had sex before the age of 13 with a partner at least 4 years older, felt hurt by the experience, and were unwilling participants. These men were more likely than individuals in the other two groups to engage in receptive anal sex and to do so without protection.

Internalized Homophobia

The following set of studies again seem to indicate the need for therapists to continually assist sexual minority clients in addressing their internalization of societal heterosexism and the disclosure of their homosexuality. Internalized homophobia and extent of disclosure are thought to play a role in immune statue and AIDS-related risk-taking behaviors (Jurek, 1999; Zuckerman, 1999), but "this relationship may be complex and . . . a variety of intervening processes might be at work under different circumstances" (Meyer & Dean, 1998, p. 180). For example, in summarizing preliminary findings from the Sacramento Men's Health Study ($n = 96$), Herek and Glunt (1995) noted that "to the extent that men are out of the closet, have positive feelings about their sexual orientation, and feel a sense of connection to other gay and bisexual men, they are more likely to perceive social support for safe-sex practices and to feel empowered to practice safe sex with their partner, and are less likely to perceive interpersonal barriers to safe sex" (p. 69). The investigators also found the converse to be true for the men sampled: that is, those who manifested a higher degree of internalized homophobia lacked the personal empowerment to practice safe sex because of their expectation that sexual partners would refuse to cooperate and that their social world would not support safe-sex practices. Results of other studies reflected that the interpersonal situation (Sacco & Rickman, 1996), behavioral skills (Boldero, Sanitioso, & Brain, 1999), and presence of a safety strategy negotiated between the men (Kippax, Noble, Prestage, & Crawford, 1997) play major roles in decisions to use condoms during sex.

Meyer and Dean (1998) provided an alternative explanation using data from the Longitudinal AIDS Impact Project (n = 912). They found that internalized homophobia was a predictor of mental health and intimacy problems, as well as of AIDS-related risk-taking behavior. This difficulty in accepting one's homosexuality appears to be associated with adjustment and mental health problems that, when combined with anxiety about AIDS and depressive symptoms, leads to escapist behaviors, such as the use of alcohol and drugs during sex, and may result in high-risk behavior.

Support for the relationship between internalized homophobia and psychosexual adjustment was found by Dupras (1994) in a study of 261 adult gay men, ages 19 to 62. Participants completed a survey of attitudes toward homosexuality and the Multidimensional Sexuality Questionnaire. Those who had difficulty accepting their sexual orientation rated themselves higher on sexual anxiety, sexual depression, fear of sexuality, and concern about sexual image. Conversely, they rated themselves lower on internal sexual control, sexual esteem, and sexual satisfaction. No significant differences were found, however, between HIV-positive and HIV-negative participants. In contrast, participants with AIDS (n = 22) in another study (n = 57) reported higher levels of homophobia and lower levels of self-esteem than did their counterparts (Lima, Lo Presto, Sherman, & Sobelman, 1993).

Hypermasculinity

A study of Cuban American, Puerto Rician, African American, and Anglo gay men was conducted, and findings reflected that the meanings the men attributed to their sexual behaviors were constructed in response to inherited masculinity norms, as well as to the hypermasculinity structure of the gay male sexual culture (Kurtz, 1999). In his research, Kurtz found that the men who had engaged in unprotected anal intercourse with casual partners during the previous 12 months tended to have grown up without their fathers in the home, had been teased for effeminacy during childhood, were defensive about their masculinity, did not trust men, had been cheated on by boyfriends, and believed that long-term gay male relationships were problematic.

Specifically in reference to Latino gay men, Diaz (1997) explained the high incidence of unprotected intercourse in this population. He cited six specific sociocultural factors that undermine safe-sex practices: machismo, homophobia, family cohesion, sexual silence, poverty, and racism (see Chapter 10 for detailed discussion). Many of these concepts also were considered by Schifter and Madrigal (2000) when they described the sexual construction of Latino youth and the related implications for the spread of HIV infection in this population.

Living with HIV Infection

Remien and Rabkin (1995) conducted in-depth interviews with 53 gay men and 10 women who had been diagnosed with an AIDS-defining opportunistic infection at least 3 years earlier. The longitudinal study began with the gay men and later added the women, who were from much more varied backgrounds than were the men. In spite of multiple illnesses, stressors, losses, and a wide range of physical impairments, the survivors exhibited low rates of mood and psychiatric disorders. Symptoms of depression, anxiety, hostility, and hopelessness were mild and unrelated to the degree of physical impairment, but the more physically challenged individuals were less optimistic about the future. The participants reported that confronting their own mortality was the hardest part about being diagnosed with AIDS.

Other concerns of those 63 individuals who were living with AIDS included disclosures to family and friends, physical restrictions imposed by the illness, being dependent on others, and the difficulties raised by the continual need for medical care and the related problems with insurance reimbursement. Their most prominent fear was of future illness, and the respondents noted three conditions they would find extremely problematic: dementia, pain, and incontinence. Several cited suicide an option should their medical condition become intolerable. These individuals generally felt that a close and trusting relationship with their physician contributed to their physical and mental health. As had been found in numerous other studies, social supports were "positively associated with hope and overall psychological functioning and negatively associated with depressive symptoms" (Remien & Rabkin, 1995, p. 177). The support of other infected individuals was important to the respondents, as was continuing to have a sense of humor, even in the wake of multiple losses. Loneliness was a problem, however, particularly in the area of romantic relationships. Feelings of being "tainted" and experiences of being rejected and stigmatized were reported.

Stigma

Due to social misperceptions and taboos against homosexuality, disease, and death, HIV-infected gay men are stigmatized repeatedly and feel an intense amount of shame at having incurred the virus (Cadwell, 1991; Demarco, 1999; Ostrow, 1996). Bennett (1990) interviewed 10 gay men with AIDS, ages 29 to 34 years, in order to explore their perceptions of stigmatization. All respondents described experiences of rejection that included subtle avoidance from others and displacement from employment, housing, and their families. These feelings of isolation resulted in participants not discussing their disease and possible death with many others.

By understanding the effect of the multiple stigmata, clinicians can increase their awareness of possible prejudice in the therapeutic relationship, as it can manifest itself in both transference and countertransference. In fact, many HIV-positive patients have reported feeling stigmatized rather than mirrored by their healthcare providers, as well as by society (Paradis, 1993). In addition, the farther removed they are from the average physician's comprehension (e.g., gay, Hispanic, and HIV-positive), the more marginalized they often feel (Wainberg, 1999).

Ethnicity

The results of some studies suggest that HIV-positive gay and bisexual men of color are more prone to psychological stress than are their Caucasian counterparts, but the findings are mixed, perhaps because of differences in the variables that were measured. The concepts of multiple minority status and cultural clash (discussed in Chapter 10) seem to appear as commonalities, however, in that they serve to compound the trepidation inherent in an HIV-positive status. For example, in a study of 502 African American men (who were stratified by HIV serostatus, drug use, and sexual orientation), gay and bisexual men and those who were HIV-positive evidenced greater psychiatric vulnerability than did the heterosexual and HIV-negative men (Myers et al., 1997).

Siegel and Epstein (1996) additionally concluded that HIV-positive African American (n = 48) and Puerto Rican (n = 49) gay men were more stressed by factors related to their sexual orientation than were Caucasian men (n = 47). Similarly, Ceballos-Capitaine, Szapocznik, Blaney, and Morgan (1990) followed Hispanic (n = 27) and non-Hispanic (n = 49) HIV-positive gay men for 5 years and concluded that, although Hispanics were not more stressed than non-Hispanics overall, they experienced more severe stress in daily interactions related to their sexual orientation than did their Caucasian counterparts. The remarkable similarities between most other psychosocial domains was thought to be attributed to the Hispanic cohort's level of acculturation.

Given the number of oppressive conditions under which sexual minorities of color live, models for the prevention of HIV infection, as well as for treatment, must include dimensions of culture, diversity, and ethnic identity (Faryna & Morales, 2000). Specifically in reference to Chinese American and Japanese American gay men (n = 104), 31% of whom reported unprotected anal intercourse in the previous 3 months, Lai (1999) suggested the need for HIV prevention interventions to address cultural identification to improve self-esteem. Likewise, Black churches and families, gay and gay-oriented self-help organizations, and community outreach education programs are critical resources for helping reduce the spread of AIDS among African American men (Icard, Schilling, El-Bassel, & Young, 1992), but homophobia has hampered the ability of Black churches to engage in HIV prevention (Fullilove & Fullilove, 1999). Further, since access to minority community resources for AIDS-related service delivery may be limited by levels of acculturation and assertiveness, language acquisition, and immigration status, active intervention efforts are needed to overcome these barriers (Morales, 1990).

Coping Strategies and Mood

Several studies support the finding that active coping mechanisms, such as appraisal and adaptation, as well as supportive interactions with others, can contribute to improved quality of life and diminished disease progression for those who are living with HIV infection (Mulder, Antoni, Duivenvoorden, & Kauffmann, 1995; Ostrow, 1996). However, denial and passive fatalism, "use of alcohol, recreational drugs, or casual sex as distraction coping responses . . . can contribute negatively to well-being" (Ostrow, 1996, p. 862). In addition, Demarco (1999) found that the shame felt by HIV-positive gay men (n = 50) was associated with increased risk of detachment or avoidance coping, along with a decreased use of involvement coping. Further, those men who used a detachment style tended to be more depressed than those individuals who were more involved with managing their lives.

Nicholson and Long (1990) examined the relationship between self-esteem, social support, internalized homophobia, and coping strategies used by 89 HIV-positive gay men, and between coping strategies (avoidant vs. proactive) and mood states. While higher homophobia and lower self-esteem predicted avoidant coping, lower homophobia and more recent diagnosis predicted proactive coping. Less recent diagnosis, less avoidant coping, less homophobia, and higher self-esteem predicted better mood state. Given the status of current thinking, then, clinicians are urged to help HIV-positive clients cope with their disease in the most involved and proactive ways possible within the limits of their physical and other abilities. Cognitive behavioral stress management, coping effectiveness training, and therapy groups where members provide support and assistance to each other have been proven helpful (Chesney & Folkman, 1994; Guthrie, 1999; Lutgendorf, Antoni, Ironson, & Klimas, 1997)

Despite numerous psychological and medical interventions, however, a considerable number of HIV-positive clients will attempt to end their lives, and some will succeed. In one study of 167 seropositive gay men, 17% reported serious thoughts or plans to end their lives at some point in the future (Goggin et al., 2000). The authors of the study noted that, in the absence of current psychiatric disorders, plans for suicide may represent one way to maintain control and independence in the face of an uncertain future, given the unpredictable course of HIV infection.

AIDS patients have been found to request help with suicide. One hundred physicians treating these individuals were surveyed, and respondents reported a mean of 7.9 "direct" and 13.7 "indirect" requests for assistance (Slome, Mitchell, Charlebois, Benevedes, & Abrams, 1997). Further, 53% of the physicians said they had granted the request of an AIDS patient at least once. Psychotherapists working with this population thus should be prepared not only to empathize with the client's perceived unendurable psychological pain and hopelessness (A. McNaught & Spicer, 2000) but also to address their own ethical values around the issue of suicide (Kain, 1996).

Medications

With the advent of protease inhibitors and combination drug therapies, the medication regimens of many with HIV infection requires the taking of dozens of capsules and tablets a day at strictly mandated hours. The dietary restrictions often are severe; side effects, such as vomiting, nausea, diarrhea, and physical disfigurement, are frequent; and treatment noncompliance may result in the development of resistance to the drug(s) (Kauth et al., 2000; Kirby, 2000b). Adherence lapses are common. To determine reasons for noncompliance, Deboer (1999) surveyed and interviewed 70 HIV-positive gay men. Motives given by the men included forgetting to take the medications, relapsing with alcohol or drugs, needing to rebel, desiring benefits gained from an illness status, and testing to see if the treatment is truly needed to maintain a low viral load. Pretreatment and preinfection level of functioning was an important variable since men who had mastered previous developmental tasks appeared more able to devote resources toward combating the disease and planning for the future.

Because of variables such as those described here, including the expense of the medications, research trials are being conducted with structured treatment interruptions (STIs). The theory behind these STIs is that carefully scheduled and monitored "treatment interruptions might create an environment in the body whereby the immune system, through repeated raising and lowering of viral levels, learns to identity and effectively control HIV in the body" (Kirby, 2000b, p. 38). Even though there is no clear evidence to show that these "drug holidays" are beneficial, the possibility has created both excitement and confusion in many individuals who are struggling to maintain both their drug and dietary schedules, as well as the quality of their lives.

There also is controversy as to when to begin medication treatment in individuals who have been diagnosed with HIV infection. Prior thinking had HIV-positive individuals initiating drug therapy when T-cells fell to a certain level or other indicators appeared. Some authorities, however, believe that initiation of highly active antiretroviral therapy (HAART) as soon as possible after infection may alter the course of the disease. As a result, studies to test this hypothesis are being conducted. Results are meager and reflect the necessity of a trade-off between quality of life, if too much medication is administered, and reduced anti-viral efficacy, if the dosages are too low (Zinkernagel et al., 1999). This dilemma, however, exists for most of the drugs used to treat HIV infection and other diseases.

In spite of the complicated drug regimens required, the high cost of the medications, and the serious side effects, protease inhibitors and combination therapies have offered many individuals hope for an extended life. Nonetheless, this possibility of hope has caused increased distress for others who have already made numerous decisions in anticipation of death. Some have sold life insurance policies and homes, charged credit cards up to their limits, used their lifetime medical insurance benefits, and gone on permanent disability from their jobs in order to provide for medical care and living expenses. Now, they are faced not only with a future of living with HIV infection but also with the overwhelming struggles associated with reconstructing their lives.

Disclosure and Other Reactions

Reactions to testing and notification of a positive serostatus are varied and have been found to include shock, denial, depression, suicidal ideation and attempts, anxiety, somatic preoccupations, guilt, isolation, anger, and distraction coping responses such as increased use of drugs or alcohol (Ostrow, 1996). Specific concerns about the possible progression from HIV infection to AIDS increase after learning of infection, and therapists should be prepared to assist individuals in coping with a wide range of reactions across the spectrum of the disease. Clients also may need help in telling others of their HIV-positive status since this disclosure "presents an especially arduous task" (Serovich, 2000, p. 365).

Serovich (2000) outlines several steps in the process, namely: (1) making an exhaustive disclosure list of everyone in the client's social, vocational, familial, recreational, and service network; (2) evaluating the nature of each possibility in order to decide if the relationship quality is substantial enough for disclosure to occur; (3) assessing a recipient's special circumstance, including mental and physical health, age, and current crises in that person's life; (4) assessing HIV knowledge and anticipated responses; (5) identifying reasons for disclosure to each person on the list; and (6) making a decision to eliminate some individuals from the list, to tell a particular person as soon as possible, or to place others in a "wait and see" category (p. 369).

Stempel, Moulton, and Moss (1995) followed 93 gay and bisexual men from the San Francisco General Hospital Cohort for 1 year after they were notified of their HIV antibody test results to examine patterns of self-disclosure, reactions, and concerns. After 1 year, participants had told 92% of their gay friends, 82% of their primary sexual partners, 56% of their new sexual partners, 46% of their coworkers, 71% of their physicians, 37% of their dentists, 57% of their psychotherapists, and 37% of their family members. Respondents were twice as likely to inform their primary sexual partners and were more likely to self-disclose to all categories of persons, except physicians and dentists, than they anticipated before being notified of the disease. Male family members and primary sexual partners reacted least favorably to the disclosure of an HIV-positive status. Although participants were concerned about health insurance and stigmatization, fear of stigma tended to diminish over the course of a year.

S. Perry, Ryan, Fogel, and Fischman (1990) likewise interviewed 40 gay men who had learned recently that they were infected with HIV to determine the frequency with which they voluntarily disclosed their positive antibody test results to others. Some 90% of the respondents informed their personal physician, 66% informed every current sexual partner, 90% made no attempts to inform past sexual partners, and 68% informed at least one friend, but only 35% informed a family member

Among a sample of 398 gay and bisexual men (Mason, Marks, Simoni, & Ruiz, 1995), Spanish-speaking Latinos (n = 107) were more likely than English-speaking Latinos (n = 85) and Whites (n = 206) to withhold their positive HIV status and their sexual orientation from significant others, especially family members. While all three populations were likely to withhold their HIV diagnosis from their parents to avoid disturbing them rather than to prevent personal rejection, this tendency was somewhat stronger among Latinos. Among Latinos, the desire to protect family members and to maintain harmonious relations is a barrier to disclosure of HIV status (Szapocznik, 1995).

Support Systems and Stressors

HIV-infected gay and bisexual men have been shown to rely on others for advocacy and assistance as they struggle with their disease. These allies include friends, family member, and partners. The following discussion addresses each of these support networks and the dynamics involved in these relationships.

Peer and Family Support

A supportive family has been shown to benefit HIV-positive gay and bisexual men in several ways, yet the majority of studies, including those described earlier in this chapter, show various degrees of estrangement between these individuals and their families. For example, Johnston, Stall, and Smith (1995) additionally interviewed 81 gay men and 88 injection drug users who were diagnosed with AIDS about their reliance on friends and family for care. While gay men relied on friends more than did injection drug users, neither group relied primarily on their families. Catania, Turner, Choi, and Coates (1992) similarly surveyed 529 gay men every 6 months for 3 years and annually thereafter in regard to their HIV status, as well as their AIDS-related help seeking, social support, and death anxiety. Although respondents were more likely to rely on peer networks than on family systems for help in times of need, perception of positive family support was associated more strongly with lower death anxiety than was recognition of affirming peer assistance. Likewise, ethnographic and psychometric data collected from 64 gay men with various HIV-related impairments suggested that the threatening possibility of death intensified a preexisting sense of participant alienation from families (Lang, 1991).

Turner, Hays, and Coates (1993) found that social support was associated positively with gay identity acceptance and disclosure to family members about an AIDS diagnosis and was associated negatively with depression and the number of HIV-related symptoms.

Among the more symptomatic participants, family knowledge of their homosexuality was associated negatively with support. On a more positive note, in a survey of 117 gay men with HIV infection, disclosure of HIV status was associated with higher levels of support from all family members (Kadushin, 2000). Further, if family members are perceived as supportive, HIV-positive gay men are less likely to behave sexually in risky ways (Kimberly & Serovich, 1999).

Families of Origin

Parents and other family members of those infected by HIV infection face a number of unique tasks (Beckerman, 1994). These include accepting the diagnosis and perhaps the homosexuality of the afflicted individual. Family members also must make decisions about disclosure of the diagnosis to other family members and friends; must reintegrate the person into the family system, particularly if there have been strained relationships; and must cope with illness and impending loss if the disease has begun to progress. Psychosocial factors also affect the willingness of families to care for gay members with AIDS. These include caregiver resources and coping characteristics, the degree to which families hold the gay member accountable for his illness, perceptions of inadequate social support, familial obligation and affection, fears of HIV transmission and infection, perceptions of self-efficacy, the acceptance of homosexuality, and family stigma (McDonell, Abell, & Miller, 1991).

Concerns about shame and stigma are common to both HIV-infected gay and bisexual men and their families. Every member of a family is affected in some way by the revelation and must therefore make decisions about who to tell and where to receive support. An especially difficult situation involves the disclosure about an HIV-positive status by a gay or bisexual father to his children or to a heterosexual spouse (Shuster, 1996). Given the intense emotions and complicated dynamics involved, counseling for families, significant others, and friends of persons with HIV infection and AIDS is critically important to the health and wholeness of these individuals and their survivors (Williams & Stafford, 1991).

Sohier (1993) explored the grieving process of parents whose gay sons were dying from AIDS. Interview data were collected from 64 parents, ages 44 to 76 years, and 6 of their sons. Over a period of 4½ years, parents and sons were observed participating in support groups, social interactions, and volunteer hospice contacts. This filial reconstruction was said to provide closure to both generations, in that the dying son felt a psychological and spiritual freedom and parents were better prepared for a more uncomplicated bereavement after his death.

Couples

Both members of an HIV-affected couple experience a major life transition as they are confronted with multiple losses, including possible demise of the person with AIDS; disintegration of the relationship; and loss of vitality, autonomy, intimacy, and privacy (Powell-Cope, 1995). Clinical intervention with HIV-positive persons and their partners, therefore, must focus on the concerns of each individual, as well as on the dyadic issues of the couple. These may include the resurgence of internalized homophobia in one or both members, denial about impending losses, and conflicts about power and status, as well as a redefinition of roles from equals to one of caretaker and patient (R. C. Friedman, 1991; Gazarik & Fischman, 1995). Whether the couple is discordant (i.e., different HIV statuses) or concordant (i.e., both HIV positive), most will try to maintain their relationship by using either avoidance, negotiation, or acceptance to "normalize" the illness (Haas, 1999).

Kain (1996) discussed a number of additional dynamics that may occur in HIV-infected couples. For some dyads, the diagnosis serves to intensify the already strong emotional bond. Couples with dysfunctional relationships, however, may feel compelled by the illness to remain together, where otherwise they might have decided to separate. One of the major problems faced by men in serodiscordant relationships is the fear of infection of the other by the HIV-positive person. Both men may experience this consternation in a wide range of situations, including their sexual and other intimate exchanges such as the sharing of toothbrushes or dishes. Alternatively, a mutually seropositive relationship can feel comforting to the members, but the possibilities for discord also are numerous. For example, the men might fight about who infected whom or about their role in infecting their partners or allowing themselves to become infected. These couples may bring issues of guilt or blame to therapy, as well as exacerbations of unacknowledged prior dynamics.

If HIV-related illness occurs in one member of a male couple, the other member often serves as the primary caretaker. Accordingly, among urban caregivers of HIV and AIDS patients, gay and bisexual men are overrepresented. Potential consequences of this caregiving include physical and emotional stress and decreased opportunity for social and economic development (Turner, Catania, & Gagnon, 1994). Irving, Bor, and Catalan (1995) studied 38 gay men, some of whom were HIV-positive themselves, and who were providing care to a partner with AIDS. Results reflected that the majority were suffering from significant psychiatric problems, indicating that the continual and overwhelming nature of the caregiving had an adverse effect on their psychological health. The literature is replete with similar findings related to caregivers of patients with numerous other diseases. In many of these other circumstances, however, the person giving the care often is an older heterosexual spouse, or a daughter or son, all of whom have been in an emotionally close relationship with the patient for a number of years. The majority of gay and bisexual men who have contracted AIDS are in early and middle adulthood, and their caregiver partners and friends likewise are relatively young; many are unprepared developmentally and emotionally to handle the burden that has been thrust on them.

Loss and Bereavement

Multiple loss has defined the experience of many gay men since the beginning of the AIDS epidemic (Marion, 1996; Springer & Lease, 2000). Even with the advent of new drugs, the devastation continues. While those who live in urban areas generally have experienced the deaths of numerous close friends and partners, gay men in rural and nonurban areas are not immune from losses related to the epidemic. The stigma of HIV extends to them as gay men and affects their self-images, as well as relationships with other gay men and with the broader community, given its intolerance of gay male associations and sexual activity. Thus, within the context of the AIDS epidemic, many gay men struggle to integrate a positive social and sexual identity and repeatedly confront internalized homophobia as they recycle through developmental issues regarding self-disclosure and coming out (Jurek, 1999; Paradis, 1991).

Society's reluctance to validate the gay identity, the intensity of multiple loss, the lack of time between losses, and the succeeding impact on self-identity and self-esteem complicate bereavement for persons surviving the numerous deaths of persons with AIDS (Biller & Rice, 1990; Getzel & Mahony, 1990; Jurek, 1999; Springer & Lease, 2000). Gay widowers, in particular, may feel particularly invisible, isolated, and unsupported (Shernoff, 1997; Simmons, 1999) and therefore may be at increased risk for engaging in unprotected anal intercourse (Mayne, Acree, Chesney, & Folkman, 1998). In addition, many gay men and their allies have suffered progressive multiple losses, both flooding and numbing their emotions, as well as shattering their assumptions about life (Marion, 1996): "No aspect of life or identity is untouched by loss," and "the enormity of the loss is too big to grieve and too pervasive to fully comprehend" (p. 67). A large number feel powerless in the face of the epidemic, and are psychologically fatigued, depressed, ashamed, anxious, angry, drug-dependent, avoidant of intimacy, or feeling guilty that they have survived while others who participated in the same behaviors are ill or have died.

Compassion Fatigue

The HIV epidemic involves intensely painful emotions, not only for patients and their loved ones but also for the professionals who work with these individuals (McDaniel, Farber, & Summerville, 1996; Ostrow, 1996). Because of the complex and multilayered context of AIDS care, including sociocultural, medical, and psychological dimensions, the possibility of provider burnout is constantly present. Psychotherapists also can find themselves involved in unfamiliar social service and political advocacy roles with their clients, given the social and civic environments that surround AIDS care. Dual relationship issues arise more frequently than when working with other client populations, and clinicians often must make decisions about visiting ill clients in their homes or in hospitals or about attending the funerals of them or their partners. For sexual minority clinicians—in particular, those who are HIV positive, but also for empathic and supportive others—grief and loss continually are present, and strategies to manage fatigue and burnout are essential.

Cadwell (1994) investigated the experiences of 15 gay male psychotherapists who treated gay men with HIV-related disorders. Several themes emerged, including concerns about contagion, homophobia, and the possibility of overidentification. Although identification is essential to empathy, it also can distort or intensify countertransference. Cadwell described specific strategies for managing the vulnerability of clinicians to identify with AIDS patients, including behavioral and cognitive skills, as well as the development of supportive personal, organizational, and community resources and alliances.

Clinicians, therefore, must make a commitment to their own health when working with gay and bisexual men who are living either with HIV infection or its possibility. At the same time, however, they owe a responsibility to assist their clients in living the healthiest lives possible (Kauth et al., 2000; Shernoff, 1999). The Resources section contains several references and websites that can be helpful in this regard. Further, men themselves have become conscious of the need to protect and enhance their own well-being, and a considerable number of books are available to assist in this effort (Ball, 1998; Cohen, 1998; Goldstone, 1999; Penn, 1998; Shalit, 1998).

CONCLUSION

Because of the unique health and medical needs of sexual minority individuals, this entire chapter has been devoted to these issues. The discussions documented the role that stressful societal situations play in many of their physical and emotional conditions, as well as the provider bias that keeps many from seeking care. Further, this chapter, along with Chapter 4, explained the part that workplace discrimination, or employment that does not offer insurance coverage, plays in the low rate of health care use by gay, lesbian, and bisexual individuals. Assistance was provided to therapists in more effectively treating their chemically dependent clients, as well as in understanding the gender-specific health concerns of both lesbians and gay men. Websites and addresses for enhancing this affirmative care can be found in the Resources section.

13

Religious Concerns and Spiritual Development

Gay, lesbian, and bisexual individuals frequently have difficulty reconciling their sexuality with the disapproving values and teachings of traditional religion. For many, this particularly intense dilemma is often the presenting problem that brings them to psychotherapy. From the viewpoints of these clients, the conflict seems unresolvable since frequently they are bonded to a church or religion that strongly condemns both their sexual behavior and their sexual orientation. This chapter is written not only to illuminate the nature of the pain experienced by religiously oriented sexual minorities but also to assist clinicians in helping these individuals harmonize their religious faith and their sexuality. As dissonance between the two often has prevented such clients from proceeding through the phases necessary to develop positive bisexual, lesbian, or gay identities, resolving this discordance enables them to proceed with integrating their spiritual and sexual selves.

RELIGION AND SEXUAL MINORITIES

Many sexual minorities feel a profound sense of alienation from and toward organized religion (Duckitt & duToit, 1989; Haldeman, 1996; Morris, 2000; O'Neill & Ritter, 1992; Ritter & O'Neill, 1996), while others are quite hostile toward the Jewish or Christian traditions in which a majority were raised (J. M. Clark, Brown, & Hochstein, 1989). In an *OUT/LOOK* survey to which 648 readers of the national lesbian and gay publication responded (K. G. Lee & Busto, 1991), 83% had been raised in Christian (Protestant or Catholic) homes, 11% were from a Jewish tradition, and the remainder were provided with no particular religious influence as children. At the time of the survey, however, most individuals reported having left the religions of their youth, although some still retained their affiliations (Catholic, 6%; Protestant, 22%; Jewish, 6%), 12% currently referred to themselves as "gay Christian," and 4% indicated that they were Muslims, Buddhists, or Hindus. About 28% listed membership in 12-step recovery programs or placed themselves in the "alternative/other" category when asked to which religious or spiritual communities they now belonged.

In this *OUT/LOOK* study (which, incidentally, acknowledged the same sampling bias that plagues most research with sexual minorities), more than one-third of the respondents indicated that they no longer identified with any religious or spiritual community. Nonetheless, 84% rated *spirituality* as "very" or "somewhat" important to them, compared with 52% who considered *religion* as similarly significant in their lives. Two-thirds of the subjects said they believed in a transcendent God, while 20.5% responded that they did not. After comparing their data with both a *San Francisco Chronicle* survey and a 1988 Gallup poll of the general population, Lee and Busto (1991) suggested that "there are more atheists among lesbians and gays than in a broader sampling" (p. 83). The researchers noted that their percentage data (which related to *both* spirituality and belief in God) were quite comparable to the findings of the two general population surveys. Unlike Lee and Busto (1991), however, the Gallup and *Chronicle* pollsters did not ask respondents to make a distinction between *spirituality* and *religion*. Despite a common tendency to render these two concepts synonymous, nearly one-third (32%) of 648 presumably gay, lesbian, and bisexual individuals who responded to the *OUT/LOOK* survey indicated that it was important to discriminate between the two.

Support for the fact that organized religion plays a less significant role in the lives of sexual minority individuals than it does for comparable heterosexuals was provided by L. Ellis and Wagemann (1993), who studied 285 mother–offspring pairs. Of the sons and daughters (mean age, 25.5) who were asked about their sexual orientation, 39 were gay men, 14 were bisexual males, and 28 were lesbians. A questionnaire was administered to all subjects regarding their religiosity (i.e., importance of religion, frequency of church attendance, and denominational preference). As predicted, female offspring were found to be more "religious" than males, with lesbians being substantially less religious (especially in terms of church attendance) than heterosexual women. Offspring of both sexes who were not exclusively heterosexual tended to be less "religious" than heterosexuals. Morris (2000) similarly examined the religious affiliations of 568 lesbians of color and found that 44% of the women (*n* = 250) currently were "spiritual" but were not affiliated with a formal religion. She also discerned that 88% (*n* = 496) of the participants grew up in a religion. Further, only 7% of the women attended religious services weekly, with African American lesbians showing the highest level of weekly participation (11%) and the lowest level of nonattendance (33%). A majority (42%; *n* = 235) never attended services, while 29% (*n* = 164) rarely worshiped in a church, synagogue, or mosque.

Because many sexual minority clients are hostile to organized religion or do not hold membership in majority culture churches and denominations, clinicians can be misled into thinking that religious belief and spirituality are not important to them. Some of the findings described here, however, show this to be an inaccurate assumption. "The profound emotional and existential meanings associated with religious issues for many gay men and lesbians mandate that these issues be taken seriously" by therapists (Haldeman, 1996, p. 893). Like a large number of ethnic minority clients (see Chapter 10), they feel "caught between cultures." On one hand, they may feel marginalized or judged by organized religion because of their sexual orientation. On the other hand, they may experience alienation and even criticism from the members of the gay and lesbian community because they are religiously inclined or are still bonded with the Judeo-Christian tradition rather than exploring their spirituality through more nontraditional paths.

SEXUAL MINORITIES AND THE VIABILITY OF RELIGION

As discussed earlier, the official positions of most religions have been critical of sexual minorities or their intimate behaviors, or both. In turn, these condemnations have influenced the attitudes of gay, lesbian, and bisexual people toward these communities. For many, their experiences in traditional religion have been less than life giving or viable. James (1928) contended that for a religious experience to be viable it must be philosophically reasonable, morally helpful, and spiritually illuminating. The discussion of traditional religion that follows will examine the experience of sexual minority members from each of these perspectives, as well as consider the degree of communal support that is provided by religious groups (Callahan, 1985). Ritter and O'Neill (1989) provided the framework for this discourse, which is outlined in Table 13.1.

Philosophically Reasonable

Two of the most significant beliefs of the Judeo-Christian tradition are the creation of humanity in the image of God (Genesis 1:26–27, 5:1, 9:6) and the Deity's faithfulness toward, as well as enduring and unfailing love for, those who believe (Psalms 89:1–2, 14, 24, 33; 100:5; 107). From the perspective of many sexual minorities, however, these two fundamental principles don't seem applicable to them. For example, official Catholicism describes a homosexual orientation as "intrinsically disordered" and same-sex behaviors as "acts of grave depravity" (Pope John Paul II, 1995, p. 625), and many Protestants refer to the sinfulness and sexual immorality of homosexuality (Abraham, 1993; M. McKenzie, 1993). Further, Orthodox Judaism and many within the Jewish Conservative and Reform movements, as well as within numerous Christian churches and denominations, contend that scriptural texts such as Leviticus 18:22 and 20:13 apply the terms *abomination* (*to'evah* in the Torah), *perversion,* and *detestable* specifically to homosexuality. Thus, being referred to in this manner, while at the same time being told that they have been created in the image of God, leads many lesbian, gay, and bisexual individuals to question the philosophical reasonableness of the Judeo-Christian tradition.

   An additional point in this regard relates to the concept of salvation and what many sexual minorities understand they must do in order to be saved from eternal damnation. For them to be granted redemption and a place with God in heaven, they are told they have two choices: (1) repent of their homosexuality and convert to heterosexuality; or (2) repress their sinful sexual impulses and live either a pure/chaste/holy (i.e., nonsexual) life or a heterosexual one. These untenable options lead to considerable struggle and pain. Further, the end result of both choices has individuals repeatedly denying or attempting to change their basic nature, while often feeling continually ashamed, evil, or sinful. "Thus, traditional organized religion, rather than assisting with integration and wholeness, often fragments individuals by seeming to demand that [they] change or be forgiven for their very nature" (Ritter & O'Neill, 1989, p. 10).

TABLE 13.1. Traditional Religion: Four Criteria for Viability

Philosophically reasonable

Two fundamental beliefs of Judeo-Christian tradition:
• Humans are created in God's image and likeness and are, thus, essentially good.
• God unconditionally loves each and every believer.

However, traditional religion:
• Imposes conditions on:
  – the goodness of gay, lesbian, and bisexual members.
  – their worthiness of God's love.
• Creates an untenable situation for them (approval vs. integrity):
  – *Either:* Repent or repress in order to avoid condemnation.
  – *Or:* Love according to their nature and lose favor with God.

Morally helpful

Traditional religion:
• Offers three morally acceptable choices:
  – Repentance or conversion
  – Celibacy
  – Heterosexual marriage
• Leaves bisexuals, lesbians, and gay men with no morally credible ways to express themselves sexually in intimate relationships.

Spiritually illuminating

Judeo-Christian tradition:
• Offers few models of holy men and women with a same-gender sexual orientation who have been blessed by God.
• Has failed to illuminate the central roles sexual minority people played in their traditions.

Without an illuminating spirituality, identification and inspiration are lacking for gay, lesbian, and bisexual individuals.

Communally supportive

Traditional religion sends gay, lesbian, and bisexual members a double message:
• Compassion and inclusion are preached.
• Oppression and exclusion are practiced:
  – Same-gender relationships are neither recognized nor supported.
  – Ordination of gay, lesbian, and bisexual candidates is withheld.
  – No rituals to facilitate life transitions are celebrated.
  – Congregational life assumes heterosexuality.

Note. Summarized from Ritter & O'Neill (1989).

Morally Helpful

In addition to being perceived as philosophically unreasonable, much of Judeo-Christian moral teaching in reference to matters of intimate relationships has not proven helpful to sexual minority individuals. The preponderance of "official" ethical guidance as it relates specifically to male or female partnerships is critical and generally condemns all sexual contact between people of the same sex. Further, by casting both their inclinations and their sexual behaviors in disparaging language (e.g., unnatural, degrading, or abominable), traditional religion usually leaves gay, lesbian, and bisexual people with few morally credible ways to express themselves sexually or within the context of an intimate same-sex relationship.

The ethically acceptable choices offered by most of Judeo-Christian religion (i.e., re-pentance/conversion, celibacy, or heterosexual marriage) often are experienced as unreal-istic and nonviable by lesbians, bisexuals, and gay men, given the nature of their sexual and emotional attractions. The result then is that many churches and synagogues are viewed as neither trustworthy nor particularly credible teachers of moral truth. Numer-ous writers and theologians—both Christian (Boisvert, 2000; Curran, 1983; Edwards, 1984, 1989; Fortunato, 1982; Glaser, 1988, 1990, 1991, 1998; Maguire, 1984; B. McNaught, 1988; McNeill, 1985, 1988, 1995; 1998; J. B. Nelson, 1982, 1983; O'Neill & Ritter, 1992; T. Perry, 1987; Ritter & O'Neill, 1989; Scanzoni & Mollenkott, 1994; Uhrig, 1986; J. C. White, 1995; R. Woods, 1988) and Jewish (Balka & Rose, 1989; E. T. Beck, 1989; A. Cooper, 1989; Dworkin, 1996, 1997; Y. H. Kahn, 1989; Kirschner, 1988; Marder, 1985: Matt, 1978, 1987)—have attempted to offer more positive and affirming perspectives than those advocated by orthodox religion. While these and other similar writings often have been criticized by those who base their censure of same-sex orienta-tions and relations on literal interpretations of the Bible, one of the authors listed above (John McNeill) lost his right to belong to the Jesuit order of Catholic priests because of his views and another was not permitted to teach moral theology at Catholic universities (Charles Curran). Numerous others, such as Chris Glasser, Robert Goss, Troy Perry, Craig O'Neill, Larry Uhrig, and Mel White, have been denied (or lost) the right to serve in the traditional ministry. In spite of these kinds of distressing circumstances, thousands of gay, lesbian, and bisexual individuals are reading spiritually focused literature and are being offered moral and spiritual perspectives which have the potential to be authenti-cally helpful to themselves and for their relationships.

Spiritually Illuminating

Virtually no religions, denominations, or churches offer to members examples of openly lesbian, gay, or bisexual individuals who have been affirmed or blessed by God. Nor has religion illuminated the central roles that people of same-sex orientation have played in a number of sacred traditions. Only in the last decade has writing emerged that points to the very real possibility of homosexually oriented clergy, theologians, saints, and holy people (Alyson Publications, 1993; Boswell, 1980, 1989, 1994; J. M. Clark, 1987, 1989, 1997; Curb & Manahan, 1985; Glaser, 1990; Goss, 1993; Gramick, 1989; Gramick & Nugent, 1995; A. Harvey, 1997/2002; Heyward, 1989b; Hirsh, 1989; E. C. Johnson & Johnson, 2000; McNeill, 1985, 1988, 1998; Nugent, 1984a, 1984b; Nugent & Gramick, 1992; T. Perry, 1987; Rogow, 1989; Sweasey, 1997; Wolf, 1989). Unfortunately, the (pre-sumed) sexual orientations of most of these were noted years or even centuries after their deaths. Others resigned from the clerical life and were no longer liable for censure or dis-missal when they made the nature of their sexuality known. In either case, generations of individuals were deprived of prototypes who were capable of illuminating their spiritual paths.

Lives are formed by master or shaping stories (Fowler, 1981), and individuals use these mythologies as outlines for their futures. Through stories of biblical heroes and saints, the Judeo-Christian tradition offers only two types of life plans—either heterosex-ual marriage and family life or a single state of celibacy and virginity. "Models of same-sex love and friendship such as Jesus and John (John 13:23–25, 21:7), Ruth and Naomi (Ruth 1:16–17), or David and Jonathan (I Samuel 18:1–3, 20:41; II Samuel 1:26) are few and rarely highlighted. Never is a sexually intimate relationship between two people of the same sex used as an example of perfect or divine love" (Ritter & O'Neill, 1989, p. 10). Thus, with the absence of viable shaping stories that authentically reflect and illuminate the experiences of gay, bisexual, or lesbian people, "there often seems little with which to identify or toward which to aspire" (p. 10).

With few examples of people who reconciled a minority sexual orientation with a deep commitment to their religions traditions, lesbians, bisexuals, and gay men have had difficulty imagining the possibility of such an integration or synthesis. Given the absence of role models, many have been forced either to adopt a religion that does not address them at the core of their nature or to create for themselves more harmonious spiritual experiences. Some of these alternatives are discussed throughout this chapter.

Communally Supportive

According to Judeo-Christian tradition, worship preferably occurs within a community of like-minded believers. Jews refer to a *chevra tefila* (prayer community) and to a *chavurah* (a friendship circle wherein a small group meets for prayer, study, and celebration). In spite of this heritage of communal worship, openly gay, lesbian, and bisexual individuals from Jewish or Christian traditions rarely find much support in such gatherings (Dworkin, 1996, 1997). As discussed, traditional organized religion generally has not proven itself philosophically reasonable, morally helpful, or spiritually illuminating for most sexual minorities. By further denying them ordination to roles of sacred leadership or failing to ritually celebrate their life passages (such as "coming out" or a lifetime same-sex commitment), religious communities render their gay, lesbian, and bisexual members invisible in congregational life. In this regard, virtually all religious and social events in churches and synagogues (with the exception of some of those discussed earlier) assume the heterosexuality of all participants.

The ultimate irony for many sexual minority Christians is to hear stories of Jesus reaching out with concern to the downtrodden and marginalized, while they feel like the *anawim* (forsaken outcasts) in their own churches. Similarly, Jews aspire to fulfillment of Judaism's highest goals—*mishpat, tzedakah, u-gmilut hasadim* (justice, charity, and acts of loving kindness)—yet many homosexually and bisexually oriented people sense they are not among those to whom this hospitality and graciousness is to be extended. The best-case scenario for gay, lesbian, and bisexual individuals in most synagogues and churches is to be treated as invisible in regard to the intimate nature of their lives and relationships. For many, however, their worst fears come true and they are disfellowshipped, excommunicated, or ostracized by the faith community of which they once considered themselves a part. It is often this pain that they bring to psychotherapy.

RELIGION-BASED CONVERSION

Some of the primary proponents of change in sexual orientation have been pastors and religiously oriented laity (Haldeman, 1991). Haldeman (1991, 1994, 1995), who chaired the 1995 project on Conversion Therapy for the Committee on Lesbian and Gay Concerns of the American Psychological Association, contends that conversion treatments are "thriving," sometimes with support from psychologists and other mental health professionals who serve as referral sources to evangelical and fundamentalist Christian individuals and groups promising to change sexual orientation.

Psychotherapists and Paraprofessionals

In this regard, 206 psychotherapists who practice sexual conversion therapy were surveyed, and 187 of them (90.7%) said they believed conversion to be an effective and ethical treatment option (Nicolosi, Byrd, & Potts, 2000). As a group, the clinicians also concluded that their clients benefited from the therapy, experiencing both changes in sexual orientation and improved psychological functioning. Along these same lines, 193 psychiatrists who were members of the Christian Psychiatry Movement (CPM) were surveyed (Galanter, Larson, & Rubenstone, 1991) to assess the role of religious belief in their practices. Nearly all of the CPM clinicians reported having been "born again," after which they experienced a decrease in emotional distress. They generally considered psychotropic medication the most effective treatment for acute schizophrenic or manic episodes, but rated the Bible and prayer more highly for suicidal intent, grief reaction, sociopathy, and alcoholism. In addition to discouraging abortion and premarital sex, 49% said they also would dissuade strongly religious patients from homosexual acts and 28% said they also would deter other patients from same-sex behaviors.

Oordt (1990) randomly surveyed 200 of the 1,700 members of the Christian Association for Psychological Studies (CAPS). Questionnaires regarding their ethical beliefs and behaviors were returned by 69 respondents (34.5%). According to Oordt, "the data indicate that Christian psychologists are effectively understanding and implementing the ethical guidelines of the American Psychological Association although guidance may be needed regarding finances and homosexuality" (p. 255). In regard to the latter, "treating homosexuality per se as pathological" was found to constitute a "difficult judgment" and to present a "critical dilemma" for many CAPS members. On one hand, they must exist in the church that generally regards homosexuality as deviant and, on the other, follow the ethical code of the American Psychological Association (1992), which mandates that members respect the rights and dignity of all people, including those with minority sexuality orientations. Oordt (1990) concluded that "psychologists who are facing both of these influences are likely to be left without much guidance [presumably from other Christians] on integrating their Christian values with professional standards" (p. 259).

Materials from one organization, the American Association of Christian Counselors (AACC), indicate that it includes among its membership (*n* = 14,000) "professionals, religious leaders, lay counselors and others who are interested in Christian counseling but who have little or no professional training." In 1995, the AACC joined with James Dobson's Focus on the Family to sponsor the International Congress on the Family. The conference brochure reflected that one of the sessions was titled "Coming Out of Homosexuality: Practical Answers for Clients." The convention flyer further noted that Focus on the Family has a daily radio broadcast heard on 4,000 stations worldwide, publishes 9 magazines sent to 2.3 million people a month, responds to nearly 50,000 letters a week, "offers professional counseling and makes referrals to a network of 1,600 therapists."

Data are lacking as to how many members of the Christian mental health organizations described actually attempt to convert or "reorient" clients to heterosexuality or refer them to others who do. Given the response to questionnaires by CPM and CAPS members, and the alliance between Focus of the Family and AACC, however, it probably is safe to assume that the number is significant. While CPM and CAPS require professional licensure for membership, associations such as AACC appear to require only an interest in Christian counseling to join. Consequently, much religion-based therapy and many conversion programs "operate under the formidable auspices of the Christian church, and outside the jurisdiction of any professional organization that might impose ethical standards of practice and accountability on them" (Haldeman, 1991, p. 159). In a review of empirical findings concerning ex-gays, Throckmorton (2000) similarly notes that "volunteer counselors often staff ex-gay ministries as opposed to licensed clinicians who conduct reorientation counseling" (p. 6). Data from a large survey (n = 882) of individuals who had tried sexual reorientation (Nicolosi et al., 2000) appeared to verify this situation. Accordingly, slightly more than half (50.5%; n = 445)) of the subjects had received help from a professional therapist, and 229 of these had seen both a professional therapist and a pastoral counselor. The remaining 437 individuals had sought assistance only from a pastoral counselor, friends, family, ex-gay ministries, or a combination. (A note of caution is offered in interpreting these data since some individuals who refer to themselves as *pastoral counselors* are certified by the 3,000-member American Association of Pastoral Counselors and thus have graduate mental health degrees, in addition to advanced religious or theological training [see Resources section].)

Conversion Groups

The website of Exodus International (1999) describes the organization as "a Christian referral and resource network founded in 1976 [whose] primary purpose is to proclaim that freedom from homosexuality is possible through repentance and faith in Jesus Christ as Savior and Lord." Within its umbrella are larger associations such as Regeneration, Homosexuals Anonymous, and PFOX (Parents and Friends of Ex-Gays), as well as approximately 150 local groups (with their own unique names) in nearly 40 states, Puerto Rico, and the District of Columbia. Some of these often listed under the Exodus International umbrella include Courage (with Roman Catholic associations), NARTH (the National Association for Research and Therapy of Homosexuality), JONAH (for Jewish individuals seeking to change their sexual orientation), Transforming Congregations (with United Methodist affiliations), and oneBYone (ministry of the Presbyterian Renewal Network).

Many, if not most, of these organizations follow a model adapted by Homosexuals Anonymous from the 12-step program of Alcoholics Anonymous, wherein, as individuals "work the program," they supposedly increase their ability to avoid the addiction of homosexual behaviors by repenting and applying biblical principles (Goss, 1993). Exodus affiliates and other similar associations produce and distribute a vast amount of literature, including videotapes, books, newsletters, and pamphlets. Teachers' manuals are available, and home study materials, including audiotapes, are sold to supplement weekly programs that last several months and are designed to help people "come out of the homosexual lifestyle." In the summer of 1998, Exodus International and 17 other organizations, including the American Family Association, the Christian Coalition, and the Family Research Council, spent millions of dollars on full-page advertisements in newspapers across the United States. These advertisements and a television campaign that followed were designed to "proclaim that hope for change is possible for those still struggling with homosexuality" (for an example, see "Toward a New National Discussion," 1998). The text further explained that "many have walked out of homosexuality . . . into sexual celibacy or even marriage. How? Often because someone cared enough to love them, despite where they were, and to confront the truth of their sexual sin."

Clients and Treatment Issues

Gay men who question the moral and religious acceptability of being gay tend to be attracted to authoritarian religious practices. They also are likely to have high degrees of internalized homophobia and low self-concepts; to see homosexuality as sinful, to fear negative reactions from others, and to feel more depressed than the general population (Ross & Rosser, 1996; M. S. Weinberg & Williams, 1974). These men (and undoubtedly women, as well) are vulnerable targets for religion-based reorientation therapies and programs. In fact, many clients who attempt conversion to heterosexuality are confused or shame-ridden and possess extremely negative attitudes in regard to gay, lesbian, and bisexual orientations and toward themselves as persons with erotic attractions toward members of their own sex (Haldeman, 1991, 1995). Because of these client's low self-esteem, fear, and precarious mental health, Haldeman (1991) believes that their testimonials for "successful conversion" should be considered suspect. Not surprisingly, however, it is upon the endorsements of these individuals that religious conversion programs base the majority of their claims for victory.

Motivations for Treatment

People enter conversion therapy for a variety of different reasons (Haldeman, 1994, 1995, 1996, 2000; Shidlo & Schroeder, 1999, 2000). Some clients seek to literally "save their souls" and desire to have all homoerotic fantasies expunged from their minds. Others are homosexually oriented and heterosexually married, and they might enter treatment to learn how to live more comfortably with their husbands or wives, to reinforce any heteroeroticism they might posses, or both. Still others are frightened adolescents or young adults whose parents insist on treatment or elimination of all same-sex desires and behaviors. A large number experience their religious affiliation so intensely that their sexual orientation is of secondary importance. In other words, they have beliefs about the morality of same-sex behavior that have been derived from their theology, and they want to live according to the prescriptions of their religion (Beckstead & Morrow, 1999; Throckmorton, 1998, 2000; Yarhouse, 1998; Yarhouse & Burkett, 2000). Because they deeply value having a place in their "church home," they are "willing to attempt to give up their sexual orientation" to remain part of a group that seems more familiar and reassuring than the gay social world (Haldeman, 1996, p. 889). Haldeman (1991) contends that the choice of conversion treatment is always based on a negative perception of homosexuality, regardless of the reason for seeking reorientation. Similarly, Drescher (1998) believes that "every gay patient comes into treatment feeling bad about being gay, either consciously, unconsciously or both. . . . Attempts to rid oneself of homosexuality are also attempts to rid oneself of self-loathing identifications (pp. 71–72). He also says that "reparative therapies will always exist as long as people have antihomosexual moral beliefs" (Drescher, 1999, p. 76).

Results of Treatment

There is no scientific evidence that successful reorientation is possible or that "reparative therapies" can functionally change a person's sexual orientation from homosexual to heterosexual (Drescher, 1999; R. C. Friedman, 1999; Haldeman, 1991, 1995; Herek, 1999b; Isay, 1988; T. F. Murphy, 1992; Stein, 1996a; Tozer & McClanahan, 1999). Despite this lack of documentation, a *Newsweek* poll indicated that 56% of the general population think that gay men and lesbians can change their sexual orientation through therapy, will power, or religious conviction (Leland & Miller, 1998). Conversely, R. Green (1988) believes that the potential for "grafting" heterosexual behavior over homosexual orientation does not mean that sexual orientation is alterable. In fact, he contends that "therapy may not be much more effective than what would be expected from attempts to reorient heterosexuals if penile–vaginal intercourse were to become (frequently) a crime, (usually) a sin, and (for several decades, at least) a mental illness" (p. 569). Claims of reorientation success usually are based on anecdotal reports, rather than on rigorous empirical studies that have been subjected to independent peer review (Haldeman, 2000; Herek, 1999b; Shidlo & Schroeder, 1999, 2000).

Ethics of Reorientation

Despite anecdotal reports of emotional anguish, depression, severe social problems, physical trauma (e.g., genital self-mutilation), and suicide that directly result from conversion therapy, religion-based or otherwise (Haldeman, 1991, 1995; Isay, 1985; Stein, 1996a; M. White, 1995), there is no compelling empirical evidence that clients are harmed by these procedures. While about 63 individuals (7.1%) of the subjects ($n = 882$) in a recent study of people who had attempted religious conversion therapy reported that they were doing worse after the intervention than before (Nicolosi et al., 2000) these self-report data do not provide objective evidence of harm, just as reports of positive change do not provide objective evidence of help. In other words, a case *against* reorientation therapy cannot be made on a scientific basis by anecdotal reports of distress any more than a case *for* conversion treatment can be made by the 20 subjects who reported success outcomes (Beckstead & Morrow, 1999) or by the large number of participants who rated their change experience as being helpful in regard to their self-acceptance, trust of the opposite sex, self-esteem, emotional stability, depression, and relationship with God (Nicolosi et al., 2000; Throckmorton, 1998, 2000).

POSITIONS OF PROFESSIONAL ASSOCIATIONS

Haldeman (1995) states that, "given the limitations of existing data, it is difficult to make a case against the right of therapists to practice conversion therapy even though its theoretical base is blatantly prejudicial" (p. 5). This lack of research to specifically address the issue of harm (and the potential legal problems that may arise from restraint of trade without just cause), prevents professional associations from legally or ethically *prohibiting* the practice of sexual reorientation counseling. Accordingly, "the professional organizations have developed policies about conversion therapy that attempt to walk the fine line between interfering with the rights of gay people to seek appropriate treatment, and the rights of the religiously-motivated" (Haldeman, 2000, p. 3). The American Psychiatric Association (1998), for example, issued a position statement on psychiatric treatment and sexual orientation that lists several potential risks of "reparative therapy" and indicates that "therapist alignment with societal prejudices against homosexuality may reinforce self-hatred already experienced by the patient." After discussing issues related to informed consent, the statement concludes with this statement: "The American Psychiatric Association recognizes that in the course of ongoing psychiatric treatment, there may be appropriate clinical indications for attempting to change sexual *behaviors*" (emphasis added). The American Counseling Association (1998) also passed a resolution that read in part: "The American Counseling Association . . . supports the dissemination of accurate information about sexual orientation, mental health, and appropriate interventions in order to counteract bias that is based in ignorance or unfounded beliefs about same-gender sexual orientation."

When the American Psychological Association (1997) passed a *Resolution of Appropriate Therapeutic Responses to Sexual Orientation*, the action did not explicitly condemn or discourage reparative or conversion therapy. Rather, the resolution cited several principles and standards of the association's Ethical Principles of Psychologists and Code of Conduct (American Psychological Association, 1992) and related these to the ethical treatment of sexual minority clients. Among other concerns, the resolution stressed that psychologists should not engage in unfair discrimination based on sexual orientation; should respect the rights of others whose views differ from their own; should respect the rights of individuals to privacy, confidentiality, self-determination and autonomy; should be aware of cultural differences due to sexual orientation; should make appropriate referrals where differences of sexual orientation would significantly affect work with individuals; should not make deceptive or false statements regarding the clinical basis for their services; and should obtain appropriate informed consent for therapy or other services.

NECESSITY OF INFORMED CONSENT

Possibly some people are misled about what reorientation and reparative therapy can offer and may hold out too high an expectation for change. Thus clinicians should inform clients about what research has demonstrated about the results of these treatments and what the potential costs are to themselves (Beckstead & Morrow, 1999; Yarhouse, 1998): "For example, if psychologists establish that change is possible, but for only about 30% or so (and that those people tend to be high on religious motivation or some other measure), then this could be an important consideration in informed consent" (Yarhouse & Burkett, 2000, p. 15). Throckmorton (1998, 2000), a psychologist and spokesperson for conservative Christians, believes that clients who desire sexual reorientation should be advised in advance that multiple views exist and that numerous courses have been pursued with a variety of outcomes. Likewise, Yarhouse and Burkett (2000) request that clinicians respect the beliefs of religiously orthodox individuals, just as they would respect any other aspect of diversity. Building on what the profession is coming to accept about the fluidity of sexual attraction and orientation, these authors contend that the wishes of religiously motivated clients to reduce or increase inclination or behaviors can be respected within the context of both current scientific knowledge and professional ethics.

Haldeman (2000) acknowledges that, for many individuals, personal spirituality may supersede concerns about sexual orientation and that the mental health profession has no right to deny these people treatment that is in accordance with their moral values. However, he cautions against coercion of sexual minority youth and adults and says that forcing such individuals into conversion therapy is an ethical violation not unlike "committing child abuse" (p. 4): "Furthermore, any individual or organization that attempts to portray lesbians and gay men as mentally ill, more inclined toward pedophilia, or less stable in relationship or vocation adjustment by virtue of their sexual orientation, is guilty of distorting the truth" (p. 4). Just as he advises orthodox religion to "play fair" with sexual minorities, he asks the gay community to "actively work to counter prejudice against religion" (p. 4).

REVITALIZING RELIGION FOR SEXUAL MINORITIES

Thus far, this chapter has addressed certain elements of the Judeo-Christian tradition that have been extremely destructive to the religious experience of lesbians, bisexuals, and gay men. The legacy of persecution, the politics of the religious right, the nonviability of Judeo-Christian religious institutions, and systematic efforts designed to reorient sexual minorities to heterosexuality were among the areas discussed. In response to this kind of prejudicial treatment, numerous religious writers have seen a need for greater compassion and a reformulation of traditional beliefs about sexual orientation, identity, and gender. Along with these individual spokespersons, affirming communities also have emerged from various religious traditions. Most of these groups were formed to provide a viable means of communal support to gay, lesbian, and bisexual members of religious denominations and to help them reconcile or integrate their faith traditions with their minority sexual orientations. Many of these organizations, their denominational origins (if applicable), addresses, and means of contacting them are listed in the Resources section.

Further efforts to revitalize religion for sexual minorities include a burgeoning body of literature that has been generated by numerous Judeo-Christian authors who are attempting to reconcile traditional beliefs with minority sexual orientations. The following sections discuss a number of these literary endeavors in order to familiarize psychotherapists and clients with the kinds of affirmative reinterpretations that are available. Additional projects that endeavor to reconceptualize religion also are described

From Protestant Traditions

Writers from Protestant heritages have recounted the struggles of sexual minority clergy and laypersons to serve the church (Comstock, 1993; Ferry, 1994; Glaser, 1988; Pennington, 1989; T. Perry, 1987; Stuart, 1998; M. White, 1995; R. Williams, 1992). A large number of Presbyterians ($n = 67$) and other "people of faith" ($n = 50$) have been quite articulate in telling their stories (Kreider, 1998; Spahr, Poethig, Berry, & McLain, 1999; Thorson-Smith, Van Wijk-Bos, Pott, & Thompson, 1997). In addition, other Protestant writers have helped gay and lesbian Christians debate homosexuality (Geis & Messer, 1994), reclaim the spirituality sacred (Frontain, 1997; Glaser, 1990, 1998), approach God in prayer (Glaser, 1991), and critique and reclaim the Bible (England, 1998; Glaser, 1994). Others have provided a Christian response to homosexuality (Scanzoni & Mollenkott, 1994) and have contributed a gay perspective on sexual and spiritual union (Uhrig, 1986).

Along these same lines, J. B. Nelson (1982) describes Christianity as an incarnational Christian faith and a sex-affirming religion with positive resources for lesbians and gay men. He also contends that "homosexuality is a Christianly valid orientation" and "homosexual genital expression should be guided by the same general ethical criteria as are appropriate for heterosexual expression, though with sensitivity to the special situation of an oppressed minority" (p. 164). Another Protestant theologian, Edwards (1989), wrote "a critique of creationist homophobia" in which he claims that the book of Genesis does not provide explicit theological evidence of homosexual practice and thus cannot be used opportunistically for the moral and religious disapproval of homosexual persons. His "liberation alternative" opposes misogynist and homophobic abuses of creation texts and proposes a liberated sexuality based on "equal regard for the rights of others" and "the love of a God who does not show partiality" (p. 115).

From the Catholic Tradition

Like their Protestant counterparts, Catholics have offered affirming theological reformulations for lesbians and gay men. J. J. McNeill, a former Jesuit priest, for example, has discussed homosexuality and the Catholic Church (1985), offered lesbians and gay men a liberating theology (1988), encouraged them to celebrate their freedom and the fullness of their lives (1995), and discussed his own spiritual journey (1998). Another priest (Helminiak, 1994) examines "historical, cultural, philosophical, psychological, sociological, medical, spiritual and personal factors" and concludes that the "the Bible supplies no real basis for the condemnation of homosexuality" (p. 14). An additional ex-Jesuit priest (Goss, 1993) developed an activist position that celebrates and integrates gay and lesbian sexuality with liberation theology. Finally, M. Fox (1984), a one-time Dominican priest, describes the spiritual journey of the homosexual, whom he referred to as "the *anawim* [oppressed, persecuted] in our midst" (p. 203).

Others from the Catholic tradition have helped lesbians and gay men reconcile their sexual orientations with the Catholic Church (Gramick, 1983b; Gramick & Nugent, 1995); understand societal, biblical-theological, pastoral, and vocational perspectives on their sexuality (Nugent, 1984a); deepen their spirituality (R. Woods, 1988); and enhance their personal faith experience (Zanotti, 1986). In particular, Sister Jeannine Gramick and Father Robert Nugent established the New Ways Ministry in 1977 "to promote the acceptance of gay and lesbian people as full and equal members of church and society" (from website; see Resources section). They collaborated on numerous projects (Gramick & Nugent, 1995; Nugent & Gramick, 1992), including the establishment of the Center for Homophobia Education through which they conducted full-day seminars in various churches and dioceses around the United States. They also organized a Catholic Parents Network to provide a forum for mothers and fathers of sexual minority children to express their concerns and needs, examine their religious beliefs and practices, and interact with other parents. After years of investigation, Gramick and Nugent were ordered by the Vatican in 1999 to permanently abandon their ministry to lesbian and gay persons and their families. In nearly 90 pages of documents, the Vatican declared their teaching "erroneous and dangerous" and specifically asked the pair to affirm that homosexuality is an "objectively disordered" condition and that homosexual acts are "intrinsically evil" (Malcolm, 1999a, 1999b). Subject to particular scrutiny was their use of the word *natural*, rather than *disordered* to describe homosexual orientation (Gramick & Nugent, 1995; Nugent & Gramick, 1992).

From Anglican, Mormon, and Jewish Traditions

In addition to Protestants and Roman Catholics, three Episcopalians have made particularly significant contributions to gay and lesbian spirituality. Psychotherapist Fortunato (1982) outlines the healing journeys of gay Christians; Heyward (1989b), an Episcopal priest and professor of theology, discusses homoeroticism as power and the love of God; and Bishop Spong (1988) offers an affirming contextual approach to biblical interpretations regarding the morality of same-sex intimate relationships. From the Mormon tradition, Feliz (1992) describes the story of a gay high priest, while others have offered a poignant collection of essays written by gay and lesbian Latter Day Saints (Schow, Schow, & Raynes, 1991).

Compared to the gay and lesbian–affirming Christian literature, there are far fewer comparable references pertaining to sexual minority Jews. One publication assists Jewish lesbians, bisexuals, and gay men in reclaiming their religious tradition, creating a gay and lesbian Jewish community, and honoring their same-sex relationships with commitment ceremonies (Balka & Rose, 1989). E. T. Beck (1989) offers an anthology of stories about Jewish lesbians, and Dworkin (1996, 1997) extends perspective and assistance to therapists working with Jewish clients who are oriented toward bisexuality, lesbianism, or both. In addition, Rabbi Kahn discusses modern teaching on Judaism and homosexuality, and Hasbany (1989) has edited a collection of scholarly writings in which A. Cooper (1989) provides insight into gay and lesbian Jewish movements. Likewise, several Jewish periodicals further discuss homosexuality and Judaism, and the World Congress of Gay, Lesbian, and Bisexual Jewish Organizations has an excellent collection of materials on its website (see Resources section).

REFORMULATING SPIRITUALITY FOR SEXUAL MINORITIES

Sexual minorities are exploring their own spiritual paths, both alongside and apart from the Judeo-Christian tradition. Shallenberger (1998) analyzes the faith journeys of several of these individuals from the perspective of various religious traditions. His reflections are well grounded in the literature on faith development and gay and lesbian spirituality and reflect a diversity of spiritual pathways. Moreover, some people are examining religious questions from a feminist or women's viewpoint (Hunt, 1990; Reilly, 1995), whereas others are focusing on the unique spiritual concerns of bisexual individuals (Dworkin, 1996; Kolodny, 2000). Many of the more nontraditional spiritual avenues often overlap, as well as intersect, and thus they defy categorization, but the following sections consider them under three broad subheadings: shamanism, Goddess (or prepatriarchal) religions, and spiritual healing and transformation.

Shamanism

As discussed in Chapter 10, individuals known as "two-spirited people," medicine men, or manly hearted women often were sacred persons or shamans in their tribal societies (J. M. Clark, 1987, 1989, 1997; A. Evans, 1978; Grahn, 1984, 1986; Jacobs, 1968, 1997; Roscoe, 1987a, 1987b). Many contemporary lesbians and gay men have been inspired by the historical accounts of these visionaries who served as intermediaries between the natural and spiritual worlds and who ushered the wisdom of nature into the tribe (Grahn,

1984). Shamans were magicians in the sense that they directed and guided the course of events by supernatural means, primarily through rites and ceremonies that were designed to influence spirits, gods, and the secrets of nature. With the help of their guardian spirits, shamans frequently slept while their dreaming egos established relations with spiritual powers (Hultkrantz, 1988).

For some bisexuals, lesbians, and gay men, the spiritual practices of shamanism are associated with "the appearance of ghosts, spirits, and gods," as well as with sojourns to "the realms of the heavenly powers and the land of the dead" and visits from spirits to whom sacrifices are offered (Hultkrantz, 1988, p. 35). Kear (1999) describes these kinds of phenomena as manifestations of reincarnations of gay and lesbian souls. Other individuals experience the living soul of shamanism in their contemporary sexual minority "tribes" (Barzan, 1995; Doore, 1988; M. Thompson, 1987, 1994, 1995). Accordingly, gatherings are held often during which group members share collective energy to empower themselves, explore their sacred heritage, and celebrate their gay and lesbian spirituality. E. C. Johnson and Johnson (2000) discuss themes in gay spirituality, one of which they refer to as Circle-Making. Kilhefner (1988) refers to these kinds of collective activities as "re-visioning" the spiritual essence of people attracted to their own sex and a celebration of their "different window on the world" (p. 129).

Goddess Religions

Many lesbian feminists (and some feminist gay men) are turning away from Judeo-Christian traditions to Goddess religions. To them, the biblical symbols of divinity have supported a hierarchical and patriarchal system which severely has restricted the power of the feminine. Thus, they are rediscovering and reviving the ancient traditions of Goddess worship and witchcraft that they believe were suppressed by the Judeo-Christian tradition. Eisler (1987) describes how a highly advanced Neolithic civilization (approximately 6,000 BCE) that developed many tools and technologies worshiped not a cruel and vengeful God but, rather, the Great Goddess who symbolized fertility, life, regeneration, and bounty. The rediscovery and revival of this powerful feminine symbolism provides the basis for contemporary religious communities that celebrate the Goddess. Akin to the shamanistic tradition, their feminist "vision of a spirituality rooted in the body and nature is an important response to the dualism of body and soul, nature and spirit that . . . is at the heart of the suppression of women [and sexual minorities] in Western religion and culture" (Christ & Plaskow, 1979, p. 197).

The Goddess is manifested cross-culturally and transhistorically as a wise intermediary (Eisler, 1995). In fact, C. Matthews (1991) contends that Sophia, Goddess of Wisdom, "appears in nearly every culture and society" and "is distinguishable from many popular forms of the Divine Feminine by the fact that she is a Black Goddess." In Lilith, for example, this Black Goddess is represented as "the fearful possessor of both wisdom and sexuality—a dynamic and, for most learned Jews, a horrific combination in a female," as well as the embodiment of "the physical and spiritual wisdoms in one figure. She is the Goddess complete within herself, an abomination to those who also fear and despise lesbian and solitary women as dangerous" (p. 45). In addition, this Divine Feminine manifests her power through seemingly opposing appearances, such as in the Egyptian Goddess Isis, who veils her glory, and in the Indian Goddess Kali, who shocks and terrifies. Among other names, she is known as Nature, Shekinah, the Hag, the Blessed

Virgin, the World-Soul, and the Queen of Heaven. Eisler (1995) specifically noted that "the Christian veneration of the Virgin Mary is directly traceable to the ancient worship of the Goddess" (p. 148).

The Wicca movement has made major contributions to feminist (and lesbian) spirituality "by reintroducing the goddess as a symbol of Immanence and radically connecting power" (Cady, Ronan, & Taussig, 1986, p. 9). According to Starhawk (1979), the first national president of the Covenant of the Goddess, "from earliest times, women have been witches, *wicce*, 'wise ones'—priestesses, diviners, midwives, poets, and singers of songs of power" (p. 260). Witchcraft, "the craft of the wise," was "an earth-centered, nature-oriented worship that venerated the Goddess" (p. 261) before the Christian era. For several hundred years, witches and Christians peacefully coexisted, while many wise women believed that the Virgin Mary was a manifestation of the Great Goddess. During the 13th and 14th centuries, however, the church began to persecute witches, along with numerous other dissenters and nonconformists, including infidels, heretics, and sexual minorities (see Chapter 2 and earlier in this chapter). According to the church, the witches' power was derived ultimately from female sexuality, and their heresy was based fundamentally in their Goddess worship (Eisler, 1987; Starhawk, 1979).

Many lesbians also are drawn to Greek myths of Amazon women who represent the power of women's bonds. Downing (1981, 1991, 1995) describes mythological traditions about groups of women who acted together against male domination and fought male oppression. These women "were so fearful to men in part because they evoked memories of more archaic female powers, the Gorgons and the Furies" (Downing, 1991, p. 188), who were associated closely with the Amazons. Amazon communities were "women-only societies ruled by a group of sisters" who "were believed to live out their sexuality mostly among themselves" and to "seek out the men of neighboring tribes for intercourse, solely for the sake of reproduction" on an annual basis (Downing, 1991, p. 190). Daly (1978, 1987) likewise writes of the *A-mazing* Amazon, "the woman-identified woman," who broke through the maze of patriarchal culture and committed herself to friendship and fidelity with women.

Starhawk (1982) identifies Judaism and Christianity with patriarchy, power over, domination, and control. Similarly, Daly (1985) contends that oppressive patriarchy has been guilty of "the enslavement and indirect murder of women by means of legislation and moral (i.e., immoral) dictates against abortion, birth control, lesbianism, and, in general, against Self-government and expansion of woman-identified be-ing/spiritual Life" (p. xxv). Many lesbians can identify with these feelings of oppression and thus are drawn to the emphases in Goddess spirituality and witchcraft on the interrelatedness of all creation, equality of all humanity, shared power, and empowerment of the feminine.

Spiritual Healing and Transformation

Shuli Goodman (1988), who with her partner, Diane Mariechild, created Keepers of the Flame, a "sacred mystery school for women," contends that all organized religion has been overtly hostile toward sexual minorities and that "the Soul of Liberation" and the spiritual healing of gay and lesbian people is being explored actively "with the passion born of unspeakable pain and grief" (p. 9). In terms of this pursuit, Goodman asserts that the gay or lesbian spiritual journey is the quest for "whatever separates us from knowing that all life is sacred"; further, it is a "path of connectedness, whereby we know the deep oneness of all life" (p. 9). Along this same vein, Benvenuti (1993b) notes that she and other sexual minorities spend their lives "on a gamble, a great leap of faith that the individual life is of intrinsic worth, that risking all to go against the rules in order to be ourselves is a faithful response to the universe, or to the God that has brought us into being" (p. 35). Writing from a cosmic perspective (Benvenuti, 1993a, 1993b), she documents her search of the universe and discovery of the Creator's abundance and generosity. Referring to the same kind of creation-centered spirituality, Struzzo (1989) affirms that "everything in creation is part of God and a source of blessing, including sexuality in its various manifestations" (p. 197). Thus, "the fundamental challenge for gays and lesbians is to appreciate and celebrate the basic goodness of all creation, including their sexuality" (p. 199). Connor (1993) speaks of this task as a process of reclaiming the connections between homoeroticism and the sacred.

Journey

The theme of journey or path permeates gay and lesbian spirituality, and this process of moving from one stage to another is reflected in many writings (K. G. Johnson, 1998; J. J. McNeill, 1998; Shallenberger, 1998). For example, Whitehead and Whitehead (1986) wrote of passages in homosexual holiness in which "the central paradox of a passage is always loss and gain, it is a time of peril and possibility" (p. 130). According to the Whiteheads, who spoke from a Christian perspective, a passage begins in disorientation and loss and ends with transformative change. The first step of the journey for lesbians and gay men is an extremely terrifying interior passage of "coming out" to self. The next stage is one of intimacy that bridges between the gay and lesbian self and others. The final passage is a public one that involves being recognized as both homosexual and Christian in the broader world. In openly integrating an identity, "life and vocation become a public witness of homosexual and Christian maturing and a gift to the next generation. . . . Closeted lives, however holy, cannot provide images and models of religious maturing. A certain public exposure and light is required for this virtue of generativity to have its effect" (p. 142).

Loss

Several others have written about the relationship between loss and spiritual growth (Fortunato, 1982; Garanzini, 1989; Hardy, 1998; O'Neill & Ritter, 1992; Ritter & O'Neill, 1989, 1996). As previously mentioned, grieving is a lifelong task for many lesbians and gay men; it entails relinquishing the images of heterosexuality to develop an affirming sexual minority identity. Fortunato (1982) contends that "spiritual growth like psychotherapy, then, is a process of grieving" (p. 72) and "the spiritual goal is atonement with the flow of the universe, which requires letting go of all that gives us comfort and a sense of determination" (p. 73). In other words, everything, especially the ego, is given over to God or cosmic consciousness. Garanzini (1989) reiterates this same theme when he proposes that pastoral care for lesbians and gay men must be sensitive to their attachments, separations, and losses. Drawing on object relations theory and self psychology, psychotherapists must work with clients in examining "the cycle of attachment, separation, loss and reattachment that characterize all important relationships" (p. 175). Like Fortunato, Garanzini (1989) contends that suffering the loss of heterosexual myths is a frightening process and that clients find themselves in the throes of separation anxiety when these nonviable images are cast aside. As clients move through the process, however, they endure a death that enables a rebirth, a lesson that "cannot be learned outside of the experience of the grief of loss" (p. 191).

Transformation

Ritter and O'Neill (1989, 1996) contend that there are three basic processes involved in helping clients spiritually transform loss: recasting religious images, reframing losses, and facilitating spiritual pathways. As mentioned previously, all individuals need spiritually illuminating images with which to identify and emulate (James, 1928). In this regard, clinicians can assist clients by upholding some of the inspiring and hope-renewing figures that were described earlier in this chapter. Accordingly, they can remind clients of shamans, goddesses, heroic biblical figures, and saints who represent examples of same-sex love and spirituality. An excellent resource in this regard is *The Essential Gay Mystics* (Harvey, 1997/2002), which includes texts from the Greeks and Romans, the Native American *berdache* tradition, the ancient Far East and the Persian Sufi traditions, as well as works of literary figures from the Renaissance to the twentieth century. Finally, the process of reframing and transforming loss was described in the preceding paragraph (Fortunato, 1982; Garanzini, 1989) and will be developed further in the following discussion of an eight-stage loss model (J. M. Schneider, 1984, 1994). Psychotherapists can facilitate pathways for spiritual healing and transformation using these kinds of reconceptualizations, as well as by directing clients to any of the religious organizations listed in the Resources section.

Stages of Spiritual Awakening

J. M. Schneider's (1984, 1994) loss model has been adapted and used to outline the spiritual journey from loss to transformation. This model is summarized in Table 13.2 and briefly is discussed here. Clinicians also are referred to *Coming Out Within* (O'Neill & Ritter, 1992) for additional details, as well as over 50 case illustrations to use in helping gay and lesbian clients through Schneider's eight stages. The first five stages (*Initial Awareness, Holding On, Letting Go, Awareness of the Loss*, and *Gaining Perspective*), in many ways, parallel the five stages of death and dying outlined by Kübler-Ross (1969) and the first four phases of identity formation described in Chapter 5 here. Chapter 9, in particular, suggested psychotherapeutic interventions to use with clients struggling with grief over the loss of a heterosexual life image.

Schneider's sixth stage, *Integrating Loss*, moves beyond accepting the loss of heterosexuality and the acquisition of a gay or lesbian identity. Consequently, it is perhaps the most critical juncture in the therapeutic process, given that it is the first proactive step toward reformulating and spiritually transforming loss. De la Huerta (1999) refers to this as coming out spiritually. Just as Whitehead and Whitehead (1986) refer to the importance of both interior and exterior passages, Schneider contends that loss cannot be resolved until an active public step of integration has occurred. Until people thus take risks and assume responsibility for themselves and their lives, the energy they have invested in their losses cannot be reinvested elsewhere. Clinicians are encouraged, therefore, to exer-

TABLE 13.2. Schneider's Loss Model

Initial Awareness (shock; numbness; disbelief)

• Daily routine is completely disrupted.

Holding On (denial; bargaining)

• Steps are taken to limit awareness or to reverse or limit the impact of the loss.
• Alternatives to the grieving process are sought.

Letting Go

• Attempts are made to diminish the true significance of the loss.
• Individuals try to convince themselves that the loss is inconsequential.
• People pull back from involvements and commitments to diminish their sense of panic that something meaningful has been taken from their lives.

Awareness of the Loss (mourning; depression; despair)

• All ways of avoiding the loss have been exhausted:
  – What is lost is gone.   – Reality is faced.
  – There is no way out.   – Exhaustion and grieving persist.

Gaining Perspective (detachment)

• A time for solitude, healing, and acceptance.
  – There is no longer a sense of struggle.
  – Patience is needed.
• Many people foreclose on the loss process here:
  – They believe they can't tolerate any further suffering and reminders.
  – Many remain forever detached or return to strategies to limit awareness.

Integrating Loss (finishing business)

• An active public step of integration has occurred.
• Energy is freed to be reinvested elsewhere.
• People are then able to resume responsibility for their lives:
  – Restitution   – Testing/risk taking
  – Reintegration   – Restoration of continuity

Reformulating Loss

• Some type of integration has occurred.
• New energy is freed for a change in perceptual set.
• A new sense of purpose emerges.
• Limits are reformulated as potential, coping as growth, problems as challenges, tragedies as freeing:
  – A new identity is gained.   – Reorganization and renewal occur.
  – Humor returns.   – Reframing begins.

Transforming Loss (transcendence; integration)

• Sense of self can transcend time, person, and place.
• Grief has come to be viewed as a unifying rather than alienating experience.
• Transformed loss is seeing the loss as altering rather than completely severing relationships.
• Connection to all things is through cycles of continuity with the past, present, and future.
• The world is seen as symbolic.

Note. Summarized from J. M. Schneider (1984, 1994).

cise their creativity, trusting that some form of client action must occur in order for therapeutic progress to result.

Once this public step has been taken, a seventh stage, *Reformulating Loss*, usually ensues, enabling clients to see their losses from fresher perspectives. As discussed earlier, psychotherapists (often with the assistance of clergy and spiritual directors) can help clients reframe loss by helping them recast religious images and by facilitating their spiritual passages from death to life. What happens next is outside the scope of this chapter, as well as beyond the influence of the clinician. Once clients have transformed loss (an eighth stage) and are developing a transcendent spirituality, they often have more to offer psychotherapists than ever can be returned in kind.

CONCLUSION

Affirmative practice requires that clinicians understand and respect the value systems of clients, including their beliefs about religion and spirituality. Religiously inclined sexual minorities frequently experience considerable distress in reconciling their faith with their sexual inclinations and therapists can do much to help them resolve this dissonance. This chapter provides assistance in helping clients understand and objectify much of organized religion's condemnation of their sexual orientations, and the pressures directed toward them to orient toward heterosexuality. Most importantly, however, it describes the efforts of many in traditional and nontraditional religion to recast the messages of faith such that sexual minorities feel affirmed and validated, as well as help in the reformulation of their spirituality. The information in the Resources section can also support and enhance this process.

Part IV

WORKING WITH COUPLES AND FAMILIES

14

Families of Origin and Coming-Out Issues

Gay men and lesbians belong to families, both those from which they originated and those established in adulthood. The remaining chapters examine these familial configurations from a number of different perspectives, as well as explore the sociocultural influences on each element in the system. This chapter discusses the dynamics of these systems from the points of view of parents and others in the families of origin of gay men and lesbians. Chapter 15 describes numerous issues involving same-sex couples, and Chapter 16 elucidates sex therapy with these gay and lesbian pairs. Finally, Part IV concludes with discussions of parenting partners and children of sexual minorities in Chapter 17.

FAMILIES OF ORIGIN

Family members of sexual minorities usually have internalized the same homophobic attitudes and heterosexist assumptions as have their lesbian and gay loved ones (Beeler & DiProva, 1999; Laird, 1998). Consequently, the amount of emotional support they are able to provide homosexually oriented individuals within their family system often is less than that given to heterosexual members (Kurdek & Schmitt, 1986b, 1987a, 1987b). Most lesbians, bisexuals, and gay men are aware of this potential negative consequence and thus often place family of origin among the last groups to which they typically come out or from whom support is received (L. S. Brown, 1989a; Bryant & Demian, 1995; Wells-Lurie, 1996). One study of 407 lesbians indicated that 54.3% ($n = 221$) of the subjects came out initially to other lesbians, while only 7.9% ($n = 32$) first disclosed their sexual orientation to family members before all others (Radonsky & Borders, 1995). Similarly, in a survey of 1,749 lesbians and gay men, parents were rated below the mean for both populations in terms of perceived sources of support (Bryant & Demian, 1995). On a 7-point scale, with a rating of 1 indicating "strong support" and 7 indicating a "hostile" response from the parent, mothers were given a mean rating of 3.34 by lesbians, compared with 3.71 for their fathers (the overall rating for a list of several choices was 2.64). The average rating of the gay men surveyed was 2.65 (which was virtually identical to the 2.64 of the lesbian population), but their mean ratings in the cases of both mothers (2.98) and fathers (3.37) were higher than those given by the women. In this survey, then, gay men perceived more parental support than did lesbians. This point will be discussed in more detail later in the chapter.

Sometimes fears of manifest homophobia and rejection are based in reality (Beeler & DiProva, 1999; Berg-Cross, 1988; Gottlieb, 2000); thus, many "lesbians and gay men strike a devil's bargain in which a stilted or distant relationship is weighed against the possibility of no relationship at all" (L. S. Brown, 1989a, p. 67). Brown has observed three patterns for juggling the closet and the family of origin (pp. 68–69):

1. *The maintenance of rigid geographical and emotional distance from the family.* In this situation, contact is reduced to a bare minimum, and sexual minorities may lie or evade when asked about intimate details of their lives. They feel estranged from family members who, in turn, may suffer a sense of rejection or loss without being able to understand the "coldness" of their loved one.

2. *The "I know you know" pattern.* An unspoken agreement exists in which all parties agree not to talk about the personal lives of lesbian, gay, or bisexual family members or to mention the "L" ("G" or "B") word(s) in familial conversation (Laird, 1998). Denial may become an essential feature of the familial script, and although interaction occurs, sexual minorities with partners frequently may be treated as if they are uncoupled. For example, sometimes they are introduced to "single" individuals of the other sex, significant others are referred to as "friends" or "roommates," and lovers are assigned separate bedrooms when they visit a family home. Lesbians and gay men often maintain that such duplicity is the price necessary for the maintenance of family relationships.

3. *The "don't tell your father" scenario.* In these kinds of situations, sexual minorities are out to the more supportive parent or sibling(s) who have determined that the information metaphorically "will kill your father" and thus collude together not to tell the other parent, an uncle, a grandparent, or another relative. This situation resembles the "I know you know" pattern, except that the formation of subsystems around information about the sexual orientation of one member adds another dimension to the family secret.

Some of the stress that lesbian, gay, and bisexual clients report in therapy often has at least some of its etiology in the hidden agendas and interactions described here. L. S. Brown (1989a) contends that this is true even when clients believe that being unknown to family members is not problematic and that conspiracies of silence surrounding nondisclosure are normative for them. She alleges that the acceptance of such an arrangement as the standard is a reflection of internalized homophobia. Previous chapters have discussed the almost universal existence of this phenomenon in bisexual, lesbian, and gay male populations, as well as the pervasive effect of internalized homophobia on all aspects of relationships, including the number of people to whom a minority sexual orientation is disclosed (Baker, 1998; Radonsky & Borders, 1995).

Influences on the Family System

The reactions of family members to a disclosure of homosexuality reveals much about the nature of relationships and patterns of interaction within that system (Laird, 1998;

Strommen, 1989b; Zitter, 1987). For example, some perceive that having a lesbian, bisexual, or gay relative violates existing familial roles. Further, as noted previously, coalitions may form, rigidify, or realign based on the willingness of individual family members to embrace a sexual minority daughter, son, sister, brother, niece, nephew, parent, aunt, uncle, grandparent, or grandchild. Often these reconfigurations result in cutoff between family members (Laird, 1998; LaSala, 2000). Brown (1989a) describes several other scenarios that also may ensue. For example, old divisions or triangulations might reappear, with their focus being that of sexual orientation rather than another theme around which the subsystems previously coalesced. If there has been abuse, incest, chemical abuse, or illegitimacy in the family, old wounds and secrets may be exposed as members attempt to explain the reason for this homosexual "psychopathology" in the system. Blaming, animosity, and familial disruptions may occur.

Zitter (1987) also discussed the tension and disruption in the parental subsystem that may result when a couple finds out that their son is gay or their daughter is lesbian. For example, the parents may become stronger allies, or even allies for the first time, if they join together against their homosexual offspring. If either parent has a stronger bond than the other with the daughter or son, the child may have come out to that parent first—which may create or strengthen a split between parents. The situation is exacerbated if one parent is asked not to tell the other or if one parent accepts the gay or lesbian child with more ease than the other parent does. In cases of single-parent families, and at times when two parents are present in the home, a friend, relative, clergyperson, or even another child can be triangulated into the parental subsystem against the lesbian daughter or gay son.

Scapegoating as described here is not uncommon and can take many forms. For example, a member's lesbianism may become the family "red herring" (Laird, 1998), or if the gay offspring historically has served the family in a scapegoat role (i.e., the "bad" or deviant child), this position often is reinforced further after the disclosure (Zitter, 1987). However, if another sibling occupied that position, the coming out may shift the role to the lesbian, gay, or bisexual member. This situation allows the former scapegoat's relationship with the parent(s) to improve, while at the same time increasing that person's investment (either singularly or in collusion with parents or other family members) in continuing to preserve the outcast status of the homosexual individual.

On the external level, the boundaries of the family system sometimes are tightened as in preparation for an attack, and typical reactions include fusion, pseudomutuality, and shame (L. S. Brown, 1989a). Because they are anxious, fearful, and suspicious about others knowing their family secret, members may withdraw socially from friends and community, as well as from each other. In many ways their reactions of embarrassment and isolation replicate that of their gay, lesbian, and bisexual loved ones in that they, too, feel stereotyped and stigmatized. Likewise, they exhibit similar "traits due to victimization" (see Chapter 1 and Allport, 1954) because they are victims of "the same external and cultural manifestations of homophobia" (L. S. Brown, 1989a, p. 71). Unlike sexual minorities, however, families often lack a supportive community with whom to share their distress.

Helping Clients Disclose to Family of Origin

Clients contemplating disclosing their homosexuality to family members are generally anxious and uncertain, and frequently they experience anticipatory grief in the expectation that others will respond negatively and confirm their worst fears of loss and rejection (Berg-Cross, 1988; L. S. Brown, 1989a; LaSala, 2000). They may need to be reminded that the ways in which their families respond to this news probably will be similar to their responses in other stressful situations. For example, Laird (1998) explains that families who tend to be inflexible about rules for behavior are inclined to be inflexible about many things; those who have difficulty talking about sensitive or controversial issues undoubtedly will have trouble discussing a child's homosexuality; and families who cannot allow their children to grow up or differentiate can use their child's sexual orientation to insist on loyalty to their social, religious, or political views. If clients can come to see the possible reactions of their loved ones in this context, their increased objectivity may assist them in planning more carefully for the upcoming disclosure.

In addition to this information about possible reactions, clients may need to be reminded about the need for patience in giving family members time to adjust to the new situation, or they may be coached to maintain noncombative communication even if contacts initially are brief and superficial (B. E. Bernstein, 1990; Krestan, 1987; LaSala, 2000). Those persons with ineffective communication skills, poor self-esteem, and unresolved anger or grief tend to have a particularly difficult time (Borhek, 1988); therefore, clinicians first may need to address these concerns in order to prepare clients for the experience of revealing their minority sexual orientation. Those lacking in assertiveness, or who have limited verbal skills, may need special help in developing the resources necessary to communicate their thoughts, feelings, and needs clearly.

Some of the problems with disclosure might be lessened if parents could be educated about homosexuality before the revelation. Ben-Ari (1995) conducted in-depth interviews with 32 gay and lesbian young adults and 27 parents and found that, if parents were first introduced to homosexuality before finding out that their child is gay or lesbian, their adjustment to the discovery could be eased and emotional dynamics within the family could be improved. The results of this study also revealed that family dynamics before homosexuality was revealed were related to their experiences after coming out on the parts of both parents and children. Again, clients need be given this understanding so that their disclosure can be as informed and objective as possible.

PARENTS

Parental acceptance is important to most individuals, regardless of sexual orientation. Further, some research has demonstrated that male homosexuals as a group are more approval-dependent than are heterosexual men (Milic & Crowne, 1986; Siegelman, 1974, 1981). The reasons for this dependency are unclear, but the previously discussed perception of parental rejection appears to play a part. Accordingly, studies of 214 gay and 103 lesbian youth (ages 14 to 23) found that, when parental attitudes toward homosexuality were perceived as positive, subjects tended to feel comfortable with their sexual orientations (Savin-Williams, 1989a, 1989c). Subjects who reported satisfying relationships with their mothers tended to have the highest levels of self-esteem. Lesbians were most comfortable with themselves when they reported that their parents accepted their homosexuality. Further, those who described satisfying relationships with relatively young parents were more likely to have disclosed their sexual orientation to them. For the male subjects, those who were out to their mothers, and who had satisfying but infrequent relationships with their fathers, were most likely to report high self-esteem. In addition, acceptance by parents predicted their comfort with being gay if the parents were also seen as important contributors to their self-worth.

A. J. Bernstein (1997) studied the perceived parental attachment of 108 gay men and lesbians and found a consistent relationship between this attachment and emotional well-being. Maternal attachment was positively associated with homosexual identity formation at the higher developmental stages, but paternal attachment was seen to decline at these stages. Surprisingly, parent attachment factors did not vary whether a parent was aware of a child's sexual orientation or not, even though relationships between the two generations deteriorated initially after parental awareness. Most improved over time, however, and eventually returned to pre-awareness levels.

In another study, 20 lesbians in committed cohabiting relationships of at least 2 years' duration completed questionnaires that asked about parental attitudes toward their partners and their lesbianism and the effect of these attitudes on the couple (B. C. Murphy, 1989). Half of the subjects reported that *both* the affirming and rejecting attitudes of parents had "helped" their relationships. Those who felt parental acceptance said that it assisted the couple by encouraging the women to be more self-accepting. Conversely, disapproval of a daughter's lesbianism was found to be hurtful to the degree that the rejection was internalized and affected her ability to be vulnerable and close with a partner. Others reported that the secretiveness, withholding, and deception associated with relating to critical parents spilled over into their lesbian relationships and negatively influenced couple communication and intimacy. Interesting, however, was the finding that, of the 70% who reported parental disapproval of their lesbianism, some said that the parental rejection "helped" in drawing the couple closer together and that the adverse consequences of that dissatisfaction were outshone by the benefits to the couple. B. C. Murphy (1989) notes that this rationalization may reflect the use of a cognitive dissonance reduction technique known as *bolstering*, in which individuals magnify or emphasize favorable features, thus making negative consequences "more acceptable because they have been overshadowed or drowned out by the positive ones" (p. 49).

Parental Reactions to Sexual Minority Offspring

The bulk of the literature on parental perspectives is descriptive in nature and is written by and for parents of gay, lesbian, and bisexual children. It includes such topics as the feelings, experiences, attitudes, and needs of parents who are coping with an offspring's minority sexual orientation; personal reports of the children describing their parents' reactions; advice on how to come out to parents; suggestions for parents after children reveal their homosexuality; and information to and from mental health professionals about working with families in which a member is lesbian, bisexual, or gay (B. E. Bernstein, 1990; Wells-Lurie, 1996). In the following sections, several of these topics are discussed.

Themes of Responses

B. E. Bernstein (1990) conducted in-depth interviews with 62 parents of a gay son or lesbian daughter regarding their feelings, attitudes, behavior, and experiences, as related to their child's minority sexual orientation. Five themes emerged from her interviews. These are outlined briefly here and are expanded on throughout the remainder of this section.

1. *Social stigma.* The major obstacle to accepting their child's homosexuality was the fear of social stigma because of being seen either as inadequate parents or as having a sick and deviant daughter or son. Many parents felt humiliated, ashamed, or embarrassed because of the possible perceptions of others and subsequent judgment by friends, family, and community. Many experienced a reduced level of self-esteem due to their child's homosexuality, and shame often affected their relationships with others inasmuch as they tended to distance themselves from possible criticism or negative opinion.

2. *Self- and/or spouse-blame.* Most parents believed that psychological factors were responsible for a homosexual orientation and either blamed themselves, the other parent, or outside people and influences for their child's perceived difficulty. Possible reasons given for their offspring's homosexuality included negative experiences with the opposite sex; the influence of gay or lesbian companions; "spotting" during pregnancy; allowing the child in bed with the parents; a divorce; or the belief that they were or the other parent was too strict, harsh, critical, alcoholic, unavailable, preoccupied, verbally or physically explosive and abusive, neglectful, too close, or otherwise an insufficient male–female role model.

3. *Parental losses.* The greatest disappointment for many parents was their belief that they would not have grandchildren from their lesbian daughter or gay son. They recalled feeling close to their own parents because of the common experience of parenthood, and regretted not having (or being able to have) this bond with their homosexual offspring. A considerable number were distressed by the loss of a traditional family life for their child and reported that they would miss sharing with a new generation important rituals such as weddings, anniversaries, and births. In this regard, some writers (Beeler, & DiProva, 1999; L. S. Brown, 1989a; LaSala, 2000) believe that parents must first grieve the lost fantasy of a heterosexual child before being able to embrace a real-life lesbian daughter or gay son.

4. *Fears and concerns for their child.* Three major worries seemed to concern parents. For those with gay sons, AIDS and the related illness and death was their greatest apprehension. Further, nearly all parents believed that a daughter or son would not have the experiences essential for happiness, such as marriage and family, since they feared that she or he would be lonely throughout life without these opportunities. A final worry concerned discrimination and rejection by society. Anxieties in this regard included possible harassment at work, career obstacles and limitations, prejudice in the legal and social arenas, being the subject of jokes and ridicule, isolation from the mainstream, and the possibility of being victimized by violence.

5. *Fear of losing their son or daughter.* Many parents were apprehensive about showing any negative feelings about their daughter's or son's homosexuality for fear of alienating her or him. They felt isolated from their offspring, as if a "barrier had come up between them and their gay [or lesbian] child" (B. E. Bernstein, 1990, p. 43). Since they lacked adequate information for talking about the sexual minority subculture, they avoided questions or discussions about most aspects of their child's life for fear of having their interest taken as criticism or intrusion.

Living with a Lesbian or Gay Child

While Bernstein (1990) was concerned with the feelings, attitudes, experiences, and behaviors related to having a homosexual child, Muller (1987) was interested in examining the ways in which parents lived with their daughter's or son's same-sex orientation. Accordingly, she interviewed 61 lesbians and gay men, along with 10 parents, who together told the stories of 111 relationships between a parent and an adult lesbian or gay child. Slightly over half of these relationships (52%) were parent–daughter, 48% were parent–son, and 17% of those interviewed were Black. From these interviews, four different types of relationships were identified: two that Muller viewed as positive (Loving Open and Loving Denial) and two that she considered negative (Resentful Denial and Hostile Recognition). Table 14.1 shows these styles of relationship and the percentage of daughters and sons in each.

1. *Loving Open.* In these situations, the parents exhibited little denial about the sexual orientation of their sons and daughters and were fairly open and positive about it with family, friends, and others. Interactions between them and their offspring and his or her friends and lover were favorable. All the relationships were described as having been loving before the disclosures. This description characterized 5% of parent–daughter and 17% of parent–son relationships.

2. *Loving Denial.* Parents generally remained closeted with information about the sexual orientation of their daughter or son, but positive contact was maintained between parents and offspring and often included a lover. Parental acceptance was conditional, however, in that overt recognition of homosexuality rarely was tolerated. Gay and lesbian children contributed to the denial by monitoring words and actions when in the presence of their parents, but most were satisfied with their level of acceptance. This category included 42% of parent–daughter and 55% of parent–son relationships.

3. *Resentful Denial.* The parents remained closeted and limited contact with their children based on a negative view of a daughter or son's sexual orientation. Of the few who acknowledged their child's homosexuality, they did so infrequently and in a disapproving manner. This classification accounted for 48% of parent–daughter and 23% of parent–son relationships.

4. *Hostile Recognition.* All relationships in this group were estranged, and parental animosity focused on the sexual orientation of the offspring. In all situations described by Muller, connections were poor before the disclosures and alcoholism, neglect, or abuse (or a combination) were a part of the family background. Parent–daughter and parent–son relationships each constituted 5% of this group.

TABLE 14.1. Postdisclosure Parent–Child Relationship Types

	Percent responding in each category	
	Parent–daughter ($n = 58$)	Parent–son ($n = 53$)
Positive relationships		
Loving Open	5	17
Loving Denial	42	55
Negative relationships		
Resentful Denial	48	23
Hostile Recognition	5	5

Note. Summarized from Muller (1987).

As can be seen from the percentages listed in Table 14.1, Muller (1987) found that parents and gay sons had more positive relationships (72%) than did parents and lesbian daughters (46%). Conversely, she considered 28% of parent–son interactions as negative, compared with 54% for parents and their lesbian offspring (due to rounding off, the sums of percentages differ by 1% for lesbians and their parents). Of all the variables examined, *mutual appreciation* was much less the experience of daughters compared with sons and their parents. In fact, results indicated that "relationships [characterized by mutual appreciation] between parents and sons outnumbered those between parents and daughters three to one" (p. 61). In other words, the manner in which parents of homosexual children interacted with their offspring was more related to the biological sex of the child than to other influences.

Muller's (1987) finding that gay sons generally fare better in relation to their parents than lesbian daughters appears to be related to the concept of gender role socialization, which has been discussed frequently throughout this book. In this regard, she contends that "sex roles, probably more than anything else, are the unrecognized, stubborn dandelion root of conflict between lesbians, gay men, and their parents" (p. 89). Lesbian and gay offspring pose a threat to traditional gender roles, and hence to sexist and heterosexist constructs that determine appropriate ways of parenting and relating to children based on biological sex. Given that gender socialization has contributed to a somewhat different constellation of dynamics for the two sexes, the following discussion is divided into separate sections, one dealing with parental relationships with sons and another with daughters.

Relationships with Gay Sons

In one study in which gender role socialization and heterosexism appear to be factors (Cramer & Roach, 1988), 93 gay men were surveyed, most of whom reported that their parents initially reacted negatively to the disclosure of homosexuality but became more accepting over time. The majority of subjects described having more positive relations with their mothers than with their fathers, both before and after coming out. The change in parent–son relationships after the disclosure was related to parental values, as well as to the characteristics associated with heterosexism and homophobia (see Chapter 1). This phenomenon undoubtedly can be attributed to Herek's findings (also Chapter 1), which suggest that attitudes of heterosexual males toward homosexuality often are more negative than are those of heterosexual women (1988) because gender nonconformity in men tends to threaten male core gender identity (1986a).

Similar to the Cramer and Roach (1988) study, Muller (1987) found that sons had more positive relationships with their mothers (76%) than with their fathers (65%). She also noted that the alliances with fathers had not always been characterized so favorably (see Table 14.2). In fact, 47% of the sons described these relationships as negative when they were growing up, compared with 35% when the study was conducted. Those boys who had deviated from their father's expectations regarding sex roles had particularly antagonistic childhood paternal relationships: "The intensity of the father–son conflict varied in accordance with both the extent of the father's insistence on sex-role conformity and the extent of the son's nonconformity" (p. 93).

In any case, whether the conflict was overt or whether fathers acted in line with masculine gender role conditioning and withdrew, leaving the childrearing to their wives,

TABLE 14.2. Parent–Gay Son Relationships

	Percent responding in each category	
	As sons were growing up	Now
Fathers		
Positive	53	65
Negative	47	35
Mothers		
Positive	73	76
Negative	27	24

Note. Summarized from Muller (1987).

mothers often stepped in to rescue gay sons from rejection. As primary caretakers of the children and communicators between them and their fathers, maternal instincts prompted mothers to protect the young boys because, like themselves, the male children were "being penalized for differentiating from the male idealization" (Muller, 1987, p. 95). After the sons disclosed their sexual orientation, however, Muller found that a common pattern occurred in those families whose relationships she described as positive. Mother–son alliances were likely to continue, but father–son conflicts lessened (see Table 14.2). It was as if many fathers had resigned themselves to having gay offspring; they may not have known how to relate to sons any better than before, but the disclosure provided consistency to their relationships inasmuch as fathers generally ceased trying to change them. If sons were over 22 years old when they came out and if 5 or more years had passed since the disclosure, fathers tended to have more confidence that they were truly gay (and not just going through a phase). More important, however, fathers were able to take pride in their children's adult accomplishments. Unfortunately, this favorable turn of events did not occur for many of Muller's interviewees; she described 35% of current father–son relationships as negative, compared with 24% for mothers and gay sons.

On a more positive note, Gottlieb (2000) interviewed the fathers of 12 gay sons and describes how each became more comfortable with their sons' homosexuality. Gottlieb drew from literary sources and psychoanalytic theory to highlight the obstacles that such fathers must overcome to understand and identify with a gay son. Each father struggled in some way to respect and appreciate his child, and these conflicts often revolved around such issues as values, biases, concepts of masculinity, and closeness between men. Similarly, a psychologist and the mother of two gay sons, Baker (1998) describes how unprepared she was emotionally for the homosexuality of both her children, in spite of being professionally knowledgeable about homosexuality. In her narrative, Baker discusses how she and her family learned to accept one another and overcome their fears and prejudices. Her book, unfortunately, ends with the death of one of the sons to AIDS, but her efforts to understand herself and her children are illuminating, nonetheless.

Relationships with Lesbian Daughters

Often lesbians who felt same-sex inclinations as a child realized, on some level, that their feelings were not mirrored back by parents or by society. Sometimes they were given messages that what they were feeling was bad, wrong, or inappropriate, and during the daughters' adolescence relationships with both parents were quite conflicted (Kleinberg & Zorn, 1995; A. E. Schwartz, 1998). As discussed earlier in this chapter (Bryant & Demian, 1995; Muller, 1987), lesbians have reported more overall negative relationships with their parents than have gay sons, and in Muller's (1987) study, these percentages were 54% and 28%, respectively. Further, Table 14.3 indicates that the maternal alliances perceived by lesbians both when they were growing up (52%) and at the time of the study (50%) were more negative than those of gay sons and their mothers (27% and 24%, past and present, respectively; see Table 14.2). Current father–daughter relationships were described as negative in 58% of the cases (compared with 35% for gay sons) and were the most negative group of all parent–child alliances. Only in childhood did lesbian daughters fare better than gay sons, with 65% reporting positive relationships with their fathers, compared with 53% positive for boys. The relationships between mothers and both lesbian daughters and gay sons, therefore, tended to remain somewhat consistent over time, and those between gay sons and their fathers generally improved (as discussed), but those between lesbians and their fathers became much more negative (see Table 14.3).

FATHERS

This decrease in appreciation and approval after daughters disclosed their lesbianism is thought be related to the fathers' notions of appropriate sex roles and views of women as objects of sexual desire (Muller, 1987; A. E. Schwartz, 1998). As was discussed in Chapter 3, most lesbians report that parents supported their tomboy nature in childhood but insisted on feminine behaviors and attitudes when they reached adolescence (Pearlman, 1995; A. E. Schwartz, 1998). Accordingly, 65% of the women in Muller's (1987) study reported that "paternalism" characterized their early father–daughter relationships. In this regard, fathers often protected and rescued their daughters from the displeasure of their mothers, a dynamic not unlike that described above in reference to the mothers of gay sons and the alliances they formed with their offsprings against critical fathers.

The love–hate relationship between many lesbians and their mothers was discussed in Chapter 3 (Eisenbud, 1986; Pearlman, 1995) and has been referred to as a "tug-of-love" (Muller, 1987, p. 105) wherein mothers attempt to socialize their daughters into their concept of the feminine gender role. Eisenbud and Pearlman note the frequency with

TABLE 14.3. Parent–Lesbian Daughter Relationships

	Percent responding in each category	
	As daughters were growing up	Now
Fathers		
Positive	65	42
Negative	35	58
Mothers		
Positive	48	50
Negative	52	50

Note. Summarized from Muller (1987).

which lesbians as children look to their fathers for an ally in the mother–daughter strug-gle. In Muller's research, 65% of the men were able to respond favorably to their gender-nonconforming daughters when they were young, whereas only 42% could do so when the offspring were adults (see Table 14.3). Apparently, a large number found the similar-ity between themselves and their young daughters in play, dress, and socialization (Whitam & Mathy, 1991) as characteristics with which they could identify. After the chil-dren reached adolescence or adulthood and declared their lesbianism, however, the heterosexism and gender role socialization typical for non-gay males (Herek, 1986a; Kurdek, 1988a) took over and fathers withdrew their appreciation and approval. Many, in fact, simply withdrew from their daughters; 91% of those who stayed connected had at least one other daughter who was heterosexual (Muller, 1987). A. E. Schwartz (1998) found that "for young girls whose relationships with father in reality or fantasy have been based on collusion, the fall from grace is devastating" (p. 37).

MOTHERS

Regarding relationships between lesbians and their mothers, Muller (1987) found that maternal nonacceptance remained fairly constant throughout the lifespan of the daugh-ters, with 52% reporting negative relationships when they were growing up and 51% de-scribing them as negative at the present time (see Table 14.3). Others also have noted that mother–daughter relationships appear to be especially strained for many lesbians (Rosen, 1992; A. E. Schwartz, 1998; Zitter, 1987). According to the tenet of both sexism and heterosexism, the role of mothers in this culture is to "pass the baton of the traditional woman's role to their daughters" (Rosen, 1992, p. 5). A mother, therefore, tends to have difficulty being receptive to a gender-role discordant daughter when that image is neither culturally permissible nor congruent with the social values of the larger system, female role expectancies, or her own sense of personal order. Due to the power of this precept, a mother unavoidably misses cues regarding the sexuality of a lesbian daughter and is selec-tively inattentive and minimally attuned to her emotional manifestations. She is, hence, "unable to serve as an empathic resource for her daughter in this aspect of her growth" (Rosen, 1992, p. 6). Lesbian daughters also may fail their mothers empathically because, by defying the cultural prescription for women and not identifying with the mother as fe-male, they are not providing a comfortable "fit" with societal-dictated maternal require-ments for sameness (Rosen, 1992; A. E. Schwartz, 1998). Consequently, the sexist and heterosexist underpinning of the culture "violates the relationship between the lesbian and her mother, and, in most cases, ensures the lack of mutual empathy between them" (Rosen, 1992, p. 6). A form of "relational compromise" usually occurs, but not without significant mutual loss and grief for both women.

Zitter (1987) speculates that another part of the reason maternal reaction to a daughter's lesbianism frequently is negative resides in the cultural myth that, while a mother expects to lose a son to another woman, a daughter is hers "for the rest of her life" (p. 179). For lesbians, however, their mothers aren't the only women to whom they feel attached and closely connected, and this often results in their mothers feeling re-placed, rejected, or even jealous and resentful. For some, it is as if a daughter's attraction to other women is a repudiation of her values, her "failure to teach the role of woman-hood" (p. 185), and, most importantly, of *her*. However, if the lesbian daughter is also a mother, her relationship with her parents often improves or becomes closer (Clunis &

Green, 1995; Gartrell et al., 1999; Lewin, 1993; Martin, 1993). Having had a child of her own, for these individuals, makes the lesbian daughter more like the mother, so, in a sense, the mother's role in her daughter's life is validated. Further, the lesbian daughter's identification and sense of commonality with her own mother is increased.

ANOTHER VIEW OF PARENTAL RELATIONSHIPS

Laird (1998) offers another perspective on the relationship of lesbians with their parents. She contends that most lesbians are not cut off from their parents—"not forever rejected, isolated, disinherited" (p. 198). She further notes that the nature of these connections is virtually unexplored in the professional literature; when the relationships are described, they usually are viewed as "tortured." Accordingly, she conducted interviews with 19 Caucasian lesbians from various socioeconomic backgrounds. The participants ranged in age from 26 to 68, and their stories reflected different eras and changed social contexts for lesbianism. The women were not cut off from their families entirely, but each subject "remains very much in complex connection with her family of origin" (p. 210). There had been periods of conflict and distancing, especially during the coming-out process, for some, as well as brief periods of alienation and emotional separation. The issues around which these struggles revolved, however, were "powerful enough, over the long haul, to supersede the importance of family connection" (p. 211). Like the lesbian mothers in Lewin's (1993) study, neither the daughters nor the parents could endure permanent ruptures since family ties were so profound.

Many of the women whom Laird (1998) interviewed wished for a qualitatively different relationship with their parents, one in which "they could do more than often reluctantly accept the inevitable" (p. 220). They frequently wanted their families to more openly admire and affirm them, but most forgave family members "for their failures to stand up against social homophobia because they know how hard it was for them" (p. 220). Laird emphasized the importance of clinicians listening as objectively as possible to each lesbian client as she describes the nature of her relationship with her parents. On the one hand, clinicians can assume that the alliance will consist of many of the negative elements described here and fail to appreciate the strength of the bond between parent and child. On the other hand, however, therapists must be attuned to the complexity inherent in most of these relationships.

Coming Out for Parents

Integrating the reality of a homosexually oriented family member involves a series of events much like the identity formation process for sexual minorities (see Chapters 5 and 9) in that relatives must also form new identities as the parents, grandparents, siblings, aunts, uncles, and cousins of lesbian, gay, and bisexual individuals. A long and stressful sequence of events is usually involved for parents, many of which have been discussed throughout this chapter. Four general stages have been outlined by three parents of gay sons (Griffin, Wirth, & Wirth, 1986) after they conducted in-depth interviews with 23 other parents of lesbians and gay men. The interviewees were midwestern, White, middle-class adults (ages 40 to 70) from varying religious, educational, and vocational backgrounds. Further, they all were long-term members of PFLAG (Parents, Families and Friends of Lesbians and Gays; see the Resources section), had worked together in the self-help group for some time, and had been through all four stages themselves. Table 14.4 summarizes some of the common processes they described.

In addition to shock, disappointment, blame, loss, and fear (B. E. Bernstein, 1990; LaSala, 2000; Wells-Lurie, 1996), the initial reactions of the parents interviewed by Griffin et al. (1986) to the disclosure of their children's homosexuality included grief, anger, sadness, guilt, failure, and shame. The parents responded to the news in several ways, all of which generally parallel the responses of lesbians, bisexuals, and gay men as they navigate through the process of forming their sexual minority identity. Some parents physically or emotionally separated themselves from friends and family, while others attempted to change or reorient their child to heterosexuality. A large number used verbal persuasion for this purpose, and some enlisted the help of others, such as clergy and psychotherapists. Denial was a common theme, and acknowledgment was the initial response of only a few.

Wells-Lurie (1996), the mother of a gay son and a lesbian daughter, surveyed a number of parents with sexual minority children and noted the disengagement of these individuals from others. The interviewees spoke of being treated differently when others learned of the sexual orientation of their daughter or son, of divided family loyalties, of generational differences in their families, and of innuendoes from coworkers about gays or lesbians: "Be it with friends, coworkers, or even within families, it is not uncommon for parents of gay children to report that people never even mention the gay child to

---

TABLE 14.4. Stages of Coming Out for Parents of Gay and Lesbian Children

Finding out

- Emotional reactions
- Cutoff
- Conversion strategies
- Denial
- Acknowledgment

Communicating with others

- Telling friends
- Getting help from gay or lesbian children
- Listening to other gay men and lesbians
- Learning from counselors
- Receiving support from other parents

Changing inner perceptions

- Opening up to feelings
- Moving toward acceptance
- Taking the step beyond

Taking a stand and telling others

- Confronting homophobia
- "Coming out" as parents
- Speaking up and out in public
- Educating critics
- Allying with other parents

Note. Summarized from Griffin, Wirth, & Wirth (1986) and Muller (1987).

them. This leaves the parent feeling as if the child has died so far as others are concerned" (p. 163).

Parents who eventually are able to accept the minority sexual orientation of their offspring at some point begin to share the information with others and, in the course of these disclosures, receive affirmation and support for themselves. Most of the 23 PFLAG parents in the Griffin et al. (1986) survey described feeling acceptance from numerous sources, including friends, their children and other lesbians and gay men, therapists, and fellow parents. As a result of their efforts to learn and understand, their inner perspectives began to change, and they started moving toward acceptance of their children and of themselves as parents. Having been forced to confront their inner prejudice, as well as the heterosexism of society, they reported a shift in the focus of their thinking from themselves to their offspring. Many described feeling a deeper appreciation for their gay and lesbian children, an increased pride in them, and a commitment to do something about the problem of oppression.

All of the 23 parents described here collaborated with other parents and joined a chapter of PFLAG. Through this group effort, they were able to offer the same support and affirmation for others as had been given to them. Further, the organization gave them a forum through which they could provide advocacy and education of behalf of sexual minorities. K. R. Allen (1999) discusses the concept of _resiliency_ in relation to parents such as these. In her interviews with older parents of gay and lesbian children, she describes their efforts to keep their families together in the face of a nonnormative lifecourse transition. For her subjects, love for their children prompted them to behave in ways they never would have thought possible before the disclosure of their child's homosexuality.

Tasks of the Therapist

The stages delineated by Griffin et al. (1986) appear roughly parallel to the phases of sexual minority identity formation (Chapter 9) because parents, like their gay, lesbian, and bisexual children, also participate in a cycle of attachment, separation, loss, and reattachment (Garanzini, 1989; O'Neill & Ritter, 1992; J. M. Schneider, 1984, 1994) and are challenged with the formation of new identities. Hence, much of the material discussed previously concerning therapeutic interventions to facilitate identity formation relative to assisting clients in grieving a heterosexual life image (Chapters 9 and 13), is applicable to the current topic. Because Table 14.5 summarizes some of this information, previous discussions are not elucidated in any detail.

Helping to Move through Loss

Helping family members ventilate their rage and grief while confronting the homophobic stereotypes that are at the root of their anguish is a difficult task. During this catharsis, therapists must be supportive and yet careful not to collude with the family's hopes that sexual orientation is changeable; members need to be discouraged from falsely anticipating that their loved one can achieve a shift to heterosexuality. In this regard, information can help counter inaccurate beliefs about the nature of homosexuality and the family's reactions to it (see the Resources section). Sex-role stereotypes, as well as religious beliefs and issues, also may need to be addressed. Throughout the entire process, individuals might require reassurance, hope, new narratives, and a vision of a positive outcome, both

TABLE 14.5. Stage-Specific Psychotherapeutic Interventions for Parents

Finding out

- Reflect emotional reactions
- Increase range of affective responses
- Avoid collusion with bargaining
- Gently challenge denial

Communicating with others

- Bibliotherapy; education about homosexuality
- Superego modification
- Role play and rehearsal for telling others
- Encourage parents to overcome fear

Changing inner perceptions

- Facilitate grieving the loss of a heterosexual child
- Help parents recognize heterosexism in society and its effects on their children
- Assist mourning of personal losses

Taking a stand and telling others

- Facilitate selective and progressive disclosure
- Role play and rehearsal for handling situations
- Help parents move beyond fear
- Refer parents to PFLAG

Note. Summarized from B. E. Bernstein (1990) and Hanley-Hackenbruck (1989).

for themselves and for their gay, lesbian, or bisexual family members (Beeler & DiProva, 1999; B. E. Bernstein, 1990; Borhek, 1988; L. S. Brown, 1989a; Holtzen & Agresti, 1990; Laird, 1998; Myers, 1982).

Energy is freed for more productive use when parents engage in the public step of communicating with others (J. M. Schneider, 1984, 1994). Clients may need supportive challenging at this point as fear usually prevents productive action. Role playing and rehearsal of disclosures of their child's homosexuality are often helpful, as is the modification of rigid superego introjects (Hanley-Hackenbruck, 1989); in the case of parents, these usually are related to shame, guilt, and stigma. Once parents have begun to disclose and communicate their secrets and accompanying emotions, they are able to shift their perception and reformulate their loss (O'Neill & Ritter, 1992; J. M. Schneider, 1984, 1994).

As with any developmental model, not all individuals will progress to the higher stages. In the case of the 23 parents who were interviewed by Griffin et al. (1986), all were able to transform their losses such that they were able to join PFLAG, educate and support others, and take public stands on behalf of their children. While these kinds of activities might be the desirable outcome for many parent clients, others will need ongoing support and assistance in managing their perceived stigma, disclosing to a few select individuals, or dealing with the conflict that has arisen in their families due to the homosexuality of a member. Some parents, especially those who hold traditional values related to religion, marriage, and children, tend to have a particularly difficult time adjusting to having a gay, lesbian, or bisexual offspring (Beeler & DiProva, 1999; Berg-Cross, 1988; M. J. Kahn, 1991; Kahn & McNutt, 1991; Laird, 1998; Newman & Muzzonigro, 1993) and may require referrals to other sources, such as affirming clergy (see Chapter 13 and the Resources section). Further, marital or family therapy might be the treatment of choice if the family structure is exceptionally rigid or fused, or if severe conflict or dysfunction has arisen since the minority sexual orientation of a member became known. Finally, parents and other family members in all stages of identity formation can be referred to PFLAG for education, support, and mirroring (see the Resources section).

Facilitating Adaptation to a Disclosure

Families can be helped in other ways to integrate a lesbian, bisexual, or gay member into the family. Beeler and DiProva (1999), for example, identified 12 themes that were observed in individual interviews with 16 members of 4 families as they came to terms with having a sexual minority son, daughter, sister, brother, or other relative. The unstructured interviews were broad in scope and included conversations about such topics as family history, characteristic patterns of interacting, perception of other members, and reactions to the disclosure. The investigators detected 12 themes that recurred, not in any sequence, interwoven with the context of events in the lives of the interviewees. These themes also might be conceptualized as therapeutic tasks that clinicians could use as guidelines for intervention with family members and are described here for that purpose. Elaboration is given only in cases where the concept or dynamics have not been discussed elsewhere in this chapter.

• *Establishing rules for discussing homosexuality.* Prerogatives and limits should be negotiated for gay-related topics once an individual has disclosed. Unless some rules are established, the boundaries around the topic of homosexuality can become either extremely rigid or quite permeable to the point where conversations about the subject are continuous or intrusive.

• *Seeking information about homosexuality and the gay community from gay-positive sources.*

• *Second-guessing the sexuality of others: The "who else?" syndrome.* These kinds of speculations can be productive in that observations previously overlooked or attributed to different causes, now might be related to homosexuality. This potential in others makes the concept "seem more palpable and less a flight of fancy" (p. 449).

• *Exposure to gays and lesbians living "gay and lesbian lives."* Family members can become more comfortable with a homosexual relative as they become more familiar with the lives of lesbian and gay individuals.

• *Making homosexuality less exotic.* The family can be helped to integrate a member's homosexuality into its day-to-day interactions. As the values and wishes of all members are incorporated into the daily life of the family, the gay or lesbian member is perceived as more "normal" to others in the network.

• *Including gay and lesbian friends in the family.* Parents and siblings should be encouraged to meet a homosexual member's friends and include them in the family activities, rather than simply hearing them described—or not mentioned at all.

• *Dealing with the heterosexual world's institutions and conventions.* "Even the most accepting and accommodating family is going to have to figure out the details of how best to be supportive" (p. 450), since there are endless practical decisions to be made after disclosure.

• *Working through feelings of sadness, loss, and blame.*

- *Managing the family coming out.* Deciding whom, when, and how to tell is an important process that occurs over a lengthy period of time.
- *Developing alternative visions of the future.* Despite the fact that new family options are available to sexual minority individuals and couples (see Chapter 17), parents and other relatives will need to refashion their vision of what constitutes a family and how that family fits into the larger extrafamilial heterosexual world.
- *Managing stigma.* The issue of specifically how to respond to homophobic comments arises continually for family members of bisexuals, lesbians, and gay men: "The task of stigma management is exacerbated if the person making the offending remark is a family member" (p. 452).
- *Developing narrative coherency.* Therapists can assist families to construct a coherent "story" surrounding sexual minority members and to give new meaning to past events and future transpirings. By developing chronicle consistency, families can build bridges between the tale of disclosure and other life stories and experiences. In other words, they need to integrate the homosexual story into their lives (Laird, 1998).

By means of education and support, clinicians can enable families to view the identity of the lesbian, bisexual, or gay member more positively and to create a place for this person within the family system (Baker, 1998; Beeler & DiProva, 1999; Gottlieb, 2000; Hammersmith, 1987; Laird, 1998; Strommen, 1989a). This task will be more or less difficult depending on the nature of the familial structure and the dimensions of the correlates of heterosexism present (Herek, 1984). As discussed in Chapter 1 and in this chapter, these variables would include such factors as traditional attitudes toward gender roles, peers with negative attitudes toward homosexuality, little contact with sexual minorities, rural location of residence, and religious conservatism. In any case, if the sexual minority identity of a member is not in some way overtly integrated into a family's definition of itself, the system will remain dysfunctional and fragmented.

CONCLUSION

This first chapter in Part IV addressed the families of origin of sexual minority individuals and the difficulties many of these families have in accepting the homosexuality or bisexuality of members. Various family patterns and parental reactions were discussed, specifically ways in which families respond to a family member's disclosure of homosexuality both in regard to their internal dynamics, as well as ways of managing the information outside the family. Gender-specific responses of both parents and their bisexual, gay, or lesbian offspring also were described. The chapter included numerous suggestions for therapists to help them facilitate the adaptation process for family members, as well as provide a context for affirmative psychotherapy with these individuals.

15

Understanding Same-Sex Couples

Because same-sex partners are units within extended kinship networks (Laird & Green, 1996), this chapter examines various factors relative to these relationships, including societal influences, socialization factors, unique dynamics, relationship stages, and therapeutic considerations. As is true throughout this book, much of the literature on same-sex couple relationships is based on the clinical experience of therapists rather than on empirical data. Cabaj and Klinger (1996), in fact, note that "at this point, no formal treatment outcomes studies on psychotherapy with gay and lesbian couples have been completed" (p. 498).

Homosexual and heterosexual couples, nevertheless, are thought to share many commonalties since all partners bring to these relationships numerous developmental variables, behavioral repertoires, and family-of-origin issues (Bepko & Johnson, 2000; Mackey, O'Brien, & Mackey, 1997; Peplau, Veniegas, & Campbell, 1996). Otherwise, the fundamental differences between same-sex couples and their heterosexual counterparts are associated primarily with the social context of their lives, given the unique influences of both heterosexism and gender role socialization on their relationship dynamics. The effects of these two critical elements are described in the following sections.

HETEROSEXISM

Chapter 5 addressed the impact of heterosexism on sexual minority identity development. Whether lesbians and gay men form their identities before to their first relationships or within the context of their primary partnerships, societal prejudice affects their ability to establish and maintain same-sex intimacy. The extent to which this bias oppresses gay and lesbian couples depends on (1) the degree to which such relationships experience a lack of family, legal, religious, economic, financial, and social support; and (2) the magnitude of societal homophobia that is internalized by each of the partners. These two correlates of heterosexist oppression are described under separate subheadings herein. After the discussions, we review studies that demonstrate the viability of satisfying same-sex relationships that bridge partner differences in age, ethnicity, income, and residence in spite of pervasive sexual prejudice (Herek, 1998b).

Lack of Support

Heterosexual couples benefit from numerous social and institutional supports that are not available to same-sex pairs (Bepko & Johnson, 2000; Peplau et al., 1996). The effects of heterosexist influence on gay and lesbian couples vary in intensity according to the perceived lack of sustenance and encouragement that are provided for these relationships. The following discussion addresses several critical areas where support may be lacking.

Family and Friends

Families internalize the same heterosexist assumptions and sexual prejudice that encumber their gay, lesbian, and bisexual members, and, as a result, the kinship networks that commonly sustain heterosexual relationships are lacking for many homosexual partnerships (Bryant & Demian, 1995; Cabaj & Klinger, 1996; J. Meyer, 1989). In fact, heterosexually married couples have been reported to perceive more emotional support from family members than same-sex pairs experience (Kurdek & Schmitt, 1986b, 1987a, 1987b). This lack of family sustenance can cause considerable tension in gay and lesbian relationships, some specifics of which will be discussed in this and the following chapter. However, same-sex couples often are sustained by the support and gratification they receive from their friends, in spite of the sometimes negative familial attitudes toward their relationships. Kurdek and Schmitt (1986b, 1987a, 1987b), for example, studied 106 homosexual dyads (50 gay and 56 lesbian) and found that those who reported high degrees of emotional support from friends were less psychologically distressed than were those who did not.

Social support from both friends and families (and even coworkers) was found to be related to psychological adjustment for 69 gay and 50 lesbian pairs (Kurdek, 1988b). In this study, however, *differences* between partner satisfaction with social support were related to low relationship quality, especially for lesbians. Another survey of 156 cohabitating gay male couples (R. B. Smith & Brown, 1997) indicated that advocacy for their partnerships from family members and friends was positively related to the quality of the dyadic relationship. The authors carefully note that social support for the couple is more predictive of relationship quality than is support for an individual member of the pair. Berger (1990b) found an additional link to social support when he studied the impact of passing as heterosexual on relationship quality in 143 lesbians and gay men (ages 21 to 68). Those whose sexual orientation was known by significant others (i.e., parents, siblings, best friends, and employers) were found to be more satisfied with their intimate relationship. Whether from friends or from family, then, emotional support seems important for relationship satisfaction.

Legal and Religious

Homosexual pairs often are not taken as seriously as heterosexual couples because of the absence of legal and religious recognition, as well as a lack of public acknowledgment of their relationships (Cabaj & Klinger, 1996; Cabaj & Purcell, 1998; Peplau et al., 1996). Increasing numbers of lesbian and gay couples hold commitment ceremonies, and several excellent planning guides currently are available (Ayers & Brown, 1999; Cherry & Sherwood, 1995; Haldeman, 1998; S. E. James & Murphy, 1998; "Questions for Couples," 1989). These events are open and joyous events in many cases, with the extended family and broader community invited to celebrate the couplehood. Often, however, rites are held in private with only small groups of close lesbian and gay friends present. Although intimate, these isolated rituals sometimes serve to reinforce the notion that same-sex unions are less meaningful than the openly celebrated mergers of their heterosexual counterparts.

Data from a survey of 1,749 individuals representing 706 lesbian and 560 gay male couples (n = 1,266 pairs) revealed that a minority of the pairs (19% of the lesbian couples and 11% of the male couples) surveyed had held relationship ceremonies (Bryant & Demian, 1995). Others indicated they had ritualized their relationship in some other way (12% of the women and 9% of the men), and 57% of the female couples and 38% of the male couples wore a ring or some other symbol of commitment. Even though only a few of the 92 male couples studied by Berger (1990a) held a commitment ceremony, many others reported wanting a service if one were possible. Similarly, 23% of the 78 lesbians and gay men surveyed by Engel and Saracino (1986) believed that "it is important for a love relationship to be formally acknowledged in a religious and/or legal ceremony" (p. 249). With few exceptions, however, organized religions refuse to endorse unions between lesbian and gay couples, whether or not they are formalized with commitment ceremonies, and almost all governmental entities worldwide refuse to recognize the legality of homosexual partnerships. Oppressive heterosexism, in these ways, restricts the needs of sexual minority pairs for legitimacy, validation, and public affirmation.

Economic, Financial, and Social

As already implied, same-sex couples frequently hide their relationships for many reasons, including the avoidance of stigma and the maintenance of employment. Although 41% of 400 coupled gay and lesbian *OUT/LOOK* readers ("Questions for Couples," 1989) reported that they wear rings or other symbols of commitment, thousands of others are far less open about displaying any sign or expression of their relationship, such as a partner's picture at their workstation or a kiss good-bye at the bus stop. Some even avoid living together in order to maintain secrecy about being lesbian or gay (Harry, 1983; S. E. James & Murphy, 1998). Homosexual pairs, compared with heterosexual couples, also experience financial disadvantages and unequal opportunities, such as the limitation to spouses who are legally married, the issuance of health and life insurance benefits, credit applications, and discounted "family" memberships in credit unions and health clubs (Bryant & Demian, 1995; Spielman & Winfeld, 1996). Findings in two studies even noted differential treatment between homosexual and heterosexual couples in terms of the attitudes and responsiveness of salespersons in retail stores (Walters & Curran, 1996) and in hotel reservation policies (D. A. Jones, 1996). Heterosexism, in these varied ways, thus deprives same-sex couples of the family and social support, legal and religious recognition, economic and financial privileges, and social courtesies that are extended to heterosexual pairs (S. E. James & Murphy, 1998; I. H. Meyer & Dean, 1998; M. S. Schneider, 1986).

Internalized Homophobia

To the degree that lesbians and gay men adopt popular heterosexist attitudes and beliefs, homophobia and shame become embedded intrapsychically in the formation of a positive sexual identity (Canarelli, Cole, & Rizzuto, 1999; Forstein, 1986; Linde, 1998; I. H. Meyer & Dean, 1998). Shidlo (1994a), in fact, contended that this internalization is so widespread that many writers view it "as a normative developmental event, whereby almost all gay men and lesbians adopt negative attitudes toward homosexuality early in their developmental history" (p. 178). Malyon (1982) believed that this "internalized homophobic content becomes an aspect of the ego, functioning as both an unconscious introject, and as a conscious system of attitudes and accompanying affects" (p. 60). He explained further that, because sexual minority adolescents are forced by societal expectations to develop a false heterosexual identity, "the maturation of erotic and intimate capacities is confounded by a socialized predisposition which makes them ego alien and militates against their integration" (p. 60). When lesbians and gay men enter into intimate relationships, they often do so with fragmented egos that are laden with anxiety-binding psychological defenses. The interactions between these two unformed individual identities "may be mostly pathological, attempting to bind more primitive anxieties of separation, abandonment, and social alienation" (Forstein, 1986, pp. 114–115).

Bonding is especially difficult for male couples, given the effects of masculine gender role socialization in combination with the powerful, negative intrapsychic forces of homophobia (Bepko & Johnson, 2000). In fact, "the more conflicted a gay man is about his homosexuality, the more rigid and stereotyped his gender role identity is likely to be" (Forstein, 1986, p. 113). This excessive masculine socialization, along with the effects of internalized heterosexism on personality and identity formation, often has detrimental consequences for intimate relationships. McWhirter and Mattison (1982) contend that these "anti-homosexual attitudes" (p. 87) are present overtly or covertly in every gay male couple with whom they work and must be addressed by as many adjuncts to therapy as possible (i.e., books, articles, videotapes, lectures, and support groups). They also suggest that if affirmative identity formation has been compromised severely for one or both partners, individual therapy may be warranted, either prior to or concurrent with couples work, particularly when dealing with the stage-related issues of separation and individuation.

Stigmatizing homophobia also affects every lesbian relationship (Kleinberg & Zorn, 1995) and must be addressed openly by clinicians if relationship or sex therapy is to be something more than "an attempt to start a fire with wet kindling" (Hall, 1987, p. 140). L. S. Brown (1986) notes that "internalized oppression" has both direct and indirect effects on sexual functioning and satisfaction (p. 100). She also believes that, for lesbians, internalized oppression involves both misogyny and homophobia. In other words, the widespread devaluation of women that permeates most Western societies reinforces heterosexism (Gagnon, 1990). Because the two usually exist concurrently, addressing both in therapy often leads to a reduction in homophobia, as well as to an increase in lesbians valuing both themselves as women and the femininity of their partners.

Relationship Viability

Heterosexism inherently assumes that relationships between men and women are qualitatively superior and more satisfying than same-sex partnerships. As introduced in Chapter

1 and reiterated throughout this book, these assumptions pervade the broader society and are deeply held by the majority of heterosexuals. They likewise have been internalized by many sexual minorities and serve to create negative attitudes toward their own couple-hoods (Eldridge, 1987; George & Behrendt, 1987; M. S. Schneider, 1986).

Relationship Quality and Satisfaction

Numerous studies (some of which are described next) have examined relationship satisfaction in female–male and same-sex partnerships and have found that individuals in lesbian and gay relationships are at least as content as their heterosexual counterparts. Relationship satisfaction for all three combinations of couples additionally seems influenced more by feminine gender role socialization than by sexual orientation, as well as by low levels of neuroticism and depression.

ASSESSMENTS INVOLVING SAME-SEX AND HETEROSEXUAL COUPLES

To assess perceived relationship quality and satisfaction, Kurdek and Schmitt (1986b, 1987a) studied 79 heterosexual (44 married and 35 cohabitating), 50 gay, and 56 lesbian couples. They subsequently found that gay and lesbian couples, as well as heterosexually married pairs, reported more satisfaction with their relationships than cohabitating heterosexuals; and that partners across all couple categories differed equally in their assessments of relationship quality when asked to evaluate the nature of their alliances. Further, the more that mates in all categories perceived themselves as equally attached to the other, the higher they assessed the quality of their relationships.

Kurdek (1994) later matched gay, lesbian, and heterosexual couples (39 pairs in each category) and detected that relationship satisfaction for all couples was positively related to perceived rewards from the partnership, negatively related to perceived costs of the alliance, and positively related to emotional investment in the relationship. In other words, the resources invested in and benefits reaped from the partnership similarly affected both same-sex and heterosexual couples.

The relationship satisfaction of male couples in Kurdek's (1994) study, however, did not correspond to that of lesbian and heterosexual couples relative to a number of variables that are associated with feminine gender role socialization. Specifically, relationship satisfaction for male–female and female–female pairs was found to be positively related to adequate social support and perceived self-expressiveness and negatively related to anxiety, depression, and interpersonal sensitivity. Apparently, partnerships without at least one female member (i.e., male–male couples) did not rely on emotional or relational factors for mutual satisfactions as much as equity of exchange. Although social exchange theory seems to explain the nature of relationship satisfaction for many gay men, feminine gender role socialization appears to enhance the quality of women's partnerships. Along these same lines, Rosenbluth (1997) compared 90 women (ages 22 to 54 years), half in lesbian and half in heterosexual couples, and discovered that relationship values, levels of self-esteem, and capacity for intimacy were similar in the two populations. The majority in both groups, however, described their relationships with women as more emotionally and intellectually intimate than those with men.

In addition to biological sex of the partners, Kurdek (1994) found the mental health of members also was related to relationship satisfaction. He later (Kurdek, 1997b) examined the link between neuroticism in one or both mates and components of relationship commitment in 61 gay, 42 lesbian, and 155 heterosexual couples and found that neuroticism affects dedication to a relationship through both intrapersonal and interpersonal pathways in all three types of pairs. In a somewhat similar study, Kurdek (1997c) also investigated neuroticism (which he defined as being composed of the six facets: anxiety, hostility, depression, self-consciousness, impulsiveness, and vulnerability) and two dimensions of relationship commitment (attractions to the relationship and constraints against leaving) in 33 gay, 40 lesbian, and 70 heterosexual couples. He subsequently discovered that depression exerts an effect on attraction commitment in all sets of partnerships through two dimensions of attachment style (positivity of the self and positivity of the other). Finally, even in separated partners of 26 gay, 24 lesbian, and 49 heterosexual individuals, strategies for coping with stress were found to be more significant in predicting separation distress than were relationship-related events or biological sex of the former mate (Kurdek, 1997a).

STUDIES OF GAY AND LESBIAN COUPLES

In other studies with no heterosexual comparison groups, Kurdek (1991, 1992) surveyed 136 gay and 82 lesbian cohabitating partners. Regardless of whether same-sex couples based their contentment on emotional factors or equitable exchange, the investigator found few significant differences in terms of relationship satisfaction between the male and female pairs. Couples who separated, however, exchanged more negative affect than did couples who remained together, with the latter group perceiving more rewards from their relationships and more satisfaction with, and investment in, their partnerships (Kurdek, 1992). Relational entrustment also was examined by Kurdek (1995a) in a study that involved three annual assessments of 61 gay and 42 lesbian couples. Findings indicated that changes in relationship commitment over time were explained by changes in the discrepancy between current and ideal levels of equality, as well as between current levels of attachment and current levels of autonomy. Similarly, Kurdek (1996) reported data from both partners of 60 gay and 46 lesbian couples, a subset of whom annually had completed mailed surveys over a 5-year period. Those whose relationships eventually dissolved reported a decrease in positivity, an increase in relationship conflict, and an increase in personal autonomy in the preseparation period.

In an earlier and related study, Kurdek (1988c) found that both men ($n = 65$) and women ($n = 47$) who had been living together with same-sex partners for 6 or more years reported higher liking for their partners, more intrinsic and instrumental motivations for being in the relationship, more trust, and more shared decision making. This study of gay and lesbian cohabitating couples also found that women reported higher relationship satisfaction than did men. Relatively comparable data were generated when Kurdek (1989) later surveyed 74 gay and 45 lesbian couples and found that lesbian couples and couples who had been living together 11 years or more reported greater relationship quality as defined by relationship satisfaction, love for partner, and liking for partner. Satisfaction with social support, high expressiveness, and few beliefs that disagreement is destructive to a relationship also significantly predicted positive relationship quality.

Partner Differences

Large demographic differences are present in some same-sex couples, and Kurdek (1995b) explains this by noting that the homogamy principle of "like marries like" may be less true for lesbians and gay men than for heterosexual pairs because of the limited number of potential partners from which to choose (p. 246). Data verifying the actual existence of large variances are sparse, however. Similarly, empirical support is lacking for Tripp's (1975) assertion that gay and lesbian partners frequently are able to achieve compatibility with relative ease, despite having to hurdle large social barriers, such as age, ethnicity, socioeconomic status, and educational level. Accordingly, similarity of gender role socialization often facilitates an initial high rapport, meshing, and deep congeniality for same-sex partners. The quality of this harmonious union is characterized by a tendency to exaggerate common traits or perspectives to a greater degree than either partner alone would have magnified. Nichols (1990) refers to this phenomenon as "female [or male] socialization multiplied" (p. 358).

This bridging of demographic differences in same-sex couples likewise has been noted by others (Bepko & Johnson, 2000; L. S. Brown, 1994; S. E. James & Murphy, 1998), despite the lack of data supporting Tripp's contention that initial rapport enables couples to overcome social distance. Nonetheless, a few demographic studies and surveys are available that describe relationship satisfaction despite discrepancies in some of these variables. Kurdek and Schmitt (1987a), for example, examined the relationship quality in 79 heterosexual (44 married and 35 cohabiting), 50 gay, and 56 lesbian couples and found that gay male partners had the highest discrepancies in age, income, and education but that these differences had no effect on relationship satisfaction. Conversely, Peplau et al. (1982) also found that partner *similarities* in age, religion, and work status were unrelated to relationship satisfaction in gay and lesbian couples. Similar findings were detected in a study of 700 African American lesbian and gay couples. Later, Peplau et al. (1997) found that partner similarities in age, education, and type of job were unrelated to relationship satisfaction. While not denying the possibility of relationship satisfaction in couples with large cultural or other differences, Bepko and Johnson (2000) note that being of the same sex does not always mitigate different ethnic identifications, lifecycle stages, ages, educational levels, or social classes. Discrepancies in any of these areas may be potential sources of clash for a couple.

AGE

Although age-discrepant same-sex partnerships have long been recognized among both lesbians and gay men (Peplau & Cochran, 1990), Harry (1982a, 1984) suggested that age differences characterize only a minority of male couples. Furthermore, those discrepancies that do occur are relatively small (i.e., 5 to 10 years separating the ages of the two individuals). Investigating these age differences in male couples, Steinman (1990) interviewed 46 pairs with partner age discrepancies ranging from 8 to 40 years and found that the younger mates were more likely to offer or refuse sexual pleasure in order to achieve or maintain equity in their relationships. Sexual gratification, however, was not necessarily exchanged for financial resources, and the intelligence or social accomplishment of older partners was frequently as strongly appealing to younger mates as were material possessions.

ETHNICITY

Some writers (Pearlman, 1996) contend that, just as for heterosexuals, ethnic differences between same-sex partners are increasing. Pearlman also believes that these contrasts in-

clude variances in class and cultural background. In the interest of examining the perceived quality of these partnerships, *OUT/LOOK* magazine conducted a survey of their
readership (Rocchio & Merciadez, 1992). Of the respondents, 63% (*n* = 358) reported
that racial differences have had a positive effect on their relationship. One member of the
sample referred to this favorable consequence as "not only a sexual attraction, but also
an attraction of cultural differences and appreciation of different outlooks due to our different backgrounds" (p. 85). Similarly, Peplau, Cochran, and Mays (1986) studied Black
lesbians (*n* = 284 and 295) and reported no significant association between any measure
of relationship satisfaction and whether or not their partners were of the same ethnic
group. Of these women, 69.3% of their partners also were Black, 21.5% were Caucasian, and less than 10% were from Hispanic or other ethnic groups.

Peplau et al. (1997) later surveyed 398 Black women and 325 African American
men, all of whom were in a "committed, romantic/sexual relationship" with a same-sex
partner. More than one-third of the participants were in an interracial relationship, most
often with a White mate. Non-Black partners were noted by 30% of the lesbians and
42% of the gay men. Findings revealed that these interracial couples were no more or less
satisfied on the average than couples who both were African American. In other words,
ethnicity was unrelated to relationship satisfaction. Data also reflected a fair degree of demographic similarity between partners on age, educational attainment, and employment
status. The researchers commented that "this stands in marked contrast to results reported by Kurdek and Schmitt [1987a; discussed above] for White gay men and lesbians"
(p. 18) who found high discrepancies between same-sex partners in age, income, and education. They speculated that their findings of greater similarity between African American mates could be the result of ethnic, cultural, or class differences between the two
samples, or it could only be due to their greater sample size.

INCOME

With respect to income variance, women earn 76.5 cents for every dollar that men earn
(Bureau of Labor Statistics, 1999). This fact, combined with the imposed societal expectation of "mommy-track" career paths and limited vocational aspiration for wives
(Shenitz, 1999), results in predicted differences in earnings between heterosexual partners. In contrast, relatively equal income between same-sex mates might be anticipated
based on their overall rejection of heterosexist norms and their greater appreciation of
egalitarian values. Contrary to this latter expectation, an *OUT/LOOK* magazine survey
reported median differences in annual incomes within female couples as $10,200 and
within male pairs as $15,000 (Coleman & Walters, 1990). Further, 24% of the lesbian
dyads (*n* = 246) and 37% of the gay male couples (*n* = 88) disclosed income differences
between partners of more than $20,000.

Hertz and Browning (1998) believe that when one member of a gay or lesbian couple
is worth more money than the other, the relationship is fraught with more potential problems than might exist in a heterosexual marriage, because in these couplings one person
has the less-powerful and legally designated role of "wife." "For same-sex partners, income disparities may be linked to such factors as class, ability, attitude, ambition, and
personality" (Shenitz, 1999). Attorney Hertz (Shenitz, 1999) advises these couples to deal
openly with income disparities, which may mean overcoming traditional gender socialization by women learning to share less and by men becoming willing to share more. Given
the value that lesbians may assign to equality and gay men might attribute to power or

domination (Blumstein & Schwartz, 1983; Falco, 1991; S. E. James & Murphy, 1998; Julien, Arellano, & Turgeon, 1997; J. M. Lynch & Reilly, 1986; M. E. Reilly & Lynch, 1990), monetary differences potentially could result in relationship dissatisfaction if it were not for the strong presence of some mediating factors (such as the initial high rapport and compatibility to which Tripp [1975] referred).

RESIDENCE

Regarding cohabitation patterns, mixed results have been found. For example, in a 1988 national survey of 1,749 individuals representing 706 lesbian and 560 gay male couples (n = 1,266 pairs) was conducted by Bryant and Demian (1995) of the Partners Task Force for Gay and Lesbian Couples. Findings revealed that 75% of the female pairs and 82% of the male couples had lived together during the previous year of the relationship. Residences were jointly owned by 32% of the women and 36% of the men. Peplau et al. (1986) found that a lower percentage (54%, compared with the 87% and 75% found in the two studies just described) of their Black lesbian sample (n = 150) lived with lovers, and that there was no significant difference in relationship satisfaction between those who lived together and those who lived apart. Harry (1983), however, estimated that three-quarters of all female pairs live together (a figure equivalent to the Bryant and Demian lesbian data), compared with approximately half of all male couples (contrasted with 82% of the paired gay men in Bryant and Demian's investigation).

Discrepancies in the percentages cited here probably can be explained by several factors, including the eras in which the data were collected, inaccessibility of sexual minority individuals and couples at lower levels of identity formation, the clandestine conditions under which many live, and cohort differences among generations. In addition, Harry (1983) acknowledged that little is known as to why some partners elect to live together while others choose to live apart. He nonetheless offers some possible reasons for these decisions, including a rejection of a heterosexual marriage model, the requirements of jobs in different locations, the need to disguise a relationship to maintain employment, and a reluctance to pool finances. Thus, whether heterosexism is renounced or accommodated, its influence on cohabitation patterns is evident.

GENDER ROLE SOCIALIZATION

According to L. S. Brown (1994), "gender is a presence and dynamic in any intimate adult pair bond" (p. 1). Individuals are socialized into roles that are based on societal constructions of gender, and members of each sex are assumed to have similar socialization, with men being conditioned according to one set of expectations and women to another (Elise, 1998; S. E. James & Murphy, 1998; Julien et al., 1997). L. S. Brown (1994) contends, however, that this assumption is not always accurate in that few have "absorbed or complied with all the norms of gender role socialization within her or his culture of origin" (p. 1). Other issues, such as ethnicity, culture, religion, class, age cohort, and education, also contribute to the socialization process. Further, "there is a growing realization that the conception of gender identity as fixed, uniform and coherent is a conception that either pathologizes or denies multifaceted gender aspects of internalized object relations" (A. E. Schwartz, 1998, p. 21). In spite of these and other attempts to provide a more flexible and less binary concept of identity, gender nonetheless provides a popular and convenient explanation for a broad spectrum of human behaviors and a directive for how the sexes are to behave (Chodorow, 1994; Eldridge, 1987; B. Greene, 1997b).

L. S. Brown (1994) refers to these contemporary constructions of gender as "fiction" in that such conceptualizations are based on a dearth of empirical information. In fact, there even is evidence that lesbians and gay men incorporate gender constructs somewhat differently than heterosexuals do (Bailey & Dawood, 1998; R. J. Green, Bettinger, & Zacks, 1996; Julien et al. 1997). For example, Kurdek (1987) administered the Bem Sex-Role Inventory to 230 gay men, 136 lesbians, 124 heterosexual males, and 117 heterosexual women and found that gender differences on the Instrumentality, Expressiveness, and Masculinity/Femininity scales were more pronounced for the heterosexual cohorts than for the lesbians and gay men. Additionally, lesbians were more Instrumental than the other women and gay men were more Expressive than heterosexual males. Similarly, M. Cooper (1990) interviewed 15 lesbians (aged 19 to 38) and found that each refuted traditional femininity and the traditional feminine role.

In another study (Hellwege, Perry, & Dobson, 1988), the Bem Sex-Role Inventory also was administered to 39 gay men, 38 lesbians, 36 male heterosexuals, and 99 heterosexual women. Ratings on the Androgyny scale indicated that lesbians differed significantly from all other groups in how they imaged the ideal male and ideal female. Further, they categorized these ideal images in the androgynous range and were least likely to utilize traditional sex roles in organizing their perceptions. Contrary to Kurdek's (1987) study, gay men slightly tended to stereotype their concept of an ideal male.

Gender-Socialized Sex Differences

Regardless of how sexual minorities actually internalize gender roles, gay and lesbian partners still are assumed to share similar gender role socialization because they are of the same biological sex (Elise, 1998; S. E. James & Murphy, 1998; Julien et al., 1997). Further, there is thought to be enough truth in these gender-specific assumptions that they can be used as a framework for understanding homosexual partnerships (L. S. Brown, 1994; Cabaj, 1988a; S. E. James & Murphy, 1998). Gender role, in fact, is thought to influence same-sex relationships more than sexual orientation (Kurdek, 1994; Peplau, 1981).

Rusbult, Zembrodt, and Iwaniszek (1986) accordingly studied 22 heterosexual males, 28 heterosexual females, 23 gay men, and 27 lesbians, and found that, regardless of sexual orientation, psychological femininity was associated with tendencies either to attempt to improve conditions in troubled relationships or to wait for them to improve. Psychological masculinity, conversely, was correlated with proclivities toward leaving relationships or allowing conditions to deteriorate.

Along these same lines, Duffy and Rusbult (1986) compared 50 lesbians and gay men and 50 male and female heterosexuals and found that both lesbian and heterosexual women reported investing more and being more committed to maintaining their relationships than did men of either orientation. Zacks, Green, and Marrow (1988) similarly concluded that women's socialization predisposed the 52 lesbian couples they studied to form more cohesive, adaptable, and satisfying relationships than the heterosexual pairs. In other words, their significantly higher levels of cohesion, adaptability, and satisfaction were attributed more to gender role than to sexual orientation.

Gender role socialization likewise seems to influence the importance of equality and balancing of power as goals for relationships (Julien et al., 1997; Kurdek, 1994; Schreurs & Buunk, 1996; Shenitz, 1999). In this regard, Peplau and Cochran (1980) studied 50 lesbians, 50 gay men, 50 heterosexual women, and 50 male heterosexuals and discovered that all groups recognized the importance of having egalitarian relationships. Women, both lesbian and heterosexual, however, assigned equal power more importance than did men. Similarly, higher percentages of women (59% lesbian; 48% heterosexual) than men (38% gay; 40% heterosexual) reported that their current relationships were "exactly equal" in terms of power.

Monogamy

Gender-specific conditioning also seems to affect the importance assigned to sexual exclusivity (Rutter & Schwartz, 1996; Scrivner, 1997). Blumstein and Schwartz (1983), for example, found in their sample that 75% of husbands ($n = 3,635$), 62% of heterosexual male cohabitants ($n = 650$), and 35% of gay men ($n = 1,924$) believed that monogamy is important. These figures contrast with 84% of wives ($n = 3,640$) who affirmed the importance of sexual exclusively, 70% of heterosexual female cohabitants ($n = 650$), and 71% of lesbians ($n = 1,559$). Comparisons of percentages for each of the three subject categories are summarized in Table 15.1 and reveal noticeable differences in the importance that men and women assign to the exclusivity of their sexual behavior. Women in all classifications indicated a higher preference for monogamy than did men.

In addition to indicating the importance of monogamy more than twice as often as did gay men, lesbians in couple relationships of between 2 and 10 years reported instances of nonmonogamy less often than did their male counterparts (Blumstein & Schwartz, 1983). Of the lesbian respondents, 19% ($n = 706$) acknowledged at least one instance of nonmonogamy during the previous year, compared with 79% ($n = 943$) of the gay male subjects. Kurdek (1988c) also surveyed 65 gay and 47 lesbian cohabitating couples and found that all of the lesbian couples were sexually exclusive, while 47.7% ($n = 34$) of the male couples permitted sex outside the relationship. Bryant and Demian (1995) similarly asked members of 706 lesbian and 560 gay male couples about the frequency of outside sex per month; 98% of the women and 78% of the men reported none. Only 1% of the women indicated an outside encounter, compared with 10% of the gay men. Along these same lines, the *Advocate*, a popular lesbian and gay news magazine, surveyed its male readers regarding their sexuality and relationships and received 13,000 responses

TABLE 15.1. Percentage of Respondents Who Indicated How Important They Feel It Is That They Themselves Be Monogamous

	Responding "Yes" (%)		
	Heterosexually married	Heterosexually cohabitating	Lesbians and gay men
Men	75	62	35
Women	84	70	71

Note. Data from Blumstein & Schwartz (1983).

from 18% of subscribers (Lever, 1994). The sample selected for analysis consisted of every fourth questionnaire from the first 10,000 returned ($n = 2,500$). Of the men who indicated that they had a primary partner, 87% said they have a long-term commitment to the alliance. While the vast majority (71%) said they preferred long-term monogamous relationships to other arrangements, 52% were or had been sexually exclusive in their present or past union; 28% were "supposed" to be monogamous, but one or both partners had had sex with someone else; and 20% were or had been in open relationships.

The sex differences in the studies described here may be explained partially by gender-specific "sex role socialization that may teach men to value sexual variety" and by "a tendency for men to separate sexuality from emotional commitment" (Peplau & Cochran, 1990). Numerous writers (Cabaj & Klinger, 1996; Gray & Isensee, 1996; Rutter & Schwartz, 1996), in fact, believe that gender role conditioning shapes the various dynamics of gay and lesbian relationships, such as cohesion, distribution of power, and monogamy. In the following section, the specific impact of masculine socialization on the interaction patterns and processes of male couples is discussed. Afterward, the influences of gender role on female pairs is considered.

Gay Couples

Rigid stereotypic masculine gender behaviors often result in relationship problems if one or both members of a male couple have been socialized to be "competitive . . . unemotional, the best, in control, strong, capable, and independent" (George & Behrendt, 1987, p. 79). Many of the problems in gay male relationships, in fact, are thought to reflect intensified gender role conditioning in the areas of sex, aggression, achievement, and competitiveness (R. L. Hawkins, 1992; McVinney, 1998; Scrivner, 1997). These aspects of masculine socialization appear to be embedded in the earlier discussion of relationship satisfaction studies as related to male couples. Gratification with the alliance, for example, was related to the presence of dynamics that are counter to male socialization (e.g., equal attachment, Kurdek & Schmitt, 1986b, 1987a; and emotional investment, Kurdek, 1992, 1994). In other words, the less traditionally socialized the couple, the greater the degree to which members reported fulfillment in their relationship.

Other studies also appear to point in this direction. For example, Reece and Segrist (1981) studied 30 ongoing and 30 recently separated male couples and found that the pairs who remained together cooperated more than did those who separated. Along this same vein, Peplau and Cochran (1981) surveyed the intimate relationships of 128 gay men and found that the more importance partners gave to attachment values, the more love and intimacy they reported and the more they expected a future for their couplehood. After studying 132 gay men with partners, Kurdek and Schmitt (1986a) similarly concluded that high dyadic attachment and relationship quality were related. In addition, O'Brien (1992) also found that gay men ($n = 259$) in a highly satisfying alliance experienced greater well-being and tended to be less depressed than those whose partnership situation was not as favorably described.

INTIMACY ISSUES

R. L. Hawkins (1992) contends that the conditioning of gay men often leaves them ill equipped to function in relationships, given that their upbringing frequently inhibits the development of intimacy skills. Many have learned to protect themselves from pain following innumerable instances of covert and overt invalidation when their strivings for closeness and acceptance have evoked from parents and influential others responses such as distancing, rejection, devaluation, contempt, and anxiety: "For these reasons, in gay men's developmental process, attention and acceptance are traumatically severed" (Canarelli et al., 1999, p. 55)

Drescher (1998) notes that a considerable number of the gay individuals he has treated have been traumatized by heterosexual rejections throughout their lives: "Repeated attempts at closeness that are met with rejection and scorn result in dissociative tendencies in many spheres of life. The repetitive nature of this experience can sometimes generate what looks like a schizoid form of relatedness" (p. 57). It is not surprising, then, that many gay men have difficulties with closeness and intimacy (C. Friedman, 1998; Gray & Isensee, 1996) and often there develops an inability to communicate "feelings of tenderness, and feelings that, once expressed, may leave the man vulnerable" (George & Behrendt, 1987, p. 79). In this regard, Farley (1992) elucidates on the tendency of men in couple relationships to hold back from commitment for fear of losing power and control.

In discussing the treatment of identity and intimacy issues in gay men, Colgan (1988) focuses specifically on overseparation and overattachment as developmental factors. He contends that "prehomosexual boys," particularly those who are gender-nonconforming, have ample opportunity to experience rejection or emotional abandonment by primary caretakers, especially fathers who often attempt to discredit or extinguish gender-inappropriate behaviors. Perceiving these actions as desertion, the boys therefore are predisposed to develop disorders of identity and intimacy. Colgan (1988) believes that the risks for both gender-nonconforming prehomosexual boys, as well as those who are gender-conforming but also father-rejected, include a disruption of positive identity formation and "limited opportunities for healthy expressions of intimacy needs due to the perceived necessity for denial of attachment desires" (p. 109). As a result of these kinds of experiences, patterns of overseparation and distancing are strongly established in many gay men (T. W. Johnson & Keren, 1996; Stein & Cabaj, 1996). Having restricted affective involvement with other males during earlier developmental phases, these individuals often encounter difficulties in forming intimate same-sex partnerships as adults.

THERAPEUTIC CONSIDERATIONS

Colgan (1988) relates his conceptualizations to those of McWhirter and Mattison (1984) who note that each stage of couple development (which will be discussed later in this chapter) presents possibilities for negotiating separation and attachment. In other words, the establishment of an adult emotional bond frequently forms the basis of safety necessary for redressing earlier developmental wounds and for balancing independence and dependence. If couples in therapy can comprehend that the problems they are experiencing are also opportunities to ameliorate the "scar tissue of individual development" (Forstein, 1986, p. 107), they often can acquire the perspective necessary for therapeutic growth. Therapy, in fact, "provides an opportunity for the couple to work through individual and interpersonal issues, understand the developmental nature of the couple relationship, and affirm the essential nature of being gay and being coupled" (p. 136).

Gay males who bring patterns of overseparation and overattachment to the couple relationship may need specific help and suggestions in how to be intimate (Cabaj &

Klinger, 1996; Colgan, 1988). Further and even more primarily, the empathic attunement provided in the therapeutic relationship can, in and of itself, be reparative if this emotional encounter with the therapist is one that conveys respect and offers conditions of safety (Hartman, 1998). Accordingly, the clinician's modeling and "unconditional acceptance of homoerotic capacities is necessary countervalence for earlier anti-homosexual cultural conditioning" (Malyon, 1982, p. 66). All intense affective phenomena have become stigmatized, and erotic impulses have been inhibited and compartmentalized, in many gay men. These individuals have become intensely isolated from themselves, and, hence, their capacity for intimacy with others is markedly impaired. The affirmative mirroring of the therapeutic relationship can become a means by which the fragmented ego is restored to integrity so that mature mutuality and intimate couple relationships become possible.

Finally, therapists working with male couples need to focus on those variables related to masculine socialization that seem to be obstructing optimal dyadic functioning. If extreme competitiveness, aggression, fear of vulnerability, and loss of control predominate in one or both members of a couple, the chances of the alliance being problematic are high. Further, if fears of vulnerability, attachment, intimacy, or engulfment are profound and prevent commitment to the relationship, then individual therapy may be warranted before resuming couples counseling.

Lesbian Couples

Compared with gay men, lesbians are more likely to be coupled. In a survey of readers of *OUT/LOOK* magazine (n = 300; P. Nardi & Sherrod, 1990), 69% of the women (60% of the sample) and 41% of the men indicated that they currently were involved with a lover. In addition, 34% of the women, compared with 11% of the men, said that a former lover is their best friend. Lesbians tend to strive for closeness and harmony in their friendships and intimate relationships. For example, both partners of 275 lesbian couples were assessed, and the correlates of relationship satisfaction included self-esteem, power, life satisfaction, dyadic attachment, and intimacy. Role conflict and personal autonomy were found to correlate negatively with relationship satisfaction (Eldridge & Gilbert, 1990). In an attempt to test the assumption that a high degree of closeness in lesbian relationships is reached at the expense of autonomy of the partners, 119 Dutch lesbian couples were surveyed (Schreurs & Buunk, 1996). Contrary to previous findings, intimacy and equity, as well as dependency and autonomy, were independent predictors of relationship satisfaction. Autonomy was negatively related to dependency, but not at all to intimacy. In other words, the coupled women in the study described being independent from and, at the same time, close to their partners.

WOMEN'S RELATEDNESS

As discussed in Chapter 9, most women develop within the context of primary emotional connection, define themselves in association with others, and learn to experience empathically the needs of others as their own (Chodorow, 1978, 1989; Miller, 1976). This relational socialization allows women to organize their identities around the ability to maintain relationships, the first of which is the mother–daughter dyad. Since daughters are kept within this ongoing process of relatedness longer than sons, similarity and oneness between the girl and her mother enables the development of an enhanced capacity for empathy. This emotional attunement and the inner experience of another then becomes a template for all future relationships that involve cohesion and intimacy (L. S. Brown, 1994; Burch, 1993; Chodorow, 1978, 1989, 1994; Mencher, 1990). The closeness of some lesbian partners is thought to approach the intensity of the mother–daughter bond, and Burch (1987) suggests that the parallel between the lover's body and the mother's body frequently is able to evoke and recreate the deepest childhood experiences of tenderness and closeness. In addition to these sensual and romantic wishes, however, maternal transferences that are sadistic, aggressive, and moralistic may be stirred in these intimate pairs (N. O'Connor & Ryan, 1993), and other early, maternal affective experiences, including injuries, threats, and fears of reengulfment, can be brought to the surface. For some partners these unpleasant emotions reach such a high level of intensity that they erupt into fury and violence. The dynamics of these altercations in same-sex couples will be discussed in the following section.

N. O'Connor and Ryan (1993) also question why lesbian sexuality and coupling should be viewed exclusively in terms of the mother–daughter relationship at all. They consider this conceptualization too literal and contend that female partners can also be endowed with features of the father. Given that cross-gender identifications are common, to assume that same-sex relationships "deny difference" ignores important aspects of psychic reality regarding gender "in favour of what is assumed to be 'reality' in relation to gender" (p. 190). Along these same lines, Burch (1995) conducted in-depth interviews with eight individual women and four couples and noted a "history of identifications" (p. 293) in her lesbian subjects. She speculates that lesbians have a diversity of gender representations and identifications and that "there is usually an unconscious and sometimes a conscious oscillation of gender dimensions" (pp. 303–304) in their intimate relationships.

Psychoanalyst A. E. Schwartz (1998) attempts to broaden the concept of mothering, by using the concept of "mothering ones" (p. 151), which include a small number of familiar people who are in close, consistent proximity to a child and which accommodates caretakers who do not live within the context of a heterosexual matrix. The maternal functions of these individuals "are both manifest and subjectively experienced within mothering–child interactions—so as to be internalized and represented unconsciously as one aspect of self and other in relation" (p. 152). These kinesthetic and symbolic encodings, as described by Schwartz, appear to be structurally similar to other working models of attachment, except that they are not bounded by gender or heterosexist concepts of "mother."

STRENGTH OR PITFALL?

The degree of intimacy in lesbian relationships frequently has been measured by male models of development based on individuation, separation, clear emotional boundaries, and autonomy. Compared to these masculine concepts of maturity, women's relatedness has been described or pathologized as fusion (Deutsch, 1995; Elise, 1998; Klinger, 1996; Mencher, 1990; Miller, 1976). For example, classical psychoanalytic theory views experiences such as *union* and *merger* as regressive opposites of differentiation or separation of self from the other: "Merging was a dangerous form of undifferentiation, a sinking back into a sea of oneness" (Benjamin, 1988, p. 47).

Analysts N. O'Connor and Ryan (1993) believe that these preoedipal longings (including desires for fusion, merger, and enmeshment) for the "mothering ones" (after Schwartz, 1998, and in consideration of O'Connor & Ryan's reservations about the gendered concept of mother) are not the only aspects of the primary caretaker(s) that are re-created in lesbian relationships, and that other conceptualizations are possible. They acknowledge that some women's partnerships may have "powerfully symbiotic features, with all the attendant difficulties that this can entail" (p. 188), but that other forms of attraction toward the mothering figure(s) can be more mature and involve a distinction of self where the caretaker is viewed as a whole and separate person. The girl's continued search for the (degendered) "mother," in fact, implies a degree of self–object differentiation between the two individuals. The study described earlier in this section (Schreurs & Buunk, 1996)—in which the lesbian partners described their relationships as involving elements of both closeness and independence—could possibly illustrate this binary concept.

Others have attempted to depathologize female patterns of connectedness and relatedness, by redefining *merger* and *fusion* as ongoing adaptive strategies to maintain the integrity of a couple in a heterosexist environment and to counteract societal pressures that might undermine the relationship (Igartua, 1998; Klinger, 1996; McCandlish, 1982; S. McKenzie, 1992). Mencher (1990) substitutes the nonperjorative word *embeddedness* "to describe the situating of women's identity within relationships" (p. 9). Speaking from the perspective of Kohut's self psychology, Mitchell (1988) argues that flexibility and permeability of ego boundaries are essential components in all intimate relationships. Women's "ability to open the boundaries of the self, in this theory, is far from pathological. Rather, it is seen as the basis for a profound relationship and the necessary condition for psychological growth" (p. 165). Burch (1993) contends that this fluidity of ego boundaries further "lends itself to the psychological exchange found in complementary projective bonding" (p. 80), which is one of "the essential connective mechanisms for forming . . . empathic identifications" (p. 61) that are at the core of object relations theory.

When any two people are in the initial or limerence stage of their relationship, a state of fusion exists. Individual ego boundaries are crossed, and the individuals experience a state of oneness. It is only when this fusion is no longer a transient state but a prolonged one not easily altered that a problem with merger exists. Chodorow (1989) believes that "women's relational self can be both a strength or pitfall in feminine psychic life" (p. 186) in that it enables empathy, nurturance, and intimacy, as it also threatens lack of autonomy and dissolution of self into others. Closeness, in other words, only becomes problematic when it is excessive in terms of the loss of individuality in one or both members of a partnership (Klinger, 1996). The attainment of mature intimacy represents an ongoing challenge for all couples and entails a dynamic balance of closeness and distance, as well as of fusion and disengagement (R. J. Green et al., 1996; McCandlish, 1982). "If enmeshment replaces the ebb and flow of connection and separation" (Burch, 1986, p. 59), then the issue is of therapeutic concern.

Boundary regulation problems are inevitable for any couple (Elsie, 1998; Roth, 1985/1989) but are sometimes magnified in lesbians, due to the relational nature of women's psychosocial development. "However, in the absence of systematic research comparing the frequency of merger problems among lesbians and among heterosexual couples, the claim that this problem is more common among lesbians remains untested" (Peplau et al., 1996, p. 259). Clinicians thus should take care not to view the closeness of a female pair as immature and pathological, or to expect lesbian relationships to mirror masculine concepts of maturity. They need to keep in mind, nonetheless, that women's gender role socialization sometimes does result in prolonged and insidious difficulties with fusion and enmeshment in lesbian couples. The key is to remain alert to those partnerships that are fused to the point where movement between connectedness and separateness is not possible within the framework provided by the relationship.

Domestic Violence

Accurate information about the frequency of battering and physical abuse in gay and lesbian partnerships is not available, given the invisibility of the population and the fact that rarely are incidents reported to authorities (Bograd, 1999; Klinger, 1995; Klinger & Stein, 1996; Lundy & Leventhal, 1999). Most of the published studies describing selected demographics and dynamics relate to lesbian couples; few focus on abuse in male relationships (Bethea, Rexrode, Ruffo, & Washington, 1999; Fortunata, 1999; Hammond, 1989; Peplau et al., 1996; Ristock, 1998). Data from one study that concentrated on both men and women ($n = 283$) indicated that 47.5% of lesbians and 29.7% of gay men reported having been victimized by a same-sex partner (Waldner-Haugrud, Gratch, & Magruder, 1997). When asked whether they had ever been a perpetrator of relationship violence, 38% of the women and 21.8% of the men responded affirmatively. Several studies of violence in lesbian relationships have reported rates of 20% (Brand & Kidd, 1986; $n = 55$), 31% (Lockhart, White, Causby, & Isaac, 1994; $n = 284$), 40% (Waterman, Dawson, & Bologna, 1989; $n = 70$ but includes gay men who reported rates of 18%), 45% (Lie, Schilit, Bush, Montagne, & Reyes, 1991; $n = 174$), 46% (V. E. Coleman, 1994; $n = 90$), and 52% (Lie & Gentlewarrier, 1991; $n = 1,099$). Klinger and Stein (1996) contend, however, that "these studies are generally flawed by nonrandom self-selected samples (e.g., participants at women's festivals and self-definition of abuse)" (p. 810). They further note that systematic studies of the rate of violence in gay male couples are unavailable, although Island and Letellier (1991) estimate a rate between 10% and 20%. These percentages translate into about 500,000 gay men who are battered annually in the United States (Bograd, 1999; Klinger, 1995). Despite the wide range in reported findings, the prevalence and severity of lesbian and gay battering are thought to be comparable to those that occur between heterosexual partners (Burke & Follingstad, 1999; V. E. Coleman, 1997; Sarantokos, 1996).

Silent Suffering

One of the reasons for the wide disparity in terms of the pervasiveness of battering in same-sex relationships is that partners are even less likely than their heterosexual counterparts to seek help from those institutions that provide the database for much family violence research, such as shelters, police, and the medical and legal systems (Bograd, 1999; Lundy & Leventhal, 1999; S. L. Morrow & Hawxhurst, 1989). Bograd (1999) contends that the lack of statistics is not neutral; rather, "the invisibility of certain populations reflects more their social importance in the eyes of the dominant culture than the absence of domestic violence in their midst" (p. 279). Gay men, for example, often are not considered as having been battered because their relationships are viewed as neither intimate nor legitimate, because of presumptions that homosexual battering is a fight between equals, or because men rarely are described as victims (Letellier, 1994). The prevalent assumption, in fact, is that men should have the capability and freedom to simply leave an abusive relationship regardless of the circumstances (Scarce, 1997).

Gay and lesbian individuals frequently are reluctant to discuss violence in their relationships for fear of contributing to negative public opinion about homosexuality. Scarce (1997), for example, believes that many gay community leaders discourage discussions of same-sex violence and rape since it provides fodder to opponents "who are anxious for information that demonizes homosexuality when taken out of context" (p. 66). Lesbian victims usually feel extremely betrayed by their abusive partners since many have an idealized and unrealistic picture of egalitarian and loving relationships between women. Some members of the community even deny that lesbians can be cruel, violent, or brutal toward each other and thus may devaluate an announcement by of one of their sisters that she has been abused by her female partner. This minimization often is experienced as an additional betrayal by the victim of domestic violence who is looking to her lesbian kinfolk for support (Benowitz, 1986; Hammond, 1989; Klinger, 1995; S. L. Morrow & Hawxhurst, 1989; Renzetti, 1992; Renzetti & Miley, 1996).

Compounding of Trauma

Many victims feel intense shame at having either tolerated or perpetuated the abuse, experience conflict about remaining in harmful relationships, and are apprehensive about potential biased treatment or discrimination when asking for assistance (Cruz & Firestone, 1998; Lundy & Leventhal, 1999; S. L. Morrow & Hawxhurst, 1989; Peplau et al., 1996; Scarce, 1997). The trauma of domestic violence, in other words, is amplified further by distress outside the intimate relationship as the psychological consequences of battering may be compounded by the "microaggressions" (Bograd, 1999, p. 281) of racism, heterosexism, and classism. For many sexual minorities, to seek help from mainstream agencies and authorities is to solicit safely from the same individuals who are proponents of inequalities and enemies in political contexts. In essence, they believe that the anguish resulting from the battering is intensified by receiving treatment and assistance from the adversary.

The intersection of gender, race, class, culture, and sexual orientation radically shapes the experiences of domestic mistreatment, and certain men and women are more entrapped within contexts of violence than others (Almeida & Durkin, 1999). In this regard, Bograd (1999) contends that some victims are deemed more "legitimate" than others, and, consequently, services for these populations may be scarce or nonexistent. This certainly is the case with regard to programs specifically designed for lesbian and gay batterers and those whom they have injured. Given the existing state of affairs then, "some victims make the only choices possible due to constraints on many levels" (p. 284). These impediments may include the fear of having their sexual orientation exposed, losing jobs, getting or receiving custody of their children, and causing themselves or their families shame and humiliation. If therapists ignore or minimize the reality of these apprehensions, the victim's behavior can by seen as dysfunctional rather than as an adaptation to traumatic circumstances. What appears to be resistance or denial—or even possible helplessness—may actually reflect experiences related to oppression because of race, class, gender, and sexual orientation (Almeida, Woods, Messineo, & Font, 1998; McNair & Nelville, 1996).

Couple Dynamics

Abuse in intimate relationships exists in a context rather than in a vacuum (Bethea et al., 1999; Fortunata, 1999). Imbalances of power and control between partners frequently are key dynamics, but investigations into the nature of the relationship between balance of power and domestic violence have produced mixed findings: "Whether the abuser is more powerful and manifesting his or her power by battering or less powerful and aware that he or she is losing power is not clear" (Klinger & Stein, 1996, p. 811). However, one study (Landolt & Dutton, 1997) of 52 gay male couples (ages 20 to 64) found that the more frequent form of psychological abuse was significantly higher in relationships that are characterized by divided power (i.e., partners sharing decision-making authority by each making decisions in different domains). The authors thus concluded that abuse can occur in even relatively egalitarian relationships.

Renzetti (1992) found that the abusive partner in lesbian relationships tended to be overdependent and extremely jealous, pressuring the victim to separate herself from other contacts. In fact, the abuse increased when the victim tried to assert her independence. Fears of autonomy or individuation in one of the members also have been described by others as key dynamics, with anger and violence seen as attempts to restore equilibrium in the dyadic system (Berzon, 1988; Clunis & Green, 1988). The isolation of a couple also is a factor in domestic violence since many gay and lesbian partners form closed systems that insulate them from the outside world (S. E. James & Murphy, 1998; Krestan & Bepko, 1980). When jealousy and possessiveness become a part of the abuse in these impermeable relationships, the battered member of the couple becomes even more alone since the victim and abuser are highly interdependent and share common friends. If these close associates deny or minimize the extent of the problem, the alienation and betrayal of the victim is intensified.

Substance abuse frequently is associated with domestic violence (Fortunata, 1999; Scarce, 1997), but some batterers can recover from chemical dependency and continue to physically or emotionally mistreat their partners. In addition, household altercations of various sorts often are transmitted as intergenerational legacies and are passed from parents to children (Renzetti, 1992). Sometimes these inheritances accompany individuals through various partnerships. To test this, 174 self-identified lesbians (ages 21 to 59) who were then in aggressive same-sex relationships were surveyed (Lie et al., 1991). Approximately one-fourth of the subjects described themselves as victims of aggression in their current relationship, roughly two-thirds had been victimized by previous male partners, and almost three-quarters had experienced aggression by a previous female partner. Aggression in relationships between women was described most frequently as mutually aggressive, challenging the notion that victims and abusers fall into clearly distinctive categories (see also Waldner-Haugrud et al., 1997).

Psychotherapy

Therapy with gay and lesbians batterers and their partners requires a unique and careful assessment that considers the oppressive and prejudicial dimensions shaping gay and lesbian life (Renzetti, 1997). Clinicians who treat male couples also should be sensitive to the excessive masculine socialization that sets the stage for competition and aggression to erupt into physical violence (Klinger, 1995). The effects of this conditioning should be surfaced and articulated in careful detail, including environmental cues that set off the abusive behavior and cognitions that accompany it. Therapists should also explore disclosures of repeated fights; family histories of emotional, psychological, and physical abuse that may be carried over into the present relationship; couple dynamics, including whether one partner appears intimidated or frightened by the other, or is quiet during the interview; frequent physical signs of bruising or injury; and reticence to discuss any of the above (Farley, 1992).

Bograd and Mederos (1999) also recommend conducting a lethality assessment and suggest that therapists should inquire about substance abuse; past use of brutality, including a history of violent crimes and previous violations of restraining orders; use of weapons, threats of future intentions to retaliate, hurt, or kill either self or the partner; obsession with the partner; and bizarre forms of violence. Axis II pathology, particularly of the borderline, paranoid, schizoid, or antisocial variety, also must be assessed. The inquiry should include a determination of current safety, the existence of suicidal or homicidal ideation or intentions, and the availability of resources used in past instances of crisis. Moreover, a safety plan for future instances should be developed (Klinger, 1995; Klinger & Stein, 1996).

To facilitate inquiry, Hammond (1989) uses rather specific questions, such as the following: "Have you ever been afraid of any of your lovers?" "Has a lover ever kept you from leaving a room?" "Have you ever struck a lover?" (p. 101). She contends that general questions such as "Have you ever been physically or emotionally abused by a lover?" often are answered quickly in the negative due to fear, denial, or shame. Other questions might include the following from Marcus (1992, p. 277): "Does your lover try to control you through violence or the threat of violence?" "When you're with your lover, are you afraid for your safety?" "Does your lover destroy your personal property?" "Are you sexually abused or coerced in your relationship?"

Finally, couples therapy with victims and perpetrators can be inappropriate until each party receives therapy apart from the partner (preferably in a group modality). Perpetrators must become able to take responsibility for their behavior, and survivors must receive empowerment and support in order to diminish shame and isolation. Seeing both partners together prematurely commonly results in the survivor not participating in the therapy or minimizing the seriousness of the abuse out of legitimate fears of reprisal and retaliation (Farley, 1992; Klinger, 1996; Klinger & Stein, 1996). Bograd and Mederos (1999) do caution therapists not to polarize this issue since domestic violence takes many different forms and exists in many social and cultural contexts. Thus, "it is unlikely that a single treatment modality will be maximally effective" (p. 293).

Therapists may see some of the typical mental health consequences of battering, including silent suffering (Scarce, 1997) and anxiety and affective disorders. Posttraumatic stress disorder (PTSD) sometimes is associated with victimization, but most survivors do not develop the full clinical syndrome. Factors mitigating against the development of PTSD include the quality of support, rapid debriefing, and the nature of the trauma (Klinger, 1995; Klinger & Stein, 1996). As discussed here, however, affirmative assistance and expeditious questioning and discussion often are not available to gay and lesbian victims of domestic violence.

RELATIONSHIP STAGES

Same-sex couples are a recent social construct. In the past 30 years, recognition of their relationships has gone from nonexistent to the current lawful recognition of their marriages in some Scandinavian countries and legal domestic partnerships in some U. S. cities (McWhirter & Mattison, 1996). Only recently has the phenomenon of a same-sex couple emerged "with all its social, psychological, and sexual implications" (Forstein, 1986, p. 103). Essentially, then, all of the research regarding the characteristics of these dyads is relatively new. The only systematic, longitudinal inquiry into the histories of these partnerships studied male couples (McWhirter & Mattison, 1982, 1984, 1996), and other writers have conceptualized stages of lesbian relationships (Clunis & Green, 1988; Pearlman, 1988; Slater, 1995). The developmental phases of these same-sex unions are discussed in the following sections.

Gay Couples

McWhirter and Mattison (1982, 1984, 1996) conducted detailed interviews with 156 male couples whose relationships had lasted from 1 to 37 years (mean, 8.7 years). The researchers talked with the couples over a 5-year period (1974 to 1979) and used an interview schedule of 256 single items and 72 open-ended questions. Themes emerged from the conversations, and from these six clusterings or stages were formulated. These stages of gay male relationships, the general dynamics, and possible problems at each phase are summarized in Table 15.2.

Stages

McWhirter and Mattison (1982) note that "each stage has its own unique characteristics, stresses and benefits" (p. 79). As is true for all the developmental models discussed thus far, these phases are not linear. Rather, they are spiral-shaped and multidimensional, thus enabling a couple to move back and forth between stages or function at different points simultaneously (McWhirter & Mattison, 1996). The developmental stages of the McWhirter and Mattison model, as well as stage-related difficulties at each phase, are described next.

STAGE 1

Couples at this initial phase, *Blending*, tend to merge deeply and experience a high degree of sharing and "togetherness." Differences are overlooked and equality is high. For many, the resulting feelings are a marked contrast to the years of lonely "closeted" isolation during which they convinced themselves they would never find anyone who could love them unconditionally. Because initial expectations are elevated, disillusionment often is profound when the initial passion naturally diminishes. Individuals sometimes become afraid at this point and frantically try to retain the intensity of the early limerence and to prevent what they perceive may be the end of the relationship. Others withdraw from each other and employ the same protective distancing mechanisms that they developed earlier in their lifetimes to avoid the pain of personal rejection. McWhirter and Mattison

TABLE 15.2. The Male Couple: Stages, Dynamics, and Problems

Stages	Stage-related dynamics	Stage-related problems
Stage 1: *Blending* (first year)	• Intense togetherness • Similarities > differences • Shared attitude of equality • Frequent and exclusive sexual activity	• Magnifying and minimizing conflict • Disillusionment and withdrawal • Fear of intimacy • Resistance to merger
Stage 2: *Nesting* (1 to 3 years)	• Home decorating or refurbishing • Finding complementarity • Uneven reduction in limerence • Mixed feelings about relationship	• Passion declines, irritations emerge • Familiarity breeds disagreement • Failures and faults are noticed • Increase in jealous possessiveness
Stage 3: *Maintaining* (3 to 5 years)	• Individual differences reemerge • Outside liaisons or separate friends • Jealousy and differences of opinion • Steadfastness, comfort, and familiarity	• Differentiation provokes fear of loss • Separate needs are misunderstood • Risk taking generates anger or anxiety • Lack of conflict resolution skills
Stage 4: *Collaborating* (5 to 10 years)	• More security, less "processing" • New energy for generativity • Developing autonomy • Balancing individuality and intimacy	• Distancing generates fear of loss • Stage discrepancy frequently occurs (one comfortable with distance, the other dependent and clinging)
Stage 5: *Trusting* (10 to 20 years)	• Greater confidence in relationship • Mutual lack of possessiveness • Isolation and introversion of partners • Taking the partnership for granted	• Concerns of aging • Routine and monotony • Personality traits often rigidify • Struggles to change each other
Stage 6: *Repartnering* (20 years and beyond)	• Accomplishing objectives • Assuming permanence • Existential concerns • Reminiscing about relationship	• Restlessness • Withdrawal • Aimlessness • Changing partners to renew self

Note. Summarized from McWhirter & Mattison (1984).

believe that this estrangement is the most common cause of gay men ending their relationships before the end of the first year. Fear of merger or engulfment generated by the intensity of the blending (due to the previously discussed gender socialization of men to avoid intimacy and closeness) is another contributing factor.

STAGE 2

Nesting couples often focus on making a home together and finding compatibility. At the same time, however, differences become apparent and irritations are allowed to emerge. Emotional and sexual rapport naturally declines, and there often is an ambivalent mixture of positive and negative feelings about the relationship. The decline in limerence usually is not simultaneous and varies in intensity for the individual partners. Since the original high passion is no longer available to shield the couple from annoyances with each other, outside sexual interests sometimes ensue. Possessiveness and jealousies may result since these kinds of activities often are perceived as incompatible with the establishment of a permanent bond.

STAGE 3

Couples who have been together from 3 to 5 years experience a negotiation or *Maintaining* phase. To sustain their partnership, members need to balance several competing variables, such as individuation and togetherness, autonomy and dependence, conflict resolution and avoidance, and confusion and understanding. Needs for outside liaisons, separate friendships, and time spent apart can bring about misunderstandings about the needs of the mate to be separate, as well as increased fears, jealousies, and conflict. Differences and unpleasant emotions experienced at Stage 2 frequently are intensified as new angers and anxieties arise. Often only the intense blending of earlier stages enables the men to remain together. Additionally, the traditions that they have established over the years further cement the relationship, as well as facilitate their seeing the partnership as comfortable, steadfast, and dependable.

STAGE 4

McWhirter and Mattison (1982) first referred to this phase as *Collaborating* and noted that "besides the usual meaning of 'cooperation,' collaboration also implies giving aid to an occupying enemy" (1982, p. 82; 1996, p. 328). More recently (1996), they have termed the stage *Building*, presumably for a future together. The 6 to 10 years as partners frequently have resulted in declining communication between them, the making of unverified assumptions about each other, and feelings of boredom and entrapment. Some couples collude in mutual distancing or in professional activity outside the relationship in order to maintain harmony which, in turn, often leads to effective complementarity. In addition, this collaboration to maintain a degree of separateness between them helps dissipate feelings of engulfment or enmeshment, as well as provides sufficient dissimilarity to counteract apathy. Fears of loss, nevertheless, may be a consequence of this distancing, but if the efforts to preserve equanimity are successful, the energy not consumed by conflict or loss can be devoted to mutual and individual productivity, such as business partnerships, careers, and professional advancements. These kinds of efforts are facilitated by the "dependable availability of a partner for support, guidance, and affirmation" (1996, p. 328).

STAGE 5

By this stage, *Trusting* (1982, 1984) or *Releasing* (1996), couples who have been together from 11 to 20 years have come to invest confidence in each other and in the relationship. The possessiveness of earlier phases has decreased, and partners probably have developed a strong positive regard for each other. The gradual merger of money and possessions may be a manifestation of this trust. However, a possible age-related constrictedness may occur as individuals become isolated from themselves, their mates, and their friends. In addition to this tendency to become more rigid and inflexible, other concerns of aging transpire. Partners can struggle to change each other in spite of having been together for over 10 years. However, if they take each other for granted, monotony and routine can plague the relationship.

STAGE 6

McWhirter and Mattison found that these pairs (20 years and beyond) have reached a turning point in their relationship, and the twentieth anniversary appears to be a special milestone for many gay couples (1996). They often report a renewal in terms of how they relate to each other. Hence, this phase has been termed *Repartnering* (1982, 1984) or *Renewing* (1996). The mates assume they will be with each other until death, and they often spend time reminiscing about the passage of time and their years together. For many individuals and couples, their personal, financial, and professional goals have been adequately achieved, but concerns about health, security, loneliness, and death are apparent. Some men may change partners in order to alleviate feelings of restlessness, withdrawal, and aimlessness. Since the original data were collected, McWhirter and Mattison (1996) have continued to interview Stage 6 pairs and have found men who have been in coupled relationships for more than 50 years. The authors note that the development of compatibility is a lifelong task for any male couple and older mates must "continue to focus on compatibility and companionship as crucial ingredients of their ongoing commitment" (p. 334).

Considerations

A few points need to be considered regarding the use of McWhirter and Mattison (1982, 1984) stages just discussed. First, their model was based on a cross-sectional rather than a longitudinal research design and, thus, different individuals were interviewed at the six stages along the continuum. Because these subjects were from 20 to 69 years of age, the question of cohort differences arises. For example, the older men who had been in relationships for more than 20 years undoubtedly lived in quite dissimilar social and political circumstances when they were in the earlier phases of their relationships than McWhirter and Mattison's younger Stage 1 and Stage 2 subjects. McWhirter and Mattison (1996) note that Stage 6 men grew up in a much more repressed era and, hence, many of their beliefs and feelings may reflect internalized anti-gay attitudes: "Although at the present time these problems appear to be stage related, they may not be found to the same extent among gay men in the future" (p. 330). Moreover, the two researchers interviewed only couples who had lived together for at least 1 year. As discussed earlier in this chapter (see "Residence," and Harry, 1983), not all male couples share the same household, but probably more do today than in previous eras, given the somewhat more accepting societal conditions. Again, then, possible difficulties arise because of cohort differences among subjects and the problems inherent in the cross-sectional nature of the research.

McWhirter and Mattison (1982) admit that their stages are "tentative formulations needing further clinical trial and research validation" (p. 80). Since the original model was conceptualized, the authors have expanded and applied it to the psychotherapy process (Mattison & McWhirter, 1987a, 1987b). Their conceptualizations also have been used for research purposes numerous times since their presentation in the early 1980s (e.g., Deenen, 1988), and the authors believe that this stage formulation has acquired greater validity over time. They further see it "as a beginning to understanding the complex phenomenon of male couples" (McWhirter & Mattison, 1996, p. 326). Because a study on the order of the original survey never has been replicated, clinicians should use the model only as a framework for understanding the dynamics and complaints of male couples, "which in turn can lead to a better assessment of the couples' difficulties and the development of new strategies of treatment intervention" (Mattison & McWhirter, 1987b, p. 99).

Lesbian Couples

There is no model for lesbian couples comparable to the empirically based conceptualization of Mattison and McWhirter for male couples (Klinger, 1996). From their clinical and personal experiences, however, Clunis and Green (1988) blended ideas from models for heterosexual relationships (Campbell, 1980) and gay male partnerships (McWhirter & Mattison, 1982, 1984) in order to outline six stages of development for lesbian couples. Pearlman (1988) referred to similar developmental phases when she discussed the impact of distancing and connectedness on couple formation in lesbian relationships. Slater (1995) maintained that these and similar models did not extend throughout the course of the lifespan, so she proposed a 5-stage prototype that extends from the formation of the couple until the death of one of them. Borrowing from "the advantage enjoyed by researchers of heterosexual family life cycles" (p. 21), she assumed that partners came together in their 20s and remained together until old age. She accordingly refers to her model as the Lesbian Family Life Cycle as "lesbian couples constitute complete family units" (p. 32).

Table 15.3 summarizes the passages outlined by Clunis and Green and Pearlman, along with the general dynamics and possible problems encountered at each transition. Slater's conceptualizations are not included in the table as she provided her stages with unique titles, as well as contextualized her last three phases within an age-related framework. Her ideas, however, are interwoven into the following narrative discussion of the stages in Table 15.3.

Stages

STAGE 1

Clunis and Green (1988) refer to the *Prerelationship* phase of lesbian couple formation as "the 'getting to know you' stage" (p. 10). It involves two women dating and spending time together. Whether this period of time lasts a matter of weeks, days, or even hours, the primary task for the lesbian couple is making choices. During this initial phase, decisions are made based on each partner's willingness to include being sexual, as well as to invest time and energy, in the prerelationship process of getting acquainted. These options, however, often do not feel like choices when either or both of the women proceed without clarifying and communicating their expectations and intentions. In this regard, Clunis and Green (1988) identify three stage-specific barriers to clear communication: "making assumptions; mind reading; and being unsure about what is reasonable" (p. 12).

While men as well as women are inclined toward making assumptions about the nature of their dating relationships, the male-dominant culture and society teaches its fe-

TABLE 15.3. The Lesbian Couple: Stages, Dynamics, and Problems

Stages	Stage-related dynamics	Stage-related problems
Stage 1: *Prerelationship*	• Getting acquainted, dating, spending time • Deciding whether to invest time and energy • Deciding whether to include being sexual	• Making assumptions • Mind reading • Unreasonable expectations
Stage 2: *Romance/limerence*	• Merger and fusion • Loss of ego boundary and individuality • Shared dreams and fantasies • Intense emotional and sexual intimacy	• Minimizing potential irritations • Neglecting friends • Social isolation from family and community • Premature cohabitation
Stage 3: *Conflict/power or control*	• Struggles over power and dependency • Individual boundaries reestablished • Couple solidarity tested • Unrealistic expectations not fulfilled	• Feeling too close or trapped • Tension over reduced sexual frequency • Feelings of disappointment and resentment • Lack of conflict resolution skills
Stage 4: *Acceptance*	• Sense of stability and contentment • Mutual acceptance of faults and failures • Less blaming, more self-awareness • Patterns recognized, problems resolved	• Considerable unresolved conflict • Persistent power struggles • Testing of loyalties • Denial and avoidance of problems
Stage 5: *Commitment*	• Abandoning search for perfect partner • Coming to terms with contradictions • Balancing separateness and togetherness • Maintaining or recapturing passion	• Relationship stabilized around conflict • Excessive dependency • Lack of acceptable ways to be separate • Pseudomutuality
Stage 6: *Recommitment/ collaboration*	• Focusing beyond the relationship • Directing energy into joint projects • Intimacy begets generativity • Recycling through earlier stages	• Outside activities threaten connection • Failure to develop outside interests • Personal and professional stagnation • Conflicts of earlier stages

Note. Summarized from Clunis & Green (1988), and Pearlman (1988).

male members, in particular, that "mind reading is a loving communication" (Clunis & Green, 1988, p. 13). Many lesbians thus assume that if they really love each other, then both they and their partners should be able to anticipate each other's wants and needs without having to be prompted. These tendencies to make assumptions, however, often lead to feelings of betrayal, disappointment, and resentment. Additionally, most women have been taught to believe that if they just give enough of themselves, then their partners will take care of them. Consequently, they never learn to evaluate the difference between reasonable compromise and excessive sacrifice.

STAGE 2

Another early stage of lesbian relationship development has been referred to as a period of merger and fusion called *Romance* or *Limerence* (Clunis & Green, 1988; Pearlman, 1988) or *Formation of the Couple* (Slater, 1995). During this phase of evolution, individuality and ego boundaries are surrendered as partners blend and bond together, share their dreams and fantasies, and imagine a common future. This period of sexual passion, rapture, and emotional closeness is profound, especially for women with similar gender role conditioning and reciprocal feminine capacities for empathy and intimacy. Such intensity is both reinforced and reinforcing when lovers maximize their similarities and minimize their differences: "Even relatively minor disagreements can take on exaggerated significance, as they challenge the partners' subconscious fantasies that their bliss can remain uninterrupted" (Slater, 1995, p. 130). The couple therefore may complicate this early stage by not allowing for the development of skills to manage conflict between the members. Additionally, those mates who tend to rely almost exclusively on each other often forsake the very friends on whom so many sexual minorities depend for the emotional support not otherwise forthcoming from their families of origin. This kind of benign neglect frequently leads couples to premature cohabitation and social isolation, as well as negatively influences the communication and intimacy between them (S. E. James & Murphy, 1998). In addition, as with all couples who bond deeply, anxiety related to childhood or past relational rejection, hurt, and abuse can resurface. These unresolved memories and emotions intensify vulnerability, making learning to trust even more difficult (Slater, 1995).

STAGE 3

The next phase of lesbian couple formation has been called the stage of *Conflict* (Clunis & Green, 1988), *Power* or *Control* (Campbell, 1980; Pearlman, 1988), and *Ongoing Couplehood* (Slater, 1995). During this period of relationship development, the solidarity of the lesbian couple is tested as the ego boundaries that were surrendered previously in favor of merger and fusion are reestablished and members grapple over issues of power and dependency: "The partners will return to wanting distinct lives despite the more blended relational space they will continue to inhabit" (Slater, 1995, p. 127). These evolutionary struggles often feel threatening, particularly to women who reject patriarchal power relations and espouse feminist values of equality (S. E. James & Murphy, 1998; Klinger, 1996). During this difficult time of blending lives, a delicate balance exists between solidifying the relationship, while simultaneously establishing limits on that connection. Slater (1995) believes that partners must learn to distinguish manageable disappointments from basic underlying incompatibility as they struggle to blend needs for both closeness and distance, as well as desires to remain connected while still having individual boundaries and separate identities. Throughout this process, they acquire new information about their partner's personality, defensive styles, future dreams, and early lives, and this knowledge usually results in feelings of ambivalence that "break the infatuation that characterized the first life cycle stage" (Slater, 1995, p. 171).

Lesbians place particular priority on maintaining feelings of "oceanic oneness" (Slater, 1995, p. 158) with their mates. When these unrealistic expectations for the ideal egalitarian relationship are frustrated, lovers may be tempted to abandon their partnership in search of a more perfect union. In contrast, some members of Stage 3 couples begin to feel suffocated if the merger and fusion of the second phase is prolonged, but differences ensure that they will not be engulfed by each other. Overfamiliarity likewise smothers the sexual passion of the earlier stages, and, as romance and limerence decline, intense feelings of disappointment and resentment often emerge. If partners foreclose at this phase of couplehood, they risk transferring their conflict avoidance to subsequent relationships. When they maintain their connection by resolving their differences, however, feelings of trust and partnership satisfaction are strengthened.

STAGE 4

Clunis and Green (1988) describe the *Acceptance* stage of relationship development as "the calm after the storm" (p. 20). Slater (1995) refers to *The Middle Years* in keeping with her lifespan model of couple evolution, but many of the dynamics and concepts she describes are similar to those of Clunis and Green's Stages 4 and 5. At Stage 4, or in the midlife era, lesbian couples experience a sense of stability and anchoring as they see themselves moving into permanent or long-range commitment. While contentment and deepening mutual affection characterize this period, Slater (1995) contends that raising the stakes for the relationship evokes strong emotional reactions that include both joy and powerful anxiety associated with extending and deepening the investment. Since members have become more aware of the limitations of their mates over the years, some begin to worry that those realities will forever narrow their own opportunities to develop themselves if they remain with this particular partner. While most women learn to accept their own limitations and project less blame onto each other, others come to fear "relational mortality" (p. 179) to the point where they limit the intensity of their involvement or leave what they see as a (potentially) stagnant relationship: "These twin searches—for newness in a no-longer-new relationship, and for stability that does not degenerate into stagnation—constitute the primary tasks" (p. 179) of this phase of development.

The *Acceptance* phase or *The Middle Years* can be gratifying if mates are flexible enough to adapt the relationship to accommodate each woman's personal growth. Partner discrepancies in levels of relational self-differentiation, however, may be experienced as dangerous distances in lesbian relationships. If these differences are denied or avoided, there is a tendency for unresolved tensions to mount, power struggles to persist, and loyalty tests to follow. Resistance to negotiation, the submerging of negative feelings, or keeping peace at all costs may prove more damaging to the bond than the actual content of the emotions. Still, a more complex understanding of themselves, their mates, and of the relationship itself can assist members in reworking the rewards and disappointments, as well as the limits and liberations, inherent in a long-term commitment (Slater, 1995). This increased interpersonal objectivity also can help partners recognize their dysfunctional patterns of behavior and communication, thus bringing forth an enhanced perspective that enables the more effective use of negotiation skills.

STAGE 5

At this phase of couple formation, which appears to include many of the dynamics of Slater's (1995) *The Middle Years*, Clunis and Green (1988) define *Commitment* as "the decision to make choices about the relationship and be responsible for them" (p. 23).

They further contend that this quality of a partnership cannot be established before the power struggle of the *Conflict* stage or the relational self-differentiation of the *Acceptance* stage. *Commitment* involves relinquishing the quest for an ideal lover and reconciling contradictory needs for separateness and togetherness. During the *Conflict* stage, for example, partner differences can become polarized. In the *Acceptance* phase, each individual recognizes her needs for both autonomy and intimacy, but Stage 5 couples realize that these apparent contradictions are not mutually exclusive and that their relationships require a balance of both distance and closeness. To maintain this kind of stability, partners must establish liberating structures (Campbell, 1980) for meeting individual needs, as well as for enhancing their couplehood. These arrangements may include activities for maintaining passion despite sexual familiarity or for recapturing the limerence and romance of Stage 2, such as dating rituals, weekend getaways, or erotic experimentation.

According to Pearlman (1988), conflict resolution at the earlier phase of *Power* or *Control* prepares lesbian partners for "the later stages of commitment and re-commitment based on more individuality and separateness" (p. 81). When power struggles continue to persist beyond the fourth phase of *Acceptance*, Stage 5 relationships often collude to avoid and otherwise accommodate the tension around which they now stabilize. Further, partnerships held together by excessive dependency may regress to a more undifferentiated state of pseudomutuality when balancing separateness and togetherness feels too threatening (Lindenbaum, 1985; Pearlman, 1988).

STAGE 6

Successful satisfaction of previous phase-specific conditions fosters a *Recommitment* to the partnership. According to Clunis and Green (1988), *Collaboration* is the final period of relationship development, during which "women focus on something bigger than the two of them to share with the world" (p. 27) and direct the energy cultivated within the context of their intimacy into joint projects. Slater (1995) refers to this phase as *Generativity*, a time during which partners link themselves to a larger network of others to create something that will endure beyond their own finite existence. She also believes that, for many individuals and couples, this phase evolves out of a genuine crisis in which people become aware of a need to create a legacy for themselves or their couplehood in the remaining years they have together.

Couples entrenched in prolonged merger usually have fashioned their relationship such that it prevents the formation of flexible and liberating structures. Externally focused activities and interests, hence, are seen as threats to the exclusive connections of the members in the dyad. When either fear or neglect prevent the development of cooperative undertakings for the benefit of others, personal self-absorption and professional stagnation may affect one or both partners. Slater (1995) additionally believes that partnerships need shared central involvements to thrive, and lesbian couples who feel they must hide their relationship are severely compromised in their ability to build a family legacy. The need for secrecy about their partnership leaves members of these pairs only the option of pursuing separate generative commitments.

Slater (1995) ends her stages with one called *Lesbian Couples Over Sixty-Five* and this phase includes many of the issues that were discussed in Chapter 7 related to later life. Couples at this time are faced with concerns associated with retirement from work for one or both members, including the renegotiation of the blend between separateness and togetherness in their relationship. Because life is centered more at home during this phase of life, the various aspects of the women's time together and apart must be realigned. Fears of losing autonomy may resurface, which also may make sexual intimacy more threatening than previously when work gave each individual a separate identity. Accordingly, since members also may need to reestablish areas of distinctiveness, joint and individual projects may need to be reconceptualized. Present are issues common to all long-term and aging couples, such as health concerns, finances, loss of friends and family, and inevitable widowhood. If one or both mates have used isolation and compartmentalization as lifetime coping strategies for dealing with their lesbian status (which is not unusual in this age cohort), the final phase of life may be quite difficult. Alternatively, less-closeted individuals and couples may find that the social support provided by family, friends, and the lesbian community can buffer fairly well many of the effects of old age.

Considerations

Like McWhirter and Mattison (1982), Clunis and Green (1988) caution their readers to consider that "relationship development is a process, and the stages blend into each other" (p. 9). Although the phases often overlap and have features in common, each has its own specific characteristics, developmental tasks, and problems. Social class, ethnicity, and the presence of children, among other variables, also influence the extent to which this model applies to a specific lesbian partnership. Slater (1995) specifically discusses four trajectories that continually intersect to shape the developmental processes for each couple: the chronological age of each member; the stage of lesbian identity development of each (see Chapter 5), relevant issues of minority identity development for lesbians of color (see Chapter 10), and the stages of the lesbian family life cycle.

Stage Discrepancies

Movement from one stage to another is essential for growth and, as discussed previously in regard to several developmental trajectories, these processes occur over the lifetime of individuals. The situation is somewhat more complicated for same-sex couples in that two people often move through stages of identity formation at different rates, revert to characteristics of earlier phases in distinct ways, or experience unique periods of development at any given point in time. Mattison and McWhirter (1987b) note that "stage discrepancy between partners is one of the most common experiences in relationship development" and that much "psychotherapy with male couples focuses on elucidating and resolving stage-related discrepancies" (p. 92). Accordingly, they estimate that over half the couples seen in treatment are struggling with some form of stage discrepancy (McWhirter & Mattison, 1982, 1987b, 1996).

Slater (1995) similarly notes that stage discrepancies between members of a lesbian couple are virtually assured, given that "couple relationships begin before the partners have reached the final stage of incorporating their sexual identities" (p. 25). In fact, she contends that many of these partnerships begin even before the bulk of identity development work has occurred, resulting in members who grapple with their own individual growth and couple development simultaneously. A common situation in this regard occurs when one woman is more comfortable with her lesbian identity than is the other with hers and when the partner who is farther along pushes for increased exposure of the relationship. If the slower spouse hesitates or is frightened at the thought of public disclosure, the other member may perceive her mate's reluctance as an inability or an unwillingness to support them as a couple. On occasion, both parties may interpret the motives of the other as betrayal, or even as evidence that her partner is not invested in the relationship or does not love her enough to respect her wishes. Forstein (1986) discusses a comparable set of circumstances wherein a more mature person in a Stage 1 relationship becomes individuated from the dyad, while the less mature person feels isolated, rejected, and deserted: "Differences between the partners' capacity for intimacy are likely to be exacerbated as one member begins to move from one stage of development to another" (p. 115). When this occurs, the less precocious individual sometimes becomes demanding and dependent in order to defend against fears of separation and abandonment, while the more individuated member of the couple may feel intense "ambivalence about intimacy as his partner exerts a regressive pull toward merging and unindividuated attachment" (p. 116).

Other common stage-related discrepancies seen in psychotherapy with same-sex couples include the need to individuate and have separate friends or activities in Stage 3 either conflicting with the merging of a dependent mate or threatening the dependability of a Stage 4 partner; the high limerence of the initial phase, in sharp contrast with the decline in passion in the following phase; or a Stage 4 couple in which one is fairly independent and individuated while the other is confused, fearful for the future of the relationship, overly dependent and clinging desperately to his or her partner (Mattison & McWhirter, 1987b; McWhirter & Mattison, 1982, 1996).

Therapeutic Considerations

During therapy with couples, relational distress can be reduced when "behaviors, interactions, and feelings formerly considered flaws in the relationships, or individual personality defects, are seen here as merely characteristic of a certain stage" (McWhirter & Mattison, 1982, p. 80), or as a result of the "interplay of individual and relational tasks they are confronting" (Slater, 1995, p. 27). Rarely, however, will couples initially conceptualize their difficulties in terms of stage discrepancies. Rather, partners will describe behavioral manifestations of phase discordance, such as problems with intimacy, sex, power, competition, control, jealously, anger, or tenderness. If therapists can help clients see that many of their concerns do not necessarily indicate the inevitable demise of their alliance but, rather, are a by-product of correctable developmental inequities and differences in the growth of both themselves and their relationship, couples often feel considerable relief (Mattison & McWhirter, 1987b; McWhirter & Mattison, 1996; Slater, 1995). Not all stage discrepancies lend themselves to rapid improvement, but "the understanding derived from the cognitive framework of stage discrepancy makes the affective problems easier to handle and to treat" (McWhirter & Mattison, 1996, p. 331).

Cabaj and Klinger (1996) have provided guidelines for evaluation and assessment to therapists who work with same-sex couples. They conceptualize assessment as having four dimensions: clinical evaluation of each member, individual level of gay or lesbian development, staging of the relationship, and issues external to the relationship. They further suggest several diagnostic and special circumstances: presence of concurrent mental illness; presence of domestic violence in the relationship; HIV concerns of the couple;

stage discrepancies between members; and issues of intimacy, such as dynamics of merger and distance.

Finally, assigned reading can assist couples in better understanding their relationship, as well as in acquiring the skills and behaviors to help them navigate through conflict and difficulties. Fortunately, books written to improve the lives of lesbian and gay couples are continually appearing in the bookstores, and both therapists and clients are encouraged to spend time perusing the ever-expanding collection (e.g., Berzon, 1997; Driggs, 1991; M. Hall, 1998; Hanes, 1997; Isensee, 1996, 1997; Marcus, 1992, 1999; Outland, 1998).

CONCLUSION

This chapter converged around the concepts of heterosexism and gender role socialization as they affect the dynamics and relationship stages of same-sex couples. Therapeutic considerations were interspersed throughout these discussions, and Chapter 16 focuses specifically on sex therapy with lesbian and gay male partners. The same two themes again will be interwoven throughout the discourse since internalized heterosexism and masculine or feminine gender conditioning constitute the basis of many relationship and sexual difficulties for same-sex couples.

16

Sex Therapy with Gay and Lesbian Couples

Just as internalized heterosexism and gender role socialization influence the dynamics and relationships stages of lesbian and gay couples, they also affect the domain of sexual functioning. Because the ramifications of these phenomena were discussed extensively in Chapter 15, only material directly related to their influence on gay and lesbian sexuality are provided in this chapter. Due to the pervasiveness of their effects, however, these two concepts are woven through much of the following discussion.

HETEROSEXIST BIAS

The basic suppositions that underlie the field of sex therapy are heteronormative in nature (Stack, 1999). Heterosexist bias permeates the discourse, as well as the perceptions, of many sexual minorities regarding their own intimate activity (Frye, 1990; N. O'Connor & Ryan, 1993; Quinodoz, 1989; A. E. Schwartz, 1998). When commenting about the mainstream field of sex therapy, Nichols (1987a) notes the degree of subjectivity involved in diagnosis (e.g., *premature* ejaculation or *inhibited* sexual desire), as well as heterocentric assumptions that underlie most of the major sexual "dysfunctions." She contends, in this regard, that the common characteristic of many disorders appears to be the extent to which intercourse between men and women is difficult, if not impossible. Rarely, however, do lesbians complain of vaginismus or dyspareunia (painful intercourse), and some of the most common problems reported by lesbians (oral sex aversions) and gay men (anal sex difficulties) are virtually ignored (B. R. Rosser, Short, Thurmes, & Coleman, 1998). Finally, the emphasis on mutual orgasm within the field of traditional sex therapy leaves many sexual minorities feeling as if their typical style of "your turn, my turn" sex (Nichols, 1987a, p. 244) is defective or incomplete. In the following sections, other heterosexist influences on lesbian and gay male sexual attitudes

344

and functioning are discussed. Concepts related to gender role socialization are interspersed throughout this discourse.

Influences on Lesbian Sexual Relationships

Effective female sexual functioning is a social construct that has changed dramatically in the last century, and models of lesbian sexuality (in any form) have emerged only recently (L. S. Brown, 1985, 1986; Frye, 1990; M. Hall, 1998; Nichols, 1987a; N. O'Connor & Ryan, 1993; A. E. Schwartz, 1998). Most of the literature related to sexual functioning between women is observational in nature, and relies mostly on the clinical experience of therapists for its grounding. Hence, many lesbian clients who report sexual difficulties have formed inaccurate or inadequate notions of normative lesbian sexual functioning based on heterosexist or masculine notions of ideal sexual behavior.

Just as female sexuality obviously is unlike male sexuality, lesbian sexual expression is distinctly different from heterosexual coupling. Because of sexism and homophobia, lesbians frequently evaluate their sexuality against standards based on male sexual desire and experience, and they often require information about and perspective on what is natural for women who engage in intimate relations with other women (A. E. Schwartz, 1998; Slater, 1995). Frye (1990), for example, believes that many have internalized the invalidating messages that their lovemaking activities are less than complete since penile-vaginal intercourse does not occur. According to her, the rhythms of lesbian love and passion cannot be mapped on "8-minute" male definitions of sex, and typical sexual discourses include no linguistic matrix for the experiences and emotions of lesbian sexuality. L. S. Brown (1986) similarly believes that sexual desire disorders, rather than being generalized aversions, represent a fear of lesbian sexuality that is rooted in internalized heterosexism. If these beliefs devaluing relationships between women are not surfaced in therapy, they will continue to function as self-fulfilling prophecies and persist in undermining sexual functioning. The most important task of clinicians, then, is to give clients permission to see lesbian eroticism not only as normative but also as healthy and positive (Glassgold, 1995; M. Hall, 1998; B. Kassoff, 1995; Rose, 1994; Slater, 1995).

Few lesbians come to therapy prepared to discuss sex (even though they may be requesting help for sexual problems), and often therapists must request specific details regarding the history, nature, and frequency of their difficulties (Nichols, 1987a; N. O'Connor & Ryan, 1993). Due to heterosexist cultural conditioning, many clients will be fairly inexperienced in actually discussing lovemaking between women, even though they may engage in such encounters. Nevertheless, the way clients respond to the inquiry will provide insights as to their level of comfort with lesbian sexuality.

Internalized Images

L. S. Brown (1986) notes that the majority of her clients appear to have internalized images of sexual contact between women that have been gleaned from popular culture. These include portrayals of sex between lesbians as either (1) *brutal* (i.e., sexual assaults in prisons and back alleys, or experiences that occur in squalid and degrading situations in which both participants are under the influence of drugs or alcohol); or (2) "wonderful, *magical,* exciting beyond words, and remarkable as a cure-all for female sexual ills" (p. 101; emphasis added). She contends that clients who see their lesbian sexuality as debased and negative often experience problems in the desire phase of sexual arousal (discussed later in this chapter). They frequently feel anxious, humiliated, and ashamed when they become sexually aroused with other women, and they sometimes resort to drugs and alcohol to tranquilize that discomfort.

In any case, L. S. Brown (1986) asserts that both of these phenomena—brutal and magical—have their psychological roots in cultural homophobia, which maintains that genital sexuality between women places those who thus engage in a "negative, marginal, and disparate lifestyle" (p. 102). To counteract this internalized heterosexism and possibly to prove that these unfavorable images are inaccurate, some lesbians establish a dichotomy in reference to their lovemaking. Now, rather than seeing their sexual activities as shaming and degrading, they have elevated them to such an idealized status that they are virtually impossible to experience. Often, the result in each of these instances is intense anxiety and inhibition during all phases of sexual functioning.

This polarization becomes fairly rigid for some women and results in what Nichols (1987b, p. 97) referred to as "P. C. [politically correct] lesbian lovemaking." According to her, this prescription for intimate activity evolved as a reaction to societal heterosexism and misogyny. The prescribed formula mandates that:

> Two women lie side by side (tops or bottoms are strictly forbidden—lesbians must be nonhierarchical); they touch each other gently and sweetly all over their bodies for several hours (lesbians are not genitally/orgasm oriented, a patriarchal mode). If women have orgasms at all—and orgasms are only marginally acceptable because, after all, we must be process, rather than goal, oriented—both orgasms must occur at exactly the same time in order to foster true equality and egalitarianism. (pp. 97–98)

While lesbian (and gay male) relationships may be more "advanced" in regard to fewer gender-based power differentials and sex role conflicts than heterosexual relationships, "what may be good politics may make for bad sex" (p. 105).

Egalitarianism

Drawing from her clinical experience, Nichols (1987b) observes that the ethic of equality or correct lesbian sex causes much stress in relationships. The valuing of egalitarianism between partners, for example, renders many lesbians reluctant to pressure a recalcitrant mate into sexual relations. These women perceive a demand for sex as a male-oriented and abusive behavior that contradicts their notion that sexual desire should flow naturally from the love within the partnership and not be activated by coercion or intimidation. Accordingly, "the conflict between agency and internalized gender role can become paralyzing, especially if it is unknown or unacknowledged" (A. E. Schwartz, 1998, p. 60). Thus, lesbian sexual expression can be compromised by gender socialization that equates taking the role of sexual aggressor as masculine rather than feminine behavior (B. Kassoff, 1995; N. O'Connor & Ryan, 1993; A. E. Schwartz, 1998; Slater, 1995). Nichols (1987a) contends that therapists must continually examine with couples their "differing, conflictual, or covert sets of expectations about how sex should be among partners" (p. 248), and clients should be reassured that there is no one way to be lesbian. Neither heterosexist conceptualizations and idealized norms nor masculine versus feminine dichotomies should determine what is right and acceptable for them if they are comfortable with any given set of behaviors.

Parenthetically, therapists should keep in mind that not all lesbians are concerned about maintaining egalitarianism in their relationships. Until recently, most of the literature on lesbian couples reflected primarily the views of White, middle-class, educated women who often advocate more feminist positions than women in general. When Royse and Clawson (1988) studied 132 self-identified feminists (from 19 to 80 years old), for example, no significant differences on the Sex-Role Egalitarianism Scale among heterosexual, bisexual, and lesbian subjects were found. In other words, the lesbians in the study advocated no more sex role egalitarianism than did bisexual or heterosexual women. Thus, unless lesbians clients also describe themselves as feminists, clinicians may not see the emphasis in their relationships on equality and "political correctness" as described here and later in this chapter (see "Power").

Influences on Gay Male Sexual Relationships

As discussed in previous chapters, gay men frequently internalize the negative societal perceptions of homosexuality and hence split off their sexuality from the rest of their selves (R. L. Hawkins, 1992; Linde, 1998). This internal rupture results in difficulties with same-sex intimacy, as well as in "struggles over issues involving body image, sexualization, body-centered externalization, and alienation from self and community" (Canarelli et al., 1999, p. 49). Further, gay males who adapt to their interpersonal environment by splitting their emotional needs and their erotic feelings frequently experience sexual difficulties since "the sexual drive which may orient one toward intimacy with another person has been transformed into a danger signal of asserting one's homosexuality" (Forstein, 1986, p. 120).

Usually because of masculine gender role socialization, shame created by lack of acceptance and mirroring that results in internalized homophobia, some gay men can tolerate only a limited level of intimacy and may find being in an emotionally close relationship extremely anxiety provoking (Canarelli et al., 1999; Vaughan, 1999). Many of these men report being able to masturbate successfully when alone, but feel extremely anxious and have difficulty maintaining an erection and reaching orgasm with a partner (C. Friedman, 1998). For some, sexual activity outside the primary bond reduces the tension that is associated with intimacy, attachment, or potential engulfment. For still others, a period of sexual exploration with multiple partners during the coming-out process, or even long-term compulsive sexual activity, facilitates the avoidance of ongoing alliances. These short-lived encounters temporarily meet their needs for closeness while, at the same time, prevent them from having to deal with the much-feared issues of trust and intimacy that are continually present in long-term relationships.

Anxiety Reduction

"The fantasies that fuel driven sex have to do with enlivening a deadened interior and soothing and consolidating the sense of a fragmented self," say Canarelli et al. (1999, p. 59). Pincu (1989) discusses gay men who have developed a habit of using sex to reduce the anxiety created by isolation, low self-esteem, and loneliness. The sexualization of this distress "distracts or alters feelings so that a person does not have to feel loneliness or the emptiness of abandonment" (p. 64). While repetitive sexual behavior relieves emotions that are nonsexual in nature, "intimacy and relationships become subservient to the very physical act of sexual expression" (p. 64). Patterns of compulsive sexuality frequently become embedded when tension is reduced, and, for some men, the orgasmic release and the accompanying alleviation of anxiety produce sufficient reinforcement to keep the cycle in motion. Other gay men, in a sense, become addicted to the validation and excitement of the chase, which Pincu describes as "a rush, a quickening heartbeat, a nervousness, and an exhilaration" (p. 64). Those men who are the most conflicted or repressed regarding their homosexuality often are able to perform sexually only if the encounters are anonymous. The intimacy of a relationship in which they are known and emotionally close to another is extremely anxiety-provoking for these individuals. Hence, they split their sexuality from their affective core.

Splitting

Rarely as they are growing up do lesbians and gay men have the opportunity to integrate the sexual aspects of their beings into the totality of their sense of self. Many gay men, therefore, have compartmentalized their sexuality and split it off from the rest of their relationships. Some have learned to sexualize their association with other men such that their "sense of desirability, value, and self may be intricately linked to sex" (Linde, 1998, p. 350).

R. L. Hawkins (1992) believes that this splitting off of affection and erotic impulses results in some gay men developing "defenses that are narcissistic (need for self-validation or validation from others) or borderline (splitting and acting out)" (p. 84). He contends that these defenses usually are personality overlays that have been developed to cope with noxious heterosexist environments, rather than symptoms of actual personality disorders. Therapists, however, should conduct a thorough diagnosis to assess the pliability and resiliency of the defenses so that true narcissistic or borderline conditions can be ruled out (see discussion in Chapter 8).

Moreover, Forstein (1986) cautions against assuming that sexual activity outside of a primary relationship is always related to pathology, defensive splitting, characterological impairment, developmental arrest, or intimacy difficulties in one or both members of a male couple. Given what has been discussed previously about masculine socialization, therapists are likely to find a higher percentage of male couples than lesbian or heterosexual pairs in which the parties agree (either overtly or covertly) to engage sexually with others. Clinicians need to understand what issues such as sexual fidelity, sexual dysfunction, and compulsive sexuality mean to each couple, rather than seeing these behaviors through the lens of psychopathology or the values of heterosexist society.

Therapeutic Focus

Regardless of the idiosyncratic meanings, however, Forstein (1986) alleges that erotic activity outside of the primary relationship "often raises associated issues of trust, self-esteem, and dependency," as well as "concerns about competition, power, and control" (p. 119). Therapists are thus advised to pursue these paths of inquiry rather than to focus exclusively on the sexual behavior. While the majority of gay men have not responded to societal heterosexism and masculine gender role conditioning by becoming sexually compulsive or engaging in anonymous or clandestine sexual experiences, many nonetheless experience other problems with erotic functioning. Three categories of these dysfunctions will be discussed later in this chapter.

Clinicians should keep in mind that because men generally are socialized to view sex as affirmation of their masculinity, gay men are particularly vulnerable to using sex as a validation of their often-discredited manhood. For many, especially those who are self-loathing or gender-discordant, little else is available. Canarelli et al. (1999) note that lack of acceptance in childhood and adulthood "can result in compensatory attention-begetting behaviors, such as driven sexuality and compulsive body building" (pp. 47–48). In other words, the pursuit of attention often becomes the pervasive way of addressing the interpersonal environment. Their inner world is filled with anxiety and shame, and there is "little ability to tolerate the kinds of complex psychological tasks and compromises that all sustained intimate relationships require" (pp. 58–59). Therapists thus must approach many of the other sexual problems of gay men from this framework in order for clients to perceive the mirroring received in the therapeutic relationship as healing and affirming (Scasta, 1998).

ASSESSMENT

All treatment of sexual difficulties should begin with a thorough sexual history, which includes attention to any medical, chemical, or emotional problems that may be causing or contributing to the reported dysfunctions (Beckman & Ackerman, 1995; Berzon, 1988; L. S. Brown, 1985, 1986; George & Behrendt, 1987; M. Hall, 1987; Loulan, 1987, 1988; Nichols, 1987b, 1989; Reece, 1982, 1987). During this assessment, all relevant medical, psychological, and psychosocial concerns, including heterosexual experiences, coming-out histories, and negative messages about gay or lesbian sex, must be addressed. Occurrences of sexual abuse or assault should be noted, given their prevalence in sexual minority (especially lesbian) populations. Medical records or a physical examination, including laboratory tests, may be requested in order to rule out sexual dysfunction due to a general medical condition (American Psychiatric Association, 1994), and to appraise any neurological, hormonal or endocrine, or metabolic abnormalities that may specifically impair sexual desire or performance. Attention should also be given to HIV status, injuries, or urological or gynecological problems that may be contributing to the sexual difficulties. (Gynecological causes of sexual problems are less common in lesbians than in heterosexual women, given that dyspareunia, or painful intercourse, is rare among women who relate sexually with other women.) Additionally, clients who are seriously depressed, suicidal, or psychotic are not likely to benefit from sex therapy and should be treated for these conditions with other therapeutic methods (Reece, 1982).

Aversions

Aversions to specific sexual acts also should be discussed in the initial history, with focus given particularly to oral and anal sex and penetration issues. Nichols (1987a) notes that this discussion should be an explicit and matter-of-fact conversation "even in the face of giggles, shuffling feet, red faces, and averted eyes" (p. 251). For some individuals, an aversion to specific acts (e.g., a partner who enjoys oral or anal sex; or has a nonsensual or genital/orgasm orientation toward sexuality; or emphasizes fantasy or role playing as opposed to personal interaction; or has an "earthy" attitude toward bodily secretions and smells) may be more the issue than a generalized lack of sexual desire (McWhirter & Mattison, 1980; Reece, 1987).

Aversion to oral sex is also an extremely common complaint in lesbian couples. Sometimes if both women are equally uncomfortable with cunnilingus *and* each believes that avoiding it does not diminish the quality of their lovemaking, then they simply can eliminate the behavior from their repertoire without experiencing much anxiety. Usually, however, one or both women believe that something is missing from their experiences together and approach the therapist for help. The deficit may not be felt as much on the physical level as on the emotional one, however. That is, some women have come to assume that committed lesbian couples *should* have oral sex as a part of their lovemaking and that their coupling is something less than "real" sex if these kinds of behaviors are forsaken (Loulan, 1984, p. 87). Others hold the view that lesbian sex is good and pure so that cunnilingus is too dirty, vulgar, or heterosexist to be a part of their coupling.

Painful receptive anal intercourse is a common, yet underacknowledged, difficulty in gay men (Rosser, Metz, Bockting, & Buroker, 1997). A study of 277 men was designed to examine the frequency and duration of pain in same-sex anal intercourse (Rosser et al., 1998). Using a 7-point Likert scale, the severity of pain appeared positively skewed, with 12% of the men rating it as too painful to continue. Inadequate lubrication, not feeling relaxed or feeling anxious, and lack of stimulation before penetration were cited as psychophysiological factors that predict pain. Other circumstances associated with a greater amount of pain were depth and rate of thrusting, lack of social comfort with being gay, and being more "closeted." The authors suggest clinical criteria for anodyspareunia similar to that used for other sexual pain disorders. In the case of anal sex aversion, then, the basis can be as much related to physical pain as to psychological and emotional factors.

Chemical Use and Abuse

Because of the high rate of chemical use or dependency among sexual minorities, clinicians should inquire about the nature and level of drug and alcohol consumption (Berzon, 1988; L. S. Brown, 1985; George & Behrendt, 1987; Nichols, 1987a, 1987b, 1989; Reece, 1982, 1987). In Loulan's survey of 1,566 lesbians (1987, 1988), 29% indicated they were recovering from substance abuse. Loulan contends that it often takes from 1 to 3 years of sobriety for individuals to regain a sense of their own bodies and to be able to function sexually while sober; therefore, assessment of sexuality and related performance must take phases of recovery into consideration. Finally, use of prescription or illicit drugs, or both, that may impair erotic interest and response similarly must be identified before the sexual aspects of a relationship are targeted for treatment (Beckman & Ackerman, 1995).

Relationship Dynamics

In the process of taking the history, clients will tell the story of their relationships, as well as discuss their individual lives (M. Hall, 1987, 1998). Therapists who encourage this storytelling contradict the cultural messages that censure descriptions of romantic love between members of the same sex. Further, facilitating the expression of these narratives legitimizes, supports, and affirms gay and lesbian partnerships.

As couples are asked to describe the course of their relationship, clinicians should observe both verbal content and nonverbal reactions, along with the dynamics between the individuals. The degree of fusion and autonomy, as well as whether there are repeated cycles of merger and separation, will become apparent as clients tell the story of their couplehood. A considerable number of individuals will have brought negative attachment histories into the dyad, given the previously discussed childhood patterns of rejection and alienation in many lesbians and gay men. Since attachment organization in couples is likely "to match, with both partners evidencing either dismissing or preoccupied attachments, or to mesh, with one partner being dismissing and the other preoccupied" (Cicchetti & Toth, 1995, p. 288), clinicians should be especially alert to these patterns.

With lesbians in particular, but also with some male couples, the increasing closeness of the dyad requires greater distance as time passes (M. Hall, 1984; Roth, 1985, 1989), and therapists should observe the distancing strategies used by each specific couple. Thus, clinicians should ask all clients whether their alliance allows for individual friends and pursuits, and they should formulate hypotheses as to what purpose these outside allegiances and activities serve both for the partners individually and for the couple. The presence of a third entity should be noted—such as whether work, a child, a friendship, or an affair has been drawn into the relationship to create distance and whether sex is avoided for the same reason. Along the same vein, attention should be paid to the way conflict is addressed or avoided, including whether the partners are permitted to interrupt or contradict each other, or even fight about details, and if conflict is allowed to explode into violence.

Reece (1987) notes the importance of a multicausal, multilevel approach to the treatment of sexual dysfunctions since there are usually numerous contributing factors involved, ranging "from simple misinformation about some aspect of human sexual response or behavior to deep transferences within the relationship which unconsciously repeat unresolved childhood conflicts" (p. 159). He contends that some problems are maintained by interactive patterns based in poor communication skills, while others exist because of "complementary psychological defenses of each partner that ward off deeper anxieties" (p. 159).

SEXUAL DYSFUNCTIONS

The three general classifications of sexual dysfunctions described in the following sections share numerous etiologies and contributing factors. Several of these commonalities will be discussed in some detail under "Sexual Desire Disorders", and those that are relevant will be cited only briefly when "Sexual Arousal Disorders" and "Orgasmic Disorders" are examined. The discussions are designed as guidelines for clinicians in determining whether sex therapy or some other form of treatment is more applicable, given the couple dynamics presented. The intent is to provide therapists with background rather than with the specific information necessary to treat various sexual dysfunctions. Clinicians are referred to additional sources for that purpose.

Sexual Desire Disorders

In order to meet DSM-IV (1994) criteria for hypoactive sexual desire disorder, an individual must exhibit "a deficiency or absence of sexual fantasies and desire for sexual activity" and "the disturbance must cause marked distress or interpersonal difficulty"

(p. 496). Low sexual desire may be generalized or situational, as well as continuous or episodic (lifelong or acquired); nevertheless, the inhibition must present serious difficulties. Rather than isolate either high or low desire as the problem, Reece (1987) prefers to focus on incompatible desire levels within a couple, or what he refers to as *desire discrepancies*. Using the same terminology as Kaplan (1977, 1979, 1983), he discusses the low-interest partner and the high-interest partner, as well as various situations that may arise as a result of the differences in their erotic appetites.

For both lesbians and gay men, common etiologies of desire and discrepancy disorders include internalized homophobia, guilt, performance anxiety, depression, sexual and gender role conditioning, separation anxiety issues including fear of intimacy, and other relationship concerns (Meyer & Dean, 1998; Nichols, 1987a; N. O'Connor & Ryan, 1993; Scasta, 1998). Therapists must avoid assessing lesbian sexuality exclusively in terms of male standards and heterosexual norms, however. To address cultural homophobia and misogyny, as well as the heterosexist and masculine orientation of current sexual assessment and treatment models, a discussion of women's dynamics is frequently necessary. Similarly, masculine gender role socialization often produces interactive patterns that are unique to sexual relationships between men. For example, almost half of a sample of 197 gay men reported some sexual difficulty over their lifetime, and more than half noted a current sexual problem (Rosser et al., 1997), yet norms for appropriate masculine functioning often keep men from discussing their sexual dilemmas. Therefore, the following discussions of the sexual dysfunctions focus on gender-specific concerns as warranted, as well as on issues common to both lesbians and gay men. Concerns of lesbians will be examined briefly before general issues regarding sexual desire and discrepancy disorders are discussed.

Lesbians

While many aspects of psychotherapy with lesbian clients have been addressed in recent years, the field of sex therapy has been sorely neglected (L. S. Brown, 1986). In addition, "no data exist on either the incidence or the prevalence of complaints of sexual dysfunction among the lesbian population" (p. 100). Because many of the sexual difficulties of lesbians cannot be classified in any of the standard classification schemas, various writers in the field of lesbian sex therapy prefer not to categorize lesbian sexual dysfunction into the typical response cycle patterns of desire, arousal, and orgasm (Nichols, 1987a). When customary terminology is used, however, it is usually applied in reference to discrepancies in sexual desire, or the absence of desire in one or both partners. Difficulties in this area are the most frequently reported sexual concerns of lesbian couples (M. Hall, 1987; Klinger, 1996; Nichols, 1982, 1987a, 1987b; Rose, 1994; A. E. Schwartz, 1998). Not only does erotic interest decline in many of these same-sex pairs, but so also does the frequency of sexual activity.

In fact, Blumstein and Schwartz (1983) found that lesbian couples have sexual relations less frequently than do either heterosexual or gay male couples. Their data also revealed that 47% of long-term lesbian couples had sex once a month or less, compared with 15% of married heterosexual couples who had been together approximately the same length of time. In a 1988 survey of 706 lesbian couples (Bryant & Demian, 1995), only 18% of the women reported "none" or one sexual encounter with their partner per month. Loulan's data (1987, 1988) revealed a figure somewhat between the findings described in these two studies. Accordingly, she asked 1,566 lesbian respondents how much partner sex they had in 1 month and was provided with the following responses: 12%, never; 11%, less than once; 7.5%, once; 35%, 2 to 5 times; 20%, 6 to 10; 11%, 11 to 20; 3%, over 20. When the percentages for the first three categories are added together, a closer inspection reveals that 30.5% of the women engaged in sexual activity once a month or less, which is twice the rate of the 15% figure for heterosexuals in the Blumstein and Schwartz (1983) study. Loulan notes that having sex more often is not necessarily essential for satisfaction for many lesbians, as 52% of her subjects indicated that they were "fairly well" or "completely" satisfied with their sex lives. Thus, she cautions clients against comparing themselves to masculine or heterosexual notions of sexual frequency, since contentment for many lesbians is related to the quality rather than the quantity of erotic activity.

Nichols (1987b) writes of the difficulty that most women have in separating love (and "marriage") from sex and believes that this gendered phenomenon partially explains why lesbians tend to enter into cohabitation arrangements after brief courtships rather than to have casual affairs. She further alleges that, because attachment and eroticism are so intertwined in this population, sexual desire is highly vulnerable to problems in the relationship; the partnership thus must be relatively free of difficulties in order for many lesbians to feel sexually responsive toward their mates. Further, due to the previously discussed high rapport and fine attunement of lesbian relationships, partners are extremely susceptible to personalizing sexual refusal (Roth, 1985, 1989). These effects of gender role conditioning result in relatively little sexual desire and activity in a considerable number of lesbian couples.

A common way for lesbian couples to deal with their sexually devitalized relationships is to begin an affair (Klinger, 1996; Nichols, 1987b). These encounters often are highly charged and erotically ardent; in some ways they resemble the emotional intensity that was experienced early in the previous relationship. De-coupling hence occurs, and a new partnership that promises better and more frequent sex is begun. Once these women are in the new relationship for a period of time, however, the obstacles to the couplehood diminish, intense merger occurs, the sparks of differences become diminished, sexual inhibitions (or political correctness) result in a minimal numbers of techniques, and this relationship, too, ends up sexually impoverished. Therapists are cautioned to avoid assuming that all instances of nonmonogamy in lesbian couples result from sexually devitalized primary relationships, however. While many affairs are related to this dynamic, others serve a boundary function by creating distance between members of the couple, and still others equalize power inequalities. Further, some are planned alternatives to monogamy rather than spontaneous solutions to relational conflicts and dissatisfactions (E. Kassoff, 1988).

In any case, each member of the couple reporting a decline in sexual frequency should be asked what this means to her. Additional questioning must be specific and formulated to detect the role of sex in the lives of the individuals, as well as of the couple. Often clinicians will find that members are comparing themselves to a hypothetical vision of an ideal lesbian relationship. M. Hall (1987) contends that the goal of the inquiry is to "normalize" the frequency of sexual relations and to let partners know that they are free to set their own standards for contact without comparing themselves or their behaviors to heterosexist or masculine norms.

Internalized Heterosexism

Just as with lesbian couples, heterosexist influences from the majority culture can affect sexual desire and frequency in male couples. Therefore, therapists likewise should consider the level of internalized heterosexism or homophobia in low-interest partners (Berzon, 1988; Buloff & Osterman, 1995; George & Behrendt, 1987; Glassgold, 1995; Reece, 1987; Rose, 1994). While on a conscious level these individuals may have come to terms with their sexual orientation, unconscious and unresolved guilt or shame could be preventing them from feeling sexual with a member of their own sex—or even from experiencing *any* sexual responses. Heterosexually influenced religious prohibitions regarding sexuality in general or homosexuality in particular—or both—also may be operating and must be considered by clinicians when couples present with concerns about sexual desire.

Several writers have discussed the internal experience of shame in sexual minority individuals due to histories of invalidation and lack of acceptance (Canarelli et al., 1999; Gair, 1995; Rose, 1994; Vaughan, 1999). This shame "usually manifests indirectly in the form of inhibition, self-doubt, depression, rage, and inhibited or exaggerated sexual desires" (Gair, 1995, p. 110). Because of gender role socialization, lesbians more typically will express the shame in inhibited sexual desire and gay men in compulsive sexuality. In any case, however, lack of mirroring and recognition has distorted the inner experience of self and resulted in substantial shame and internalized homophobia that takes life-affirming sexuality and makes it debased. Hence, the empathic attunement and mirroring provided in the therapeutic encounter is essential for those who have lived with a lifetime of shameful impulses (Buloff & Osterman, 1995; Glassgold, 1995; Rose, 1994).

Intimacy Fears

Other concerns associated with desire discrepancies in all couples include fears or problems related to intimacy and commitment (American Psychiatric Association, 1994; Berzon, 1988; C. Friedman, 1998; N. O'Connor & Ryan, 1993; Reece, 1987). Berzon (1988) discusses situations in which individuals who fear intimacy are sometimes inclined to inhibit sexual desire whenever those apprehensions are activated. Some can tolerate closeness for a period of time, but when their levels of tolerance are reached, they will do something to push their partners away (such as precipitate a conflict, become ill or otherwise distracted, or lose interest in sex). In this regard, Berzon cites cases of couples "who were passionately sexual with each other until they decided to move in together, at which time sexual desire became significantly diminished for one or both of them" (p. 224). Explaining this phenomenon psychodynamically, N. O'Connor and Ryan (1993) discuss the desire to merge and the terror this longing arouses: "This terror is in turn seen as involving a loss of self that too great a closeness can bring" (p. 233).

As discussed previously, there often are numerous impediments to lesbian and gay partnerships, mostly in the form of societal, religious, or family opposition. Further, ex-lovers, heterosexual spouses, and children can be antagonistic to the relationship. Secrecy, clandestine meetings, and barriers frequently fuel erotic passions. Once these obstacles have been somewhat conquered, excitement often lessens, and extinction of libido occurs; the sexuality that once seemed to flourish under adverse conditions declines once the couple has nested together and there are no longer the same barriers to the union (M. Hall,

1987; Tripp, 1975). In this way, the same closeness and intensity that fuel the fires of initial passion often serve to contribute to its eventual demise.

Berzon (1988) indicates that the kinds of situations described here assist her in determining if the decrease in sexual desire is related to relationship developments that symbolize growing commitment. Similarly, Reece (1987) notes that "if interest in sex declined in connection either with a deepening commitment, symbolized by moving in together or sharing a major financial obligation, or by an experience of increased emotional vulnerability, fears of intimacy may be involved" (p. 161).

Conflict Avoidance

The avoidance of dissension and conflict should be considered when dealing with couples with desire discrepancies. Internalized heterosexism, gender role socialization, or other dynamics may have led to a situation of covert warfare between the partners. Rather than dealing directly with anger, they may suppress hostility and act out in various ways, one of which is sexually.

SUPPRESSION OF DISCORD

Some gay men feel angry not only with their partners but also toward men in general, and this situation often can be related to unresolved issues with their fathers or with other men who treated them harshly. Regardless of the source, the curbing of dissension tends to contaminate a significant relationship in the interpersonal and sexual areas of relating (Berzon, 1988; Paul, 1991). Lesbian couples particularly are inclined to submerge hostility, and lack of fighting between partners may be used as a diagnostic clue to detect a low level of sexuality (B. Kassoff, 1995; Nichols, 1987b). Although conflict often creates energy that can spark eroticism, dissent is prohibited in many lesbian relationships: "The lesbian Catch 22 is: You cannot validate, support, and hold all the hope for your relationship *and* explore frustrations and conflicts at the same time" (Kleinberg & Zorn, 1995, p. 127). For many lesbians, romance is the only way to create sexual excitement since prohibitions against expressing dissension allow "no other mechanisms to generate sexual tension" (Nichols, 1987b, p. 107). Having been conditioned by society to believe that only falling in love produces sexual desire, they sometimes leave a dispassionate relationship in order to fall in love again.

Psychoanalyst A. E. Schwartz (1998) discusses the phenomenon of "lesbian bed death," which she describes as "the ongoing or impending cessation of genital sexuality as well as other forms of passionate or lustful sexual touching" (p. 59). She contends that the falling away of passion is one of the most common complaints of lesbian couples and attributes this to the fear of *ruthlessness* on the part of oneself or one's lover. She attributes some of her thinking to Bollas (1989), who asserts that ruthlessness is inherent in erotic excitement and that partners must surrender to that vindictiveness. A joint loss of consciousness, during which lovers destroy the relationship, is essential in reaching the heights of orgasmic intensity. If couples thus cannot allow this essential destructiveness, erotic intensity suffers. A. E. Schwartz (1998) contends that lesbian couples in therapy often have difficulty incorporating healthy competition and combativeness into their relationship and that "this suppression of aggression, the avoidance of ruthlessness, manifests as a diminution or deadening of the couple's libido" (p. 62).

Likewise, L. S. Brown (1985) notes that sexual ardor tends to diminish after the first 6 months as partners move into what could become the conflict phase of their relationship. Many lesbian couples attempt to skip this stage, however, and to sacrifice conflict resolution "to the appearance of tranquillity and stability" (p. 11). Rather than permitting discord and differences of opinion to surface, the women often submerge antagonistic feelings and fuse even more tightly. This suppression of friction combined with an unspoken pact of *pseudomutuality* (i.e., conflict avoidance) further extinguishes the sparks of eroticism. Brown contends that therapists must teach lesbian couples to approach dissent in a proactive and constructive manner in order to reduce "the symbolic weight plied onto sexual functioning" (p. 8). When clinicians provide normative data about the association between prohibiting differences and diminished sexuality in lesbian couples, partners frequently begin to allow disagreements and opposing views to emerge between them.

INDEPENDENT EXISTENCES

A degree of autonomous functioning and an ability to allow differences of opinion are crucial goals for both relationship and sex therapy. Accordingly, same-sex couples who fail to confront conflict in the relationship, and to develop skills for managing and resolving discordance, frequently are unable to establish mutually satisfying sexual functioning (L. S. Brown, 1985; Falco, 1991; M. Hall, 1984, 1987; Krestan & Bepko, 1980; Loulan, 1987; Nichols, 1982, 1987b; Roth, 1985, 1989). Along these same lines, M. Hall (1987) attributes the highly charged merger of lesbians early in their couplehood to the affiliative nature of women and their "gender-bound conditioning" to abandon ego boundaries and to submerge themselves "in the larger arena of the relationship" (p. 138). She contends, however, that if the partners eventually are not able to reclaim a degree of individuality, the frequency of sexual exchange plunges, "the relationship becomes stultifying, and the spark of difference that ignites eroticism disappears" (p. 138). Similarly, N. O'Connor and Ryan (1993) discuss how the frequent splits between lesbian desire and identification, along with the demands for sameness and identity, often obliterate erotic tension and desire, as well as diversity. However, they caution against assuming that only lesbians are vulnerable to symbiotic desexualized relationships since this phenomenon is also present in many heterosexual and gay male couples.

According to the "barrier theory" (i.e., barriers fuel erotic passion) discussed earlier (Tripp, 1975), excessive intimacy actually hurts sexual desire in lesbian relationships. In other words, "as intimacy increases and individual differences decrease, so may the very distance, mystery, and unpredictability necessary to maintain sexual tension" (Nichols, 1987b, p. 107). Paradoxically, Nichols (1987b) believes that the more successful couples are in obliterating differences between them, the more compatible they are as roommates who can live together easily because they are so much alike. She contends that the other side of the coin is that the two women make "lousy lovers." M. Hall (1987) challenges this pseudomutuality whenever she has the opportunity, even from the beginning of therapy when she arranges three chairs in the form of an equilateral triangle. This prevents lesbian couples from sitting in their typical "us-against-the world" (p. 141) positions together across from the expert therapist. By splitting the dyad, therapists can form temporary alliances with either partner. Unbalancing the merged union further can uncover conspiracies of silence that were designed to preserve the stability of the relationship and the "muffled various disappointments, sex among them, under layers of compromise and denial." Hall cautions, however, against attempting to assign individual activities too early in therapy, since the couple frequently has developed strong "anti-outsider defenses" and will resist this overt attempt at differentiation. Rather than risk individuation (and possible separation), the women often opt instead to tighten even further the boundaries around their couplehood.

Power

Power differences affect erotic desire for both lesbian and gay couples, as "less powerful" partners frequently withhold or otherwise manipulate the sexual relationship in order to maintain the balance of power. While the perceived (or actual) inequality may result from differences in age, education, income, attractiveness, or social status, the dynamics associated with the imbalance are usually similar (Reece, 1987). Although differences in influence and authority exist in all intimate relationships, including those involving same-sex couples, women often are inclined to reject this notion because of its association with heterosexism and patriarchy. In fact, feminist ideals of equality may lead members of lesbian pairs to deny power disproportions between them.

Many lesbians often become disillusioned with their partners when the power struggles that are common in heterosexual relationships exist in their own partnerships (Falco, 1991; Kleinberg & Zorn, 1995). To prevent discouragement and maintain their ideals, couples frequently strive to maintain an equality balance and sometimes go to elaborate lengths to equalize power in as many areas as possible, including financial sharing and decision making (J. M. Lynch & Reilly, 1986; M. E. Reilly & Lynch, 1990). Contrasts in income or status often are suppressed in conversation, but nonetheless present as problems in the sexual arena. The first step in therapy is to have these differences and the concomitant resentment rise to the surface since "if the less powerful partner cannot replace sexual refusal with another power source of her [or his] own, either external or intrapsychic, it is unlikely that the imbalance in the bedroom can be corrected" (M. Hall, 1987, p. 148).

Communication Difficulties

Communication problems also might be associated with desire discrepancies in couples. Accordingly, individuals with inadequate or limited conversational skills might find it difficult to initiate or refuse sex, or otherwise to discuss issues that may be causing problems in their relationship (Berzon, 1988; George & Behrendt, 1987; Reece, 1987; Scasta, 1998). E. Coleman (1981/1982) and Grace (1992) describe numerous interpersonal difficulties that occur for sexual minorities before and during the identity formation process due to having grown up in an oppressive society (see Chapters 5 and 9). Because many lesbians and gay men enter relationships with low self-esteem, poor interpersonal skills, concerns about attractiveness, and social awkwardness, communication problems frequently arise in all these aspects of the relationship, including the sexual dimension.

Abuse

Trauma, such as sexual or physical mistreatment, may inhibit the ability of survivors to access their erotic impulses and can serve to deeroticize same-sex relationships. Experiences of rape or of childhood incest or sexual abuse, which are relatively high in sexual minority populations (especially for lesbians), can contaminate sexual expression throughout the lifespan (L. S. Brown, 1985; M. Hall, 1987; Loulan, 1984, 1987, 1988; Nichols, 1987a, 1987b; Robinson & Parks, 1999; Scarce, 1997; Weingourt, 1998). Loulan (1987, 1988), for example, surveyed 1,566 lesbians and found that 38% had been sexually abused before the age of 18, a figure she contends is comparable to that of women in the general population. Further, 32% of Loulan's subjects reported that the experiences occurred before they were 5 years old. Visual, emotional, and kinesthetic memories from sexual traumas, both early in life and in adolescence, can be elicited by a wide range of cues—some so explicit that they are readily discernible, and others so subtle that they may be unidentifiable or even unconscious. In any case, however, the resulting cognitions, affects, images, sensations, or behaviors can serve to inhibit sexual desire and functioning. In contrast, even positive past sexual experiences can have a detrimental effect, especially if they are being compared to the present state of living in a sexless or passionless union.

Chemical Use

Finally, drug and alcohol use and abuse, both past and present, must be considered when assessing disorders of sexual desire, arousal, or orgasm with same-sex couples (Beckman & Ackerman, 1995; Berzon, 1988; J. Paul, 1991; Spencer, 1991). If problems with substances are ongoing, sexual dysfunctions in all phases may result. If one or both partners are recovering from chemical abuse, other difficulties may emerge upon sobriety. For example, the negative introjects, feelings, or experiences that the substances were used to contain, moderate, or abate may surface. Memories of abuse, homophobic messages, feelings of inadequacy, fears of intimacy and lack of control, and religious prohibitions can return and adversely impact sexual functioning on all levels, including desire.

Summary

Psychoanalysts N. O'Connor and Ryan (1993) believe that the traditional (heterosexist) psychoanalytic position regarding the Oedipus Complex must be reconceptualized in order for sexual desire to become activated in some lesbians (and, perhaps, gay men). According to the theory, mature individuals eventually come to identify with the same-sex parent and desire the parent of the opposite sex, thus allowing for a gendered split "between who is identified with (same-sex) and who is desired (different sex)" (p. 268). Rather than seeing these as mutually exclusive, psychotherapy with sexual minorities entails reformulating conceptualizations of male/masculine and female/feminine identifications (A. E. Schwartz, 1998). This expansion in the breadth and diversity of gender role taxonomy, thus, can promote an individual's ability both to identify with and to desire a person of the same biological sex. By reconstructing the role of identification in relation to desire, splits between the two can be resolved and sexual feelings can be permitted to develop toward a person with whom one identifies.

Sexual Arousal Disorders

Like all phase-specific sexual dysfunctions, sexual arousal disorders must cause marked distress or interpersonal difficulty. Additionally, individuals must have an inability to attain, or maintain until completion of the sexual activity, an adequate lubrication–swelling response of sexual excitement (women) or an adequate erection (men) (American Psychiatric Association, 1994). The DSM-IV (American Psychiatric Association, 1994) refers to sexual arousal disorders in men as male erectile disorders and indicates that these difficulties "are frequently associated with sexual anxiety, fear of failure, concerns about sexual performance, and a decreased subjective sense of sexual excitement and pleasure" (p. 503). For women, they are referred to as female sexual arousal disorders, and "limited evidence" suggests that such conditions are often accompanied by difficulties in the desire and orgasmic phases of sexual response (p. 501).

Nonetheless, virtually all of the literature that considers sexual arousal concerns in lesbians also discusses difficulties in the areas of desire and orgasm. In fact, few writings are available that concentrate exclusively on arousal problems. Because of availability and focus, then, the majority of the following discussion of these concerns deals with gay men. Much of the material described earlier in reference to desire disorders or discrepancies in lesbians, however, is relevant to their difficulties with sexual arousal. Similarly, the next section, which focuses on orgasmic issues in female couples, contains information applicable to the arousal phase of the sexual response cycle.

Gay Men

Inhibited sexual excitement is somewhat common in gay male clients, and several New York and San Francisco sex therapists estimate that half their caseloads involve erection problems (Reece, 1982). In this regard, Reece (1982) conducted group therapy for 31 gay men with sexual dysfunctions who presented a total of 50 complaints, half of which involved the inability to have or maintain an erection. Predictably, few of his clients had lifelong erectile difficulties, and almost all reported erections in some situations. These episodes generally occurred when the clients were alone or were engaged in nongenital intimacy with another person. When they were sexually involved with partners, however, erections either were absent or, if present, faded soon after attempts at intercourse.

GENDER ROLE CONDITIONING

George and Behrendt (1987) believe that masculine gender role socialization is a major factor that contributes to inhibited sexual excitement in gay men and can help explain why many are able to have erections when they are alone or in nonsexual interpersonal situations, but not when they are with a male partner whom they may imagine is rating their competency, masculinity, potency, or virility. Apparently, the anxiety associated with these kinds of encounters, alone or in combination with fears of feeling exposed or humiliated, results in erectile failure.

Having been conditioned to compete and achieve, many men evaluate the proficiency of their erotic performances. Fracher and Kimmel (1989) believe that the male sexual script (i.e., the normative construction of sexuality) "contains dicta for sexual distancing, objectification, phallocentrism, and a pressure to become and remain erect without ejaculation for as long as possible" (p. 477). Hence, for gay and heterosexual men alike, both of whom are socialized to have "male sex" (p. 478), the successful execution of these prescriptions is an indication of masculinity and sexual potency. Thus conditioned to believe that sexual problems are an indication of damaged gender (i.e., masculine) identity, many gay men become extremely anxious about the quality of their sexual performances (Scasta, 1998). During sex, these individuals continually monitor their behavior and that of the other person, questioning themselves, and watching their every move for possible defects: "They spectate rather than participate in the sexual activity, are constantly grading themselves or believe that they are being graded by their partner on how well they are doing sexually, and very rarely abandon themselves in a sexual act" (George & Behrendt, 1987, p. 85).

OTHER ISSUES

In addition to issues about masculine socialization, several other considerations discussed earlier must be taken into account when treating sexual arousal disorders. For example, traumas such as childhood sexual abuse, rape, or a religious environment that equated sex, especially homosexual intimacy, with sin can hinder erectile functioning (Scarce, 1997; Spencer, 1991). Likewise, clients with mood disorders and substance-related disorders often report problems with sexual arousal. These conditions particularly affect the ability of sexual minority men to attain or maintain erections. With regard to mood disorders in particular, some sexual dysfunctions may be secondary to a serious depression; in other cases, clients may become depressed as a result of erectile problems that have negatively affected their intimate relationships (Paul, 1991). Therefore, this aspect of the sexual history should be especially detailed. In addition, because there are different patterns of erectile dysfunction, clinical interviewing should attempt to determine the specific conditions under which problems with erections occur, as well as the emotions that accompany these various events. Finally, clinicians should inquire about antidepressant medications as many of them produce side effects that include diminished sexual desire and erectile difficulties (Pillard, 1991a; Spencer, 1991).

HIV INFECTION

Paul (1991) also asks his gay male clients their concerns and attitudes about AIDS. Those who are HIV-positive often fear exposing their partners, and individuals who have tested negative for HIV worry about contracting the virus. Fears of possible infection have kept many other gay and bisexual men from presenting themselves for antibody testing. Even people who are in denial about the seriousness of the AIDS epidemic feasibly have some level of anxiety about the disease. In one study of 197 gay men (Rosser et al., 1997), almost half of the respondents reported that HIV infection had a negative effect on their sexual functioning, with most noting a heightened fear of sex as the major negative outcome. Thus, for many individuals, every sexual encounter has the potential for eliciting apprehension sufficient to interfere with sexual desire, erection/arousal, or orgasmic response (Marion, 1996; Paul et al., 1995). Chapter 12 provided a detailed discussion about gay men and the AIDS epidemic.

Clients may need accurate information about safer sex or a clinician's assistance in developing the personal limits or communication skills, or both, necessary to negotiate safer and more anxiety-free sexual encounters. One of the primary goals of couples therapy, relationship adjustment, appears to be related to safer sex practices, both inside and outside of the primary relationship (Julien, Chartrand, & Begin, 1996). Among 41 cohabiting male couples, those who reduced their exposure to HIV infection reported greater adaptation to the relationship. Not surprising, however, was the finding that the members who practiced safer sex had lower relationship satisfaction when their primary partner practiced unprotected sex. Another set of findings poses a more difficult dilemma for therapists. Questionnaires were given to 45 male couples, and results indicated that the more partners idealized each other, the more satisfied they were with their relationship; moreover, as their level of excitement increased, condom use decreased (McNeal, 1997). While these intimacy and erotic factors thus seem to have a positive effect on relationship satisfaction, they also may be associated with unsafe sexual practices among gay male couples. In other words, the intensity experienced in the partnership may prevail over the possibility that they may be risking their lives.

Summary

Berzon (1988) believes that for both lesbians and gay men with difficulties of sexual arousal or excitement, performance anxiety is an important ingredient since "it is easier not to meet the challenge at all than to have to face the pain of rejection for a flawed performance" (p. 218). For example, women who adhere to the "lesbian-sex-is-magical" model (L. S. Brown, 1986, p. 102) may set themselves up for self-criticism and performance anxiety, which can lead to problems in either the arousal or orgasm phases of sexual activity. Similarly, gay men often engage in spectatoring and self-monitoring, which generates anxiety and fear sufficient to inhibit sexual arousal (Berzon, 1988; George & Behrendt, 1987; Scasta, 1998).

Therapy for these men not only must address the multiple issues related to erectile dysfunction but also should invite clients to examine the excessive masculine gender-role socialization that underlies much of their performance anxiety. Further, they (and lesbians with arousal concerns) need to be taught how "to identify performance anxiety in themselves and to replace it with an awareness of pleasurable sensations, either through sensate focus skills, focus on the partner's pleasurable response, or fantasy material" (Reece, 1982, p. 122). Nichols (1987a) and Loulan (1984) describe their process of teaching clients how to concentrate on pleasurable sensations, rather than on performance, and to increase their ability to fantasize so that apprehension related to sexual arousal may be overcome. Pillard (1991a) contends that "repeated failure to perform sexually has a circular and devastating effect; anxiety about previous failures increases the probability of yet another 'complete disaster' " (p. 3). Vigorous intervention is needed to interrupt this cycle, often in the form of therapy directed toward the performance-focused thinking and cognitive distortions that are perpetuating the process. Focus on the here-and-now and thought substitution is often helpful in this regard (Berzon, 1988).

Orgasmic Disorders

DSM-IV (American Psychiatric Association, 1994) indicates that the essential feature of a female or male orgasmic disorder involves a persistent or recurrent delay in, or absence of, orgasm following a normal sexual excitement phase. As with other sexual disorders, marked distress or interpersonal difficulty must result. Clinicians are free to use their judgment in determining whether the orgasmic capacity of individuals is less than would be reasonable for their age, sexual experience, and the adequacy of stimulation. Couples therapists also might consider the quality and affective climate of the relationship. Because orgasmic disorders involve considerably different dynamics in gay men than in lesbians, the concerns of these populations are discussed separately.

Gay Men

In the study discussed above related to group treatment of sexual dysfunction in gay men (Reece, 1982), the second highest frequency of complaints (after excitement phase or erectile disorders) was inhibited ejaculation (30% of the 50 complaints; $n = 15$). Of these 15 concerns, 12 accompanied erectile difficulties and, for most of these, inhibited ejaculation pre-dated the development of secondary erectile dysfunction. In other words, when gay male clients present with arousal or excitement phase disorders, clinicians need to inquire further to determine if the concerns about inhibited ejaculation may have led to the performance anxiety that is often associated with inhibited erectile functioning. If this is the case, the ejaculatory or orgasmic difficulty must be treated if the therapy for the arousal phase disorder is to succeed.

Reece (1982) compared his frequency percentages with those of Masters and Johnson (1970) related to presumably heterosexual populations. Both sets of data revealed that approximately 50% of complaints were for excitement or sexual arousal disorders. In contrast, comparatively few gay men (10%) reported rapid or premature ejaculation difficulties, whereas 41.5% of Masters and Johnson's male subjects were treated for this concern. Conversely, 4% of the heterosexual subjects described inhibited or retarded ejaculation, compared with 30% of the complaints that were presented to Reece.

GENDER ROLE SOCIALIZATION

Noting that other sex therapists, including McWhirter and Mattison (1980), also have detected these percentage discrepancies between gay and heterosexual males, Reece (1982) speculated as to possible causes. In this regard, he asserts that "the apparent higher frequency of complaints of inhibited ejaculation among gay men, as opposed to heterosexual men, has to do with issues of male–male intimacy and with the male's acceptance of his own homosexual identity" (p. 119). He further conjectures that the socialization of men to be competitive, defensive, and emotionally inexpressive creates difficulties in the orgasm phase of sexual functioning, as well as in the desire and arousal or excitement stages. For some gay men, the intimacy of orgasm brings about the previously discussed fear of vulnerability. Having worked hard most of their life to remain composed and in control, they dread the unguarded state that accompanies orgasm. The closeness of an intense sexual experience leaves them feeling unprotected and defenseless and, hence, they do not permit themselves this degree of emotional exposure. Again, rigid masculine socialization affects not only the quality of their intimate relationships but also their orgasmic functioning.

INTERNALIZED HETEROSEXISM

Meyer and Dean (1998) examined data from a 7-year longitudinal project that interviewed more than 1,000 gay and bisexual men. Findings suggested that "men with high levels of internalized homophobia were almost four times more likely to report sex problems than men with low levels of internalized homophobia" (p. 171). Similarly, those men in the original cohort who described high levels of heterosexist attitudes were about twice as likely to report sex problems, including inhibited sexual desire, excitement, or orgasm in the year before the interview. Two studies discussed previously in this chapter point to somewhat similar findings. Accordingly, the men ($n = 197$) who reported having higher levels of sexual satisfaction (and presumably had fewer sexual difficulties) had more liberal attitudes toward human sexuality, greater comfort with sexual attractions to other men, lower levels of homophobia, and greater satisfaction with their relationship status (Rosser et al., 1997). In a similar vein, the participants in another project who experienced pain in anal intercourse so severe that they could not continue (12% of 277 men) tended to be "closeted" or lacked social comfort with being gay or bisexual (Rosser et al., 1998).

Many gay men are convinced that allowing themselves to experience the intense feelings that accompany ejaculation and orgasm opens them to the possibility of an intimate relationship with another man (C. Friedman, 1998; George & Behrendt, 1987; Reece, 1982). Those who are particularly homophobic and conflicted about their sexual orientation often experience inhibited orgasm. From their point of view, the withholding of climax or ejaculation allows them to retain the illusion of a heterosexual identity; to become orgasmic or emotionally intimate would force them to acknowledge that they are sexually oriented toward other males. Believing on some level that homosexuality is wrong and they should not be having sex with another man, they have difficulties surrendering themselves in intimate and sexual relationships. Reading in the area of male sexuality may help them reformulate their notions of intimate relationships between men (e.g., Goldstone, 1999; Hart, 1998; Palerno, 1999; Shalit, 1998; C. Silverstein, 1993).

Lesbians

Loulan (1987, 1988) reported that 14% of her lesbian sample ($N = 1,566$) indicated that they were occasionally or never orgasmic with masturbation, and 19% said that they were occasionally or never orgasmic with a partner. Many of these women described their infrequent orgasmic response as a locus of anxiety and friction in their relationships. Internalized heterosexist norms that suggest sex is either over, complete, or satisfying only with the achievement of orgasm were cited as the major source of this conflict. Since society defines all of sex except intercourse as "foreplay," lesbians erroneously learn to replace the word *intercourse* with *orgasm*, thus further compromising the range of their sexual response (Loulan, 1984). Therapists, however, can educate these women regarding the homophobic nature of their sexual conditioning with its goal of orgasm as the only acceptable culmination of intimate activity.

OVERCOMING HETEROSEXIST CONDITIONING

Loulan (1984) tells her clients that "not experiencing orgasm does not make you cold, frigid, or unresponsive. It simply means that you do not experience orgasm, nothing more, nothing less" (p. 73). For those who wish to become orgasmic, however, she recommends desensitization with masturbation, use of vibrators, and her own exercises, but she also stresses that lesbian sexual encounters are permissible and undiminished in any form that fulfills the needs of both partners. Further, therapists can help reduce the pressure to reach orgasm by helping couples focus on the sensations present in any activity that is found mutually pleasing.

Openness to sexual experiences is difficult for many lesbians, but desire and excitement are frightening. Erotic emotions often trigger painful memories of sexual abuse or of non-gratifying encounters with men or former female partners (Loulan, 1988; A. E. Schwartz, 1998). Excitement and engorgement are also distressing because they arouse previously forbidden feelings of shame and guilt, as well as a fear of vulnerability. Many women stop having sex when these negative emotions arise, and these clients may need education and desensitization experiences to counteract prior conditioning. Loulan (1988) contends that, in order to overcome their tendency not to recognize sexual desire, lesbian clients often must be taught to make sex a more conscious part of their lives. In other words, they must *will* sexuality without waiting for desire or excitement, or even an invitation. Loulan's (1984) model of the traditional sexual responses cycle (desire, excitement, engorgement, and orgasm), thus, is preceded by an initial stage of willingness.

TREATMENT CONSIDERATIONS

With highly fused lesbian couples, short-term sex therapy approaches are often contraindicated initially since the women cannot yet tolerate sufficient autonomy and contrast to spark sexual responsiveness. With women who are each other's best friend, political ally, support network, and often business partner, the lack of sexual contact is their way of establishing distance (Hall, 1987). In other words, emotional camaraderie takes the place of sex, and the relationship cannot tolerate further closeness without collapse. Thus, prescribing sexual activity or even additional time spent together in order to rekindle intimacy often elicits fears of engulfment that provoke the termination of therapy.

Once intimacy fears have been addressed and some degree of autonomy has been established, however, therapy techniques to heighten eroticism can be employed. Sensate focus exercises that introduce a series of gradually more sexually pleasurable activities can be used, as well as in vivo desensitization, which Nichols (1987a) contends is the therapy of choice for lesbians with oral sex phobias. Further, since many lesbians have never felt free to imagine and visualize sexually, exercises and readings can be assigned to help these clients develop this ability (Loulan [1984] describes a number of these exercises for this and various other purposes). Specifically in regard to imagination, however, Nichols (1987a) believes that erotic desire in women is related to the frequency with which they think about sex and that lesbians must learn to fantasize sexually with regularity. They also need to attend consciously to their sexual feelings and acknowledge them as such, rather than continuing to reframe them as relational desires or translate them into traditional notions of love and marriage (M. Hall, 1998; Slater, 1995). Because women often consider intimacy and sharing to be serious concerns, lesbians tend to view issues related to their sexual orientation as matters of considerable consequence. Hence, to see sexuality as light, fun, and playful is quite difficult. To many lesbians, "talking dirty" with their partners, using props or mood enhancers, or reading or viewing lesbian erotica is simply incompatible with their notions of love between women. Likewise, as discussed previously (A. E. Schwartz, 1998), the idea of behaving ruthlessly or selfishly, or even angrily, with each other may create cognitive and affective dissonance, or even seem abhorrent. Thinking creatively and in terms of new contextualizations can help liberate clients from past conceptualizations of (lesbian) sexuality and create therapeutic movement (M. Hall, 1998; Kleinberg & Zorn, 1995). Reading some of the many books and other publications that address lesbian sexuality may also help facilitate this effort (e.g., Caster, 1993; F. Newman, 1999).

Like Nichols, Loulan (1987) invites each member of a lesbian couple to examine her sexual introjects by making a list of all the "sex rules" she lives by. She contends that couples often are surprised by the number of these regulations and how significantly they affect their relationship and sexual functioning. Among the most common she finds are rules relating to the sacredness of sex between women and the spiritual dimension it brings to their relationships; those regarding the frequency, nature, and quality of each act of lovemaking; and prohibitions against fun, play, fantasy, and artificial devices when engaging in serious and loving lesbian sex. Much of Loulan's therapy involves challenging these kinds of notions and offering alternative perspectives, as well as providing couples with ideas and activities that can enlarge their sexual, behavioral, and cognitive repertoire.

In this same regard, Nichols (1987a) encourages therapists to help lesbian clients become somewhat "male" in their orientation toward sex by placing more emphasis on sex and less on romance. There is probably a fine line in this regard, however. The discussions earlier in this and in the previous chapter indicate that excessive masculine socialization in gay male couples is detrimental to effective coupling. The same was found for 111 lesbians after they completed a battery of measures, including the Bem Sex-Role Inventory and the Hudson Index of Sexual Satisfaction (Rosenzweig & Lebow, 1992). Subjects tended to view themselves significantly more feminine when they interacted sexually than with their overall sex role perceptions in general. Further, those women who saw themselves as either androgynous or feminine in a sexual context had a higher level of sexual satisfaction and dyadic adjustment than did other sex role groups. Thus, lesbians may need to adopt some stereotypically masculine modes of thinking if their sex lives are to improve, but not to the point of developing some of the characteristics that keep gay male couples from achieving gratification in their relationships.

CONCLUSION

This chapter focused on the heterosexist and masculine gender bias in the field of human sexuality and the influences of this skewed perspective as it affects sexual minorities. The effects of feminine and masculine gender role socialization on the sexual functioning of gay male and lesbian couples also was discussed. DSM-IV (American Psychiatric Association, 1994) sexual disorder subcategories of desire, arousal, and orgasm were reformulated to apply to sexual minorities; dynamics unique to male and female pairs in each of these areas were described. Therapists were encouraged to take a multicausal and multilevel approach to the treatment of sexual problems in their lesbian and gay clients and to avoid viewing their difficulties through heterosexist and misogynist frames of reference.

Finally, as when focusing on the sexual experiences of all clients but especially for those who behave intimately with their own biological sex, clinicians are cautioned about the possibility of countertransference issues clouding their objectivity (R. C. Friedman, 1999; Vaughan, 1999). The material presented may be threatening to therapists of all sexual orientations, either because the content arouses personal concerns and anxieties or because it is so foreign to them. In either case, they might be tempted to overreinforce boundary and framework issues, to allow too much intellectualization of the clients' difficulties, or to avoid discussion of sexual material (B. Greene, 1997a; . O'Connor & Ryan, 1993). Likewise, clinicians may too easily accept the erotic disinterest of clients due to their own insecurities about sexual expression or fears of not being able to contain the transference. These and similar concerns "are not in themselves unusual, and may have parallels with other forms of erotic transference" (N. O'Connor & Ryan, 1993, p. 184), but they are striking only in a context of virtual silence in conversation and professional literature about the sexual experiences of same-sex couples.

17

Families with a Gay,
Lesbian, or Bisexual Parent

This final chapter discusses families from the perspective of lesbian and gay parents and from the viewpoints of their children and the differing familial circumstances of their births. The formation of lesbian and gay families is explored, and research regarding their dynamics and the development of their children is summarized. Possibly because of the greater socialization of women toward relationships and families, the majority of the research in this area has been about lesbian mothers and their children. Because these studies are fairly recent, the conclusions are tentative, and comparatively few are available that relate to gay fathers and their children. Since the observations appear to point in the same direction (Fitzgerald, 1999; Golombok, 1999; Patterson, 1992, 1994, 1995a, 1995b, 1996, 1997a, 1998), however, suggestions for therapists are provided at several points in this chapter.

Lesbians and gay men have always been a part of family life; they are sons, daughters, sisters, brothers, nieces, nephews, and grandchildren. They also have forged family bonds with each other, and they parent (or are parenting) children conceived of previous heterosexual unions and those offspring who are born, adopted, or raised after their coming out. Clunis and Green (1988) described these families in three categories: "*nuclear*, with children who are born to or adopted by the couple; *blended*, where children are included who came originally from their mother's [or father's] prior relationship; and *extrablended*, where children come from both sources" (p. 112). These units challenge the model of the traditional family "at its core, raising fundamental questions about the relation between gender and parenting, the significance of biological versus social connections, and the role of the state in family life" (Benkov, 1994, p. 6). In any case, nuclear families exist in many forms and include the relationships lesbians and gay men create, both with their partners and with their children (Ariel & McPherson, 2000; Drucker, 1998; R. J. Green, 2000; Kirby, 1999b; Patterson, 1995a; Ricketts & Achtenberg, 1989; Savin-Williams & Esterberg, 2000; Sullivan & Dawidoff, 1999). These families have problems similar to those of heterosexual families, and some have difficulties that stem from the parents' homosexuality. Ethical mental health practice necessitates that clinicians be able to differentiate between the two since many families of gay men and lesbians present in therapy with problems that are unrelated, or tangential, to the sexual orientation of the parents (Baptiste, 1987b; Carlson, 1996; Clunis & Green, 1995; G. D. Green & Bozett, 1991).

Before the mid-1970s, virtually no psychological investigations of families with children headed by a lesbian or gay parent were available, and the few that existed were conducted during the 1970s in response to an increasing number of child custody and visitation battles. Almost all of the studies involving this population, therefore, have been conducted in recent years, and the majority involve primarily small samples of White, educated, urban lesbian mothers (and a few gay fathers) and their children. Most of this research involving families headed by gay men or lesbian women has been conducted to refute the charges and assumptions of the courts and mainstream culture about homosexuality. Accordingly, empirical evidence continues to be essential in defending sexual minority parents and their children against the heterosexist bias of the culture and the legal system (Benkov, 1994; Bigner & Jacobsen, 1992; Buxton, 1999; G. D. Green & Bozett, 1991; Patterson, 1992, 1995a, 1995b, 1998; Scrivner & Benkov, 1995).

FORMATION OF FAMILIES

Heterosexual marriage is the most common way through which sexual minority parents acquire children. A large number of individuals remain in these relationships and either acknowledge their homosexuality or remain closeted. Many eventually divorce, and some of these become the custodial parent, while others do not. With a high degree of intentionality, lesbians also conceive children through artificial insemination, using sperm from both known and unknown donors, including sperm banks (Chabot, 1999). Gay men become parents by donating sperm to lesbians and heterosexual women or by enlisting the help of surrogate donors or women who will carry the child for them. Some gay fathers participate actively in the raising of their offspring, and a few of these men cohabit with the mother(s), but most live separately either with or without a partner. Finally, both gay men and lesbians adopt children or become foster parents, but heterosexist assumptions on the part of governmental or adoption agencies, as well as continual legal challenges from religious conservatives, often make these efforts challenging, expensive, and difficult (Clunis & Green, 1995; Demian, 2000; G. D. Green & Bozett, 1991; Patterson, 1995a, 1998: Rochman, 1999b; L. B. Silverstein, 1996). Chapter 4 contained an extensive discussion of the legal dimensions of the issues related to gay and lesbian families.

When working with lesbian or gay couples around issues that are related to acquiring children, therapists are advised to help them resolve as many legal questions as possible before committing themselves to parenting. Agreements, contracts, and wills should be drafted, whether a child is adopted, conceived through sexual intercourse or donor insemination, or carried by a surrogate mother. Without these protections, given the climate of courts even in the best of circumstances for sexual minority parents and separating same-sex partners, one or both undoubtedly will lose (Gideonse, 1999; Morton, 1998; Scrivner & Benkov, 1995). The information provided in this chapter, as well as in

Chapter 4 and in the Resources section, may prove helpful to these individuals. Referral to appropriate legal counsel also may be warranted.

Adoption and Foster Parenting

In spite of numerous logistical and legal obstacles, many sexual minorities, nevertheless, choose to become foster parents or adopt children of their own. *Gay adoption* is a concept that defies easy definition since it "can involve single parents or partners; orphans, children in foster care, or the offspring of surrogate mothers and sperm donors; infants or adolescents; and lawyers, social workers, and agencies here and abroad" (Woog, 1998, p. 69). Because women have the option of bearing children and men do not, about 80% of gay adoptive parents are male. Independent adoptions and those through private agencies often are more costly ($12,000 to $30,000, depending on expenses for the birth mother and legal fees) than are those that are arranged through public agencies, but these latter types can get delayed or prevented altogether because of bureaucratic and state restrictions on adoptions by sexual minorities (Gideonse, 1999; Woog, 1998; also see Chapter 4). Some individuals openly declare themselves as lesbian or gay when applying, while others allow officials to believe they are single in order to avoid undue complications.

To avoid the kinds of problems described here, and because of availability, many gay men and lesbians are adopting children from other countries. In fact, same-sex couples may account for a large percentage of the increase in overseas adoptions. These procedures usually are facilitated by private adoption agencies, take place in the country of the child's birth, and are quite expensive (sometimes $25,000, including travel expenses and fees for intermediaries). There is little fear of losing the child to the birth mother, however, as sometimes happens when attempts at adoption are made in the United States (Woog, 1998). A consideration for prospective parents as they are deciding to adopt internationally, however, is whether they are willing to assume the additional difficulties that will arise for both children and parents because they are members of an interracial adoptive family (Clunis & Green, 1995). In spite of these complications, a number of lesbians who have a strong preference for a daughter have adopted girls from China (B. R. Rich, 2000). Some make this choice, given that conception from donor insemination results in a male fetus about 65% of the time, which is partially due to the amount of time that has lapsed between ejaculation and fertilization. Another variable is that insemination often is attempted when there are indications that ovulation has occurred (e.g., using a thermometer or increased mucus production) and the faster male-producing (Y chromosome) sperm are able to unite with the egg first (Clunis & Green, 1995; Martin, 1993; B. R. Rich, 2000; Rohrbaugh, 1988; Wells, 1997).

Pregnancy with a Known Donor

Although current research, however limited, suggests that lesbian mothers, gay fathers, and their children are well adjusted and functioning normally (Patterson, 1998; Wells, 1997), some lesbians feel a father figure is important to a child and may want to know the donor of the sperm (Martin, 1993; Rohrbaugh, 1988). The man chosen may be a friend, relative, or acquaintance. The danger is that the donor later may assert his legal rights as biological father and want custody or visitation, or he could come to desire a more active role in the child's life than was initially envisioned by any of the parties involved (Clunis & Green, 1995; Demian, 2000; N. A. Friedman, 1999; Martin, 1993). Therefore, trust in this person is critical. This expansion of the lesbian family, notwithstanding, to include a third adult with whom the couple seldom has a history of intimacy almost always is problematic and involves a great deal of emotional investment to make the arrangement viable. Difficulties of this nature can occur whether the conception took place through sexual intercourse or by means of insemination with fresh sperm from a man known to the women.

Gay men are having children with surrogate women, but not in the same numbers that lesbians are reproducing through donor insemination (Martin, 1993; Patterson & Chan, 1996). In this process, a woman is hired to carry a baby for a couple, either gay or heterosexual. When both partners are male, one of the men donates a sperm to a woman who will carry the child for the couple. If the same woman who donates the egg also is pregnant with the fetus, the method is referred to as *traditional surrogacy*. Sometimes the men will elect *gestational surrogacy*, which is a set of procedures in which one woman donates an egg that later is united with sperm from one of the men and a second woman carries the baby during the pregnancy. "With the egg donor not involved in the pregnancy and the surrogate not biologically related to the embryo, there [is] less emotional risk for both women" (Gideonse, 1999, p. 87). The risk for the men as co-parents also is reduced since the two women's legal standing as the *one* biological mother is less clear. Further, as with women and donor issues, the male couples need to consider the fact that only one of the men is the biological father of the child and the nonbiological parent could be denied access to the child should a separation between the partners occur (Demian, 2000). Obviously, couples and individuals are advised not to enter into these kinds of potentially complicated legal and biological situations without consulting legal counsel before they consent to any agreements. Choice of birth mothers, including their health status and reliability, also is crucial since these mothers have been known to take money from the prospective fathers and are never heard from again; others have returned after the birth to ask for visitation or even custody (Martin, 1993). Growing Generations, the first company devoted to managing surrogacy exclusively for gay men, both couples and individuals, was formed to assist people through these complex processes. This company estimates that total surrogacy costs are between $50,000 and $70,000—a price that restricts the procedure to only the most affluent (Gideonse, 1999).

Insemination with an Unknown Donor

Many in mainstream society see lesbian parenting as undermining traditional notions of the family and the heterosexual monopoly on reproduction (G. A. Dunne, 2000). In spite of this bias, a large number of lesbians are electing conception by means of donor or alternative insemination rather than by relying on male partners or men they may know. By choosing anonymous donors through sperm banks, these women can minimize the risk that a donor later will insist on parental rights with the child (Demian, 2000; N. A. Friedman, 1999). Donors usually are selected on the basis of such characteristics as ethnicity, education, age, religion, occupation, hair color, complexion, bone structure, and height (Kirkpatrick 1996; Leiblum, Palmer, & Spector, 1995; Martin, 1993). If the potential mothers elect to use fresh sperm, an intermediary, such as a discerning friend, physician, or sperm bank can provide assistance. Using frozen sperm is more convenient, available, and often less expensive, but the procedure is associated with lower pregnancy rates, fewer motile sperm, and a higher male birth rate (Martin, 1993; Rohrbaugh, 1988). This higher male birth rate has resulted in a large number of sons being raised by lesbian mothers and numerous publications directed toward these family units (Wells, 1997). In all cases, whether the sperm is fresh or frozen, or the donors are unknown or known, the men involved should be checked for health and HIV status, and a medical history should be obtained in case the child develops health problems at some point in life.

Martin (1993) notes that some lesbians have become mothers via surrogates, especially in situations where one or another (if a couple is involved) is either unable to become pregnant or unwilling to carry a child. In these cases, a prospective mother contributes her egg for fertilization with the sperm of a known or unknown donor and then hires a surrogate to carry the pregnancy: "There are lesbian couples where one partner is implanted with an embryo created by her lover's ovum and donor sperm. That partner, technically a surrogate, then gets to give birth to her lover's baby" (p. 369).

Many children born to lesbian mothers will be curious about their conception, and they often give indications of missing the fathers that their friends talk about. When they are old enough to understand their place in the dominant culture, donor-inseminated children may ask questions about their biological father, such as where or who he is (Carlson, 1996; Martin, 1993). Some of these youngsters are angry or embarrassed about the circumstances of their birth. The distress of their children usually is painful to lesbian mothers, and they may need the assistance of a therapist in sorting through their concerns and working through feelings of guilt they may experience about not being able "to provide a family closer to the sterotypical cultural ideal" (p. 65). Prospective mothers may want to consider selecting semen from donors who have indicated that they are willing to be contacted by children who result from insemination once the offspring are 18 years old (Kirkpatrick, 1996; Martin, 1993), thus providing youngsters with the assurance that they someday may meet the person whose genetics they carry. Regardless, "with little cultural or social support, the lesbian mother must deal here with a complex and difficult issue that will most likely extend over many years of her children's lives" (Loulan, 1986, p. 185).

Several studies have shown that lesbian parents are becoming more inclined to be honest with their children surrounding the use of a donor, but many nevertheless worry about how their child will deal with the absence of a known father (Brewaeys, Ponjaert-Kristoffersen, Van Steirteghem, & Devroey, 1993; Leiblum et al., 1995). In one investigation, 115 coupled lesbian and heterosexual women received donor insemination (Wendland, Burn, & Hill, 1996). Married couples were less likely than lesbian couples to tell others, including the child, of the nature of his or her conception, and to support disclosing identifying data about the donor to the child. Unlike the heterosexual couples ($n = 28$), all lesbian participants ($n = 14$) in another study (Leiblum et al., 1995) planned to disclose the donor insemination to their offspring. Similarly, 25 lesbian and 25 heterosexual parents were surveyed, and findings revealed that the lesbians intended to inform their children that they were conceived by donor insemination. Further, 40% of these women preferred that the identity of the donor be registered. Heterosexual couples, on the other hand, chose secrecy and donor anonymity (Brewaeys et al., 1993). The registration of a donor as the biological contributor of the sperm used in conception, presumably for later genetic purposes, is controversial. The recording of this information has implications for the children when they are old enough to acquire this information, but also for lesbian families and nonbiological mothers who might later have their rights as parents challenged legally. Accordingly, in one study, 56% of the sample of lesbian mothers (n = 100) wanted the identity of the donor of their child registered, but opinions differed in 12 of the 50 couples in the study. In these cases, the biological mother was in favor of the registration while the co-mother was not (Brewaeys, Devroey, Helmerhorst, Van Hall, & Ponjaert, 1995).

SEXUAL MINORITY PARENTS

Gay and lesbian parents are by no means rare, but estimates of the number of these individuals in the United States are imprecise. Many do not publicly reveal their sexual orientation for fear of losing child custody or visitation privileges, and heterosexism, homophobia, and fear of discrimination cause many others to remain closeted (Bigner & Jacobsen, 1992; Drucker, 1998; Patterson, 1996; L. B. Silverstein, 1996). Appraisals of the sum total of these parents range from 2 million to 8 million; some sources conjecture that the number of gay fathers is between 1 and 3 million and the number of lesbian mothers is between 1.5 and 5 million (Ariel & McPherson, 2000; Demian, 2000; G. D. Green & Bozett, 1991; Patterson, 1992, 1995a). Further, approximately 20% of gay men and up to one-third of lesbian women have been married and are parents of at least one child (Bigner & Jacobsen, 1992; Cabaj, 1995; Kirkpatrick, 1996). Because of cultural differences, the rates of childbearing in lesbians may differ by ethnicity. Morris (2000), for example, found that of the 568 lesbians of color in her study, 36% of Native American women were mothers, compared with 32% of African American participants, 20% of the Latina subjects, and 8% of the Asian American lesbians.

Stepfamily Concerns

A large number of lesbians and a much smaller number of gay men are custodial parents. Many of these individuals live in committed relationships, sometimes with a partner who also has custody of her or his children (Erera & Fredriksen, 1999). J. M. Lynch and Murray (2000) studied 23 lesbian and gay custodial stepfamilies and concluded that these kinds of families represent a unique type of familial unit, distinct from heterosexual stepfamilies and from lesbian and gay families who have children within the context of a lesbian or gay relationship. In addition to the usual strains that exist in stepfamilies, such as rejection of the stepparent by the partner's children and children's competition for parental attention, a lack of clarity regarding the role of a lesbian or gay stepparent is not uncommon. These individuals, for example, sometimes are not introduced as a parent's partner to the children and, hence, are not perceived by them to be functioning in a role similar to the stepparents of their friends. In addition, gay and lesbian stepparents often complain, much like their heterosexual counterparts, that they have no authority with the children, have no place in their partner's family, and are neglected by their mate because of the children (Baptiste, 1987a; Barret & Robinson, 1990; Bozett, 1990; Loulan, 1986; Wright, 1998). Given the complexity of these dynamics, even a seemingly simple question as to what to call stepparents can be extremely problematic (Slater, 1995). Issues of secrecy, homophobia, and inclusion arise when mates try to decide on a form of address to use within the family, with the children, and when referring to each other. The situation can become even more controversial when attempting to *mutually* select a form of reference to use with friends, coworkers, neighbors, school personnel, and families of origin.

These concerns, incidentally, can arise in all of the gay and lesbian household configurations described earlier in this chapter (J. M. Lynch & Murray, 2000).

One study assessed aspects of functioning that are associated with family happiness in 48 stepfamilies with gay fathers, their partners, and at least one child who either lives with them or visits (Crosbie-Burnett & Helmbrecht, 1993). Not surprisingly, the best predictors of family happiness on the part of gay fathers and their children related to the integration and inclusion of the stepfathers. Clunis and Green (1995) made this same point in reference to lesbian mother stepfamilies when they noted that "when children have to compete with their mother's new partner for attention, they are not likely to welcome her into the family" (p. 47). Slater (1995) discussed the need for parents to learn "to sustain their intimacy with less time, less uninterrupted attention, and less energy available for their connection as lovers" (p. 95). This is especially important in stepfamily situations, in relationships where the nonbiological parent may feel particularly left out of the parent–child bond, or in lesbian couples whose relationships may have been built on "much time alone together, reciprocal emotional nurturing, and an intense exclusivity within the couple relationship" (p. 95). These dynamics of lesbian parental couples will be discussed in more detail in a later section of this chapter.

Prolonged custody disputes are not uncommon since former spouses may have no where else to take their struggles except to the legal system (Carlson, 1996). Children always are affected by these contentions, and they, too, may act out their pain. Unlike custody battles that involve heterosexual former couples, however, the sexual orientation of a parent may be a focal point in the battle for both previous spouses and children. Buxton (1991), a heterosexual parent who was married for 25 years to a gay man, believes that the straight parent's attitude toward the lesbian mother or gay father is a key factor in how the children will accept the minority sexual orientation of a parent. In order for children not to feel as if they have lost either parent after a divorce or a disclosure of homosexuality, she advocates that the former spouse of a lesbian or gay man continue to be seen as a part of the family. While this is "easier said than done," given the amount of animosity often present in these situations, therapists can sometimes be of assistance in keeping open the lines of communication between all parties in these diverse and complicated families. Clunis and Green (1995) likewise believe that having biological parents disappear or be minimally involved with their children causes damage to the youngsters. Correspondingly, they note that "even when a father undermines a lesbian mother's relationships with her child, the mother may still want to support the father–child connection—for her child's sake" (p. 50).

Dalton and Bielby (2000) interviewed 14 coupled lesbian mothers and revealed how these women and their partners reinscribed gendered understandings in constructing and maintaining family roles and relations. Wright (1998) used ethnographic research methodology in interviewing five lesbian stepfamilies and noted the importance of a stepmother and a legal mother negotiating and organizing parenting and homemaking tasks, as well as defining and creating the stepmother's role with the children. Clunis and Green (1995) noted that these understandings are easier and less cumbersome if the partner's parenting style and values are similar to what the children are accustomed to.

Societal Concerns of Lesbian and Gay Parents

The dominant culture assumes that parents are heterosexual, and gay and lesbian parents often feel caught in a cultural clash, much like the experience of sexual minorities of color described in Chapter 10. Once they become parents, or sometimes when they assume custody of their children, they no longer fit well into the childless sexual minority community (Carlson, 1996). In contrast, the parenting culture of sports, ballet lessons, girl and boy scouts, and school functions is strongly heterosexual, and they may feel like anomalies at these events, whether or not they have revealed their sexual orientation to others: "A firm gay or lesbian identity may be disarmed during this transition" (p. 66). They and their children may feel as if they are straddling two contradictory worlds, and, as will be discussed later in this chapter, they may feel as if they continually are faced with the decisions about disclosure of the family configuration or secrecy about their lives.

Sometimes parents are in the early stages of identity formation (see Chapter 5) and are struggling either to foreclose on a sexual minority orientation or to come out. Their own concerns at the time may be so predominant that they have few resources left for parenting or to be the strong focal point their children need (Carlson, 1996): "This period can be particularly disruptive to family life in that it may not be possible to put the child's needs first" (p. 70). Therapeutic intervention may prove helpful to these parents and families, especially if the parent is having difficulty reconciling or integrating the identities of gay and father (or lesbian and mother) (Bigner & Bozett, 1989). Superego modification (Hanley-Hackenbruck, 1989; see Chapter 9) could prove useful to these mothers and fathers since frequently their own internalized homophobia has been replaced by perfectionism. Many feel guilty for being an inadequate parent, because of either their sexual orientation or their emotional confusion. Some feel they do not deserve to have children, in spite of having struggled hard to either acquire or keep them, and this self-criticism and perfectionism should be addressed in therapy.

Despite the high number of stressors in their lives, however, the studies relating to the mental health of lesbian mothers indicate that they score at least as high as divorced heterosexual mothers on assessments of psychological functioning and overall adjustment. Further, there appears to be no major differences between the two groups of mothers in terms of their self-concepts, happiness levels, or psychiatric status, but "no published studies of gay fathers make such comparisons with heterosexual fathers" (Patterson, 1995a, p. 270). The family lives of 45 lesbian parents were studied, and findings revealed that these women were aware of the impact of their sexual orientation on their children (Lott-Whitehead & Tully, 1993). Consequently, the mothers were vigilant about maintaining the integrity of their families and reported that the stress this entailed was buffered by support networks. Maintaining these systems, however, is especially difficult for lesbian parents, both single and coupled, if they live in rural areas. The stresses of these women often are exacerbated by the combination of their sexual minority status and their social and geographic isolation (L. J. Friedman, 1997; McCarthy, 2000). This situation probably is similar for gay fathers who live in rural areas, as well.

Issues with Families of Origin

If gay men and lesbians have not disclosed their sexual orientation to their parents, even during the pregnancy or adoption, the stress on a couple is intensified after the arrival of a child. The invisibility of coparents is increased since they are often perceived as close friends of their daughter or son rather than as a member of the family. In the case of lesbians, becoming a parent frequently brings the birth mother into closer contact with her family of origin, while the parents of the co-mother sometimes do not consider the baby their grandchild (McCandlish, 1987; Patterson, 1998; Slater, 1995). The situation is complicated even further in the case of gay couples when one is the biological father of a child carried by a surrogate. These issues of lineage intensify the difference between the two extended families since, on the surface, one has no legal or familial relationship to the child (Hequembourg & Farrell, 1999; Rohrbaugh, 1988, 1992). The circumstances become more stressful over the years as the youngster (if acquired as an infant) learns to talk and describe people by name and their relationship to each other and to her or him. In other words, lesbian or gay parents continually run the risk of being "outed" by their own child.

Grandparents who may have rejected their lesbian or gay children are often torn between their disapproval of the sexual orientation of their offspring and a need to see their grandchildren (Slater, 1995). Baptiste (1987a) notes that many grandparents have resolved this dilemma by compartmentalizing the two sets of relationships; they continue to ostracize their own child, while lavishing attention on the grandchildren who must live in an "unhealthy" (p. 123) situation. Some even verbally denigrate the stepfamily living arrangements directly to their grandchildren.

Lesbian Couples Who Are Mothers

For all lesbian couples who are considering motherhood, the *"daddy question* (or 'no-daddy dilemma,' as it is sometimes called)" arises (Baum, 1996, p. 118). Clunis and Green (1995) refer to this as "the great lesbian sperm chase" (p. 24). The couple must first decide how the child will be brought into their family, whether through foster parenting, adoption, or biological childbirth (Kirkpatrick, 1996; Slater, 1995). If the latter is chosen, they must then determine which of them will carry the child and be considered the legal mother of the baby. "Feelings of competition are aroused here, along with issues of control. Who will be more central in the relationship as a parent? Whose work schedule will be most disrupted by parenting?" (Rohrbaugh, 1988, p. 53). If their relationship already is fraught with control and competition struggles, motherhood is "a perfect arena to play out these issues" (p. 53).

Couple Dynamics

Stiglitz (1990) explored what happens to the dynamics of a lesbian couple when a child is introduced into the system. She reviewed the literature, as well as surveyed 12 couples (7 lesbian and 5 heterosexual), and concluded that the lesbian pairs experienced dissatisfaction with the amount and depth of their intimacy and sharing, and discord as they attempted to balance issues of merger and separation (see Chapter 15). If this power balance between the members was not relatively stable and equal before the birth, the women tended to compete for power as they struggled with their fear of being overpowered by the relationship of the other with the child. Many of these issues are not unique to lesbian mother families, however. For example, relationships in 30 lesbian families created through donor insemination were compared with 38 donor-inseminated heterosexual families and with 30 heterosexual families that were created through sexual intercourse (Brewaeys, Ponjaert, Van Hall, & Golombok, 1997). Findings revealed that the quality of the couples' relationship and that of the mother–child interaction did not differ between the three populations. Further, the nonbiological mother in lesbian families was regarded by her children to be as much of a "parent" as was the father in both types of heterosexual families, and her interaction with the children was superior to that of the biological fathers. Similarly, 55 families headed by lesbian mothers were compared with 25 heterosexual families (Chan, Raboy, & Patterson, 1998). These included 50 families with two parents and 30 with one parent. The adjustment of the children in all these combinations of situations was unrelated to parental sexual orientation or the number of parents in the household. Lesbian parents, however, reported sharing unpaid child-care tasks more equally than did heterosexual counterparts. Probably most importantly, *coupled* parents—both lesbian and heterosexual—who were experiencing higher levels of stress and conflict and lower levels of love for each other, had children who exhibited more behavior problems.

Lesbian couples often struggle in other ways after the birth of a child since pregnancy, nursing, and biological motherhood create asymmetries in their parental relationship (Carlson, 1996; N. A. Friedman, 1999; Hequembourg & Farrell, 1999; Martin, 1993; McCandlish, 1987; Rohrbaugh, 1988, 1992; Scrivner & Benkov, 1995). The nonbiological mother role in relation to the child is far less visible than is that of the birth mother and is even more invisible if she is closeted and has few of her own sources of support. Sometimes she is envious of the birth mother's closeness with the child, who, in turn, often is jealous of the other mother's freedom. Further, the biological and nonbiological mothers have unequal legal status as parents (see Chapter 4); the fact that the children usually bear the surname of the biological or adoptive mother underscores this (Patterson, 1994, 1998). Therapists can assist couples in helping their child(ren) make a developmental shift from primary mother attachment to an emotional connection to both lesbian parents (McCandlish, 1987). Intervention can also help partners examine their couple dynamics when sexual intimacy is reduced or ceases altogether and "the birth of a child seems to cause a crack in the couple's fantasy of sameness" (p. 33).

Resiliency

In spite of the many possible difficulties described here, literature cited throughout this chapter attests to the fact that lesbian families fare as well as heterosexual families on virtually all of the variables measured. One study, in particular, analyzed the perceptions of 59 mothers (24 lesbian and 35 heterosexual) by asking them to complete a questionnaire comprised of four scales: the Index of Family Relations, the Index of Parental Attitudes, the Family Awareness Scale, and the Dyadic Adjustment Scale (McNeill, Rienzi, & Kposowa, 1998). The mean scores for both sets of mothers were remarkably similar and reflected few differences on self-reported stress, adjustment, competence, and the quality of relationship with their families.

CHILDREN

Somewhere between 3 and 14 million children in the United States are estimated to live with a lesbian or gay parent (Ariel & McPherson, 2000; Demian, 2000; Drucker, 1998; Patterson, 1996). As with their parents, estimates vary greatly since their numbers are hidden due to fear of discrimination and sociocultural norms for family life. Most of these children are the biological offspring of one of the parents and were born within the context of heterosexual relationships. Because of the legal bias in favor of heterosexuality, much of the impetus for research about these children has come from judicial concerns about their welfare if they live with their gay or lesbian parents (Patterson, 1995a, 1995b, 1996). More of these parents than ever before are living openly, however, and record numbers of them, particularly lesbians, are having or adopting children as single parents or within the context of same-sex relationships (Bull, 1999b; Clunis & Green, 1995; Slater, 1995; Tasker & Golombok, 1997). Consequently, more children raised in openly gay and lesbian households are available for research and are willing to tell their stories. Often these are tales of ostracism, of harassment, or of being the objects of intense curiosity as the youths struggle with pressures to fit in and to be like everyone else. Sometimes, refreshingly, these narratives sound much like those of children raised by heterosexual parents and are about not only the problems but also the advantages of growing up in their families and the values and wisdom learned from their parents (Kirby, 1999b; McGuire, 1996; Raab, 2000).

Unfortunately, many of the first studies (in the 1970s and 1980s) focused on the gender role appropriateness of the offspring. The underlying presumption was that, if children behaved according to the gender stereotypes of their biological sex, they were presumed to be heterosexual (i.e., the gay or lesbian parent had not influenced the child abnormally toward homosexuality). The personal development, psychiatric and behavior problems, personality, self-concept, locus of control, moral judgment, intelligence, and social relationships of the children were other foci of research (Patterson, 1995a). Recent studies have continued to examine these themes, as well as others within the parameters of child development. The purpose of much of this research, however, appears to have shifted from that of providing information to be used in the courts to one that attempts to objectively describe the personalities of children who are raised in different family and parental circumstances. An illustration of this is a report describing a series of longitudinal investigations of psychological adjustment of European children who were conceived by sexual intercourse compared with those conceived by assisted reproduction, as well as those reared in lesbian households contrasted with those raised by single heterosexual mothers (Golombok, 1999).

While many of the studies of lesbians and gay men and their children have a number of methodological difficulties, the accumulation of findings still can be meaningful (Kirkpatrick, 1996; Patterson, 1995a, 1995b). The sample sizes often are small; control groups are not always used when needed; samples have been composed largely of White, urban, well-educated individuals; and no longitudinal studies have been conducted. Also, "no information is yet available on differences stemming from race or ethnicity, family economic circumstances, cultural environments, or related variables" (Patterson, 1995a, p. 281). Several issues—such as whether parents currently are coupled or single, or were at the time of the child's birth, the sex of the parents, and the kinds of households into which the children were born—are confounded in many studies. In spite of these limitations, however, the conclusions that "common stereotypes are not supported by the data"(Patterson, 1995b, p. 1) are quite uniform.

Sexist Bias

Bias toward the development of children raised in gay and lesbian families is apparent other than in research efforts and legal opinion since the heterosexist and sexist prejudice of the culture influences public policy, as well. For example, units headed by lesbian mothers suffer from misogyny, which sees "families without fathers as deficient, inherently pathological environments for child development" (L. B. Silverstein, 1996, p. 6). L. B. Silverstein (1996) also asserts that, given the growing body of research that demonstrates normal developmental outcomes for children of lesbian mothers (to be discussed later in this section), a family headed by a lesbian mother should not automatically be considered inferior to one with two heterosexual parents. She admits, however, that numerous studies have demonstrated that children who are raised in households headed by *mothers* [both lesbian and heterosexual] tend to have poorer developmental outcomes than those who live with both biological parents, but she contends that an undue emphasis has been placed on the sex of the parents rather than on other sociopolitical considerations that affect mother-headed families (e.g., poverty, a second adult to assist with childrearing, or the effects of divorce). In commenting about findings of this nature, Steckel (1987) notes that "mother aloneness, rather than father absence, was shown to predispose children to difficulties in development and adaptation" (p. 83).

The findings of the following study appear to support Steckel's observation. In an investigation that was designed to examine the family functioning and the psychological development of children raised in fatherless homes, 30 lesbian mother families were compared with 42 families headed by a single heterosexual mother, and 41 two-parent heterosexual families were interviewed (Golombok, Tasker, & Murray, 1997). Results showed that children raised in homes without a father from infancy experienced greater warmth and interaction with their mother and were more securely attached to her. They perceived themselves to be less cognitively and physically competent than their peers from father-present families, however. No differences were identified between families headed by the two groups of mothers, except that there was greater mother–child interaction in lesbian mother families.

Just as with families headed by lesbian mothers, bias also exists toward those headed by gay fathers, and these units often are evaluated from both heterosexist and sexist perspectives. In this instance, however, the sexism is reversed and the children frequently are thought to be affected negatively by the lack of a mother's role. L. B. Silverstein (1996) contends that "research suggests that neither a female parent nor a male parent is *necessary* for positive developmental outcomes, gender identity formation, sex role socialization, or the development of a heterosexual orientation in children of either sex" (p. 12). In any case, Scrivner and Benkov (1995) caution against automatically assuming stigma, which can exist in all forms and on a continuum, for children of sexual minorities.

Summary of Findings

Most studies of children raised by sexual minority parents concentrate on those either with lesbian mothers or with gay fathers, although only a few are available that focus on the latter population. To illustrate the kind of work being done in this area, a few of these gender-specific studies are discussed in later sections of this chapter. First, however, some conclusions regarding the combined body of this research are provided. Fitzgerald (1999), for example, reviewed the literature from 1972 to 1997 that focused on the development of children with gay and lesbian parents. She included studies of offspring of divorced lesbian and gay parents, as well as those conducted with "planned" children who lived in gay and lesbian families. She noted that the body of research generally determines that children from both sets of circumstances are developing psychologically, intellectually, behaviorally, and emotionally in normative directions and that the sexual orientation of parents is not an effective or important predictor of successful child development. Patterson (1995a, 1996, 1997a) similarly summarized studies on the personal and social development of children of gay and lesbian parents. She also examined the mediating effects of divorce and adoption compared with biological birth and found that youngsters in all groups were progressing normally. In an earlier summary, she noted that "if, as would appear to be the case, neither parents nor children in lesbian and gay families have any special risk of maladjustment or other psychosocial problems, then a good rationale for prejudice and discrimination is more difficult to provide." Until such a day when bias toward such units no longer exists, however, these families will have "a broad range of special needs" (Patterson, 1996, p. 292).

Children of Lesbian Mothers

Studies of children of lesbian mothers appear to cluster into two categories (Patterson, 1994): characteristics of those children conceived in heterosexual relationships, and traits of children born or adopted in the context of their mothers' lives as lesbians. The following discussion summarizes research in terms of these two types. Precise estimates as to the number of lesbians with children in both groups are not available, but "the rise in births among openly lesbian women in the United States has been so dramatic that many observers have labeled it a lesbian baby boom" (p. 156).

Children Born to Heterosexual Couples

Probably the largest group of children with gay or lesbian parents are those born within the context of heterosexual relationships (Patterson, 1996). This is a relatively diverse group and includes offspring whose parents either divorced after a disclosure of homosexuality or decided not to divorce. Lesbian or gay parents may be single or in a relationship with a partner who may or may not act as a stepparent to the children. If the partner has children, the offspring may be in stepsibling relationships with one another. A number of studies have compared children of lesbian mothers and heterosexual mothers, all born within the context of heterosexual relationships, and found few differences in terms of mental health, psychological well-being, personal characteristics, social relationships, self-esteem, cognitive functioning, behavioral adjustment, gender role development, sex role behavior, and sexual orientation or identity between the two groups (Falk, 1989; Flaks, Ficher, Masterpasqua, & Joseph, 1995; Gibbs, 1989; Golombok & Tasker, 1996; Gottman, 1990; R. Green, 1986; Huggins, 1989; Kirkpatrick, 1996; Mooney-Somers & Golombok, 2000; Patterson, 1992, 1995a, 1996, 1998; S. B. Pennington, 1987; Tasker & Golombok, 1995, 1997).

Despite these favorable research findings, anecdotal reports from participants often describe stresses in these households that are related to the children's noncustodial biological parent. These are not unique to lesbian families, however, but involve dynamics similar to those of divorced heterosexual women and their former spouses, the fathers of their children (Kirkpatrick, 1996; L. B. Silverstein, 1996). Some fathers blame all the difficulties of separation on the mother's lesbian identity, and this can result in vindictiveness, threats, or legal and custodial battles. For the lesbian parent, "the sense of the father's presence as a sort of heterosexual policemen of her activities can be quite painful and damaging" (Loulan, 1986, p. 185). As in the case of all separated families, parental strife can be quite distressing to children.

Children Acquired by Lesbian Mothers

Studies of children born to, or raised by, lesbian mothers reveal findings similar to those conducted with children born to heterosexual couples; that is, they were well adjusted, and normal attainment had been reached on a number of developmental milestones (Brewaeys et al., 1997; Brewaeys & Van Hall, 1997; Chan et al., 1998; McCandlish, 1987). In one of the first systematic studies in this regard, Steckel (1985, 1987) compared three behavior indicators of the developmental tasks of separation–individuation (independence, ego functions, and object relations) of 3- and 4-year-old children born to 11 coupled lesbian mothers with those born to 11 married heterosexual mothers. She found considerable similarity in the development of the children from both populations, but also some striking differences. For example, children of heterosexual couples "had a more aggressively tinged separation process, seeing themselves as more aggressive and being seen by parents and teachers as more bossy and domineering, more active in asserting themselves, more negativistic, and more involved in power struggles" (Steckel, 1987, p. 81). Conversely, children of lesbian mothers demonstrated a more lovable self-image, expressed more helplessness, and were seen by parents and teachers as more affectionate, responsive, and protective toward younger children than were the offspring of heterosexual mothers. Steckel concluded that the presence of a female coparent, as compared with a father, does not negatively affect a child's separation–individuation process, but does establish a qualitatively different experience. Because the fathers in this study participated less than the lesbian coparents in the daily care of the children, the children living with heterosexual couples had to separate more forcefully from the mother–child dyad and in an aggressive manner they may have modeled from their male parent.

Children of Gay Fathers

The largest group of gay fathers is divorced, having entered into a heterosexual marriage before declaring a gay identity. Because courts usually favor mothers over fathers, and heterosexual over homosexual, most of these fathers are nonresidential parents and do not live in the same household as their children (Patterson, 1995a; Patterson & Chan, 1996). Gay father family configurations exist in many forms, however, and Barret and Robinson (1990) described eight of them:

Unmarried Gay Fathers

This kind of family configuration can evolve for many reasons. The father and mother may or may not love each other, and the pregnancy could have been unplanned or was preplanned as a means for both parties to have biological children. The parents may or may not live together. In some cases the mother was inseminated with the gay man's sperm. In all cases, however, the dynamics are complicated and involve custody, visitation, and financial arrangements, but also what to tell children and other sexual partners, what surnames to give the children, and how their family is to be defined.

Single, Adoptive Gay Fathers

The number of gay men who are adopting children is rising, and some of these youngsters are acquired from orphanages in other countries. Most of these adoptees, however, are older children who often are considered "hard to place," given their age, ethnicity, or histories of abandonment, mental and physical disabilities, abuse, or delinquency (Barret & Robinson, 1990; Patterson & Chan, 1996). One report states: "Surprisingly though, past history in dealing with life's problems often makes it easier for these children to understand and accept their adopted father's homosexuality" (Barret & Robinson, 1990, p. 63).

Gay Fathers with Intact Marriages

The spouse in these families may not know of her husband's homosexuality, and psychotherapy may include concerns revolving around disclosure. Other considerations can involve negotiating mutually acceptable arrangements to live together, to live separately, or to divorce. Buxton's (1991) work describes the coming-out process to heterosexual spouses and offers ideas for negotiating the complex relationship issues that are involved.

Sole-Custody, Single Gay Fathers

These families usually were constituted as a result of maternal death or the mother's willingness to give custody of the children to the father. While painful for children, these situations are extremely stressful for fathers because they face the stigma that results from being a "double minority" (i.e., a single custodial father and a gay man).

Joint-Custody, Single Gay Fathers

These men are separated or divorced from the biological mother of their children. A considerable number of them conceal their sexual orientation from either their former spouse, their children, or both, due to fear of losing parental rights or to unresolved internalized homophobia. Stressors include joint custody decisions, along with issues that involve the father's sexual orientation on the part of his ex-wife, his children, or himself.

Gay Father Stepfamilies

Several concerns of lesbian and gay stepfamilies were discussed earlier in this chapter. Additional difficulties of these gay male families may involve other dynamics, such as a former wife's boyfriend or husband who dislikes gay men; or mothers who worry about the safety from sexual molestation of their children while in the company of two gay men; or the concern of mothers over the development or gender identity of their children due to having spent time with a gay couple.

Separated or Divorced and Estranged Gay Fathers

These fathers have little or no contact with their children, often as a result of prolonged and stressful custody battles. Therapy involves resolution of the father's possible feelings of rejection, alienation, isolation, and bitterness. Since grieving the loss of a relationship with children is extremely painful, support groups composed of sexual minority parents in similar situations or sympathetic websites might be helpful (see the Resources section).

Two Gay Fathers and Lesbian Mother

This newer configuration of families is found mostly in urban areas with large concentrations of lesbians and gay men. In these situations, a woman is inseminated with mixed sperm from two gay men. Most of these parental threesomes do not cohabitate as a family unit, but some do reside together with their child(ren). These arrangements have been referred to as *quadra-parenting* if four people (a lesbian couple and a gay couple) are involved in the creation of the family (Patterson & Chan, 1996, p. 374). In these cases, the child(ren) might spend part of the time in one home and the remainder of the time in the other. Variations on this situation might include one or a pair of gay men (one or both of whom might donate a sperm) with a single heterosexual or lesbian woman, or a gay man donating a sperm to a lesbian couple. Obviously, in all cases, the legal, custodial, financial, and logistical arrangements are complicated and may need either legal or therapeutic intervention for resolution.

Summary

Research on gay fathers and their children is quite new and relatively sparse, especially when compared with that relating to lesbian mothers and their children (Bigner, 1996; Bozett, 1989; Bozett & Hanson, 1991; Patterson, 1995a; Patterson & Chan, 1996). Almost all of what is available focuses on divorced gay fathers, rather than men who have become parents within the context of a gay identity. Finally, the majority of empirical research is nearly a decade old or more.

As mentioned previously, most of the early studies on gay fathers were motivated by prejudicial societal attitudes and the need to provide a reasoned defense against them (Patterson, 1995a). Investigations of gay fathers, for example, demonstrated that their offspring identified themselves as gay in the same percentage range as children of heterosexual parents (Bailey, 1995; Bailey, Bobrow, Wolfe, & Mikash, 1995; Bozett, 1989; Patterson, 1995a). In a large investigation of the sexual orientation of sons of gay fathers (82 adult sons of 55 gay fathers), 9% of sons were reported to be gay or bisexual (Bailey, 1995). The sexual orientation of the offspring was not related to the number of years the father and son lived in the same household, to the frequency of contact between them, or to the quality of their relationship. Other research attempted to refute the fallacy that children of sexual minority parents are at a heightened risk for sexual abuse (Patterson, 1992, 1995a, 1996; Patterson & Chan, 1996). In this regard, Barret and Robinson (1990) noted that children who reside with lesbian or gay parents appear to be *less* at risk for sexual abuse than are children who live with heterosexual parents. Most other aspects of the personal and social development of children of gay fathers have not been studied, and the majority of what is available describes the attitudes and behaviors of fathers, rather than the impact of the fathers' sexual orientation on the development of their children (Bigner, 1996; Patterson & Chan, 1996; Ross & Arrindell, 1988).

Disclosure and Children

Some children do not know the sexual orientation of their gay or lesbian parents, but most eventually find out. In one study of 34 lesbian mothers and 32 gay fathers (Wyers, 1987), almost all of the mothers (32; 94.1%) and over half of the fathers (17; 53.1%) reported that their children had knowledge of their sexual orientation. Conversely, only one mother and slightly more than one-third of the fathers (11; 34.4%) reported that their children did not know of their sexual orientation. One mother and one father additionally acknowledged that their children probably knew about their sexual orientation, although they had not disclosed or discussed it with them. Some of the variance between the gay and lesbian parents in their children's knowledge of their sexual orientation may be attributed to child custody. Children of 53% of the lesbian mothers lived with them, but children of 90% of the gay fathers lived with their mothers. These data further suggest that lesbian mothers may be more open about their sexual orientation with their children, while gay fathers may be more tentative about disclosing their sexual orientation to their children (Wyers, 1987). Children's initial reactions to finding out ranged from positive to negative, including anger and confusion.

Effects of Secrecy

Not disclosing a homosexual orientation creates the same inauthenticity and distance between sexual minority parents and their offspring as between gay and lesbian children and their parents (discussed previously in Chapter 14). Just as in the latter case, the cost of holding a secret is severe to gay fathers and lesbian mothers (Baptiste, 1987a; Bozett, 1990; Carl, 1990; Clunis & Green, 1988, 1995; E. J. Dunne, 1987). Often in their own homes, they hide their identities from their children and constantly monitor their behaviors and friendships. Further, they forego participation in the lesbian and gay community, thus depriving themselves of needed social support. Fear of accidental disclosure of their sexual orientation is always present, both when they are with their children and when they are away from them. This secrecy can be confusing for the children, as well as quite difficult for couples who hide the nature of their relationship from those with whom they share a residence. "The compromises needed to maintain the illusion of heterosexuality in the presence of the children places the entire family, but especially the adults, under tremendous pressure" (Baptiste, 1987a, p. 128).

Children who know of the sexual orientation of their parents may feel the pressure of the family secret in their relationships with their noncustodial (usually heterosexual and biological) parent, both sets of grandparents, and other relatives (Baptiste, 1987a). Because lesbian and gay parents often fear losing custody of their children, they sometimes attempt to prevent an ex-spouse from knowing of their sexual orientation or their same-sex relationship, or both. Visits to noncustodial parents and grandparents often are strained as children engage in "many subterfugal maneuvers" (p. 122) to keep the secret from being exposed.

Stepsibling relationships create difficulties, as well. The lack of legal ties between parents in lesbian and gay stepfamilies often create confusion between the children of the partners as to the nature of their relationships to each other. This ambiguous situation often leads to resentment of their parents and the rejection of requests for cooperation between them (Baptiste, 1987b). Sometimes they may behave like (step)brothers and sisters while at home, but are reluctant to do so with people outside of the immediate family for fear of removing the "veil of secrecy" (p. 231) and exposing the family to negative sanctions from the school, peer group, community, church, and other biological parent.

These children frequently feel isolated from peers, the neighborhood community, and the broader society as a consequence of the secrecy that surrounds the lifestyle of the adults in the family (Ariel & McPherson, 2000; Bozett, 1990; Kirkpatrick, 1996). In other words, they live with a secret and spend considerable energy protecting it. Adolescents, in particular, may be reluctant to bring home dates and friends for fear of discovery, and they may fear being asked probing questions about their family (Baptiste, 1987a, 1987b). This point was made in a study of 48 gay father stepfamilies in which 54% of the adolescent children reported that their heterosexual friends did not know about their father's sexual orientation (Crosbie-Bennett & Helmbrecht, 1993). These teenagers also described receiving little support from their nongay friends.

Discussing Homosexuality with Children

In preparing parents to disclose their homosexuality to their children, E. J. Dunne (1987) suggests therapists conceptualize two aspects of the conversation(s): proactive and reactive. He then helps clients role-play situations in these two categories. Examples of proactive situations include answering generic and personal questions about sexuality and homosexuality, enlisting the assistance of the child's parent, and helping children deal with schoolmates' attitudes about having a lesbian or gay parent. Sample reactive situations involve scenarios such as, "Your child(ren) saw you being affectionate with your lover," "Your child(ren)'s mother tells your child(ren) about your sexual orientation without your consent," and "Your lover insists you tell your child(ren) about your sexual [orientation]" (p. 218). Table 17.1 summarizes some of the considerations addressed by Dunne and others in helping clients disclose their sexual orientation to their children.

Helping Children Understand

Lesbian mothers and gay fathers often are extremely concerned that their children will react negatively to the confirmation of parental homosexuality. Sometimes their worst fear is that their offspring will reject them completely and never speak to them again, which, as with their own parents, rarely occurs. Others are apprehensive that their children will be angry or disillusioned with them; will be confused or sad about the entire situation; or will retaliate, possibly by asking to live with a noncustodial parent. These kinds of situations do occur, but generally they are temporary and eventually diminish in intensity. Table 17.2 provides guidelines for both therapists and parents in assisting children through the process of integrating the sexual orientation of their parents into the totality of their lives.

Parents may need reassurance that favorable relationships with their children are possible after disclosure. For example, in one study, most of the 10 gay fathers and 11 lesbian mothers, with 37 children between them, reported that their children accepted their homosexuality better than anticipated, and they described overall positive relationships between them (R. H. Turner, Scadden, & Harris, 1990). The children appeared to have few long-term problems because of the sexual orientation of their parents; in fact, paren-

TABLE 17.1. Gay and Lesbian Parents: Coming Out to Children

Help gay and lesbian parents . . .

- Come to terms with their sexual orientation before disclosing to their children
  - Self-acceptance increases the likelihood that children will react positively.
  - Shame increases the likelihood that children will react negatively.

- Plan for self-disclosure
  - Parents need to tell their children before they hear from others.
  - Children rarely initiate a discussion of the topic.
  - Time and place of disclosure should be planned in advance.

- Prepare conversation
  - Disclosure should be positive and sincere, and not apologetic.
  - Reassure children that loving relationship with parents will not change.

- Cast self-disclosure in age-appropriate language
  - Parents should disclose to children as early as possible.
  - Children are never too young to be told.
  - Details should be confined to child's level of understanding.

- Prepare for possible questions
  - Why are you telling me?
  - What does being gay (or lesbian) mean?
  - What makes a person gay (or lesbian)?
  - Will I be gay (or lesbian), too?
  - Don't you like women (or men)?
  - What should I tell my friends?

- Prepare for the child to withdraw for a while

- Stay calm

Note. Summarized from Barret & Robinson (1990), Bozett (1990), Buxton (1991), Clunis & Green (1988, 1995), and Schulenburg (1985).

tal homosexuality appeared to be of little consequence in the overall alliance between these children and their parents. As discussed previously, many of the problems of the lesbian mothers were somewhat unrelated to their sexual orientation and were similar to those of single heterosexual mothers in that they were more economically depressed than were gay fathers, felt greater role strain, and had poorer relationships with ex-spouses than did the men with their former mates.

After conversations with about 100 gay fathers in Germany, Büntzly (1993) concluded that most of the problems encountered by the children of these men occur when the offspring are old enough to have contacts outside the family and hence are exposed to the value judgments of society. He suggests that the best way for homosexual parents to minimize this situation for their children is to counteract it with a "social frame" (p. 111) that consists of a number of lesbians and gay men, as well as supportive heterosexuals, so that the young people can see various forms of stable relationships in numerous individuals whom they have come to value. In addition to providing this social frame, Büntzly (1993) advocates that parents disclose their minority sexual orientation when their children are young (9 to 12 years old at the latest) so that the offspring have time to integrate the parental homosexuality in a natural and positive manner before they hear the status of their parent demeaned by others. Some children raised as such have been known to become both defenders and advocates not only of their parents but also of other sexual minorities.

TABLE 17.2. Helping Children Understand Their Gay and Lesbian Parents

Help children . . .

- Separate issues of sexual orientation and divorce
  – Sexual orientation and concerns regarding separation from parent(s) need to be discussed independently.
  – Relationships with both/all parents should be encouraged.
  – Routines should be maintained to assure predictability.

- Grieve the loss of the heterosexual parent
  – Nuclear family images and issues often are intertwined.
  – Ongoing nature of the adjustment process should be explained.

- Resolve conflict between inner feelings and social standards
  – Children will need permission to express negative emotions.
  – Redefining the concept of family may be useful.
  – Age-appropriate information can facilitate understanding.

- Examine their own sexuality
  – Children's fear of being gay or lesbian may need to be discussed.
  – Information may need to be provided about the variety of relationships between the same and different sexes.

- Disclose selectively to others
  – Tradeoff between carrying a secret and risking humiliation should be discussed.
  – Children may need to be provided with the skills for telling others.

- Network with other children
  – Healthy role models are essential.
  – Peer socialization reverses isolation.
  – Interacting with other families can normalize experiences.

Note. Summarized from Barret & Robinson (1990), Baum, (1996), Bozett (1989), Buxton (1991), Clunis & Green (1988, 1995), Dunne (1987), and Pennington (1987).

Suggestions for Psychotherapists

Therapists can be helpful to gay and lesbian parents in many ways (Ariel & McPherson, 2000; Baum, 1996; Büntzly, 1993; Gibbs, 1989). Mothers and fathers can learn how to help their children cope with any tension, anxiety, or stress related to being in a gay or lesbian family. They can be assisted in actively preparing their offspring for uncomfortable situations that arise in their interactions with others, including teasing and ridicule from friends and classmates. These parents also can learn to remain as objective and empathic as possible when their children verbalize feelings of anger or sadness about their families being "different" from those of peers. Finally, just as with their parents, children can benefit from social and educational groups that foster a sense of pride in their families, while offering support.

Lesbian mothers and gay fathers often need assistance in discussing with their children what they are allowed to tell peers and how to cope with harassment by neighbors, schoolmates, or teachers about the sexual orientation of their parents (Wyers, 1987). To help alleviate these problems at school, parents should know both the benefits and risks of disclosing their sexual orientation to their children's teachers and administrators and the best methods to use to do this (Casper & Schultz, 1996; Casper, Schultz, & Wickens, 1992). Parents should also know that having children probably will increase the need to disclose their homosexuality to numerous others, such as school personnel, pediatricians, babysitters, and neighbors (Shidlo, 1994b). Youngsters, further, may need a listening ear if they experience distress about their grandparents' unwillingness to be involved with them or their gay or lesbian parent (Loulan, 1986). Similarly, therapists can provide support and perspective to parents and angry adolescent children who may focus on the sexual orientation of their parents as being the source of many of their difficulties. Daughters of lesbians may fight with their mothers, and sons may withdraw during their teenage years (Clunis & Green, 1995). Clinicians can offer information to parents about normal adolescent separation behaviors that, in these instances, may appear to focus on parental sexual orientation. At stressful times such as described here, it might be necessary to bring the entire family together in therapy to discuss these issues (Bigner, 1996) or to refer them to other services especially designed for gay or lesbian families (Patterson, 1996).

McCandlish (1987) believes it is important to clarify specifically the external stresses on the family, including their legal and social vulnerability. Both biological and non-biological parents may need information about the health of their children and "clear support for their legitimacy as parents" (p. 33). Children should be included in these discussions in an age-appropriate way and should be allowed to have a part in defining the nature of their particular family. All members should be encouraged to develop a support system that enables each to have safe others with whom to discuss his or her family (Barret, 1996; Patterson, 1996; Shidlo, 1994b).

Finally, clinicians should encourage the making of legal arrangements for the protection of the family, primarily since children raised in lesbian mother and gay father families "find that the expected correspondences of social, biological, and legal aspects of parent–child relationships do not hold for them" (Patterson, 1998, p. 162). Chapter 4 included discussions that may be helpful in this regard, and the Resources section contains appropriate legal and family sources of information. Fortunately, books that address the concerns of gay and lesbian families are being published continually, and these often include references, sample documents, and various agreements (Benkov, 1994; Clunis & Green, 1995; Martin, 1993; T. R. Sullivan & Dawidoff, 1999).

CONCLUSION

Families of gay, lesbian, and bisexual individuals were the focus of this final chapter. The formation of these unique familial configurations was discussed in sufficient detail to assist both therapists and clients in comprehending the numerous and complex dynamics often embedded in the family relationship. A separate section addressed various concerns of sexual minority parents, including the incorporation of a stepparent into a family, relationships with the families of origin of both the biological and nonbiological parent, and the interactions of the same-sex parental couple. The chapter concluded with a discussion of the children of lesbian mothers and gay fathers and offered suggestions to therapists for enhancing the lives and relationships of all members of these families.

Resources

BISEXUALITY

BiNet USA
4201 Wilson Boulevard, #110-311
Arlington VA 22203
Phone: (202) 986-7186
E-mail: BiNetUSA@aol.com
Website: http://www.binetusa.org

Formed in 1987, collects and distributes information about bisexuality, facilitates community development, and works for equal rights. Publishes a quarterly newsletter, operates an information clearinghouse, holds conferences and workshops, has created a media press kit, and is a presence in the nation's capitol.

Bi.Org
Website: http://www.bi.org

This website serves the worldwide bisexual community by providing a free Internet presence for individuals, groups, and nonprofit organizations. Contains numerous links, resources, and guides.

Bisexual.Org
Website: http://www.bisexual.org

A listing of Internet resources aimed specifically at bisexual women and men. Contains websites, meeting locations, newsgroups, e-mail, and more.

BOOKSTORES AND PUBLISHERS

Alyson Publications
Phone: (800) 5-ALYSON (800-525-9766)

E-mail: bookstore@alyson.com
Website: http://www.alyson.com

A source of books for gay teens and lesbians and gay men and their children. Publications explore
the political, legal, financial, medical, spiritual, social, and sexual aspects of gay and lesbian life.
Read reviews with authors or excerpts from chapters on the website. Order by phone or online.
Special features and gifts also available.

Chi Rho Press, Inc.
P.O. Box 7864
Gaithersburg, MD 20898
Phone/Fax: (301) 926-1208
E-Mail: ChiRhoPress@aol.com
Website: http://www.members.aol.com/ChiRhoPrss

A gay/lesbian/bisexual/transgendered religious publisher, a special work of the Metropolitan Community Churches. Has books, tapes, and other materials and resources. Order directly from Chi
Rho Press.

A Different Light Bookstores
8853 Santa Monica Boulevard
West Hollywood, CA 90069
Phone: (310) 854-6601
Fax: (310) 854-6603
E-Mail: adlwh@adlbooks.com

489 Castro Street
San Francisco, CA 94114
Phone: (415) 431-0891
Fax: (415) 431-0874
E-Mail: adlsf@adlbooks.com
Website: http://www.adlbooks.com

Specializes in gay and lesbian literature.

Lambda Rising Bookstore
Phone: (800) 621-6969

Specializes in gay and lesbian literature. Has no website but orders can be placed by phone or a catalog can be requested.

CHEMICAL DEPENDENCY

Alternatives
Phone: (800) DIAL GAY (342-5429)
Website: http://www.alternativesinc.com

Alternatives is a alcohol, drug, and mental health recovery program for lesbian, gay, bisexual, and
transgendered adults. It also specializes in treating HIV/AIDS-related grief and loss.

Hazelden Foundation
P.O. Box 11, CO3
Center City, MN 55012-0011
Phone: (800) 257-7810
E-Mail: info@hazelden.org
Website: http://www.hazelden.org

An inpatient and outpatient treatment center for chemical dependency with clinics in Center City, MN, and Florida, Illinois, and New York. Publishes a wide range of materials related to treatment, recovery, and other topics. Several of Hazelden's publications are written for sexual minority clients and their therapists.

National Association of Lesbian and Gay Addictions Professionals (NALGAP)
901 North Washington Street, Suite 600
Arlington, VA 22314
Phone: (703) 465-0539
Fax: (703) 741-6989
E-Mail: membership@nalgap.org (membership questions)
clinical@nalgap.org (clinical information and resources)
Website: http://www.nalgap.org

NALGAP publishes a quarterly newsletter.

Pride Institute
Phone: (800) 54-PRIDE (547-7433)

Specializes in addictions and mental health treatment to lesbian, gay, bisexual, and transgendered clients. Offers residential, outpatient, and halfway house services in various parts of the country, as well as a referral network to supportive therapists located in geographical areas not served by Pride Institute facilities and programs.

CULTURALLY SPECIFIC RESOURCES

The Blackstripe
Website: http://www.blackstripe.com/about.html

A website resource for "news, information, and culture effecting lesbian, gay, bisexual, and transgendered people of African descent." In keeping with Blackstripe's educational mission, this site is "child friendly" and strives to support young people who often use the web in their search for identity. Contains numerous links.

Gay Asian Pacific Alliance (GAPA)
P.O. Box 421884
San Francisco, CA 94142-1884
Phone: (415) 282-GAPA (282-4272)
E-Mail: info@gapa.org
Website: http://www.gapa.org

An organization dedicated to furthering the interests of gay and bisexual Asian/Pacific Islander men. Addresses the social, cultural, and political issues affecting this community. Most GAPA social events are held around the San Francisco area.

National Institute for Gay, Lesbian, Bisexual and Transgender Education
3932 Broadway, Box 45600
Kansas City, MO 64171
Phone: (816) 960-7200
E-Mail: info@thenationalinstitute.org
Website: http://thenationalinstitute.org

The National Institute is dedicated to providing comprehensive educational programs to assist individuals, families, communities of faith, corporations, and professionals facing GLBT issues. The Resource Center of the website contains an extensive listing of national organizations and a national directory with links, several of which are to groups for sexual minorities of color.

National Latina/o Lesbian, Gay, Bisexual and Transgender Organization (LLEGO)
1420 K Street NW, Suite 200
Washington, DC 20006
Phone: (202) 408-5380
Fax: (202) 408-8478
Website: http://www.llego.org

LLEGO works with more than 170 affiliates and allies throughout the United States and Puerto Rico. Provides assistance to community-based Latina/o LGBT organizations in the areas of health and wellness services, organization building, and the development of cultural, political, and community resources. Also involved in the political process at the national and international level. The website includes resources and links.

Two Spirit
Website: http://spiritgatherings.org/pages/two-spirit

A website dedicated to sharing the knowledge and teachings of the "Two-Spirit" tradition. Honors all ways (Native and non-Native) and can be helpful for gays and lesbians to hear the call of the Great Mystery.

Utopia
E-Mail: info@utopia-asia.com
Website: http://www.utopia-asia.com

The Utopia website contains Asian/Pacific Gay and Lesbian resources for more than a dozen countries in Asia. Most of these also have links to U.S. organizations for individuals from these heritages. The website also has a women's space.

Vietnamese Lesbians, Gays, Bisexuals, Transgenders (VLGBT)
(formerly Queer American Vietnamese Association)
P.O. Box 51679
San Jose, CA 95151
Phone: (408) 453-2139 (women)

(408) 251-2643 (men)
Website: http://www.gayviet.com/vlgbtindex.htm

Promotes and advocates for the visibility, rights, needs, and empowerment of the gay, lesbian, bisexual, transgender, and questioning self-identified Vietnamese communities.

Youth Resource
Website: http://www.youthresource.com

A website with webpages for lesbian, gay, bisexual, and transgender youth of color. Contains links to websites and resources for Black, Asian and Pacific Islander, Latina and Latino, and Native American youth.

FAMILY

Alyson Bookstore (Books for Children)
Phone: (800) 5-ALYSON (800-525-9766)
E-Mail: bookstore@alyson.com
Website: http://store.yahoo.com/alysonbooks/kids.html

Children of Lesbians and Gays Everywhere (COLAGE)
3543 18th Street, #1
San Francisco, CA 94110
Phone: (415) 861-KIDS (861-5437)
Fax: (415) 255-8345
E-mail: colage@colage.org
Website: http://www.colage.org

COLAGE is a support and advocacy organization for daughters and sons of lesbian, gay, bisexual, and transgendered parents. Publishes a newsletter for parents and offers an outreach for their children. The Kids' Club features games, stories, articles, and interviews.

Family Pride Coalition (FPC)
(formerly Gay and Lesbian Parents Coalition International)
P.O. Box 34337
San Diego, CA 92163
Phone: (619) 296-0199
Fax: (619) 296-0699
E-Mail: pride@familypride.org
Website: http://www.glpci.com

FPC exists to advance the well being of lesbian, gay, bisexual, and transgendered parents and their families through mutual support, community collaboration, and public understanding. Has parents' groups in the United States and overseas. Offers information related to adoptions and other issues and provides listservs for lesbian mothers, gay fathers, and prospective parents.

Parents, Families and Friends of Lesbians and Gays (PFLAG)
1726 M Street NW, Suite 400
Washington, DC 20036
Phone: (202) 467-8180
Fax: (202) 467-8194
E-Mail: info@pflag.org
Website: http://www.pflag.org

PFLAG is an international federation of national, local and regional chapters with headquarters in Washington, DC.

Partners Task Force for Gay and Lesbian Couples
P.O. Box 9685
Seattle, WA 98109-0685
Phone: (206) 935-1206
E-Mail: demian@buddybuddy.com
Website: http://www.buddybuddy.com

A national resource for same-sex couples. The constantly updated website contains more than 200 essays, surveys, legal articles, and resources on legal marriage, ceremonies, domestic partner benefits, adoptions, relationship tips, parenting, and immigration.

Straight Spouse Network (SSN)
Amity Pierce Buxton, PhD
8215 Terrace Drive
El Cerrito, CA 94530-3058
Phone: (510) 525-0200
E-Mail: dir@ssnetwk.org
Website: http://www.ssnetwk.org

An international organization of heterosexual spouses and partners whose current or former mates are gay, lesbian, bisexual, or transgendered. Members provide confidential support and resource information to spouses and partners nationwide and abroad. The network also offers information about spouse issues and resources to other family members, professionals, and community organizations.

LEGAL AND ADVOCACY

American Civil Liberties Union (ACLU)
ACLU Lesbian and Gay Rights Project
125 Broad Street
New York, NY 10004
Phone: (212) 549-2627
Website: http://www.aclu.org/issues/gay/aboutgl.html#aboutlgrp

American Psychological Association (APA)
APA Public Interest Policy Office/APA Public Interest Directorate
750 First Street NE
Washington, DC 20002

Phone: (202) 336-6050
E-Mail: publicinterest@apa.org
Website: http://www.apa.org/pi/policy.html

Gay and Lesbian Alliance Against Defamation (GLAAD)
Phone: (800) GAY-MEDIA
E-Mail: glaad@glaad.org
Website: http://www.glaad.org

GLAAD in the only national organization that works to combat hatred and intolerance in all forms of media, promoting fair, accurate, and inclusive representations of individuals and events regardless of sexual orientation or identity. Serves as a community resource and a resource to journalists, a media advocate, and a local activist. Has offices in Atlanta, Kansas City, Los Angeles, New York, San Francisco, and Washington, DC.

Human Rights Campaign (HRC)
919 18th Street NW, Suite 800
Washington, DC 20006
Phone: (202) 628-4160
Fax: (202) 347-5323
E-Mail: hrc@hrc.org
Website: http://www.hrc.org

HRC's WorkNet webpages provide news, advice, sample forms, and hard data aimed at helping employees and employers implement fair and inclusive policies for GLBT workers. Included is a list of insurance companies that write policies covering domestic partners, as well as a guide on transgender issues and transitioning in the workplace. The HRC website also offers a current database of employers with written nondiscrimination policies, GLBT employee groups, and domestic partner benefits.

Lambda Legal Defense and Education Fund (LLDEF)
National Headquarters
120 Wall Street, Suite 1500
New York, NY 10005-3904
Phone: (212) 809-8585
Fax: (212) 809-0055

Western Regional Office
6030 Wilshire Boulevard
Los Angeles, CA 90036-3617
Phone: (323) 937-2728
Fax: (323) 937-0601

Midwest Regional Office
11 East Adams, Suite 1008
Chicago, IL 60603-6303
Phone: (312) 663-4413
Fax: (312) 663-4307

Southern Regional Office
1447 Peachtree Street NE, Suite 1004
Atlanta, GA 30309-3027
Phone: (404) 897-1880
Fax: (404) 897-1884
E-Mail: lambda@lambdalegal.org
Website: http://www.lambdalegal.org

Founded in 1973, LLDEF is a not-for-profit, tax-exempt national organization committed to achieving full recognition of the civil rights of lesbians, gay men, and people with HIV/AIDS, through impact litigation, education, and public policy work. A number of publications are available by mail and on the website.

Lesbian Mothers National Defense Fund
P.O. Box 21567
Seattle, WA 98111
Phone: (206) 325-2643

National Center for Lesbian Rights (NCLR)
870 Market Street, Suite 570
San Francisco, CA 94102
Phone: (415) 392-6257
Fax: (415) 392-8442
E-Mail: info@nclrights.org
Website: http://www.nclrights.org

An organization dedicated to ensuring the rights of lesbians by providing legal advice and information, supplying public education, and creating new laws and policies in the areas of partner benefits, child custody and visitation, adoption, donor insemination, civil rights, employment, housing, immigration and asylum, and youth rights. NCLR publishes more than 20 booklets, fact sheets, bibliographies, and manuals that include the following lesbian legal issues:

- Partnership Protection Documents: A Sampler of Forms
- Model Documents for Second Parent Adoption
- Lesbian Health Overview: Recommendations and Report of Advocacy Efforts

National Gay and Lesbian Task Force (NGLTF)
1700 Kalorama Road NW
Washington, DC 20009-2624
Phone: (202) 332-6483
Fax: (202) 332-0207
TTY: (202) 332-6219
Website: http://www.ngltf.org

NGLTF works to eliminate prejudice, violence, and injustice against gay, lesbian, bisexual, and transgendered people at the local, state, and national level. The website contains a listing of NGLTF's vast collection of publications, as well as updated maps of state legislation related to sodomy, marriage, hate crimes, and civil rights.

National Lesbian and Gay Law Association (NLGLA)
P.O. Box 180417
Boston, MA 02118
Phone/Fax: (508) 982-8290
E-Mail: NLGLA@aol.com
Website: http://www.nlgla.org

An association of lawyers, judges and other legal professionals, law students and affiliated lesbian, gay, bisexual, and transgender (LGBT) legal organizations. An affiliate of the American Bar Association.

Other Legal Resources
Curry, H., Clifford, D., Leonard, R., & Hertz, F. (Eds.). (2001). *A legal guide for lesbian and gay couples* (10th ed.). Berkeley, CA: Nolo Press. (Updated annually)
Hertz, F., & Browning, F. (1998). *Legal affairs: Essential advice for same-sex couples.* New York: Henry Holt/Owl Books.

Sexual Orientation: Science, Education, and Policy
Website: http://www.psychology.ucdavis.edu/rainbow

An electronic source of information about hate crimes, AIDS stigma, homophobia, critical reviews of videos targeting gay and bisexual men, etc.

NATIONAL PUBLICATIONS

The Advocate
P.O. Box 4371
Los Angeles, CA 90078
Phone: (323) 871-1225
Fax: (323) 467-0173
E-Mail: postmaster@advocate.com
Website: http://www.advocate.com

Biweekly magazine for lesbians and gay men, with national and international news, features, health coverage, letters to the editor, arts and entertainment reviews, and opinion columns. The website contains links to numerous GLBT resources.

Gay and Lesbian Online: Your Indispensable Guide to Cruising the Queer Web (4th ed.)

Encyclopedic in scope, this book charts the entire spectrum of gay and lesbian interests on the Internet. Lists several thousand websites. An Alyson publication (www. alyson.com). Revised in 2000.

Gayellow Pages
P.O. Box 533, Village Station
New York, NY 10014-0533
Phone: (212) 674-0120
Fax: (212) 420-1126

E-Mail: gayellowpages@earthlink.net
Website: http://gayellowpages.com

A national index of gay, lesbian, and bisexual businesses, organizations, resources, and more. Updated annually.

Gay Parent
P.O. Box 750852
Forest Hills, NY 11375-0852
Phone: (718) 997-0392
E-Mail: info@gayparentmag.com
Website: http://www.gayparentmag.com

This magazine is published every 2 months online and in newsprint. Includes articles, resources for families, parenting information, camps, classes, and links.

In the Family
P.O. Box 5387
Takoma Park, MD 20913
Phone: (301) 270-4771
Fax: (301) 270-4660
E-mail: LMarkowitz@aol.com

A quarterly family magazine that examines the complexities of same-sex family relationships, including couples and intimacy, money, sex, extended families, parenting, and other related topics. Readers include therapists of all sexual orientations, as well as lesbians, gay men, bisexual individuals, and their family members.

Proud Parenting
Proud Parenting, Inc.
P.O. Box 8272
Van Nuys, CA 91409-8272
Phone: (818) 909-0314
E-Mail: info@proudparenting.com
Website: http://www.proudparenting.com

A magazine for gay, lesbian, bisexual, and transgendered parents and their families. Contains a Business Directory and a Resource Guide that include information about adoptions, parenting, and finances, as well as articles, advice, and columns.

PROFESSIONAL JOURNALS

The Haworth Press
10 Alice Street
Binghamton, NY 13904-1580
Phone: (800) 429-6784
Fax: (800) 895-0582
E-Mail: getinfo@haworthpressinc.com
Website: http://www.haworthpressinc.com

Journal of Bisexuality
Journal of Gay and Lesbian Psychotherapy
Journal of Gay and Lesbian Social Services
Journal of Homosexuality
Journal of Lesbian Studies

PROFESSIONAL ORGANIZATIONS

APA Committee on Lesbian, Gay, and Bisexual Concerns
APA Public Interest Policy Office/APA Public Interest Directorate
750 First Street NE
Washington, DC 20002
Phone: (202) 336-6050
E-Mail: publicinterest@apa.org
Website: http://www.apa.org/pi/lgbc/clgbc/homepage.html

Association for Gay, Lesbian, and Bisexual Issues in Counseling (AGLBIC)
American Counseling Association
5999 Stevenson Avenue
Alexandria, VA 22304
Phone: (800) 347-6647
Fax: (703) 823-0252
Website: http://www.aglbic.org

Association of Gay and Lesbian Psychiatrists (AGLP)
4514 Chester Avenue
Philadelphia, PA 19143-3707
Phone: (215) 222-2800
Fax: (215) 222-3881
E-Mail: aglp@algp.org
Website: http://www.aglp.org

National Association of Lesbian and Gay Addictions Professionals (NALGAP)
901 North Washington Street, Suite 600
Arlington, VA 22314
Phone: (703) 465-0539
Fax: (703) 741-6989
E-Mail: membership@nalgap.org (membership questions)
clinical@nalgap.org (clinical information and resources)
Website: http://www.nalgap.org

NALGAP publishes a quarterly newsletter.

The Society for the Psychological Study of Lesbian, Gay, and Bisexual Issues (Division 44)
American Psychological Association (APA)
750 First Street NE
Washington, DC 20002

Phone: (202) 336-5500
E-Mail: div44@apa.org
Website: http://www.apa.org/divisions/div44

RELIGIOUS ORGANIZATIONS

Affirmation (Gay and Lesbian Mormons)
P.O. Box 46022
Los Angeles, CA 90046-0022
Phone: (323) 255-7251
Website: http://www.affirmation.org

A social, educational, and support organization for gay, lesbian, and bisexual Mormons (LDS) and their family and friends. The goal is understanding of sexual minorities as full and equal members of society and the church. The website contains numerous links to local chapters and other groups and resources.

Affirmation (United Methodists for GLBT Concerns)
P.O. Box 1021
Evanston, IL 60204
Phone: (847) 733-9590
E-Mail: umaffirmation@yahoo.com
Website: http://www.umaffirm.org

Al-Fatiha Foundation, USA
P.O. Box 33532
Washington, DC 20033
E-Mail: gaymuslims@yahoo.com
Website: http://www.al-fatiha.net

An international organization dedicated to Muslims who are lesbian, gay, bisexual, transgendered, those questioning their sexual orientation, and/or gender identity, as well as their families, friends, partners, and allies.

American Association of Pastoral Counselors
9504A Lee Highway
Fairfax, VA 22031-2303
Phone: (703) 385-6967
Fax: (703) 352-7725
E-Mail: info@aapc.org
Website: http://www.aapc.org

An association of 3,000 pastoral counselors who have graduate mental health degrees and religious or theological training. The website contains an online directory of Certified Pastoral Counselors.

American Baptists Concerned for Sexual Minorities
Website: http://www.rainbowbaptists.org/ambaptists.htm

Axios (Eastern and Orthodox Christian Gay Men and Women)
Website: http://www.eskimo.com/~nickz/axios.html

Brethren/Mennonite Council for Lesbian and Gay Concerns
Box 6300
Minneapolis, MN 55406
Phone: (612) 722-6906
E-Mail: BMCouncil@aol.com
Website: http://www.webcom.com/bmc

Cathedral of Hope
5910 Cedar Springs Road
P.O. Box 35466
Dallas, TX 75235
Phone: (214) 351-1901
(800) 501-HOPE
Fax: (214) 351-6099
E-Mail: hope@cathedralofhope.com
Website: http://www.cathedralofhope.com

This large Dallas church provides opportunities to be involved in its ministry regardless of geographical location. Internet worship is broadcast four times a week. The website includes sermons, news, resources, spiritual information, and links. Affiliated with the Universal Fellowship of Metropolitan Community Churches.

Common Bond (A GLBT Support Group for Former and Current Jehovah's Witnesses)
Websites: http://www.lagayxjw.org (Los Angeles/Orange County)
http://www.geocities.com/commonbondeast/nyc/index.html (NYC)
http://www.gayxjw.org (San Francisco)

Conference of Catholic Lesbians
P.O. Box 436
Planetarium Station
New York, NY 10024
E-Mail: info@catholiclesbians.org
Website: http://www.catholiclesbians.org

The website includes resources, links, events, liturgies, conferences, and stories.

Dignity/USA (Catholic)
1500 Massachusetts Avenue NW, Suite 11
Washington, DC 20005-1894
Phone: (202) 861-0017
(800) 877-8797
Fax: (202) 429-9808
E-Mail: dignity@aol.com
Website: http://www.dignityusa.org

Dignity works for education, for the reform of the Catholic Church's teachings and pastoral practices toward sexual minorities, and for the acceptance of all people as full members of the Catholic
Church. The website includes links, resources, and local chapters.

Evangelicals Concerned
311 East 72nd Street
New York, NY 10021
(212) 517-3171
E-Mail: ecinc.org
Website: http://www.ecinc.org

A task force network for evangelical gay, lesbian, bisexual, and transgendered (GLBT) Christians.

Evangelicals Concerned Western Region, Inc.
P.O. Box 19734
Seattle, WA 98109-6734
Phone: (206) 621-8960
Website: http://www.ecwr.org

A nationwide ministry of Bible-believing GLBT Christians whose primary purpose is to provide
reconciliation, integration, and opportunities for Christian growth. Includes listings of resources,
conferences, and local area chapters.

Friends for Lesbian and Gay Concerns (Quakers)
143 Campbell Avenue
Ithica, NY 14850

An association of lesbian, gay, bisexual, transgender, and non-gay Friends (Quakers) who seek spiritual community within the Religious Society of Friends. The FLGC newsletter is published four
times a year.

Gay Bahai
Website: http://www.gaybahai.homestead.com/index~ns4.html

GayChristian.Net
Website: http://www.gaychristian.net

A "starting point" page for gay Christian sites all over the web. Every site relevant to being gay and
Christian is reviewed before it is listed.

Gays for God
Website: http://www.gaysforgod.org

A collection of gay-affirming religious websites. Contains links to many resources, including news,
events, conferences, protests, and groups.

Gay, Lesbian and Affirming Disciples (GLAD) Alliance (Disciples of Christ)
P.O. Box 44400
Indianapolis, IN 46244-0400
E-Mail: glad@gladalliance.org
Website: http://www.gladalliance.org

Honesty (Support and Education for Gay, Lesbian Southern Baptists)
E-Mail: honesty@rainbowbaptists.org
Website: http://www.rainbowbaptists.org/honesty.html

Honesty is an association of local groups that provide support, education, and advocacy for gay, lesbian, bisexual, and transgender Baptists with a Southern Baptist background. Believing that gay men, lesbians, bisexual, and transgender persons are wholly loved and accepted as they are by our Creator, Honesty groups bring a voice of enlightenment, hope, and encouragement to all Baptists.

Integrity (Episcopalian)
1718 M Street NW
PM Box 148
Washington, DC 20036
Phone: (202) 462-9193
Fax: (202) 588-1486
E-Mail: info@integrityusa.org
Website: http://www.integrityusa.org

Interweave (Unitarian Universalists for LGBT Concerns)
167 Milk Street, #406
Boston, MA 02109-4339
Website: http://qrd.tcp.com/qrd/www/orgs/uua/uu-interweave.html

Lesbian, Gay, and Bisexual Catholic Handbook
Website: http://www.bway.net/~halsall/lgbh/

A handbook of information, resources, and links. The 12 chapters include church documents, theological, biblical, and ethical discussions; Catholic organizations and Dignity chapters; and facts about the religious right. Includes many links.

Lesbian, Gay, Bisexual and Transgendered Christian Scientists
Website: http://www.cslesbigay.org

Lutherans Concerned North America
Box 10461, Fort Dearborn Station
Chicago, IL 60610-0461
E-Mail: luthconc@aol.com
Website: http://www.lcna.org

More Light Presbyterians (Presbyterian Church, USA)
PMB 246
4737 County Road 101
Minnetonka, MN 55345-2634
Website: http://www.mlp.org

A pro-gay movement among Presbyterian congregations. Evolved since 1974 from the Presbyterians for Lesbian and Gay Concerns (PLGC) that has encouraged full participation of sexual minorities in the church.

National Gay Pentecostal Alliance
P.O. Box 20428
Ferndale, MI 48220
Website: http://www.ameritech.net/users/lighthse84/ngpa.html

New Ways Ministry (Catholic)
4012 29th Street
Mt. Rainier, MD 20712
Phone: (301) 277-5674
Fax: (301) 864-6948
E-Mail: newwaysm@aol.com
Website: http://www.members.aol.com/NewWaysM

Provides a gay-positive ministry of advocacy for gay and lesbian Catholics. Has links and resources. Publishes *Bondings*, a seasonal newspaper.

Reconciling Ministries Network (United Methodist)
3801 North Keeler Avenue
Chicago, IL 60641
Phone: (773) 736-5526
Fax: (773) 736-5475
Website: http://www.rmnetwork.org

Open Hands is an award-winning quarterly of ecumenical ministries that affirm the diversity of human sexuality. Initiated by the Reconciling Congregation Program (United Methodist) and published cooperatively with affirming movements within the United Church of Christ, the Evangelical
Lutheran Church in America, Presbyterian Church USA, American Baptist Church, the Christian
Church (Disciples of Christ), and the United Church of Canada (Website: http://www.rcp.org/
openhands)

Seventh Day Adventist (SDA) Kinship International, Inc. (Kinship)
P.O. Box 7320
Laguna Niguel, CA 92607
Phone: (949) 248-1299
E-Mail: sdakinship@aol.com
Website: http://www.sdakinship.org

Soulforce, Inc.
P.O. Box 4467
Laguna Beach, CA 92652
Fax: (949) 455-0959
Website: http://www.soulforce.org

The website describes Soulforce as a "network of friends learning nonviolence from Gandhi and
King seeking justice for God's lesbian, gay, bisexual and transgendered children."

Tumescence
P.O. Box 461144
Los Angeles, CA 90046-1144
Phone: (323) 874-9561
E-Mail: webmaster@tumescence.org
Website: http://www.tumescence.org

A nonprofit organization dedicated to encouraging and supporting Gay Soul Making by gay men. Focus is on the development of gay-centered psychospiritual consciousness.

United Church of Christ Coalition for LGBT Concerns
PMB 230, 800 Village Walk
Guilford, CT 06437-2740
Phone: (800) 653-0799
Website: http://www.ucccoalition.org

Universal Fellowship of Metropolitan Community Churches
8704 Santa Monica Boulevard, 2nd Floor
West Hollywood, CA 90069-4548
Phone: (310) 360-8640
Fax: (310) 360-8680
E-Mail: info@ufmcchq.com
Website: http://www.ufmcc.com

Welcoming and Affirming Baptists (ABC/USA)
Website: http://www.wabaptists.org

World Congress of Gay, Lesbian, and Bisexual Jewish Organizations
P.O. Box 23379
Washington, DC 20026-3379
Phone: (202) 452-7424
E-Mail: info@wcgljo.org
Website: http://www.wcgljo.org

SEXUAL MINORITY HEALTH

AIDS Clinical Trials Information Services (ACTIS)
Phone: (800) 874-2572
E-Mail: actis@actis.org
Website: http://www.actis.org

A service of the U.S. Department of Health and Human Services. A central resource for federally and privately funded HIV/AIDS clinical trials information.

AIDS Research Alliance
621-A North San Vicente Boulevard
West Hollywood, CA 90069
Phone: (310) 358-2423

Fax: (310) 358-2431
E-mail: info@aidsresearch.org
Website: http://www.aidsresearch.org

An aggressive leader in HIV/AIDS research with a national reputation for identifying and pursuing the newest and most promising treatments for HIV; operates the nation's first and only free-standing facility dedicated to fast-track, AIDS clinical trials, providing enrollment to trials regardless of race, gender, age, or ability to pay for medical care; publishes *Searchlight*, a quarterly news journal.

AIDS Treatment News
Phone: (800) 873-2812
E-Mail: aidsnews@aidsnews.org
Website: http://www.aidsnews.org

American Psychological Association Office on AIDS
APA Public Interest Directorate
750 First Street NE
Washington, DC 20002
Phone: (202) 336-6050
E-mail: publicinterest@apa.org
Website: http://www.apa.org/pi/aids.html

Publishes *Psychology & AIDS Exchange*, a newsletter that includes articles on research, treatment, federally funded projects, legislation, and public policy issues related to HIV. The projects of the Office on AIDS include an HIV/AIDS training program for mental health professionals.

Center for Disease Control National AIDS Hotline
Phone: (800) 342-AIDS (342-2437)
(800) 344-7432 (Spanish)
TTY: (800) 243-7889

Gay Men's Health Crisis (GMHC)
119 West 24th Street
New York, NY 10011
Hotline: (800) AIDS-NYC (243-7692)
E-Mail: hotline@gmhc.org
Website: http://www.thebody.com/gmhc/gmhcpage.html

Treatment Issues, a newsletter of experimental AIDS therapies, is published 12 times a year by GMHC.

GLBT Health Access Project
100 Boylston Street, Suite 815
Boston, MA 02116
Phone: (617) 988-2605
Fax: (617) 988-8708
Email: access@jri.org
Website: http://www.glbthealth.org

A website containing information about health issues relevant to lesbian, gay, bisexual, and transgendered individuals.

HIV InSite
Website: http://hivinsite.ucsf.edu/InSite

An electronic source of information on HIV/AIDS clinical trials, Centers for Disease Control surveillance data, and a state-by-state guide to HIV/AIDS information and resources.

The Lambda Center
4228 Wisconsin Avenue NW
Washington, DC 20016
Phone: (877) 2LAMBDA (252-6232)
E-Mail: contact@lambdacenter.com
Website: http://www.lambdacenter.com

Behavioral healthcare programs for the gay, lesbian, bisexual, and transgender communities. A partnership between the Psychiatric Institute of Washington and Whitman–Walker Clinic that assists in overcoming problems with substance abuse, relationship issues, and HIV and AIDS.

Lesbian Health Foundation
Phone: (510) 883-0778
Fax: (510) 883-0848
E-Mail: info@lesbianhealthfoundation.org
Website: http://www.lesbianhealthfoundation.org

Developed to increase awareness and understanding of the special health needs of lesbian, bisexual, and transgendered women among policymakers, healthcare professionals, researchers, and the public. The website includes health information and services. Provides a Speaker's Bureau, as well as education and training for healthcare professionals.

The Mautner Project for Lesbians with Cancer
1707 L Street NW, Suite 500
Washington, DC 20036
Phone/TTY: (202) 332-5536
Fax: (202) 332-0662
E-Mail: mautner@mautnerproject.org
Website: http://www.mautnerproject.org

A national organization dedicated to lesbians with cancer, their partners, and caregivers. Provides direct services, education and information to the lesbian and healthcare communities, and advocacy on lesbian health issues in national and local arenas.

National Minority AIDS Council (NMAC)
1931 13th Street NW
Washington, DC 20009
Phone: (202) 483-6622
Fax: (202) 483-1135

E-Mail: info@nmac.org
Website: http://www.nmac.org

Provides demographic, research, and treatment information for people of color living with HIV and AIDS. The website includes a national listing of HIV/AIDS-related employment opportunities as well as *The Patients' Guide to HIV Medicines* in English, Spanish, and French editions.

POZ *Magazine and* POZ en Español
Phone: (800) READ-POZ (973-2376)
E-Mail: subscription@poz.com
Website: http://www.poz.com

A magazine and website providing HIV/AIDS information; published in English and in Spanish.

Project Inform
205 13th Street, Suite 2001
San Francisco, CA 94103-2461
Phone: (415) 558-8669
Fax: (415) 558-0684
Hotline: (800) 822-7422
Hotline: (415) 558-9051 (in the San Francisco Bay area and internationally)
E-Mail: info@projectinform.org
Website: http://www.projectinform.org

Provides medical information and advocacy for persons living with HIV disease. Publishes *Project Inform Perspective*, a newsletter summarizing the latest in research and treatment, three times a year.

Wellness Health Care Information Resources
Website: http://www-hsl.mcmaster.ca/tomflem/gay.html

The foregoing website contains a large number of gay, lesbian, and bisexual health links.

SEXUAL MINORITY SENIORS

Gay and Lesbian Association of Retiring Persons, Inc. (GLARP)
10940 Wilshire Boulevard, Suite 1600
Los Angeles, CA 90024
Phone: (310) 966-1500
E-Mail: glarp@earthlink.net
Website: http://www.gaylesbianretiring.org

GLARP is a new nonprofit corporation dedicated to encourage gay and lesbian individuals and businesses to give financially and of their time and talent to enhance the aging experience of all retiring gays and lesbians in exchange for tax and other benefits.

Lesbian and Gay Aging Issues Network (LGAIN)
American Society on Aging
833 Market Street, Suite 511

San Francisco, CA 94103
E-Mail: info@asaging.org
Website: http://www.asaging.org/lgain.html

The LGAIN website provides extensive links to articles and agencies related to housing, health care, social services, and gay retirement communities, as well as other information.

Pride Senior Network
356 West 18th Street
New York, NY 10011
Phone: (212) 271-7288
Fax: (646) 336-6685
Voicemail: (212) 757-3203
E-mail: pridesr@erols.com
Website: http://www.pridesenior.org

Pride Senior Network is a young organization preparing to become the full-range resource network of services advocating for older lesbians and gay men, starting in the New York metropolitan area.

Ripe Magazine
Website: http://www.ripemag.com

An online and print magazine for gay, lesbian, and transgender individuals in midlife and older.

Senior Action in a Gay Environment (SAGE)
305 Seventh Avenue, 16th Floor
New York, NY 10011
Phone: (212) 741-2247
Fax: (212) 366-1947
E-Mail: sageusa@aol.com
Website: http://www.sageusa.org

SEXUAL MINORITY YOUTH

Gay and Lesbian Adolescent Social Services (GLASS)
650 North Robertson Boulevard, Suite A
West Hollywood, CA 90069
Phone: (310) 358-8727
Fax: (310) 358-8721
Website: http://www.glassla.org

GLASS provides a complete range of psychosocial services, including crisis intervention, job skills training, health care, foster family placement, and intensive residential services.

Gay, Lesbian, and Straight Education Network (GLSEN)
121 West 27th Street, Suite 804
New York, NY 10001
Phone: (212) 727-0135
E-Mail: glsen@glsen.org
Website: http://www.glsen.org

GLSEN is a national network of more than 700 local chapters and groups that brings together teachers, parents, students, and concerned citizens to work together to combat anti-gay bias in K–12 schools. Curriculum materials and training programs for educators, *Safe Schools* and other videos, and books for children and adolescents are available. These may be ordered by e-mail or from the website. Information on local chapters is available from the New York office. A booklet, *Just the Facts About Sexual Orientation and Youth*, was sent to 15,000 school superintendents in 1999.

Gay/Straight Alliances
Massachusetts Department of Education
350 Main Street
Malden, MA 02148-5023
Phone: (781) 388-3000
Website: http://www.doe.mass.edu/lss/GSA

Gay/Straight Alliances (GSAs) are school-based support groups that help to reduce anti-gay violence, harassment, and discrimination by educating the school community about homophobia and enhancing the understanding of students and school personnel. The groups also give all students a safe place to discuss their feelings and fears related to sexual orientation. For more information, call the Massachusetts Department of Education's Safe Schools Program for Gay and Lesbian Students.

The Hetrick–Martin Institute, Inc. (IPLGY)
2 Astor Place
New York, NY 10003
Phone: (212) 674-2400
Fax: (212) 674-8650
TTY: (212) 674-8695
E-Mail: info@hmi.org
Website: http://www.hmi.org

The Hetrick–Martin Institute, Inc. is a national clearinghouse for sexual minority youth services, and operates Harvey Milk alternative high school for gay and lesbian teens in cooperation with the New York public school system.

Los Angeles Gay and Lesbian Center
(formerly Gay and Lesbian Community Center)
1625 North Schrader Boulevard
Los Angeles, CA 90028
Phone: (323) 993-7400
TDD: (323) 993-7698
Website: http://www.laglc.org

The Los Angeles Gay and Lesbian Center's Youth Services Department has provided shelter and meals, material support, and supportive services as components of comprehensive life stabilization efforts for more than 15 years.

National Runaway Switchboard
3080 North Lincoln Avenue
Chicago, IL 60657
Phone: (773) 880-9860
Fax: (773) 929-5150
Information: (800) 344-2785
Email: info@nrscrisisline.org
Website: http://www.nrscrisisline.org

Oasis Magazine
Website: http://www.oasismag.com

An online magazine for lesbian, gay, bisexual, and transgendered youth, and for those questioning their sexuality. Written by and for people between the ages of 12 and 22. Includes support resources and age appropriate links.

PROJECT 10
115 West California Boulevard, #116
Pasadena, CA 91105
Phone: (626) 577-4553
Website: http://www.project10.org

PROJECT 10 is the nation's first public school program dedicated to providing *on-site* educational support services to gay, lesbian, bisexual, transgender, and questioning youth. PROJECT 10 began in 1984 at Fairfax High School in the Los Angeles Unified School District. This website was developed to give teachers, counselors, and administrators assistance in providing similar services in their own schools or school districts.

Sexual Minority Youth Assistance League (SMYAL)
410 7th Street SE
Washington, DC 20003-2707
Phone: (202) 546-5940
Fax: (202) 544-1306
TTY: (202) 546-7796

SMYAL offers directed group sessions, support, and assistance to sexual minority youth (ages 13 to 21).

Student Pride USA
121 West 27th Street, Suite 804
New York, NY 10001
Phone: (212) 727-0135
E-Mail: studentpride@glsen.org
Website: http://www.studentprideUSA.org

A "for and by" youth project working to support the creation and maintenance of Gay Straight Alliances and similar youth groups across the nation. Provides resources, materials, education and training.

Youth Resource
Website: http://www.youthresource.com

A project of Advocates for Youth containing a large number of resources and links. Topics in the online library include coming-out resources (in both English and Spanish), health and HIV information, facts about the military, videos, hotlines, books, safe schools programs, college and university safe zone programs, and general resources.

VIOLENCE AND HARASSMENT

Several cities have hotlines that offer services to gay and lesbian domestic violence victims. These include:

Boston [men only] (800) 832-1901
Chicago (773) 871-CARE
Denver (303) 852-5094
Los Angeles (800) 373-2227
New York City (212) 714-1141
San Francisco (415) 333-HELP

Los Angeles Gay and Lesbian Center
(formerly Gay and Lesbian Community Center)
1625 North Schrader Boulevard
Los Angeles, CA 90028
Phone: (323) 993-7400
TDD: (323) 993-7698
Website: http://www.laglc.org

The world's largest gay and lesbian organization. Provides such services as addiction recovery, counseling, primary medical care, HIV-related assistance, youth services and housing, classes, employment training and placement, and cultural and seniors programming. The Legal Services Department has an Anti-Violence Project that provides legal assistance and advocacy within the criminal justice system to people who are targets of violence, attack, or harassment. Phone: 1-800-373-2227.

References

Abbott, L. J. (1998). The use of alcohol by lesbians: A review and research agenda. *Substance Use and Misuse, 33*(13), 2647–2663.

Able v. USA, U.S. Court of Appeals for the Second Circuit, 95-9111 (L) (1996).

Abraham, K. (1993). *Stand up and fight back: A young person's guide to spiritual warfare.* Ann Arbor, MI: Servant.

Acuff, C., Cerbone, A., & Shidlo, A. (1996). *Interventions in psychotherapy with lesbians and gay men: A review of the literature.* Paper presented at the 104th annual meeting of the American Psychological Association, Toronto.

Adam, B. D. (1985). Age, structure, and sexuality: Reflections on the anthropological evidence on homosexual relations. *Journal of Homosexuality, 11*(3–4), 19–33.

Adams, L. A., Jr., & Kimmel, D. C. (1997). Exploring the lives of older African American gay men. In B. Greene (Ed.), *Ethnic and cultural diversity among lesbians and gay men* (pp. 132–151). Thousand Oaks, CA: Sage.

Adelman, M. (1980). Adjustment to aging and styles of being gay: A study of elderly gay men and lesbians. *Dissertation Abstracts International, 41*(2-B), 679.

Adelman, M. (1986). *Long time passing: Lives of older lesbians.* Boston: Alyson.

Adelman, M. (1990). Stigma, gay lifestyles, and adjustment to aging: A study of later life gay men and lesbians. *Journal of Homosexuality, 20*(3–4), 7–32.

Albarran, J. W., & Salmon, D. (2000). Lesbian, gay and bisexual experiences within critical care nursing, 1988–1998: A survey of the literature. *International Journal of Nursing Studies, 37*(5), 445–455.

Allen, K. R. (1999). Reflexivity in qualitative analysis: Toward an understanding of resiliency among older parents with adult gay children. In H. I. McCubbin & E. A. Thompson (Eds.), *The dynamics of resilient families: Vol. 4. Resiliency in families* (pp. 71–98). Thousand Oaks, CA: Sage.

Allen, P. G. (1986). *The sacred hoop: Recovering the feminine in American Indian traditions.* Boston: Beacon Press.

Allport, G. (1954). *The nature of prejudice.* Reading, MA: Addison-Wesley.

Almeida, R., Woods, R., Messineo, T., & Font, R. (1998). Cultural context model: Revisioning family therapy, race, culture, gender, and sexual orientation in clinical practice. In M. McGoldrick, J. Giordano, & J. K. Pearce (Eds.), *Ethnicity and family therapy* (2nd ed., pp. 414–431). New York: Guilford Press.

Almeida, R. V., & Durkin, T. (1999). The cultural context model: Therapy for couples with domestic violence. *Journal of Marital and Family Therapy, 25*(3), 313–324.

Almvig, C. (1982). *The invisible minority: Aging and lesbianism.* New York: Utica College of Syracuse University Press.

413

Alyson Publications. (1990). *The Alyson almanac: A treasury of information for the gay and lesbian community.* Boston: Author.

Alyson Publications. (1993). *The Alyson almanac: The fact book of the lesbian and gay community.* Boston: Author.

American Counseling Association. (1998). *Resolution with respect of sexual orientation and mental health.* Alexandria, VA: Author.

American Medical Association. (1996). Health care needs of gay men and lesbians in the United States. *Journal of the American Medical Association, 275*(17), 1354–1359.

American Psychiatric Association. (1952). *Diagnostic and statistical manual of mental disorders.* Washington, DC: Author.

American Psychiatric Association. (1968). *Diagnostic and statistical manual of mental disorders* (2nd ed.). Washington, DC: Author.

American Psychiatric Association. (1980). *Diagnostic and statistical manual of mental disorders* (3rd ed.). Washington, DC: Author.

American Psychiatric Association. (1987). *Diagnostic and statistical manual of mental disorders* (3rd ed., rev.). Washington, DC: Author.

American Psychiatric Association. (1994). *Diagnostic and statistical manual of mental disorders* (4th ed.). Washington, DC: Author.

American Psychiatric Association. (1998). *Position statement on psychiatric treatment and sexual orientation.* Washington, DC: Author.

American Psychological Association. (1992). *Ethical principles of psychologists and code of conduct.* Washington, DC: Author.

American Psychological Association. (1997). *Resolution on appropriate therapeutic responses to sexual orientation.* Washington, DC: Author.

American Psychological Association. (2000). Guidelines for psychotherapy with lesbian, gay, and bisexual clients. *American Psychologist, 55*(12), 1440–1451. [Online]. Available: http://www.apa.org/pi/lgbc/guidelines.html.

Anderson, S. C. (1996). Addressing heterosexist bias in the treatment of lesbian couples with chemical dependency. In J. Laird & R. J. Green (Eds.), *Lesbian and gay couples and families: A handbook for therapists* (pp. 316–340). San Francisco: Jossey-Bass.

Anhalt, K., & Morris, T. L. (1998). Developmental and adjustment issues of gay, lesbian, and bisexual adolescents: A review of the empirical literature. *Clinical Child and Family Psychology Review, 1*(4), 215–230.

Anti-gay bias barred in schools in Mass. (1993, December 11). *The Philadelphia Inquirer*, p. 1.

Ariel, J., & McPherson, D. W. (2000). Therapy with lesbian and gay parents and their children. *Journal of Marital and Family Therapy, 26*(4), 421–432.

Armon, V. (1960). Some personality variables in overt female homosexuality. *Journal of Projective Techniques and Personality Assessment, 24,* 292–309.

Astin, H. S. (1985). The meaning of work in women's lives: A sociopsychological model of career choice and work behavior. *Counseling Psychologist, 12*(4), 117–128.

Atkinson, D. R., & Hackett, G. (1995). *Counseling diverse populations.* Dubuque, IA: Brown.

Atkinson, D. R., Morten, G., & Sue, D. W. (1993). *Counseling American minorities: A cross-cultural perspective* (4th ed.). Dubuque, IA: Brown.

Atkinson, L. (1993, July 4) Mass. begins teacher training on helping support gay students. *The Boston Sunday Globe*, p. 1.

Ayers, T., & Brown, P. (1999). *The essential guide to lesbian and gay weddings.* Boston: Alyson.

Badgett, M. V. L. (1996). Employment and sexual orientation: Disclosure and discrimination in the workplace. In A. L. Ellis & E. D. B. Riggle (Eds.), *Sexual identity on the job: Issues and services* (pp. 29–52). New York: Haworth Press.

Badgett, M. V. L. (1999). *Lesbians' access to healthcare coverage.* Paper presented at the 107th annual meeting of the American Psychological Association, Boston.

Baggett, C. R. (1992). Sexual orientation: Should it affect child custody rulings? *Law and Psychology Review, 16,* 189–200.

Bailey, J. M. (1995). Biological perspectives on sexual orientation. In A. R. D'Augelli & C. J. Patterson

(Eds.), *Lesbian, gay, and bisexual identities over the lifespan: Psychological perspectives* (pp. 102–135). New York: Oxford University Press.

Bailey, J. M. (1996). Gender identity. In R. C. Savin-Williams & K. M. Cohen (Eds.), *The lives of lesbians, gays, and bisexuals: Children to adults* (pp. 71–93). Ft. Worth, TX: Harcourt Brace.

Bailey, J. M., & Benishay, D. S. (1993). Familial aggregation of female sexual orientation. *American Journal of Psychiatry, 150*(2), 272–277.

Bailey, J. M., Bobrow, D., Wolfe, M., & Mikash, S. (1995). Sexual orientation of adult sons of gay fathers. *Developmental Psychology, 31*, 124–129.

Bailey, J. M., & Dawood, K. (1998). Behavioral genetics, sexual orientation, and the family. In C. J. Patterson & A. R. D'Augelli (Eds.), *Lesbian, gay, and bisexual identities in families: Psychological perspectives* (pp. 3–18). New York: Oxford University Press.

Bailey, J. M., & Pillard, R. C. (1991). A genetic study of male sexual orientation. *Archives of General Psychiatry, 48*, 1089–1096.

Bailey, J. M., Willerman, L., & Parks, C. (1991). A test of the maternal stress theory of human male homosexuality. *Archives of Sexual Behavior, 20*(3), 277–293.

Bailey, J. M., & Zucker, K. J. (1995). Childhood sex-typed behavior and sexual orientation: A conceptual analysis and quantitative review. *Developmental Psychology, 31*(1), 43–55.

Bailey, J. V., Kavanagh, J., Owen, C., McLean, K. A., & Skinner, C. J. (2000). Lesbians and cervical cancer. *British Journal of General Practice, 50*(455), 481–482.

Baker, J. M. (1998). Family secrets: Gay sons—A mother's story. Binghamton, NY: Haworth Press.

Balka, C., & Rose, A. (Eds.). (1989). *Twice blessed: On being lesbian or gay and Jewish.* Boston: Beacon Press.

Ball, S. (Ed.). (1998). *The HIV-negative gay man: Developing strategies for survival and emotional well-being.* Binghamton, NY: Haworth Press.

Bancroft, J. (1990). Commentary: Biological contributions to sexual orientation. In D. P. McWhirter, S. A. Sanders, & J. M. Reinisch (Eds.). *Homosexuality/heterosexuality: Concepts of sexual orientation* (pp. 101–111). New York: Oxford University Press.

Baptiste, D. A. (1987a). The gay and lesbian stepparent family. In F. W. Bozett (Ed.), *Gay and lesbian parents* (pp. 112–137). New York: Praeger.

Baptiste, D. A. (1987b). Psychotherapy with gay/lesbian couples and their children in "stepfamilies": A challenge for marriage and family therapists. In E. Coleman (Ed.), *Integrated identity for gay men and lesbians: Psychotherapeutic approaches for emotional well-being* (pp. 223–238). New York: Harrington Park Press.

Baptiste, D. A. (1990). Night terrors as a defense against feelings of homosexual panic: A case report. *Journal of Gay and Lesbian Psychotherapy, 1*(3), 121–131.

Baron, J. (1996). Some issues in psychotherapy with gay and lesbian clients. *Psychotherapy, 33*(4), 611–616.

Barret, R. L. (1996). Gay fathers in groups. In M. P. Andronico (Ed.), *Men in groups: Insights, interventions, and psychoeducational work* (pp. 257–268). Washington, DC: American Psychological Association.

Barret, R. L., & Robinson, B. E. (1990). *Gay fathers.* Lexington, MA: Lexington Books.

Barrett, J. (2000, April 11). Youth quakes. *The Advocate,* p. 30.

Bartholow, B. N., Doll, L. S., Joy, D., Douglas, J. M. Jr., Bolan, G., Harrison, J. S., Moss, P. M., & McKirnan, D. (1994). Emotional, behavioral, and HIV risks associated with sexual abuse among adult homosexual and bisexual men. *Child Abuse and Neglect, 18*(9), 747–761.

Barzan, R. (Ed.). (1995). *Sex and spirit: Exploring gay men's spirituality.* San Francisco: White Crane Press [Also Online]. Available: www.whitecranejournal.com/wc01003.htm.

Bass, E., & Kaufman, K. (1996). *Free your mind: The book for gay, lesbian, and bisexual youth and their allies.* New York: HarperCollins.

Baum, M. I. (1996). Gays and lesbians choosing to be parents. In C. J. Alexander (Ed.), *Gay and lesbian mental health: A sourcebook for practitioners* (pp. 115–126). New York: Harrington Park Press.

Beard, J., & Glickauf-Hughes, C. (1994). Gay identity and sense of self: Rethinking male homosexuality. *Journal of Gay and Lesbian Psychotherapy, 2*(2), 21–37.

Beatty, R. L., Geckle, M. O., Huggins, J., Kapner, C., Lewis, K., & Sandstrom, D. J. (1999). Gay men, lesbians, and bisexuals. In B. S. McCrady & E. E. Epstein (Eds.), *Addictions: A comprehensive guidebook* (pp. 542–551). New York: Oxford University Press.

Beck, E. T. (Ed.). (1989). *Nice Jewish girls: A lesbian anthology.* Boston: Beacon Press. (Original work published 1982, Watertown, MA: Persephone Press)

Beck, J., & Rosenbaum, M. (1994). *Pursuit of ecstasy: The MDMA experience.* Albany: State University of New York Press.

Beckerman, N. L. (1994). Psychosocial tasks facing parents whose adult child has AIDS. *Family Therapy, 21*(3), 209–216.

Beckman, L. J., & Ackerman, K. T. (1995). Women, alcohol, and sexuality. *Recent Developments in Alcoholism, 12,* 267–285.

Beckstead, A. L., & Morrow, S. L. (1999). *"Gay is not me": Seeking congruence through sexual reorientation therapy.* Paper presented at the 107th annual meeting of the American Psychological Association, Boston.

Beeler, J., & DiProva, V. (1999). Family adjustment following disclosure of homosexuality by a member: Themes discerned in narrative accounts. *Journal of Marital and Family Therapy, 25*(4), 443–459.

Bell, A. P., & Weinberg, M. S. (1978). *Homosexualities: A study of diversity among men and women.* New York: Simon & Schuster.

Bem, D. J. (1996). Exotic becomes erotic: A developmental theory of sexual orientation. *Psychological Review, 103,* 320–335.

Bem, D. J. (1997, August). *Exotic becomes erotic: Explaining the enigma of sexual orientation.* Invited address presented at the 105th annual meeting of the American Psychological Association, Chicago.

Bem, S. L. (1993). *The lens of gender: Transforming the debate on sexual inequality.* New Haven: Yale University Press.

Ben-Ari, A. (1995). The discovery that an offspring is gay: Parents', gay men's, and lesbians' perspectives. *Journal of Homosexuality, 30*(1), 89–112.

Benjamin, J. (1988). *The bonds of love: Psychoanalysis, feminism, and the problem of domination.* New York: Pantheon Books.

Benkov, L. (1994). *Reinventing the family: The emerging story of lesbian and gay parents.* New York: Crown.

Bennett, M. J. (1990). Stigmatization: Experiences of persons with AIDS. *Issues in Mental Health Nursing, 11*(2), 141–154.

Benowitz, M. (1986). How homophobia affects lesbians' response to violence in lesbian relationships. In K. Lobel (Ed.), *Naming the violence: Speaking out about lesbian battering* (pp. 198–201). Seattle: Seal Press.

Benvenuti, A. (1993a). The remoralization of a people: Part one. *Creation Spirituality, 9*(1), 24–27.

Benvenuti, A. (1993b). The remoralization of a people: Part two. *Creation Spirituality, 9*(2), 32–35.

Bepko, C., & Johnson, T. (2000). Gay and lesbian couples in therapy: Perspectives for the contemporary family therapist. *Journal of Marital and Family Therapy, 26*(4), 409–419.

Berenbaum, S. A., & Hines, M. (1992). Early androgens are related to childhood sex-typed toy preferences. *Psychological Science, 3,* 203–206.

Berg-Cross, L. (1988). Lesbians, family process and individuation. *Journal of College Student Psychotherapy, 3*(1), 97–112.

Berger, R. M. (1980). Psychological adaptation of the older homosexual male. *Journal of Homosexuality, 5*(5), 161–175.

Berger, R. M. (1982a). *Gay and grey: The older homosexual man.* Urbana: University of Illinois Press.

Berger, R. M. (1982b). The unseen minority: Older gays and lesbians. *Social Work, 27,* 236–242.

Berger, R. M. (1983). What is a homosexual? A definitional model. *Social Work, 28,* 132–135.

Berger, R. M. (1990a). Men together: Understanding the gay couple. *Journal of Homosexuality, 19*(3), 31–49.

Berger, R. M. (1990b). Passing: Impact on the quality of same-sex relationships. *Social Work, 35*(4), 328–332.

Berger, R. M. (1992a). Passing and social support among gay men. *Journal of Homosexuality, 23*(3), 85–97.

Berger, R. M. (1992b). Research on older gay men: What we know, what we need to know. In N. J. Woodman (Ed.), *Lesbian and gay lifestyles: A guide for counseling and education* (pp. 217–234). New York: Irvington.

Berger, R. M. (1995). *Gay and grey: The older homosexual man* (2nd ed.). Binghamton, NY: Haworth Press.

Berger, R. M., & Kelly, J. J. (1986). Working with homosexuals of the older population. *Social Casework, 67*(4), 203–210.

Berger, R. M., & Kelly, J. J. (1996). Gay men and lesbians grown older. In R. P. Cabaj & T. S. Stein (Eds.), *Textbook of homosexuality and mental health* (pp. 305–316). Washington, DC: American Psychiatric Press.

Bergmark, K. H. (1999). Drinking in the Swedish gay and lesbian community. *Drug and Alcohol Dependence, 56*(2), 133–143.

Berkey, B. R., Perelman-Hall, T., & Kurdek, L. A. (1990). The multidimensional scale of sexuality. *Journal of Homosexuality, 19*(4), 67–87.

Bernhard, L. A. (2000). Physical and sexual violence experienced by lesbian and heterosexual women. *Violence Against Women, 6*(1), 68–79.

Bernhard, L. A., & Applegate, J. M. (1999). Comparison of stress and stress management strategies between lesbian and heterosexual women. *Health Care for Women International, 20*(4), 335–347.

Bernstein, A. C. (2000). Straight therapists working with lesbians and gays in family therapy. *Journal of Marital and Family Therapy, 26*(4), 443–454.

Bernstein, A. J. (1997). The relationship between perceived parent attachment, homosexual identity formation, psychological adjustment and parent awareness of gay and lesbian young adults. *Dissertation Abstracts International, 57*(9-A), 4145. (University Microfilms No. AAM97–06942)

Bernstein, B. E. (1990). Attitudes and issues of parents of gay men and lesbians and implications for therapy. *Journal of Gay and Lesbian Psychotherapy, 1*(3), 37–53.

Bersoff, D. N., & Ogden, D. W. (1991). APA amicus curiae briefs: Furthering lesbian and gay male civil rights. *American Psychologist, 46*(9), 950–956.

Berzon, B. (1988). *Permanent partners: Building gay and lesbian relationships that last.* New York: Dutton.

Berzon, B. (1997). *The intimacy dance: A guide to long-term success in gay and lesbian relationships.* New York: Plume.

Bethea, A. R., Rexrode, K. R., Ruffo, A. C., & Washington, S. D. (1999). *Violence in lesbian relationships: A narrative analysis.* Poster session presented at the 107th annual meeting of the American Psychological Association, Boston.

Betz, N. E., & Fitzgerald, L. F. (1995). Career assessment and interventions with racial and ethnic minorities. In F. T. Leong (Ed.), *Career development and vocational behavior of racial and ethnic minorities* (pp. 263–279). Mahwah, NJ: Erlbaum.

Bhugra, D. (1987). Homophobia: A review of the literature. *Sexual and Marital Therapy, 2*(2), 169–177.

Biaggio, M., Roades, L. A., McCaffery, D., Cardinali, J., & Duffy, R. (1996). *Clinical Evaluations: Impact of Sexual Orientation, Gender, and Gender Role.* Paper presented at the 104th annual meeting of the American Psychological Association, Toronto.

Bieber, I., & Bieber, T. B. (1979). Male homosexuality. *Canadian Journal of Psychiatry, 24*(5), 409–421.

Bieschke, K. J., Eberz, A. B., Bard, C. C., & Croteau, J. M. (1998). Using social cognitive career theory to create affirmative lesbian, gay, and bisexual research training environments. *The Counseling Psychologist, 26*(5), 735–753.

Bieschke, K. J., & Matthews, C. (1996). Career counselor attitudes and behaviors toward gay, lesbian, and bisexual clients. *Journal of Vocational Behavior, 48*(2), 243–255.

Bigner, J. J. (1996). Working with gay fathers: Developmental, postdivorce parenting, and therapeutic issues. In J. Laird & R. J. Green (Eds.), *Lesbian and gay couples and families: A handbook for therapists* (pp. 370–403). San Francisco: Jossey-Bass.

Bigner, J. J., & Bozett, F. W. (1989). Parenting by gay fathers. *Marriage and Family Review, 14*(3–4), 155–175.

Bigner, J. J., & Jacobsen, R. B. (1992). Adult responses to child behavior and attitudes toward fathering: Gay and nongay fathers. *Journal of Homosexuality, 23*(3), 99–112.

Biller, R., & Rice, S. (1990). Experiencing multiple loss of persons with AIDS: Grief and bereavement issues. *Health and Social Work, 15*(4), 283–290.

Billingham, R. E., & Hockenberry, S. L. (1987). Gender conformity, masturbation fantasy, infatuation, and sexual orientation: A discriminant analysis investigation. *Journal of Sex Research, 23*(3), 368–374.

Birt, C. M., & Dion, K. L. (1987). Relative deprivation theory and responses to discrimination in a gay and lesbian sample. *British Journal of Social Psychology, 26*(2), 139–145.

Bittle, W. E. (1982). Alcoholics Anonymous and the gay alcoholic. *Journal of Homosexuality, 7*(4), 81–88.

Blair, R. (1972). *Vocational guidance and gay liberation* (The Otherwise Monograph Services, No. 19). National Task Force on Student Personnel Services and Homosexuality.

Blanchard, R., & Bogaert, A. F. (1996a). Homosexuality in men and number of older brothers. *American Journal of Psychiatry, 153*(1), 27–31.

Blanchard, R., & Bogaert, A. F. (1996b). Biodemographic comparisons of homosexual and heterosexual men in the Kinsey interview data. *Archives of Sexual Behavior, 25*(6), 551–579.

Blanchard, R., & Bogaert, A. F. (1997). Additive effects of older brothers and homosexual brothers in the prediction of marriage and cohabitation. *Behavior Genetics, 27*(1), 45–54.

Blanchard, R., & Sheridan, P. M. (1992). Sibship size, sibling sex ratio, birth order, and parental age in homosexual and nonhomosexual gender dysphorics. *Journal of Nervous and Mental Disease, 180*(1), 40–47.

Blanchard, R., Zucker, K. J., Siegelman, M., Dickey, R., & Klassen, P. (1998). The relation of birth order to sexual orientation in men and women. *Journal of Biosocial Science, 30*(4), 511–519.

Blinde, E. M., & Taub, D. E. (1992). Women athletes as falsely accused deviants: Managing the lesbian stigma. *Sociological Quarterly, 33*(4), 521–533.

Blum, A., & Pfetzing, V. (1997). Assaults to the self: The trauma of growing up gay. *Gender and Psychoanalysis, 2*(4), 427–442.

Blumenfeld, W. J., & Raymond, D. (1988). *Looking at gay and lesbian life.* Boston: Beacon Press.

Blumstein, P., & Schwartz, P. (1983). *American couples: Money, work, and sex.* New York: William Morrow.

Bogaert, A. F. (1997). Birth order and sexual orientation in women. *Behavioral Neuroscience, 111*(6), 1395–1397.

Bograd, M. (1999). Strengthening domestic violence theories: Intersections of race, class, sexual orientation, and gender. *Journal of Marital and Family Therapy, 25*(3), 275–289.

Bograd, M., & Mederos, F. (1999). Battering and couples therapy: Universal screening and selection of treatment modality. *Journal of Marital and Family Therapy, 25*(3), 291–312.

Boisvert, D. L. (2000). *Out on holy ground: Meditations on gay spirituality.* Cleveland, OH: Pilgrim Press.

Boldero, J., Sanitioso, R., & Brain, B. (1999). Gay Asian Australians' safer-sex behavior and behavioral skills: The predictive utility of the theory of planned behavior and cultural factors. *Journal of Applied Social Psychology, 29*(10), 2143–2163.

Boles, J., & Elifson, K. W. (1994). Sexual identity and HIV: The male prostitute. *Journal of Sex Research, 31*(1), 39–46.

Bollas, C. (1989). *Forces of destiny: Psychoanalysis and human idiom.* Northvale, NJ: Jason Aronson.

Bonilla, L., & Porter, J. (1990). A comparison of Latino, Black, and non-Hispanic White attitudes toward homosexuality. *Hispanic Journal of Behavioral Sciences, 12*(4), 437–452.

Borhek, M. V. (1988). Helping gay and lesbian adolescents and their families: A mother's perspective. *Journal of Adolescent Health Care, 9*(2), 123–128.

Bosga, M. B., De Wit, J. B. F., De Vroome, E. M., & Houweling, H. (1995). Differences in perception of risk for HIV infection with steady and non-steady partners among homosexual men. *AIDS Education and Prevention, 7*(2), 103–115.

Boswell, J. (1980). *Christianity, social tolerance, and homosexuality: Gay people in western Europe from the beginning of the Christian era to the fourteenth century*. Chicago: University of Chicago Press.

Boswell, J. (1989). Homosexuality and religious life: A historical approach. In J. Gramick (Ed.), *Homosexuality in the priesthood and the religious life* (pp. 3–20). New York: Crossroad.

Boswell, J. (1994). *Same-sex unions in premodern Europe*. New York: Villard Books.

Botkin, M., & Daly, J. (1987, March). *Occupational development of lesbians and gays*. Paper presented at the annual meeting of the American College Student Personnel Association, Chicago.

Botnick, M. R. (2000). Fear of contagion, fear of intimacy. *Journal of Homosexuality, 39*(4, Pt. 2), 77–101.

Bowen, D. J. (1999). *Comparing health behaviors among women of diverse sexual orientations*. Paper presented at the 107th annual meeting of the American Psychological Association, Boston.

Bowers v. Hardwick (85-140), 478 U.S. 186 (1986).

Boxer, A. M., & Cohler, B. J. (1989). The life course of gay and lesbian youth: An immodest proposal for the study of lives. *Journal of Homosexuality, 17*(3–4), 315–355.

Boxer, A. M., Cook, J. A., & Herdt, G. (1991). Double jeopardy: Identity transitions and parent–child relations among gay and lesbian youth. In K. Pillemer & K. McCartney (Eds.), *Parent–child relations throughout life* (pp. 59–92). Hillsdale, NJ: Erlbaum.

Boykin, K. (1998). *One more river to cross: Black and gay in America*. New York: Doubleday.

Bozett, F. W. (1989). Gay fathers: A review of the literature. *Journal of Homosexuality, 18*(1–2), 137–162.

Bozett, F. W. (1990). Fathers who are gay. In R. J. Kus (Ed.), *Keys to caring: Assisting your gay and lesbian clients* (pp. 106–118). Boston: Alyson.

Bozett, F. W., & Hanson, S. M. H. (1991). Cultural change and the future of fatherhood and families. In F. W. Bozett & S. M. H. Hanson (Eds.), *Focus on men: Vol. 6. Fatherhood and families in cultural context* (pp. 263–274). New York: Springer.

Bozett, F. W., & Sussman, M. B. (1989). Homosexuality and family relations: Views and research issues. *Marriage and Family Review, 14*(3–4), 1–8.

Bradford, J. B., & Ryan, C. (1988). *The national lesbian health care survey: Final report*. Washington, DC: National Lesbian and Gay Health Foundation. (Also available as Contract No. 86MO19832201D. Washington, DC: U.S. Department of Health and Human Services)

Bradford, J., & Ryan, C. (1991). Who we are: Health concerns of middle-aged lesbians. In B. Sang, J. Warshow, & A. J. Smith (Eds.), *Lesbians at midlife: The creative transition* (pp. 147–163). San Francisco: Spinsters.

Bradford, J., Ryan, C., & Rothblum, E. D. (1994). National lesbian health care survey: Implications for mental health care. *Journal of Consulting and Clinical Psychology, 62*(2), 228–242.

Brady, S., & Busse, W. J. (1994). The gay identity questionnaire: A brief measure of homosexual identity formation. *Journal of Homosexuality, 26*(4), 1–22.

Brand, P. A., & Kidd, A. H. (1986). Frequency of physical aggression in heterosexual and female homosexual dyads. *Psychological Reports, 59*, 1307–1313.

Brewaeys, A., Devroey, P., Helmerhorst, F. M., Van Hall, E. V., & Ponjaert, I. (1995). Lesbian mothers who conceived after donor insemination: A follow-up study. *Human Reproduction, 10*(10), 2731–2735.

Brewaeys, A., Ponjaert, I., Van Hall, E. V., & Golombok, S. (1997). Donor insemination: Child development and family functioning in lesbian mother families. *Human Reproduction, 12*(6), 1349–1359.

Brewaeys, A., Ponjaert-Kristoffersen, I., Van Steirteghem, A. C., & Devroey, P. (1993). Children from anonymous donors: An inquiry into homosexual and heterosexual parents' attitudes. *Journal of Psychosomatic Obstetrics and Gynaecology, 14* (Suppl.), 23–35.

Brewaeys, A., & Van Hall, E. V. (1997) Lesbian motherhood: The impact on child development and family functioning. *Journal of Psychosomatic Obstetrics and Gynaecology, 18*(1), 1–16.

Bridges, K. L., & Croteau, J. M. (1994). Once-married lesbians: Facilitating changing life patterns. *Journal of Counseling and Development, 73*(2), 134–140.

Bridget, J., & Lucille, S. (1996). Lesbian Youth Support Information Service (LYSIS): Developing a distance support agency for young lesbians. *Journal of Community and Applied Social Psychology,* *6*(5), 355–364.

Britton, D. M. (1990). Homophobia and homosociality: An analysis of boundary maintenance. *Sociological Quarterly, 31*(3), 423–439.

Brown, D., & Brooks, L. (Eds.). (1996). *Career choice and development* (3rd ed.). San Francisco: Jossey-Bass.

Brown, L. B. (Ed.). (1997). *Two spirit people: American Indian lesbian women and gay men.* Binghamton, NY: Haworth Press.

Brown, L. S. (1985). *Sexual issues in the development of lesbian couples.* Paper presented at the 93rd annual meeting of the American Psychological Association, Los Angeles.

Brown, L. S. (1986). Confronting internalized oppression in sex therapy with lesbians. In M. Kehoe (Ed.), *Historical, literary, and erotic aspects of lesbianism* (pp. 99–107). New York: Harrington Park Press.

Brown, L. S. (1989a). Lesbians, gay men and their families: Common clinical issues. *Journal of Gay and Lesbian Psychotherapy, 1*(1), 65–77.

Brown, L. S. (1989b). New voices, new visions: Toward a lesbian/gay paradigm for psychology. *Psychology of Women Quarterly, 13*(4), 445–458.

Brown, L. S. (1994). *Gender issues in lesbian relationships: Strengths and struggles.* Paper presented at the 102nd annual meeting of the American Psychological Association, Los Angeles.

Brown, L. S. (1996). Ethical concerns with sexual minority patients. In R. P. Cabaj & T. S. Stein (Eds.), *Textbook of homosexuality and mental health* (pp. 897–916). Washington, DC: American Psychiatric Press.

Brown, L. S. (2000). Foreword. In R. M. Perez, K. A. DeBord, & K. J. Bieschke (Eds.), *Handbook of counseling and psychotherapy with lesbian, gay, and bisexual clients* (pp. xi-xiii). Washington, DC: American Psychological Association.

Browning, C. (1987). Therapeutic issues and intervention strategies with young adult lesbian clients: A developmental approach. *Journal of Homosexuality, 14*(1–2), 45–52.

Browning, C. (1988). Therapeutic issues and intervention strategies with young adult lesbian clients: A developmental approach. In E. Coleman (Ed.), *Integrated identity for gay men and lesbians: Psychotherapeutic approaches for emotional well-being* (pp. 45–52). New York: Harrington Park Press.

Browning, C., Reynolds, A. L., & Dworkin, S. H. (1991). Affirmative psychotherapy for lesbian women. *Counseling Psychologist, 19*(2), 177–196.

Brownsworth, V. A. (1992, March 24). America's worst-kept secret: AIDS is devastating the nation's teenagers, and gay kids are dying by the thousands. *The Advocate,* pp. 38–46.

Brunette, M. F., Rosenberg, S. D., Goodman, L. A., Mueser, K T., Osher, F. C., Vidaver, R., Auciello, P., Wolford, G. L., & Drake, R. E. (1999). HIV risk factors among people with severe mental illness in urban and rural areas. *Psychiatric Service, 50*(4), 556–558.

Bryant, S., & Demian. (1995). *Partners national survey of lesbian and gay couples* [Online]. Available: www.eskimo.com/-demian/survey.html (Survey data used with permission; see also Resources).

Buckel, D. (1999, Fall). Youth bring gay rights movement to school. *The Lambda Update, 16*(3), 6–7.

Buenting, J. A. (1992). Health life-styles of lesbian and heterosexual women. *Health Care for Women International, 13*(2), 165–171.

Buhrich, N., Bailey, J. M., & Martin, N. J. (1991). Sexual orientation, sexual identity, and sex-dimorphic behaviors in male twins. *Behavior Genetics, 21*(1), 75–96.

Bull, C. (1994, April 5). Suicidal tendencies. *The Advocate,* pp. 35–42.

Bull, C. (1999a, April 13). The state of hate: Special report. *The Advocate,* p. 23.

Bull, C. (1999b, June 22), The new activism. *The Advocate,* pp. 53–60.

Bull, C. (1999c, August 31). Connect the dots. *The Advocate,* pp. 25–29.

Bull, C. (2000a, April 11). Ahead of the class. *The Advocate,* pp. 25, 27.

Bull, C. (2000b, June 20). Pride across America. *The Advocate,* pp. 65–66.

Buloff, B., & Osterman, M. (1995). Queer reflections: Mirroring and the lesbian experience of self. In J.

M. Glassgold & S. Iasenza (Eds.), *Lesbians and psychoanalysis: Revolutions in theory and practice* (pp. 93–106). New York: Free Press.

Büntzly, G. (1993). Gay fathers in straight marriages. *Journal of Homosexuality, 24*(3–4), 107–114.

Burch, B. (1986). Psychotherapy and the dynamics of merger in lesbian couples. In T. S. Stein & C. J. Cohen (Eds.), *Contemporary perspectives on psychotherapy with lesbians and gay men* (pp. 57–71). New York: Plenum.

Burch, B. (1987). Barriers to intimacy: Conflicts over power, dependency, and nurturing in lesbian relationships. In Boston Lesbian Psychologies Collective (Ed.), *Lesbian psychologies: Explorations and challenges* (pp. 126–141). Urbana: University of Illinois Press.

Burch, B. (1993). *On intimate terms: The psychology of difference in lesbian relationships*. Urbana: University of Illinois Press.

Burch, B. (1995). Gender identities, lesbianism, and potential space. In J. M. Glassgold & S. Iasenza (Eds.), *Lesbians and psychoanalysis: Revolutions in theory and practice* (pp. 287–307). New York: Free Press.

Bureau of Labor Statistics. (1999). *Usual weekly earnings summary*. Washington, DC: U.S. Department of Labor.

Burke, L. K., & Follingstad, D. R. (1999). Violence in lesbian and gay relationships: Theory, prevalence, and correlational factors. *Clinical Psychology Review, 19*(5), 487–512.

Burnett, C. B., Steakley, C. S., Slack, R., Roth, J., & Lerman, C. (1999). Patterns of breast cancer screening among lesbians at increased risk for breast cancer. *Women and Health, 29*(4), 35–55.

Burr, C. (1993, March). Homosexuality and biology. *The Atlantic Monthly*, pp. 47–65.

Bux, D. A. (1996). The epidemiology of problem drinking in gay men and lesbians: A critical review. *Clinical Psychology Review, 16*(4), 277–298.

Buxton, A. P. (1991). *The other side of the closet: The coming-out crisis for straight spouses*. Santa Monica, CA: IBS Press.

Buxton, A. P. (1999). The best interest of children of gay and lesbian parents. In R. M. Galatzer-Levy & L. Kraus (Eds.), *The scientific basis of child custody decisions* (pp. 319–356). New York: Wiley.

Byne, W. (1994, May). The biological evidence challenged. *Scientific American*, pp. 50–55.

Byne, W. (1995). Science and belief: Psychobiological research on sexual orientation. *Journal of Homosexuality, 28*, 303–344.

Byne, W. (1996). Biology and homosexuality: Implications of neuroendocrinological and neuroanatomical studies. In R. P. Cabaj & T. S. Stein (Eds.), *Textbook of homosexuality and mental health* (pp. 129–146). Washington, DC: American Psychiatric Press.

Byne, W., & Parsons, B. (1993). Human sexual orientation: The biologic theories reappraised. *Archives of General Psychiatry, 50*, 228–239.

Cabaj, R. P. (1988a). Gay and lesbian couples: Lessons on human intimacy. *Psychiatric Annals, 18*(1), 21–25.

Cabaj, R. P. (1988b). Homosexuality and neurosis: Considerations for psychotherapy. *Journal of Homosexuality, 15*(1–2). 13–23.

Cabaj, R. P. (1995). Sexual orientation and the addictions. *Journal of Gay and Lesbian Psychotherapy, 2*(3), 97–117.

Cabaj, R. P. (1996a). Gay, lesbian, and bisexual mental health professionals and their colleagues. In R. P. Cabaj & T. S. Stein (Eds.), *Textbook of homosexuality and mental health* (pp. 33–39). Washington, DC: American Psychiatric Press.

Cabaj, R. P. (1996b). Sexual orientation of the therapist. In R. P. Cabaj & T. S. Stein (Eds.), *Textbook of homosexuality and mental health* (pp. 513–524). Washington, DC: American Psychiatric Press.

Cabaj, R. P. (1996c). Substance abuse in gay men, lesbians, and bisexuals. In R. P. Cabaj & T. S. Stein (Eds.), *Textbook of homosexuality and mental health* (pp. 783–799). Washington, DC: American Psychiatric Press.

Cabaj, R. P., & Klinger, R. L. (1996). Psychotherapeutic interventions with lesbians and gay couples. In R. P. Cabaj & T. S. Stein (Eds.), *Textbook of homosexuality and mental health* (pp. 485–501). Washington, DC: American Psychiatric Press.

Cabaj, R. P., & Purcell D. W. (Eds.). (1998). *On the road to same-sex marriage: A supportive guide to psychological, political, and legal issues.* San Francisco: Jossey-Bass.

Cadwell, S. (1991). Twice removed: The stigma suffered by gay men with AIDS. *Smith College Studies in Social Work, 61*(3), 236–246.

Cadwell, S. A. (1994). Over-identification with HIV clients. *Journal of Gay and Lesbian Psychotherapy, 2*(2), 77–99.

Cady, S., Ronan, M., & Taussig, H. (1986). *Sophia: The future of feminist spirituality.* San Francisco: Harper & Row.

Cain, R. (1991a). Stigma management and gay identity development. *Social Work, 36*(1), 67–73.

Cain, R. (1991b). Relational contexts and information management among gay men. *Families in Society, 72*(6), 344–352.

Callahan, S. (1985). The laity and alienated Catholics. In M. Glazier (Ed.), *Where we are: American Catholics in the 1980's* (pp. 51–63). Wilmington, DE: Michael Glazier.

Cameron, P., & Cameron, K. (1995). Does incest cause homosexuality? *Psychological Reports, 76,* 611–621.

Cameron, P., & Cameron, K. (1996a). Do homosexual teachers pose a risk to pupils? *Journal of Psychology, 130,* 603–613.

Cameron, P., & Cameron, K. (1996b). Homosexual parents. *Adolescence, 31,* 757–776.

Campbell, S. M. (1980). *The couple's journey: Intimacy as a path to wholeness.* San Luis Obispo, CA: Impact.

Canarelli, J., Cole, G., & Rizzuto, C. (1999). Attention vs. acceptance: Some dynamic issues in gay male development. *Gender and Psychoanalysis, 4*(1), 47–70.

Capitanio, J. P. (1995). Black heterosexuals' attitudes toward lesbians and gay men in the United States. *Journal of Sex Research, 32*(2), 95–105.

Carballo-Dieguez, A. (1989). Hispanic culture, gay male culture, and AIDS: Counseling implications. *Journal of Counseling and Development, 68*(1), 26–30.

Carballo-Dieguez, A., & Dolezal, C. (1995). Association between history of childhood sexual abuse and adult HIV-risk sexual behavior in Puerto Rican men who have sex with men. *Child Abuse and Neglect, 19*(5), 595–605.

Carl, D. (1990). Parenting/blended family issues. In D. Carl (Ed.), *Counseling same-sex couples* (pp. 91–106). New York: Norton.

Carlson, K. (1996). Gay and lesbian families. In M. Harway (Ed.), *Treating the changing family: Handling normative and unusual events* (pp. 62–76). New York: Wiley.

Carpenter, E. (1987). Selected insights. In M. Thompson (Ed.), *Gay spirit: Myth and meaning* (pp. 152–164). New York: St. Martin's Press.

Carrier, J. M. (1986). Childhood cross-gender behavior and adult homosexuality. *Archives of Sexual Behavior, 15*(1), 89–93.

Carroll, N. M. (1999). Optimal gynecologic and obstetric care for lesbians. *Obstetrics and Gynecology, 93*(4), 611–613.

Case, P. (1999). *Social context of HIV risk among IDU women in New York.* Paper presented at the 107th annual meeting of the American Psychological Association, Boston.

Casper, V., & Schultz, S., (1996). Lesbian and gay parents encounter educators: Initiating conversations. In R. C. Savin-Williams & K. M. Cohen (Eds.), *The lives of lesbians, gays, and bisexuals: Children to adults* (pp. 303–330). Fort Worth, TX: Harcourt Brace.

Casper, V., Schultz, S., & Wickens, E. (1992). Breaking the silence: Lesbian and gay parents and the schools. *Teachers College Record, 94*(1), 109–137.

Cass, V. C. (1979). Homosexual identity formation: A theoretical model. *Journal of Homosexuality, 4,* 219–235.

Cass, V. C. (1983/1984). Homosexual identity: A concept in need of definition. *Journal of Homosexuality, 9,* 105–126.

Cass, V. C. (1984). Homosexual identity formation: Testing a theoretical model. *Journal of Sex Research, 20,* 143–167.

Cass, V. C. (1990). The implications of homosexual identity formation for the Kinsey model and scale of sexual preference. In D. P. McWhirter, S. A. Sanders, & J. M. Reinisch (Eds.), *Homosexuality/heterosexuality: Concepts of sexual orientation* (pp. 239–266). New York: Oxford University Press.

Caster, W. (1993). *The lesbian sex book*. Boston: Alyson.

Catania, J. A., Turner, H. A., Choi, K., & Coates, T. J. (1992). Coping with death anxiety: Help-seeking and social support among gay men with various HIV diagnoses. *AIDS, 6*(9), 999–1005.

Cates, J. A. (1989). Adolescent male prostitution by choice. *Child and Adolescent Social Work Journal, 6*(2), 151–156.

Ceballos-Capitaine, A., Szapocznik, J., Blaney, N. T., & Morgan, R. O. (1990). Ethnicity, emotional distress, stress-related disruption, and coping among HIV seropositive gay males. *Hispanic Journal of Behavioral Sciences, 12*(2), 135–152.

Chabot, J. M. (1999). Transition to parenthood: Lesbian couples' experiences with donor insemination. *Dissertation Abstracts International, 59*(10-A), 3976. (University Microfilms No. AAM99–09272)

Chaimowitz, G. A. (1991). Homophobia among psychiatric residents, family practice residents and psychiatric faculty. *Canadian Journal of Psychiatry, 36*(3), 206–209.

Chan, C. S. (1989). Issues of identity development among Asian American lesbians and gay men. *Journal of Counseling and Development, 68*(1), 16–20.

Chan, C. S. (1992). Cultural considerations in counseling Asian American lesbians and gay men. In S. H. Dworkin & F. J. Gutierrez (Eds.), *Counseling gay men and lesbians: Journey to the end of the rainbow* (pp. 115–124). Alexandria VA: American Association for Counseling and Development.

Chan, C. S. (1997). Don't ask, don't tell, don't know: The formation of a homosexual identity and sexual expression among Asian American lesbians. In B. Greene (Ed.), *Ethnic and cultural diversity among lesbians and gay men* (pp. 240–248). Thousand Oaks, CA: Sage.

Chan, R. W., Raboy, B., & Patterson, C. J. (1998). Psychosocial adjustment among children conceived via donor insemination by lesbian and heterosexual mothers. *Child Development, 69*(2), 443–457.

Chapman, B. E., & Brannock, J. C. (1987). Proposed model of lesbian identity development: An empirical examination. *Journal of Homosexuality, 14*(3–4), 69–80.

Charbonneau, C., & Lander, P. S. (1991). Redefining sexuality: Women becoming lesbian at midlife. In B. Sang, J. Warshow, & A. J. Smith (Eds.), *Lesbians at midlife: The creative transition* (pp. 35–43). San Francisco: Spinsters.

Cherry, K., & Sherwood, Z. (Eds.). (1995). *Equal rites: Lesbian and gay worship, ceremonies, and celebrations*. Louisville, KY: Westminster/John Knox Press.

Chesney, M. A., Barrett, D. C., & Stall, R. (1998). Histories of substance use and risk behavior: Precursors to HIV seroconversion in homosexual men. *American Journal of Public Health, 88*(1), 113–116.

Chesney, M. A., & Folkman, S. (1994). Psychological impact of HIV disease and implications for intervention. *Psychiatric Clinics of North America, 17*(1), 163–182.

Chodorow, N. J. (1978). *The reproduction of mothering: Psychoanalysis and the sociology of gender*. Berkeley: University of California Press.

Chodorow, N. J. (1989). *Feminism and psychoanalytic theory*. New Haven, CT: Yale University Press.

Chodorow, N. J. (1992). Heterosexuality as a compromise formation: Reflections on the psychoanalytic theory of sexual development. *Psychoanalysis and Contemporary Thought, 15*(3), 267–304.

Chodorow, N. J. (1994). *Femininities, masculinities, sexualities: Freud and beyond*. Lexington: University of Kentucky Press.

Chojnacki, J. T., & Gelberg, S. (1994). Toward a conceptualization of career counseling with gay/lesbian/bisexual persons. *Journal of Career Development, 21*, 3–10.

Christ, C., & Plaskow, J. (Eds.). (1979). *Womanspirit rising: A feminist leader in religion*. San Francisco: Harper & Row.

Chuang, H. T., & Addington, D. (1988). Homosexual panic: A review of its concept. *Canadian Journal of Psychiatry, 33*(7), 613–617.

Chung, Y. B. (1995). Career decision making of lesbian, gay, and bisexual individuals. *Career Development Quarterly, 44*, 178–190.

Chung, Y. B., & Katayama, M. (1996). Assessment of sexual orientation in lesbian/gay/bisexual studies. *Journal of Homosexuality, 30*(4), 49–62.

Cicchetti, D., & Toth, S. L. (1995). Childhood maltreatment and attachment organization: Implications for intervention. In S. Goldberg, R. Muir, & J. Kerr (Eds), *Attachment theory: Social, developmental, and clinical perspectives* (pp. 279–308). Hillsdale, NJ: Analytic Press.

Clark, D. (1987). *The new loving someone gay.* Berkeley, CA: Celestial Arts.

Clark, J. M. (1987). *Gay being, divine presence: Essays in gay spirituality.* Las Colinas, TX: Tangelwuld.

Clark, J. M. (1989). *A place to start: Toward an unapologetic gay liberation theology.* Dallas: Monument Press.

Clark, J. M. (1997). *Defying the darkness: Gay theology in the shadows.* Cleveland, OH: Pilgrim Press.

Clark, J. M., Brown, J. C., & Hochstein, L. M. (1989). Institutional religion and gay/lesbian oppression. *Marriage and Family Review, 14*(3–4), 265–284.

Clark, W. M., & Serovich, J. M. (1997). Twenty years and still in the dark? Content analysis of articles pertaining to gay, lesbian, and bisexual issues in marriage and family therapy journals. *Journal of Marital and Family Therapy, 23*(3), 239–253.

Clunis, D. M., & Green, G. D. (1988). *Lesbian couples.* Seattle: Seal Press.

Clunis, D. M., & Green, G. D. (1995). *The lesbian parenting book: A guide to creating families and raising children.* Seattle: Seal Press.

Cochran, S. D. (1999). *Prevalence of mental health syndromes among homosexually active women.* Paper presented at the 107th annual meeting of the American Psychological Association, Boston.

Cochran, S. D., & Mays, V. M. (1986, August). *Sources of support in the Black lesbian community.* Paper presented at the 94th annual meeting of the American Psychological Association, Washington, DC.

Cochran, S. D., & Mays, V. M. (2000a). Lifetime prevalence of suicide symptoms and affective disorders among men reporting same-sex sexual partners: Results from NHANES III. *American Journal of Public Health, 90*(4), 573–578.

Cochran, S. D., & Mays, V. M. (2000b). Relation between psychiatric syndromes and behaviorally defined sexual orientation in a sample of the US population. *American Journal of Epidemiology, 151*(5), 516–523.

Cohen, M. R. (with Doner, K.). (1998). *The HIV wellness sourcebook.* New York: Henry Holt.

Coleman, E. (1981/1982). Developmental stages of the coming out process. *Journal of Homosexuality, 7*(2–3), 31–43.

Coleman, E. (1982). Bisexual and gay men in heterosexual marriage: Conflicts and resolutions in therapy. In J. C. Gonsiorek (Ed.), *Homosexuality and psychotherapy: A practitioner's handbook of affirmative models* (pp. 93–103). Binghamton, NY: Haworth Press.

Coleman, E. (1988). Assessment of sexual orientation. In E. Coleman (Ed.), *Integrated identity for gay men and lesbians: Psychotherapeutic approaches for emotional well-being* (pp. 9–24). New York: Harrington Park Press.

Coleman, E. (1989). The development of male prostitution activity among gay and bisexual adolescents. *Journal of Homosexuality, 17*(1–2), 131–149.

Coleman, E. (1990). Toward a synthetic understanding of sexual orientation. In D. P. McWhirter, S. A. Sanders, & J. M. Reinisch (Eds.), *Homosexuality/heterosexuality: Concepts of sexual orientation* (pp. 267–276). New York: Oxford University Press.

Coleman, E., & Remafedi, G. (1989). Gay, lesbian, and bisexual adolescents: A critical challenge to counselors. *Journal of Counseling and Development, 68*(1), 36–40.

Coleman, M. T., & Walters, J. M. (1990, Summer). Chores: The results. *OUT/LOOK, 9,* 86.

Coleman, V. E. (1994). Lesbian battering: The relationship between personality and the perpetration of violence. *Violence and Victims, 9*(2), 139–152.

Coleman, V. E. (1997). Lesbian battering: The relationship between personality and the perpetration of violence. In L. K. Hamberger & C. Renzetti (Eds.), *Domestic partner abuse* (pp. 77–101). New York: Springer.

Colgan, P. (1988). Treatment of identity and intimacy issues in gay males. In E. Coleman (Ed.), *Integrated identity for gay men and lesbians: Psychotherapeutic approaches for emotional well-being* (pp. 101–123). New York: Harrington Park Press.

Comas-Diaz, L. (1990). Hispanic/Latino communities: Psychological implications. *Journal of Training and Practice in Professional Psychology, 4*(1), 14–35.

Committee on Lesbian and Gay Concerns. (1991). *Bias in psychotherapy with lesbians and gay men.* Washington, DC: American Psychological Association.

Comstock, G. D. (1993). *Gay theology without apology.* Cleveland, OH: Pilgrim Press.

Condon, L. (2000, May 23). Outbreak. *The Advocate,* pp. 40, 43.

Connolly, C. (1998). The description of gay and lesbian families in second-parent adoption cases. *Behavioral Science and the Law, 16*(2), 225–236.

Connor, R. P. (1993). *Blossom of bone: Reclaiming the connections between homoeroticism and the sacred.* San Francisco: Harper.

Cook, A. T., & Pawlowski, W. (1991). *Youth and homosexuality.* (Issue Paper: Respect All Youth Project; Available from Parents, Families and Friends of Lesbians and Gays [PFLAG]; see Resources for ordering information.)

Cooper, A. (1989). No longer invisible: Gay and lesbian Jews build a movement. In R. Hasbany (Ed.), *Homosexuality and religion* (pp. 83–94). Binghamton, NY: Haworth Press.

Cooper, M. (1990). Rejecting "femininity": Some research notes on gender identity development in lesbians. *Deviant Behavior, 11*(4), 371–380.

Coos, C. (1991). Single lesbians speak out. In B. Sang, J. Warshow, & A. J. Smith (Eds.). *Lesbians at midlife: The creative transition* (pp. 132–140). San Francisco: Spinsters.

Corbett, K. (1996). Homosexual boyhood: Notes on girlyboys. *Gender and Psychoanalysis, 1*(4), 429–461.

Corbett, K. (1997). Speaking queer: A reply to Richard C. Friedman. *Gender and Psychoanalysis, 2*(4), 495–514.

Corbett, K. (1999). Homosexual boyhood: Notes on girlyboys. In M. Rottnek (Ed.), *Sissies and tomboys: Gender nonconformity and homosexual childhood* (pp. 107–139). New York: New York University Press.

Cornett, C. W., & Hudson, R. A. (1987). Middle adulthood and the theories of Erikson, Gould, and Vaillant: Where does the gay man fit? *Journal of Gerontological Social Work, 10*(3–4), 61–73.

Coxon, A. P. M., & McManus, T. J. (2000). How many account for how much? Concentration of high-risk sexual behavior among gay men. *Journal of Sex Research, 37*(1), 1–7.

Craib, K. J. P., Weber, A. C., Cornelisse, P. G. A., Martindale, S. L., Miller, M. L., Schechter, M. T., Strathdee, S. A., Schilder, A., & Hogg, R. S. (2000). Comparisons of sexual behaviors, unprotected sex, and substance use between two independent cohorts of gay and bisexual men. *AIDS, 14*(3), 303–311.

Cramer, D. W., & Roach, A. J. (1988). Coming out to mom and dad: A study of gay males and their relationships with their parents. *Journal of Homosexuality, 15*(3–4), 79–91.

Crawford, D. (1990). *Easing the ache: Gay men recovering from compulsive behaviors.* New York: Plume.

Crawford, I., & Solliday, E. (1996). The attitudes of undergraduate college students toward gay parenting. *Journal of Homosexuality, 30*(4), 63–77.

Cronin, D. M. (1974). Coming out among lesbians. In E. Goode and R. Troiden (Eds.), *Sexual deviance and sexual deviants* (pp. 268–277). New York: William Morrow.

Crosbie-Burnett, M., & Helbrecht, L. (1993). A descriptive empirical study of gay male stepfamilies. *Family Relations, 42,* 256–262.

Crosby, G. M., Stall, R. D., Paul, J. P., & Barrett, D. C. (1998). Alcohol and drug use patterns have declined between generations of younger gay-bisexual men in San Francisco. *Drug and Alcohol Dependence, 52*(3), 177–182.

Crosby, G. M., Stall, R. D., Paul, J. P., & Barrett, D. C. (2000). Substance use and HIV risk profile of gay/bisexual males who drop out of substance abuse treatment. *AIDS Education and Prevention, 12*(1), 38–48.

Cruikshank, M. (1991). Lavender and gray: A brief survey of lesbian and gay aging studies. In J. A. Lee (Ed.), *Gay midlife and maturity* (pp. 77–87). New York: Harrington Park Press.

Cruz, J. M., & Firestone, J. M. (1998). Exploring violence and abuse in gay male relationships. *Violence and Victims*, 13 (2), 159–173.

Curb, R., & Manahan, N. (Eds.). (1985). *Lesbian nuns: Breaking silence*. Tallahassee, FL: Naiad Press.

Curran, C. (1983). Moral theology and homosexuality. In J. Gramick (Ed.), *Homosexuality and the Catholic church* (pp. 138–168). Chicago: Thomas More Press.

Curry, H., Clifford, D., Hertz, F., & Leonard, R. (1999). *A legal guide for lesbian and gay couples* (10th ed.). Berkeley, CA: Nolo Press.

Dahir, M. (2000, May 23). State of the unions. *The Advocate*, pp. 57–58, 60–61.

Dalton, S. E., & Bielby, D. D. (2000). "That's our kind of constellation": Lesbian mothers negotiate institutionalized understandings of gender within the family. *Gender and Society*, 14(1), 36–61.

Daly, M. (1978). *Gyn/Ecology: The metaethics of radical feminism*. Boston: Beacon.

Daly, M. (1985). *The church and the second sex: With the feminist postchristian introduction and new archaic afterwords by the author*. Boston: Beacon.

Daly, M. (1987). *Webster's first new intergalactic wickedary of the English language*. Boston: Beacon.

Dancey, C. P. (1990). The influence of familial and personality variables on sexual orientation in women. *Psychological Record*, 40(3), 437–449.

Dancey, C. P. (1992). The relationship of instrumentality and expressivity to sexual orientation in women. *Journal of Homosexuality*, 23(4), 71–82.

D'Augelli, A. R. (1989a). AIDS fears and homophobia among rural nursing personnel. *AIDS Education and Prevention*, 1(4), 277–284.

D'Augelli, A. R. (1989b). Lesbian women in a rural helping network: Exploring informal helping resources. In E. D. Rothblum & E. Cole (Eds.), *Lesbianism: Affirming nontraditional roles* (pp. 119–130). Binghamton, NY: Haworth Press.

D'Augelli, A. R. (1989c). Lesbian's and gay men's experiences of discrimination and university community. *American Journal of Community Psychology*, 17(3), 317–321.

D'Augelli, A. R. (1991). Gay men in college: Identity processes and adaptations. *Journal of College Student Development*, 32(2), 140–146.

D'Augelli, A. R. (1992). Lesbian and gay male undergraduates' experiences of harassment and fear on campus. *Journal of Interpersonal Violence*, 7(3), 383–395.

D'Augelli, A. R. (1994a, January). Focus on lesbian, gay and bisexual youth. *Division 44 Newsletter*, 9(3), 16–18.

D'Augelli, A. R. (1994b). Lesbian and gay male development: Steps toward an analysis of lesbians' and gay men's lives. In B. Greene & G. M. Herek (Eds.), *Lesbian and gay psychology: Theory, research, and clinical applications* (pp. 187–210). Thousand Oaks, CA: Sage.

D'Augelli, A. R. (1998). Developmental implications of victimization of lesbian, gay, and bisexual youths. In G. M. Herek (Ed.), *Stigma and sexual orientation: Understanding prejudice against lesbians, gay men, and bisexuals* (pp. 223–255). Thousand Oaks, CA: Sage.

D'Augelli, A. R., Collins, C., & Hart, M. M. (1987). Social support patterns of lesbian women in a rural helping network. *Journal of Rural Community Psychology*, 8(1), 12–22.

D'Augelli, A. R., & Herschberger, S. L. (1993). Lesbian, gay, and bisexual youth in community settings: Personal challenges and mental health problems. *American Journal of Community Psychology*, 21(4), 421–448.

Dawis, R. V. (1996). The theory of work adjustment and person-environment-correspondence counseling. In D. Brown & L. Brooks (Eds.), *Career choice and development* (3rd ed., pp. 75–120). San Francisco: Jossey-Bass.

Dawis, R. V., & Lofquist, L. H. (1984). *A psychological theory of work adjustment*. Minneapolis: University of Minnesota Press.

Dawood, K., Pillard, R. C., Horvath, C., Revelle, W., & Bailey, J. M. (2000). Familial aspects of male homosexuality. *Archives of Sexual Behavior*, 29(2), 155–163.

Deboer, D. S. (1999). Vicissitudes of hope in the lazarus effect: Psychosocial responses of HIV-positive gay men in the post crisis-era of HIV and AIDS. *Dissertation Abstracts International*, 60(6-B), 2937. (University Microfilms No. AAI99–34042)

DeBord, K. A., Wood, P. K., Sher, K. J., & Good, G. E. (1998). The relevance of sexual orientation to substance abuse and psychological distress among college students. *Journal of College Student Development, 39*(2), 157–168.

De Cecco, J. P. (1987). Homosexuality's brief recovery: From sickness to health and back again. *Journal of Sex Research, 23*(1), 106–114.

De Cecco, J. P. (1990). Sex and more sex: A critique of the Kinsey conception of human sexuality. In D. P. McWhirter, S. A. Sanders, & J. M. Reinisch (Eds.). *Homosexuality/heterosexuality: Concepts of sexual orientation* (pp. 367–386). New York: Oxford University Press.

De Crescenzo, T. (1983/1984). Homophobia: A study of the attitudes of mental health professionals toward homosexuality. *Journal of Social Work and Human Sexuality, 2*(2–3), 115–136.

Deenen, A. (1988). Research on gay couples: Sexuality, love, and friendship. *Nordisk-Sexologi, 6*(4), 235–240.

Dejowski, E. F. (1992). Public endorsement of restrictions on three aspects of free expression by homosexuals: Socio-demographic and trends analysis 1973–1988. *Journal of Homosexuality, 23*(4), 1–18.

De La Cancela, V. (1985). Toward a sociocultural psychotherapy for low-income ethnic minorities. *Psychotherapy: Theory, Research and Practice, 22*, 427–435.

De La Huerta, C. (1999). *Coming out spiritually: The next step*. New York: Putnam.

Demarco, F. J. (1999). Coping with the stigma of AIDS: An investigation of the effects of shame, stress, control and coping on depression in HIV-positive and -negative gay men. *Dissertation Abstracts International, 59*(10-B), 5574. (University Microfilms No. AAM99–09285)

Demian. (2000). *Adoption, foster case, donor insemination, surrogating* [Online]. Available: www.eskimo.com/-demian/adoption.html (see also Resources)

de Monteflores, C. (1986). Notes on the management of difference. In T. S. Stein & C. J. Cohen (Eds.) *Contemporary perspectives on psychotherapy with lesbians and gay men* (pp. 73–101). New York: Plenum.

Deutsch, L. (1995). Out of the closet and on to the couch: A psychoanalytic exploration of lesbian development. In J. M. Glassgold & S. Iasenza (Eds.), *Lesbians and psychoanalysis: Revolutions in theory and practice* (pp. 19–37). New York: Free Press.

Diamant, A. L., Schuster, M. A., & Lever, J. (2000). Receipt of preventative health care by lesbians. *American Journal of Preventative Medicine, 19*(3), 141–148.

Diamant, A. L., Schuster, M. A., McGuigan, K., & Lever, J. (1999). Lesbians' sexual history with men: Implications for taking a sexual history. *Archives of Internal Medicine, 159*(22), 2730–2736.

Diamond-Friedman, C. (1990). A multivariant model of alcoholism specific to gay–lesbian populations. *Alcohol Treatment Quarterly, 7*(2), 111–117.

Diaz, R. M. (1997). *Latino gay men and HIV: Culture, sexuality, and risk behavior*. New York: Routledge.

Dickemann, M. (1995). Wilson's Panchreston: The inclusive fitness hypothesis of sociobiology re-examined. Special Issue: Sex, cells, and same-sex desire: The biology of sexual preference: I. *Journal of Homosexuality, 28*(1–2), 147–183.

Diggs, M. (1993). Surveying the intersection: Pathology, secrecy and the discourses of racial and sexual identity. *Journal of Homosexuality, 26*(2–3), 1–19.

DiPlacido, J. (1998). Minority stress among lesbians, gay men, and bisexuals: A consequence of heterosexism, homophobia, and stigmatization. In G. M. Herek (Ed.), *Stigma and sexual orientation: Understanding prejudice against lesbians, gay men, and bisexuals* (pp. 138–159). Thousand Oaks, CA: Sage.

DiPlacido, J. (2000). *Stress of self-concealment among lesbians and bisexual women*. Paper presented at the 108th annual meeting of the American Psychological Association, Washington, DC.

Dittmann, R. W., Kappes, M. E., & Kappes, M. H. (1992). Sexual behavior in adolescent and adult females with congenital adrenal hyperplasia. *Psychoneuroendocrinology, 17*, 153–170.

Dohrn, B. (1995, Spring). "Don't ask, don't tell" unconstitutional. *The Lambda Update, 12*(2), 1.

Doll, L. S., Harrison, J. S., Frey, R. L., & McKirnan, D. (1994). Failure to disclose HIV risk among gay and bisexual men attending sexually transmitted disease clinics. *American Journal of Preventive Medicine, 10*(3), 125–129.

Doll, L. S., Joy, D., Bartholow, B. N., & Harrison, J. S. (1992). Self-reported childhood and adolescent sexual abuse among adult homosexual and bisexual men. *Child Abuse and Neglect, 16*(6), 855–864.

Dombrowski, D., Wodarski, J. S., Smokowski, P. R., & Bricout, J. C. (1995). School-based social work interventions with gay and lesbian adolescents: Theoretical and practice guidelines. *Journal of Applied Social Science, 20*(1), 51–61.

Donovan, J. M. (1992). Homosexual, gay, and lesbian: Defining the words and sampling the populations. *Journal of Homosexuality, 24*(1–2), 27–47.

Doore, G. (Ed.). (1988). *Shaman's path: Healing, personal growth and empowerment.* Boston: Shambhala.

Downey, J., Ehrhardt, A. A., Schiffman, M., & Dyrenfurth, I. (1987). Sex hormones in lesbian and heterosexual women. *Hormones and Behavior, 21*(3), 347–357.

Downing, C. (1981). *The goddess: Mythological representations of the feminine.* New York: Crossroad.

Downing, C. (1991). *Myths and mysteries of same-sex love.* New York: Continuum.

Downing, C. (1995). An archetypal view of lesbian identity. In J. M. Glassgold & S. Iasenza (Eds.), *Lesbians and psychoanalysis: Revolutions in theory and practice* (pp. 265–285). New York: Free Press.

Doyle, J. M. (2000, Spring). From the ashes: Republican leaders kill Hate Crimes Prevention Act but HRC is determined to try again. *HRC Quarterly*, pp. 8–9.

Drescher, J. (1998). Contemporary psychoanalytic psychotherapy with gay men with a commentary on reparative therapy of homosexuality. *Journal of Gay and Lesbian Psychotherapy, 2*(4), 51–74.

Drescher, J. (1999). The therapist's authority and the patient's sexuality. *Journal of Gay and Lesbian Psychotherapy, 3*(2), 61–80.

Driggs, J. H. (with Finn, S. E., contributor). (1991). *Intimacy between men: How to find and keep gay love relationships.* New York: NAL/Dutton.

Drucker, J. (1998*). Families of value: Gay and lesbian parents and their children speak out.* New York: Insight Books/Plenum.

Duckitt, J. H., & duToit, L. (1989). Personality profiles of homosexual men and women. *Journal of Psychology, 123*(5), 497–505.

Due, L. (1995). *Joining the tribe: Growing up gay and lesbian in the 90's.* New York: Anchor/Doubleday.

Duffy, S. M., & Rusbult, C. E. (1986). Satisfaction and commitment in homosexual and heterosexual relationships. *Journal of Homosexuality, 12*(2), 1–24.

Dulit, R. A., Fyer, M. R., Miller, F. T., Sacks, M. H., & Frances, A. J. (1993). Gender differences in sexual preference and substance abuse of inpatients with borderline personality disorder. *Journal of Personality Disorders, 7*(2), 182–185.

Dunker, B. (1987). Aging lesbians: Observations and speculations. In Boston Lesbian Psychologies Collective (Ed.), *Lesbian psychologies: Explorations and challenges* (pp. 72–82). Urbana: University of Illinois Press.

Dunkle, J. H. (1994). Counseling gay male clients: A review of treatment efficacy research: 1975–present. *Journal of Gay and Lesbian Psychotherapy, 2*(2), 1–19.

Dunkle, J. H. (1996). Toward and integration of gay and lesbian identity development and Super's Life-Span Approach. *Journal of Vocational Behavior, 48*, 149–159.

Dunne, E. J. (1987). Helping gay fathers come out to their children. *Journal of Homosexuality, 14*(1–2), 213–222.

Dunne, G. A. (2000). Opting into motherhood: Lesbians blurring the boundaries and transforming the meaning of parenthood and kinship. *Gender and Society, 14*(1), 11–35.

Dupras, A. (1994). Internalized homophobia and psychosexual adjustment among gay men. *Psychological Reports, 75*(1, Pt. 1), 23–28.

Durkheim, E. (1951). *Suicide.* New York: Free Press.

Dworkin, S. H. (1996). From personal therapy to professional life: Observations of a Jewish, bisexual lesbian therapist and academic. In N. D. Davis, E. Cole, & E. D. Rothblum (Eds.), *Lesbian therapists and their therapy: From both sides of the couch* (pp. 37–46). Binghamton, NY: Harrington Park Press.

Dworkin, S. H. (1997). Female, lesbian, and Jewish: Complex and invisible. In B. Greene (Ed.), *Ethnic and cultural diversity among lesbians and gay men* (pp. 63–87). Thousand Oaks, CA: Sage.

Dworkin, S. H. (2000a). Individual therapy with lesbian, gay and bisexual clients. In R. M. Perez, K. A. DeBord, & K. J. Bieschke (Eds.), *Handbook of counseling and psychotherapy with lesbian, gay, and bisexual clients* (pp. 157–181). Washington, DC: American Psychological Association.

Dworkin, S. H. (2000b, August). *Issues of diversity in research on bisexual issues in psychology.* Paper presented at the 108th annual meeting of the American Psychological Association, Washington, DC.

Eckert, E. D., Bouchard, T. J., Bohlen, J., & Heston, L. L. (1986). Homosexuality in monozygotic twins reared apart. *British Journal of Psychiatry, 148,* 421–425.

Edwards, G. R. (1984) *Gay/lesbian liberation: A biblical perspective.* New York: Pilgrim Press.

Edwards, G. R. (1989). A critique of creationist homophobia. (pp. 95–118). In R. Hasbany (Ed.), *Homosexuality and religion.* Binghamton, NY: Haworth Press.

Ehrenberg, M. (1996). Aging and mental health: Issues in the gay and lesbian community. In C. J. Alexander (Ed.), *Gay and lesbian mental health: A sourcebook for practitioners* (pp. 189–210). New York: Harrington Park Press.

Ehrlich, H. J. (1990). The ecology of antigay violence. *Journal of Interpersonal Violence, 5*(3), 359–365.

Eisenbud, R. J. (1982). Early and later determinants of lesbian choice. *Psychoanalytic Review, 69,* 85–109.

Eisenbud, R. J. (1986). Lesbian choice: Transferences to theory. In J. L. Alpert (Ed.), *Psychoanalysis and women: Contemporary reappraisals* (pp. 215–233). Hillsdale, NJ: Analytic Press.

Eisler, R. (1987). *The chalice and the blade: Our history, our future.* San Francisco: Harper & Row.

Eisler, R. (1995). *Sacred pleasure: Sex, myth, and the politics of the body.* San Francisco: Harper.

Ekstrand, M. L., Stall, R. D., Paul, J. P., Osmond, D. H., & Coates, T. J. (1999). Gay men report high rates of unprotected anal sex with partners of unknown or discordant HIV status. *AIDS, 13*(12), 1525–1533.

Eldridge, N. S. (1987). Gender issues in counseling same-sex couples. *Professional Psychology: Research and Practice, 18*(6), 567–572.

Eldridge, N. S., & Gilbert, L. A. (1990). Correlates of relationship satisfaction in lesbian couples. *Psychology of Women Quarterly, 14*(1), 43–62.

Eliason, M., & Hughes, T. (2000). *Lesbians and alcohol: What does the research tell us?.* Paper presented at the 108th annual meeting of the American Psychological Association, Washington, DC.

Eliason, M. J., & Raheim, S. (2000). Experiences and comfort with culturally diverse groups in undergraduate pre-nursing students. *Journal of Nursing Education, 39*(4), 161–165.

Eliason, M. J., & Randall, C. E. (1991). Lesbian phobia in nursing students. *Western Journal of Nursing Research, 13*(3), 363–374.

Elise, D. (1998). Gender configurations: Relational patterns in heterosexual, lesbian, and gay male couples. *Psychoanalytic Review, 85*(2), 253–267.

Elliott, J. E. (1993). Lesbian and gay concerns in career development. In L. Diamant (Ed.), *Homosexual issues in the workplace* (pp. 25–43). Washington, DC: Taylor & Francis.

Ellis, A. L. (1996). Sexual identity issues in the workplace: Past and present. In A. L. Ellis & E. D. B. Riggle (Eds.), *Sexual identity on the job: Issues and services* (pp. 1–16). New York: Haworth Press.

Ellis, A. L. (2000). *Gay men at midlife: Age before beauty.* Binghamton, NY: Haworth Press.

Ellis, L. (1996a). The role of perinatal factors in determining sexual orientation. In R. C. Savin-Williams & K. M. Cohen (Eds.), *The lives of lesbians, gays, and bisexuals: Children to adults* (pp. 35–70). Fort Worth, TX: Harcourt Brace.

Ellis, L. (1996b). Theories of homosexuality. In R. C. Savin-Williams & K. M. Cohen (Eds.), *The lives of lesbians, gays, and bisexuals: Children to adults* (pp. 11–34). Fort Worth, TX: Harcourt Brace.

Ellis, L., & Ames, M. A. (1987). Neurohormonal functioning and sexual orientation: A theory of homosexuality-heterosexuality. *Psychological Bulletin, 101*(2), 233–258.

Ellis, L., Ames, M. A., Peckham, W., & Burke, D. (1988). Sexual orientation of human offspring may be altered by severe maternal stress during pregnancy. *Journal of Sex Research, 25*(1), 152–157.

Ellis, L., Burke, D., & Ames, M. A. (1987). Sexual orientation as a continuous variable: A comparison between the sexes. *Archives of Sexual Behavior, 16,* 523–529.

Ellis, L., & Wagemann, B. M. (1993). The religiosity of mothers and their offspring as related to the offspring's sex and sexual orientation. *Adolescence, 28*(109), 227–234.

Eminson, S., Gillett, T., & Hassanyeh, F. (1989). Homosexual erotomania. *British Journal of Psychiatry*, *155*, 128–129.

Engel, J. W., & Saracino, M. (1986). Love preferences and ideals: A comparison of homosexual, bisexual, and heterosexual groups. *Contemporary Family Therapy: An International Journal*, *8*(3), 241–250.

England, M. E. (1998). *The Bible and homosexuality* (5th ed.). Gaithersburg, MD: Chi Rho Press.

Erera, P. I., & Fredriksen, K. (1999). Lesbian stepfamilies: A unique family structure. *Families in Society*, *80*(3), 263–270.

Erikson, E. H. (1963). *Childhood and society* (rev. ed.). New York: Norton.

Erikson, E. H., & Erikson, J. M. (1981). On generativity and identity. *Harvard Education Review*, *51*, 240–278.

Ernst, F. A., Francis, R. A., Nevels, H., & Lemeh, C. A. (1991). Condemnation of homosexuality in the Black community: A gender-specific phenomenon? *Archives of Sexual Behavior*, *20*(6), 579–585.

Espin, O. M. (1984). Cultural and historical influences on sexuality in Hispanic/Latina women: Implications for psychotherapy. In C. Vance (Ed.), *Pleasure and danger: Exploring female sexuality* (pp. 149–163). London: Routledge & Kegan Paul.

Espin, O. M. (1987a). Issues of identity in the psychology of Latina lesbians. In Boston Lesbian Psychologies Collective (Eds.), *Lesbian psychologies: Explorations and challenges* (pp. 35–55). Urbana: University of Illinois Press.

Espin, O. M. (1987b). Psychological impact of migration on Latinas; Implications for psychotherapeutic practice. *Psychology of Women Quarterly*, *11*, 489–503.

Espin, O. M. (1994, August). *Crossing borders and boundaries: The life narratives of immigrant lesbians.* Paper presented at the 102nd annual meeting of the American Psychological Association, Los Angeles, CA.

Espin, O. M. (1997). *Crossing borders and boundaries: The life narratives of immigrant lesbians.* In B. Greene (Ed.), *Ethnic and cultural diversity among lesbians and gay men* (pp. 191–215). Thousand Oaks, CA: Sage.

Espin, O. M. (2000, August). *Making love in English; The interplay of language and sexuality in the life narratives of immigrant women.* Paper presented at the 108nd annual meeting of the American Psychological Association, Washington, DC.

Ettelbrick, P. L. (1991). Legal protections for lesbians. In B. Sang, J. Warshow, & A. J. Smith (Eds.), *Lesbians at midlife: The creative transition* (pp. 258–264). San Francisco: Spinsters.

Ettore, E. M. (Ed.). (1980). *Lesbians, women and society.* London: Routledge & Kegan Paul.

Evans, A. (1978). *Witchcraft and the gay counterculture.* Boston: Fag Rag Books.

Evans, N., & Levine, H. (1990). Perspectives on sexual orientation. *New Directions for Student Services*, *51*, 49–58.

Exodus International. (1999). *Exodus International* [Online]. Available: www.messiah.edu/hpages/facstaff/chase/h/exodus/.

Faderman, L. (1984). The "new gay" lesbians. *Journal of Homosexuality*, *10*(3–4), 85–95.

Faderman, L. (1991). *Odd girls and twilight lovers: A history of lesbian life in twentieth-century America.* New York: Penguin.

Faderman, L. (1997, July 22). Last word: It's not just a movie. *The Advocate*, p. 72.

Falco, K. L. (1991). *Psychotherapy with lesbian clients: Theory into practice.* New York: Brunner/Mazel.

Falco, K. L. (1996). Psychotherapy with women who love women. In R. P. Cabaj & T. S. Stein (Eds.), *Textbook of homosexuality and mental health* (pp. 397–412). Washington, DC: American Psychiatric Press.

Falk, P. J. (1989). Lesbian mothers: Psychosocial assumptions in family law. *American Psychologist*, *44*(6), 941–947.

Farley, N. (1992). Same-sex domestic violence. In S. H. Dworkin & F. J. Gutierrez (Eds.), *Counseling gay men and lesbians: Journey to the end of the rainbow* (pp. 231–242). Alexandria VA: American Association for Counseling and Development.

Faryna, E. L., & Morales, E. (2000). Self-efficacy and HIV-related risk behaviors among multiethnic adolescents. *Cultural Diversity and Ethnic Minority Psychology*, *6*(1), 42–56.

Fassinger, R. E. (1995). From invisibility to integration: Lesbian identity in the workplace. *Career Development Quarterly, 44,* 148–167.

Fassinger, R. E. (1996). Notes from the margins: Integrating lesbian experience into the vocational psychology of women. *Journal of Vocational Behavior, 48,* 160–175.

Fassinger, R. E (2000). Applying counseling theories to lesbian, gay, and bisexual clients: Pitfalls and possibilities. In R. M. Perez, K. A. DeBord, & K. J. Bieschke (Eds.), *Handbook of counseling and psychotherapy with lesbian, gay, and bisexual clients* (pp. 107–131). Washington, DC: American Psychological Association.

Feigal, A. (1983). The other side. In M. Borhek (Ed.), *Coming out to parents* (pp. 84–113). New York: Pilgrim Press.

Fein, S. B., & Nuehring, E. M. (1981). Intrapsychic effects of stigma: A process of breakdown and reconstruction of social reality. *Journal of Homosexuality, 7*(1), 3–13.

Fejes, F. (1991). Gays, lesbians, and the media: A selected bibliography. *Journal of Homosexuality, 21*(2), 261–277.

Feliz, A. A. (1992). *Out of the bishop's closet* (2nd ed.). San Francisco: Alamo Square Press.

Fergusson, D. M., Horwood, L., J., & Beautrais, A. L. (1999). Is sexual orientation related to mental health problems and suicidality in young people? *Archives of General Psychiatry, 56*(10), 876–880.

Ferrando, S., Goggin, K., Sewell, M., Evans, S., Fishman, B., & Rabkin, J. (1998). Substance use disorder in gay/bisexual men with HIV and AIDS. *American Journal on Addictions, 7*(1), 51–60.

Ferris, D. G., Batish, S., Wright, T. C., Cushing, C., & Scott, E. H. (1996). A neglected lesbian health concern: Cervical neoplasia. *Journal of Family Practice, 43*(6), 581–584.

Ferry, J. (1994). *In the courts of the Lord: A gay minister's story.* New York: Crossroad.

Ficarrotto, T. J. (1990). Racism, sexism, and erotophobia: Attitudes of heterosexuals toward homosexuals. *Journal of Homosexuality, 19*(1), 111–116.

Finn, P., & McNeil, T. (1987, October 7). *The response of the criminal justice system to bias crime: An exploratory review.* Contract report submitted to the National Institute of Justice, U.S. Department of Justice. (Available from Abt Associates, Inc., 55 Wheeler St., Cambridge, MA 02138–1168)

Finnegan, D. G., & McNally, E. B. (1987). *Dual identities: Counseling chemically dependent gay men and lesbians.* Center City, MN: Hazelden.

Finnegan, D. G., & McNally, E. B. (1989). The lonely journey: Lesbians and gay men who are co-dependent. *Alcoholism Treatment Quarterly, 6*(1), 121–134.

Finnegan, D. G., & McNally, E. B. (1990). Lesbian women. In R. C. Engs (Ed.), *Women: Alcohol and other drugs* (pp. 149–156). Dubuque, IA: Kendall/Hunt.

Firestein, B. A. (1996). Introduction. In B. A. Firestein (Ed.), *Bisexuality: The psychology and politics of an invisible minority* (pp. xix-xxvii). Thousand Oaks, CA: Sage.

Fisher, R. D., Derison, D., Polley, C. F., & Cadman, J. (1994). Religiousness, religious orientation, and attitudes towards gays and lesbians. *Journal of Applied Social Psychology, 24*(7), 614–630.

Fitzgerald, B. (1999). Children of lesbian and gay parents: A review of the literature. *Marriage and Family Review, 29*(1), 57–75.

Flaks, D. K., Ficher, I., Masterpasqua, F., & Joseph, G. (1995). Lesbians choosing motherhood: A comparative study of lesbian and heterosexual parents and their children. *Developmental Psychology, 31*(1), 105–114.

Fontaine, J. H., & Hammond, N. L. (1996). Counseling issues with gay and lesbian adolescents. *Adolescence, 31*(124), 817–830.

Forstein, M. (1986). Psychodynamic psychotherapy with gay male couples. In T. S. Stein & C. J. Cohen (Eds.), *Contemporary perspectives on psychotherapy with lesbians and gay men* (pp. 103–137). New York: Plenum.

Forstein, M. (1988). Homophobia: An overview. *Psychiatric Annals, 18*(1), 33–36.

Fortunata, B. (1999). Lesbian experience of domestic violence. *Dissertation Abstracts International, 60*(2-B), 0872. (University Microfilms No. AAM99–18488)

Fortunato, J. E. (1982). *Embracing the exile: Healing journeys of gay Christians.* New York: Harper & Row.

Fowler, J. W. (1981). *Stages of faith: The psychology of human development and the quest for meaning.* San Francisco: Harper & Row.

Fox, M. (1984). The spiritual journey of the homosexual . . . and just about everyone else. In R. Nugent (Ed.), *A challenge to love: Gay and lesbian Catholics in the Church* (pp. 189–204). New York: Crossroad.

Fox, R. C. (1993, August). *Coming-out bisexual: Identity, behavior, and sexual orientation self-disclosure.* Paper presented at the 101st annual meeting of the American Psychological Association, Toronto, Canada.

Fox, R. C. (1995). Bisexual identities. In A. R. D'Augelli & C. J. Patterson (Eds.), *Lesbian, gay, and bisexual identities over the lifespan: Psychological perspectives* (pp. 48–86). New York: Oxford University Press.

Fox, R. C. (1996a). Bisexuality: An examination of theory and research. In R. P. Cabaj & T. S. Stein (Eds.), *Textbook of homosexuality and mental health* (pp. 147–171). Washington, DC: American Psychiatric Press.

Fox, R. C. (1996b). Bisexuality in perspective: A review of theory and research. In B. A. Firestein (Ed.), *Bisexuality: The psychology and politics of an invisible minority* (pp. 3–50). Thousand Oaks, CA: Sage.

Fracher, J., & Kimmel, M. S. (1989). Hard issues and soft spots: Counseling men about sexuality. In M. S. Kimmel & M. A. Messner (Eds.), *Men's lives* (pp. 471–482). New York: Macmillan.

Franke, R., & Leary, M. R. (1991). Disclosure of sexual orientation by lesbians and gay men: A comparison of private and public processes. *Journal of Social and Clinical Psychology, 10*(3), 262–269.

Franklin, K. (1998). Unassuming motivations: Contextualizing the narratives of antigay assailants. In G. M. Herek (Ed.), *Stigma and sexual orientation: Understanding prejudice against lesbians, gay men, and bisexuals* (pp. 1–23). Thousand Oaks, CA: Sage.

Freiberg, P. (1987, September 1). Sex education and the gay issue: What are they teaching about us in schools? *The Advocate,* pp. 42–49.

Freud, S. (1953). Three essays on the theory of sexuality. In J. Strachey (Ed. and Trans.), *The standard edition of the complete psychological works of Sigmund Freud* (Vol. 7, pp. 135–243). London: Hogarth Press. (Original work published 1905)

Freud, S. (1957). On narcissism: An introduction. In J. Strachey (Ed. and Trans.), *The standard edition of the complete psychological works of Sigmund Freud* (Vol. 14, pp. 73–102). London: Hogarth Press. (Original work published 1914)

Freud, S. (1961a). The dissolution of the Oedipus complex. In J. Strachey (Ed. and Trans.), *The standard edition of the complete psychological works of Sigmund Freud* (Vol. 19, pp. 173–179). London: Hogarth Press. (Original work published 1924)

Freud, S. (1961b). Some psychical consequences of the anatomical distinction between the sexes. In J. Strachey (Ed. and Trans.), *The standard edition of the complete psychological works of Sigmund Freud* (Vol. 19, pp. 248–258). London: Hogarth Press. (Original work published 1925)

Freud, S. (1963). Introductory lectures on psychoanalysis, Part III. In J. Strachey (Ed. and Trans.), *The standard edition of the complete psychological works of Sigmund Freud* (Vol. 16, pp. 243–479). London: Hogarth Press. (Original work published 1917)

Freud, S. (1964a). An outline of psychoanalysis. In J. Strachey (Ed. and Trans.), *The standard edition of the complete psychological works of Sigmund Freud* (Vol. 23, pp. 144–207). London: Hogarth Press. (Original work published 1940)

Freud, S. (1964b). Femininity. In J. Strachey (Ed. and Trans.), *The standard edition of the complete psychological works of Sigmund Freud* (Vol. 22, pp. 112–135). London: Hogarth Press. (Original work published 1933)

Friedman, C. (1998). Eros in a gay dyad: A case presentation. *Gender and Psychoanalysis, 3*(3), 335–346.

Friedman, L. J. (1997). Rural lesbians and their families. In J. D. Smith &, R. J. Mancoske (Eds.), *Rural gays and lesbians: Building on the strenghts of communities* (pp. 73–82). New York: Harrington Park Press.

Friedman, N. A. (1999). The experience of pregnancy for lesbian couples. *Dissertation Abstracts International, 59*(8-B), 4536. (University Microfilms No. AAM99–03743)

Friedman, R. C. (1986). Male homosexuality: On the need for a multiaxial developmental model. *Israel Journal of Psychiatry and Related Sciences, 23*(1), 63–76.

Friedman, R. C. (1988). *Male homosexuality: A contemporary psychoanalytic perspective.* New Haven, CT: Yale University Press.

Friedman, R. C. (1991). Couple therapy with gay couples. *Psychiatric Annals, 21*(8), 485–490.

Friedman, R. C. (1997). Response to Ken Corbett's "homosexual boyhood: Notes on girlyboys." *Gender and Psychoanalysis, 2*(4), 487–494.

Friedman, R. C. (1999). Discussion of articles by Drs. Vaughan, Drescher, and Cohler. *Journal of Gay and Lesbian Psychotherapy, 3*(2), 91–98.

Friedman, R. M. (1986). The psychoanalytic model of male homosexuality: A historical and theoretical critique. *Psychoanalytic Review, 73*(4), 483–519.

Friend, R. A. (1980). GAYging: Adjustment and the older gay male. *Alternative Lifestyles, 3*(2), 231–248.

Friend, R. A. (1987). The individual and social psychology of aging: Clinical implications for lesbians and gay men. *Journal of Homosexuality, 14*(1–2), 307–331.

Friend, R. A. (1989). Older lesbian and gay people: Responding to homophobia. *Marriage and Family Review, 14*(3–4), 241–263.

Friend, R. A. (1990). Older lesbian and gay people: A theory of successful aging. *Journal of Homosexuality, 20*(3–4), 99–118.

Frommer, M. S. (1994). Homosexuality and psychoanalysis: Technical considerations revisited. *Psychoanalytic Dialogues, 4*(2), 215–233.

Frontain, R. J. (Ed.). (1997). *Reclaiming the sacred: The Bible in gay and lesbian culture.* Binghamton, NY: Haworth Press.

Frost, J. C. (1997). Group psychotherapy with the aging gay male: Treatment of choice. *Group, 21*(3), 267–285.

Frye, M. (1990). Lesbian "sex." In J. Allen (Ed.), *Lesbian philosophies and cultures* (pp. 305–316). Albany: State University of New York Press.

Fullilove, M. T., & Fullilove, R. E. III. (1999). Stigma as an obstacle to AIDS action: The case of the African American community. *American Behavioral Scientist, 42*(7), 1117–1129.

Gagnon, J. H. (1990). Gender preferences in erotic relations: The Kinsey scale and sexual scripts. In D. P. McWhirter, S. A. Sanders, & J. M. Reinisch (Eds.), *Homosexuality/heterosexuality: Concepts of sexual orientation* (pp. 177–207). New York: Oxford University Press.

Gair, S. R. (1995). The false self, shame, and the challenge of self-cohesion. In J. M. Glassgold & S. Iasenza (Eds.), *Lesbians and psychoanalysis: Revolutions in theory and practice* (pp. 107–123). New York: Free Press.

Galanter, M., Larson, D., & Rubenstone, E. (1991). Christian psychiatry: The impact of evangelical belief on clinical practice. *American Journal of Psychiatry, 148*(1), 90–95.

Gallagher, J. (1997a, September 30). Lesbian plague? *The Advocate*, pp. 20–26.

Gallagher, J. (1997b, September 30). The fight against breast cancer: Will gay men be there? *The Advocate*, p. 27.

Gallagher, J. (1998, February 17). Gay for the thrill of it. *The Advocate*, pp. 33–39.

Garanzini, M. J. (1989). Psychodynamic theory and pastoral theology: An integrated model. In R. Hasbany (Ed.), *Homosexuality and religion* (pp. 175–194). Binghamton, NY: Haworth Press.

Garnets, L., Hancock, K., Cochran, S. D., Goodchilds, J., & Peplau, L. A. (1991). Issues in psychotherapy with lesbians and gay men: A survey of psychologists. *American Psychologist, 46*(9), 964–972.

Garnets, L., & Kimmel, D. (1991). Lesbian and gay male dimensions in the psychological study of human diversity. In J.D. Goodchilds (Ed.), *Psychological perspectives on human diversity in America* (pp. 137–192). Washington, DC: American Psychological Association.

Garofalo, R., Wolf, R. C., Kessel, S., Palfrey, S. J., & DuRant, R. H. (1998). The association between health risk behaviors and sexual orientation among a school-based sample of adolescents. *Pediatrics, 101*(5), 895–902.

Garofalo, R., Wolf, R. C., Wissow, L. S., Woods, E. R., & Goodman, E. (1999). *Archives of Pediatric Adolescent Medicine, 153*(5), 487–493.

Gartrell, N., Banks, A., Hamilton, J., Reed, N., Bishop, H., & Rodas, C. (1999). The national lesbian family study: II. Interviews with mothers of toddlers. *American Journal of Orthopsychiatry, 69*(3), 362–369.

Gay, Lesbian and Straight Education Network. (1999). *GLSEN's national school climate survey.* [Online]. Available: http://www:glsen.org/pages/sections/news/natlnews/1999/sep/survey.

Gazarik, R., & Fischman, D. (1995). A time-limited group for patients with HIV infection and their partners. *Group, 19*(3), 173–182.

Geis, S. B., & Messer, D. E. (1994). *Caught in the crossfire: Helping Christians debate homosexuality.* Nashville, TN: Abingdon Press.

Gelberg, S., & Chojnacki, J. T. (1996). *Career and life planning with gay, lesbian, and bisexual persons.* Alexandria, VA: American Counseling Association.

Gelso, C. J., Fassinger, R. E., Gomez, M. J., & Latts, M. G. (1995). Countertransference reactions to lesbian clients: The role of homophobia, counselor gender, and countertransference management. *Journal of Counseling Psychology, 42*(3), 356–364.

General Accounting Office. (1990). *AIDS education, public school programs require more student information and teacher training* (GAO Publication No. HRD 90–103). Washington, DC: Author.

Gentry, C. S. (1987). Social distance regarding male and female homosexuals. *Journal of Social Psychology, 127*(2), 199–208.

Genuis, M., Thomlison, B., & Bagley, C. (1991, Fall). Male victims of child sexual abuse: A brief overview of pertinent findings. *Journal of Child and Youth Care,* 1–6.

George, K. D., & Behrendt, A. E. (1987). Therapy for male couples experiencing relationship problems and sexual problems. *Journal of Homosexuality, 14*(1–2), 77–88.

Gerstel, C. J., Feraios, A. J., & Herdt, G. (1989). Widening circles: An ethnographic profile of a youth group. *Journal of Homosexuality, 17*(1–2), 75–92.

Getzel, G. S., & Mahony, K. F. (1990). Confronting human finitude: Group work with people with AIDS (PWAs). *Journal of Gay and Lesbian Psychotherapy, 1*(3), 105–120.

Gewirtzman, D. (2000, Winter). Advanced planning: Easier than you think. *The Lambda Update,* p. 14.

Ghindia, D. J., & Kola, L. A. (1996). Co-factors affecting substance abuse among homosexual men: An investigation within a midwestern gay community. *Drug and Alcohol Dependence, 41*(3), 167–177.

Gibbs, E. D. (1989). Psychosocial development of children raised by lesbian mothers: A review of research. *Women and Therapy, 8,* 55–75.

Gibson, P. (1989). Gay male and lesbian youth suicide. In U.S. Department of Health and Human Services (Ed.), *Report of the Secretary's Task Force on Youth Suicide* (pp. 3–110 to 3–142) (DHHS Publication No. ADM 89–1623). Washington, DC: U.S. Department of Health and Human Services.

Gideonse, T. (1999, June 22). Baby by proxy. *The Advocate,* pp. 83–91.

Gilligan, C. (1982). *In a different voice: Psychological theory and women's development.* Cambridge, MA: Harvard University Press.

Gladue, B. A. (1987). Psychobiological contributions. In L. Diamant (Ed.), *Male and female homosexuality: Psychological approaches. The series in clinical and community psychology* (pp. 129–153). Washington, DC: Hemisphere.

Gladue, B. A. (1988). Biological influences upon the development of sexual orientation. In E.E. Filsinger (Ed.), *Sage focus editions: Vol. 96. Biological perspectives on the family* (pp. 61–92). Newbury Park, CA: Sage.

Glaser, C. (1988). *Uncommon calling: A gay man's struggle to serve the church.* San Francisco: Harper & Row.

Glaser, C. (1990). *Come home! Reclaiming spirituality and community as gay men and lesbians.* San Francisco: Harper & Row.

Glaser, C. (1991). *Coming out to God: Prayers for lesbians and gay men, their families and friends.* Louisville, KY: Westminster/John Knox Press.

Glaser, C. (1994). *The word is out: The Bible reclaimed for lesbians and gay men.* San Francisco: Harper.

Glaser, C. (1998). *Come home! Reclaiming spirituality and community as gay men and lesbians* (2nd ed.). Gaithersburg, MD: Chi Rho Press.

Glassgold, J. M. (1995). Psychoanalysis with lesbians: Self-reflection and agency. In J. M. Glassgold & S. Iasenza (Eds.), *Lesbians and psychoanalysis: Revolutions in theory and practice* (pp. 203–228). New York: Free Press.

Glassgold, J. M., & Iasenza, S. (1995). Introduction. In J. M. Glassgold & S. Iasenza (Eds.), *Lesbians and psychoanalysis: Revolutions in theory and practice* (pp. xxiii–xxx). New York: Free Press.

Glaus, K. O. (1988). Alcoholism, chemical dependency and the lesbian client. *Women and Therapy, 8*(1–2), 131–144.

Gock, T. S. (1996, August). Integrating ethnicity and sexual orientation in psychotherapy: Beyond lip service. In A. R. Cerbone (Chair), *Psychotherapy guidelines with lesbians, gays, and bisexuals: A literature review.* Symposium presented at the 104th annual meeting of the American Psychological Association, Toronto.

Goff, J. L. (1990). Sexual confusion among certain college males. *Adolescence, 25*(99), 599–614.

Goffman, E. (1963). *Stigma: Notes on the management of spoiled identity.* Englewood Cliffs, NJ: Prentice-Hall.

Goggin, K., Sewell, M., Ferrando, S., Evans, S., Fishman, B., & Rabkin, J. (2000). Plans to hasten death among gay men with HIV/AIDS: Relationship to psychological adjustment. *AIDS Care, 12*(2), 125–136.

Golden, C. (1987). Diversity and variability in women's sexual identities. In Boston Lesbian Psychologies Collective (Ed.), *Lesbian psychologies: Explorations and challenges* (pp. 19–34). Urbana: University of Illinois Press.

Goldstone, S. E. (1999). *The ins and outs of gay sex: A medical handbook for men.* New York: Dell.

Golombok S. (1999). New family forms: Children raised in solo mother families, lesbian mother families, and in families created by assisted reproduction. In L. Balter & Tamis-LeMonda, C. S. (Eds.), *Child psychology: A handbook of contemporary issues* (pp. 429–446). Philadelphia: Psychology Press/Taylor and Francis.

Golombok S., & Tasker, F. (1996). Do parents influence the sexual orientation of their children? Findings from a longitudinal study of lesbian families. *Developmental Psychology, 32*(1), 3–11.

Golombok S., Tasker, F., & Murray, C. (1997). Children raised in fatherless families from infancy: Family relationships and the socioemotional development of children of lesbian and single heterosexual mothers. *Journal of Child Psychology and Psychiatry, 38*(7), 783–791.

Gonsiorek, J. C. (1982). The use of diagnostic concepts in working with gay and lesbian populations. *Journal of Homosexuality, 7*(2–3), 9–20.

Gonsiorek, J. C. (1988). Mental health issues of gay and lesbian adolescents. *Journal of Adolescent Health Care, 9*(2), 114–122.

Gonsiorek, J. C. (1991). The empirical basis for the demise of the illness model of homosexuality. In J. C. Gonsiorek & J. D. Weinrich (Eds.), *Homosexuality: Research implications for public policy* (pp. 115–136). Newbury Park, CA: Sage.

Gonsiorek, J. C. (1993). Threat, stress, and adjustment: Mental health and the workplace for gay and lesbian individuals. In L. Diamant (Ed.), *Homosexual issues in the workplace* (pp. 243–264). Washington, DC: Taylor & Francis.

Gonsiorek, J. C. (1994). Foreword. In B. Greene, & G. M. Herek (Eds.), *Lesbian and gay psychology: Theory, research, and clinical applications* (pp. vi–ix). Thousand Oaks, CA: Sage.

Gonsiorek, J. C., & Rudolph, J. R. (1991). Homosexual identity: Coming out and other developmental events. In J. C. Gonsiorek & J. D. Weinrich (Eds.). *Homosexuality: Research implications for public policy* (pp. 161–176). Newbury Park, CA: Sage.

Gonsiorek, J. C., Sell, R. L., & Weinrich, J. D. (1995). Definition and measurement of sexual orientation. *Suicide and Life-Threatening Behavior, 25*(Suppl.), 40–51.

Gonsiorek, J. C., & Weinrich, J. D. (1991). The definition and scope of sexual orientation. In J. C. Gonsiorek & J. D. Weinrich (Eds.), *Homosexuality: Research implications for public policy* (pp. 1–12). Newbury Park, CA: Sage.

Gonzalez, F. J., & Espin, O. M. (1996). Latino men, women, and homosexuality. In R. P. Cabaj & T. S.

Stein (Eds.), *Textbook of homosexuality and mental health* (pp. 583–601). Washington, DC: American Psychiatric Press.

Goode, E. E., & Wagner, B. (1993, July 5). Intimate friendships. *U.S. News & World Report*, pp. 49–52.

Goodenow, C., & Hack, T. (1998). *Risks facing gay, lesbian, and bisexual high school adolescents: The Massachusetts Youth Risk Behavior Survey.* Paper presented at the 106th annual meeting of the American Psychological Association, San Francisco.

Goodman, S. (1988). The soul of liberation: The emergence of a gay and lesbian spirituality. *Lambda Rising Book Report, 1*(6), 1, 9.

Gooren, L. (1990). Biomedical theories of sexual orientation: A critical examination. In D. P. McWhirter, S. A. Sanders, & J. M. Reinisch (Eds.), *Homosexuality/heterosexuality: Concepts of sexual orientation* (pp. 71–87). New York: Oxford University Press.

Gorman, E. M. (2000). *Ethnographic perspectives on drug use among gay and bisexual men.* Paper presented at the 108th annual meeting of the American Psychological Association, Washington, DC.

Gorski, R. A., Gordon, J. H., Shryne, J. E., & Southam, A. M. (1978). Evidence for a morphological sex difference within the medial preoptic area of the rat brain. *Brain Research, 148*(2), 333–346.

Goss, R. (1993). *Jesus acted up: A gay and lesbian manifesto.* New York: HarperCollins.

Gottfredson, L. S. (1981). Circumscription and compromise: A developmental theory of occupational aspirations. *Journal of Counseling Psychology, 28,* 545–579.

Gottfredson, L. S. (1996). Gottfredson's theory of circumscription and compromise. In D. Brown & L. Brooks (Eds.), *Career choice and development* (3rd ed., pp. 179–232). San Francisco: Jossey-Bass.

Gottlieb, A. R. (2000). *Out of the twilight: Fathers of gay men speak.* Binghamton, NY: Haworth Press.

Gottman, J. S. (1990). Children of gay and lesbian parents. *Marriage and Family Review, 14*(3–4), 177–196.

Gottsfield, R. L. (1985). Child custody and sexual lifestyle. *Conciliation Courts Review, 23*(1), 43–46.

Gould, D. (1995). A critical examination of the notion of pathology in psychoanalysis. In J. M. Glassgold & S. Iasenza (Eds.), *Lesbians and psychoanalysis: Revolutions in theory and practice* (pp. 3– 17). New York: Free Press.

Gov. Weld asks schools to aid gay students. (1993, July 4). *The New York Times,* p. 1.

Governor's Commission on Gay and Lesbian Youth. (1993). *Making schools safe for gay and lesbian youth: Breaking the silence in schools and in families.* (Publication No. 17296–60–500–2/93–C.R.). Boston, MA: Author.

Grace, J. (1979, November). *Coming out alive.* Paper presented at the sixth biennial Professional Symposium of the National Association of Social Workers, San Antonio, TX.

Grace, J. (1992). Affirming gay and lesbian adulthood. In N. J. Woodman (Ed.), *Lesbian and gay lifestyles: A guide for counseling and education* (pp. 33–47). New York: Irvington.

Grahn, J. (1984). *Another mother tongue: Gay words, gay worlds.* Boston: Beacon.

Grahn, J. (1986). Strange country this: Lesbianism and North American Indian tribes. In M. Kehoe (Ed.), *Historical, literary, and erotic aspects of lesbianism* (pp. 43–57). New York: Harrington Park Press. [Also published in 1986 in the *Journal of Homosexuality, 12*(3–4), 43–57]

Gramick, J. (1983a). Homophobia: A new challenge. *Social Work, 28,* 137–141.

Gramick, J. (1983b). *Homosexuality and the Catholic church.* Mt. Rainier, MD: New Ways Ministry.

Gramick, J. (Ed.). (1989). *Homosexuality in the priesthood and the religious life.* New York: Crossroad.

Gramick, J., & Nugent, R. (Eds.). (1995). *Voices of hope: A collection of positive Catholic writings on gay and lesbian issues.* Mt. Rainier, MD: New Ways Ministry (or Center for Homophobia Education, P. O. Box 1985, New York, NY, 10159).

Gray, D., & Isensee, R. (1996). Balancing autonomy and intimacy in lesbian and gay relationships. In C. J. Alexander (Ed.), *Gay and lesbian mental health: A sourcebook for practitioners* (pp. 95–114). New York: Harrington Park Press/Haworth Press.

Green, G. D. (1990). Is separation really so great? *Women and Therapy, 9*(1–2), 87–104.

Green, G. D., & Bozett, F. W. (1991). Lesbian mothers and gay fathers. In J. C. Gonsiorek & J. D. Weinrich (Eds.), *Homosexuality: Research implications for public policy* (pp. 197–214). Newbury Park, CA: Sage.

Green, R. (1985). Gender identity in childhood and later sexual orientation: Follow-up of 78 males. *American Journal of Psychiatry, 142*(3), 339–341.

Green, R. (1986). Lesbian mothers and their children: A comparison with solo parent heterosexual mothers and their children. *Archives of Sexual Behavior, 15*(2), 167–184.

Green, R. (1987). *The "sissy boy syndrome" and the development of homosexuality.* New Haven, CT: Yale University Press.

Green, R. (1988). The immutability of (homo)sexual orientation: Behavioral science implications for a constitutional (legal) analysis. *Journal of Psychiatry and Law, 16*(4), 537–575.

Green, R., Williams, K., & Goodman, M. (1982). Ninety-nine "tomboys" and "nontomboys": Behavioral contrasts and demographic similarities. *Archives of Sexual Behavior, 11,* 247–266.

Green, R. J. (2000). Introduction to the special section: Gay, lesbian, and bisexual issues in family therapy. *Journal of Marital and Family Therapy, 26*(4), 407–408.

Green, R. J., Bettinger, M., & Zacks, E. (1996). Are lesbian couples fused and gay male couples disengaged? Questioning gender straightjackets. In J. Laird & R. J. Green (Eds.), *Lesbian and gay couples and families: A handbook for therapists* (pp. 185–230). San Francisco: Jossey-Bass.

Greene, B. (1986). When the therapist is White and the patient is Black: Considerations for psychotherapy in the feminist heterosexual and lesbian communities. *Women and Therapy, 5*(2–3), 41–65.

Greene, B. (1994a). Lesbian and gay sexual orientations: Implications for clinical training, practice, and research. In B. Greene, & G. M. Herek (Eds.), *Lesbian and gay psychology: Theory, research, and clinical applications* (pp. 1–24). Thousand Oaks, CA: Sage.

Greene, B. (1994b). Lesbian women of color: Triple jeopardy. In L. Comas-Diaz & B. Greene (Eds.), *Women of color: Integrating ethnic and gender identities in psychotherapy* (pp. 389–427). New York: Guilford Press.

Greene, B. (1996). The legacy of ethnosexual mythology in heterosexism. In E. Rothblum & L. Bond (Eds.), *Preventing heterosexism and homophobia* (pp. 59–70). Thousand Oaks, CA: Sage.

Greene, B. (1997a). Ethnic minority lesbians and gay men: Mental health and treatment issues. In B. Greene (Ed.), *Ethnic and cultural diversity among lesbians and gay men* (pp. 216–239). Thousand Oaks, CA: Sage.

Greene, B. (1997b). Preface. In B. Greene (Ed.), *Ethnic and cultural diversity among lesbians and gay men* (pp. xi–xv). Thousand Oaks, CA: Sage.

Greene, B., & Boyd-Franklin, N. (1996a). African American lesbian couples: Ethnocultural considerations in psychotherapy. *Women and Therapy, 19*(3), 49–60.

Greene, B., & Boyd-Franklin, N. (1996b). African-American lesbians: Issues in couples therapy. In J. Laird & R. J. Green (Eds.), *Lesbian and gay couples and families: A handbook for therapists* (pp. 251–271). San Francisco: Jossey-Bass.

Greene, D., & Faltz, B. (1991). Chemical dependency and relapse in gay men with HIV infection: Issues and treatment. *Journal of Chemical Dependency Treatment, 4*(2), 79–90.

Grellert, E. A. (1989). Childhood photographs of homosexual and heterosexual men. *Psychological Reports, 65*(1), 331–336.

Griffin, C. W., Wirth, M. J., & Wirth, A. G. (1986). *Beyond acceptance: Parents of lesbians and gays talk about their experiences.* Englewood Cliffs, NJ: Prentice-Hall.

Gross, L. (1991). Out of the mainstream: Sexual minorities and the mass media. *Journal of Homosexuality, 21*(1–2), 19–46.

Grossman, A. H., D'Augelli, A. R., & Hershberger, S. L. (2000). Social support networks of lesbian, gay, and bisexual adults 60 years of age and older. *Journals of Gerontology: Series B: Psychological Sciences and Social Sciences, 55B*(3), 171–179.

Groth, A. N., & Burgess, A. W. (1980). Male rape: Offenders and victims. *American Journal of Psychiatry, 137*(7), 806–810.

Groves, P. A., & Ventura, L. A. (1983). The lesbian coming out process: Therapeutic considerations. *The Personnel and Guidance Journal, 62,* 146–149.

Guthrie, C. S. (1999). An examination of current practices in group treatment of HIV-positive gay and bisexual men. *Dissertation Abstracts International, 60*(2-B), 0830. (University Microfilms No. AAM99–20193)

Gutierrez, F. J. (1992). Eros, the aging years: Counseling older gay men. In S. H. Dworkin, & F. J. Gutierrez (Eds.), *Counseling gay men and lesbians: Journey to the end of the rainbow* (pp. 49–60). Alexandria, VA: American Association for Counseling and Development.

Gutierrez, F. J., & Dworkin, S. H. (1992). Gay, lesbian, and African American: Managing the integration of identities. In S. H. Dworkin & F. J. Gutierrez (Eds.), *Counseling gay men and lesbians: Journey to the end of the rainbow* (pp. 141–156). Alexandria, VA: American Association for Counseling and Development.

Haaga, D. A. (1991). "Homophobia"? *Journal of Social Behavior and Personality, 6*(1), 171–174.

Haas, S. M. (1999). Relationship maintenance in gay male couples coping with HIV/AIDS. *Dissertation Abstracts International, 60*(5-A), 1395. (University Microfilms No. AEH99–31609)

Haber, S. (Ed.), with Acuff, C., Ayers, L., Freeman, E. L., Goodheart, C., Kieffer, C. C., Lubin, L. B., Mikesell, S. G., Siegel, M., & Wainrib., B. R. (1995). *Breast cancer: A psychological treatment manual.* New York: Springer.

Haldeman, D. C. (1991). Sexual orientation conversion therapy for gay men and lesbians; A scientific examination. In J. C. Gonsiorek & J. D. Weinrich (Eds.), *Homosexuality: Research implications for public policy* (pp. 149–160). Newbury Park, CA: Sage.

Haldeman, D. C. (1994). The practice and ethics of sexual orientation conversion therapy. *Journal of Consulting and Clinical Psychology, 62*(2), 221–227.

Haldeman, D. C. (1995). Sexual orientation conversion therapy update. *Division 44 Newsletter, 11*(1), 4–6.

Haldeman, D. C. (1996). Spirituality and religion in the lives of lesbians and gay men. In R. P. Cabaj & T. S. Stein (Eds.), *Textbook of homosexuality and mental health* (pp. 881–896). Washington, DC: American Psychiatric Press.

Haldeman, D. C. (1998). Ceremonies and religion in same-sex marriage. In R. P. Cabaj & D. W. Purcell (Eds.), *On the road to same-sex marriage: A supportive guide to psychological, political, and legal issues* (pp. 141–164). San Francisco: Jossey-Bass.

Haldeman, D. C. (2000). *Gay rights, patient rights: The implications of sexual orientation conversion therapy.* Paper presented at the 108th annual meeting of the American Psychological Association, Washington, DC.

Halkitis, P. N. (2000). *Sexual practices of combined methamphetamine and nitrate users.* Paper presented at the 108th annual meeting of the American Psychological Association, Washington, DC.

Hall, J. M. (1994a). Lesbians recovering from alcohol problems: An ethnographic study of health care experiences. *Nursing Research, 43*(4), 238–244.

Hall, J. M. (1994b). The experiences of lesbians in Alcoholics Anonymous. *Western Journal of Nursing Research, 16*(5), 556–576.

Hall, J. M. (1996). Pervasive effects of childhood sexual abuse in lesbians' recovery from alcohol problems. *Substance Use and Misuse, 31*(2), 225–239.

Hall, J. M. (1998). Lesbians surviving childhood sexual abuse: Pivotal experiences related to sexual orientation, gender, and race. In C. M. Ponticelli (Ed.), *Gateways to improving lesbian health and health care: Opening doors* (pp. 7–28). New York: Harrington Park Press.

Hall, J. M. (1999). Lesbians in alcohol recovery surviving childhood sexual abuse and parental substance misuse. *International Journal of Psychiatric Nursing Research, 5*(1), 507–515.

Hall, M. (1984). Lesbians, limerence and longterm relationships. In J. Loulan, *Lesbian sex* (pp. 141–150). San Francisco: Spinsters.

Hall, M. (1986). The lesbian corporate experience. *Journal of Homosexuality, 12*(3–4), 59–75.

Hall, M. (1987). Sex therapy with lesbian couples: A four stage approach. *Journal of Homosexuality, 14*(1–2), 137–156.

Hall, M. (1998). *The lesbian love companion: How to survive everything from heartthrob the heartbreak.* San Francisco: Harper.

Hall, M., & Gregory, A. (1991). Subtle balances: Love and work in lesbian relationships. In B. Sang, J. Warshow, & A. J. Smith (Eds.), *Lesbians at midlife: The creative transition* (pp. 122–131). San Francisco: Spinsters.

Hamer, D, & Copeland, P. (1998). *Living with our genes: Why they matter more than you think.* New York: Doubleday.

Hammelman, T. L. (1993). Gay and lesbian youth: Contributing factors to serious attempts or considerations of suicide. *Journal of Gay and Lesbian Psychotherapy, 2*(1), 77–89.

Hammersmith, S. K. (1987). A sociological approach to counseling homosexual clients and their families. *Journal of Homosexuality, 14*(1–2), 173–190.

Hammond, N. (1989). Lesbian victims of relationship violence. In E. D. Rothblum, & E. Cole (Eds.), *Lesbianism: Affirming nontraditional roles* (pp. 89–105). Binghamton, NY: Haworth Press.

Hancock, K. A. (1995). Psychotherapy with lesbians and gay men. In A. R. D'Augelli (Ed.), *Lesbian, gay, and bisexual identities over the lifespan* (pp. 398–432). New York: Oxford University Press.

Hanes, K. (1997). *The gay guy's guide to love: The dos, don'ts, and definite maybes of dating and mating.* Victoria, BC: Crown.

Hanley-Hackenbruck, P. (1988). "Coming out" and psychotherapy. *Psychiatric Annals, 18*(1), 29–32.

Hanley-Hackenbruck, P. (1989). Psychotherapy and the "coming out" process. *Journal of Gay and Lesbian Psychotherapy, 1*(1), 21–39.

Hansen, B. (1989). American physicians' earliest writings about homosexuals, 1880–1900. *Milbank Quarterly, 67*(1), 92–108.

Harbeck, K. M. (1992). Gay and lesbian educators: Past history/future prospects. In K. M. Harbeck (Ed.), *Coming out of the classroom closet: Gay and lesbian students, teachers, and curricula* (pp. 121–140). New York: Harrington Park Press.

Hardy, R. P. (1998). *Loving men, gay partners, spirituality, and AIDS.* New York: Continuum.

Harley, D. A., Hall, M., & Savage, T. A. (2000). Working with gay and lesbian consumers with disabilities: Helping practitioners understand another frontier of diversity. *Journal of Applied Rehabilitation Counseling, 31*(1), 4–11.

Harrison, A. E. (1996). Primary care of lesbian and gay patients: Educating ourselves and our students. *Family Medicine, 28*(1), 10–23.

Harrison, A. E., & Silenzio, V. M. (1996). Comprehensive care of lesbian and gay patients and families. *Primary Care, 23*(1), 31–46.

Harry, J. (1982a). Decision making and age differences among gay male couples. *Journal of Homosexuality, 8*(2), 9–22.

Harry, J. (1982b). *Gay children grown up: Gender culture and gender deviance.* New York: Praeger.

Harry, J. (1983). Gay male and lesbian relationships. In E. Macklin & R. Rubin (Eds.), *Contemporary families and alternative lifestyles: Handbook on research and theory* (pp. 216–234). Beverly Hills, CA: Sage.

Harry, J. (1984). *Gay couples.* New York: Praeger.

Harry, J. (1986). Sampling gay men. *Journal of Sex Research, 22*(1), 21–34.

Harry, J. (1989). Sexual identity issues. In U.S. Department of Health and Human Services (Ed.), *Report of the Secretary's Task Force on Youth Suicide* (pp. 2–131 to 2–142) (DHHS Publication No. ADM 89–1623). Washington, DC: U.S. Department of Health and Human Services.

Harry, J. (1993). Being out: A general model. *Journal of Homosexuality, 26*(1), 25–39.

Hart, J. (1998). *Gay sex: A manual for men who love men* (rev. ed.). Boston: Alyson.

Hartman, L. (1998). Discussion: Eros in a gay dyad. *Gender and Psychoanalysis, 3*(3), 361–369.

Harvey, A. (Ed.). (1997/2002). *The essential gay mystics.* San Francisco: Harper.

Hasbany, R. (Ed.). (1989). *Homosexuality and religion.* Binghamton, NY: Haworth Press.

Hawkins, D., Herron, W. G., Gibson, W., & Hoban, G. (1988). Homosexual and heterosexual sex-role orientation on six sex-role scales. *Perceptual and Motor Skills, 66*(3), 863–871.

Hawkins, R. L. (1992). Therapy with the male couple. In S. H. Dworkin & F. J. Gutierrez (Eds.), *Counseling gay men and lesbians: Journey to the end of the rainbow* (pp. 81–94). Alexandria, VA: American Association for Counseling and Development (now the American Counseling Association).

Heckman, T. G., Kelly, J. A., Roffman, R. A., Sikkema, K. J., Perry, M. J., Solomon, L. J., Winett, R. A., Norman, A. D., Hoffman, R. G., & Stevenson, L. Y. (1995). Psychosocial differences between recently HIV tested and non-tested gay men who reside in smaller US cities. *International Journal of STD and AIDS, 6*(6), 436–440.

Heffernan, K. (1998a). Binge eating, substance use, and coping styles in a lesbian sample. *Dissertation Abstracts International, 58*(7-B), 3924. (University Microfilms No. AAM98–00262)

Heffernan, K. (1998b). The nature and predictors of substance use among lesbians. *Addictive Behavior, 23*(4), 517–528.

Hellman, R. E., Stanton, M., Lee, J., Tytun, A., & Vachon, R. (1989). Treatment of homosexual alcoholics in government-funded agencies: Provider training and attitudes. *Hospital and Community Psychiatry, 40*(11), 1163–1168.

Helminiak, D. A. (1994). *What the Bible really says about homosexuality: Recent findings by top scholars offer a radical new view.* San Francisco: Alamo Square Press.

Hendin, H. (1978). Homosexuality: The psychosocial dimension. *Journal of the American Academy of Psychoanalysis, 6*(4), 479–496.

Hellwege, D. R., Perry, K., & Dobson, J. (1988). Perceptual differences in gender ideals among heterosexual and homosexual males and females. *Sex Roles, 19*(11–12), 735–746.

Henry, G. W. (1941). *Sex variants: A study of homosexual patterns.* New York: Hoeber.

Hequembourg, A. L., & Farrell, M. P. (1999). Lesbian motherhood: Negotiating marginal mainstream identities. *Gender and Society, 13*(4), 540–557.

Herdt, G. (1988). Cross-cultural forms of homosexuality and the concept "gay." *Psychiatric Annals, 18*(1), 37–39.

Herdt, G. (1990). Cross-cultural issues in the development of bisexuality and homosexuality. In M. E. Perry (Ed.), *Handbook of sexology* (Vol. 7). Amsterdam: Elsevier Science.

Herdt, G. H. (1992). "Coming out" as a rite of passage: A Chicago study. In G. H. Herdt (Ed.), *Gay culture in America: Essays from the field* (pp. 29–67). Boston: Beacon Press.

Herek, G. M. (1984). Beyond "homophobia": A social psychological perspective on attitudes toward lesbians and gay men. *Journal of Homosexuality, 10*(1–2), 2–17.

Herek, G. M. (1986a). On heterosexual masculinity: Some psychical consequences of the social construction of gender and sexuality. *American Behavioral Scientist, 29*(5), 563–577.

Herek, G. M. (1986b). The social psychology of homophobia: Toward a practical theory. *Review of Law and Social Change, 14*(4), 923–934.

Herek, G. M. (1987). Religious orientation and prejudice: A comparison of racial and sexual attitudes. *Personality and Social Psychology Bulletin, 13*(1), 34–44.

Herek, G. M. (1988). Heterosexuals' attitudes toward lesbians and gay men: Correlates and gender differences. *Journal of Sex Research, 25*(4), 451–477.

Herek, G. M. (1989). Hate crimes against lesbians and gay men. *American Psychologist, 44*(6), 948–955.

Herek, G. M. (1991). Stigma, prejudice, and violence against lesbians and gay men. In J. C. Gonsiorek & J. D. Weinrich (Eds.), *Homosexuality: Research implications for public policy* (pp. 60–80). Newbury Park, CA: Sage.

Herek, G. M. (1996). Heterosexism and homophobia. In R. P. Cabaj & T. S. Stein (Eds.), *Textbook of homosexuality and mental health* (pp. 101–113). Washington, DC: American Psychiatric Press.

Herek, G. M. (1998a). Bad science in the service of stigma: A critique of the Cameron Group's survey studies. In G. M. Herek (Ed.), *Stigma and sexual orientation: Understanding prejudice against lesbians, gay men, and bisexuals* (pp. 223–255). Thousand Oaks, CA: Sage.

Herek, G. M. (1998b, August). *Sexual prejudice: The social psychology of homophobias and heterosexisms.* Invited address presented at the 106th annual meeting of the American Psychological Association, San Francisco.

Herek, G. M. (1999a). AIDS and stigma. *American Behavioral Scientist, 42*(7), 1106–1116.

Herek, G. M. (1999b). *"Reparative Therapy" and other attempts to alter sexual orientation: A background paper* [Online]. Available: http://psychology.ucdavis.edu/rainbow/html/facts_changing.html.

Herek, G. M., & Berrill, K. T. (Eds.). (1991). *Hate crimes: Confronting violence against lesbians and gay men* (2nd ed.). Newbury Park, CA: Sage.

Herek, G. M., & Capitanio, J. P. (1996). "Some of my best friends": Intergroup contact, concealable stigma, and heterosexuals' attitudes toward gay men and lesbians. *Personality and Social Psychology Bulletin, 22*(4), 412–424.

Herek, G. M., Cogan, J. C., & Gillis, J. R. (2000). Psychological well-being and commitment to lesbian, gay, and bisexual identities. Paper presented at the 108th annual meeting of the American Psychological Association, Washington, DC.

Herek, G. M., & Glunt, E. K. (1993). Interpersonal contact and heterosexuals' attitudes toward gay men: Results from a national survey. *Journal of Sex Research, 30*(3), 239–244.

Herek, G. M., & Glunt, E. K. (1995). Identity and community among gay and bisexual men in the AIDS era: Preliminary findings from the Sacramento Men's Health Study. In G. M. Herek & B. Greene (Eds.), *AIDS, identity, and community: The HIV epidemic and lesbians and gay men* (pp. 55–84). Thousand Oaks, CA: Sage.

Heron, A. (Ed.). (1983). *One teenager in ten: Writings by gay and lesbian youth.* Boston: Alyson.

Hersch, P. (1991). Secret lives. *The Family Therapy Networker, 15*(1), 36–43.

Hertz, F., & Browning, F. (1998). *Legal affairs: Essential advice for same-sex couples.* New York: Henry Holt/Owl Books.

Herzog, D., Newman, K., Yeh, C., & Warshaw, M. (1992). Body image satisfaction in homosexual and heterosexual women. *International Journal of Eating Disorders, 11*, 391.

Hetherington, C., Hillerbrand, E., & Etringer, B. D. (1989). Career counseling with gay men: Issues and recommendations for research. *Journal of Counseling and Development, 67*(8), 452–454.

Hetherington, C., & Orzek, A. (1989). Career counseling and life planning with lesbian women. *Journal of Counseling and Development, 68*(1), 52–57.

Hetrick, E. S., & Martin, A. D. (1987). Developmental issues and their resolution for gay and lesbian adolescents. *Journal of Homosexuality, 14*(1–2), 25–43.

Heyward, C. (1989a). *Coming out and relational empowerment: A lesbian feminist theological perspective* (Work in Progress No. 38). Wellesley, MA: Wellesley College, the Stone Center.

Heyward, C. (1989b). *Touching our strength: The erotic as power and the love of God.* San Francisco: Harper & Row.

Hidalgo, H., & Hidalgo-Christensen, E. (1976). The Puerto-Rican lesbian and the Puerto-Rican community. *Journal of Homosexuality, 2*, 109–121.

Hill, I. (Ed.) (1987). *The bisexual spouse: Different dimensions in human sexuality.* McLean, VA: Barlina Books.

Hirsh J. (1989). In search of role models. In C Balka & A. Rose (Eds.), *Twice blessed: On being lesbian or gay and Jewish* (pp. 83–91). Boston: Beacon Press.

Hockenberry, S. L., & Billingham, R. E. (1987). Sexual orientation and boyhood gender identity: Development of the Boyhood Gender Conformity Scale (BGCS). *Archives of Sexual Behavior, 16*(6), 475–492.

Hogan, R. A., Fox, A. N., & Kirchner, J. H. (1977). Attitudes, opinions, and sexual development of 205 homosexual women. *Journal of Homosexuality, 3*(2), 123–136.

Hogan, R. A., Kirchner, J. H., Hogan, K. A., & Fox, A. N. (1980). The only child factor in homosexual development. *Psychology: A Quarterly Journal of Human Behavior, 17*(1), 19–33.

Holland, J. L. (1992). *Making vocational choices: A theory of vocational personalities and work environments* (2nd ed.). Odessa, FL: Psychological Assessment Resources.

Holtzen, D. W., & Agresti, A. A. (1990). Parental responses to gay and lesbian children: Differences in homophobia, self-esteem, and sex-role stereotyping. *Journal of Social and Clinical Psychology, 9*(3), 390–399.

Hooker, E. (1993). Reflections of a 40–year exploration: A scientific view on homosexuality. *American Psychologist, 48*(4), 450–453.

Hopcke, R. H. (1992). Midlife, gay men, and the AIDS epidemic. *Quadrant, 25*(1), 101–109.

Hotchkiss, L., & Borow, H. (1996). Sociological perspective on work and career development. In D. Brown & L. Brooks (Eds.), *Career choice and development* (3rd ed., pp. 281–334). San Francisco: Jossey-Bass.

Huggins, S. L. (1989). A comparative study of self-esteem of adolescent children of divorced lesbian mothers and divorced heterosexual mothers. *Journal of Homosexuality, 18*(1–2), 123–135.

Hughes, T. L., Haas, A. P., Razzano, L., Cassidy, R., & Matthews, A. (2000). Comparing lesbians' and heterosexual women's mental health: A multi-site survey. *Journal of Gay and Lesbian Social Services, 11*(1) 57–76.

Hughes, T. L., & Wilsnack, S. C. (1997). Use of alcohol among lesbians: Research and clinical implications. *American Journal of Orthopsychiatry, 67*(1), 20–36.

Hultkrantz, A. (1988). Shamanism: A religious phenomenon? In G. Doore (Ed.), *Shaman's path: Healing, personal growth and empowerment.* Boston: Shambhala.

Human Rights Campaign. (2001). *HRC Worknet* [Online]. Available: www.hrc.org/worknet/index.asp.

Humphreys, L. (1972). *Out of the closets: The sociology of homosexual liberation.* Englewood Cliffs, NJ: Prentice-Hall.

Hunsberger, B. (1996). Religious fundamentalism, right-wing authoritarianism, and hostility toward homosexuals in non-Christian religious groups. *International Journal for the Psychology of Religion, 6*(1), 39–49.

Hunt, M. (1990). *Fierce tenderness: A feminist theology of friendship:* New York: Crossroad.

Hunter, J. (1990). Violence against lesbian and gay male youths. *Journal of Interpersonal Violence, 5*(3), 295–300.

Hunter, J., & Schaecher, R. (1987). Stresses on lesbian and gay adolescents in schools. *Social Work in Education, 9*(3), 180–190.

Hunter, J., & Schaecher, R. (1990). Lesbian and gay youth. In M. J. Rotheram-Borus, J. Bradley, & N. Obolensky (Eds.), *Planning to live: Evaluating and treating suicidal teens in community settings* (pp. 297–316). Tulsa: University of Oklahoma Press.

Hyman, B. (2000). The economic consequences of child sexual abuse for adult lesbian women. *Journal of Marriage and the Family, 62*(1), 199–211.

Icard, L. (1985/1986). Black gay men and conflicting social identities: Sexual orientation versus racial identity. *Journal of Social Work and Human Sexuality, 4*(1–2), 83–93.

Icard, L. D., Schilling, R. F., El-Bassel, N., & Young, D. (1992). Preventing AIDS among Black gay men and Black gay and heterosexual male intravenous drug users. *Social Work, 37*(5), 440–445.

Icard, L., & Traunstein, D. M. (1987). Black, gay, alcoholic men: Their character and treatment. *Social Casework, 68*(5), 267–272.

Igartua, K. J. (1998). Therapy with lesbian couples: The issues and the interventions. *Canadian Journal of Psychiatry, 43*(4), 391–396.

Innala, S. M., & Ernulf, K. E. (1994). When gay is pretty: Physical attractiveness and low homophobia. *Psychological Reports, 74*(3, Pt. 1), 827–831.

Irving, G. A., Bor, R., & Catalan, J. (1995). Psychological distress among gay men supporting a lover or partner with AIDS: A pilot study. *AIDS Care, 7*(5), 605–617.

Isay, R. A. (1985). On the analytic therapy of homosexual men. *Psychoanalytic Study of the Child, 40,* 235–254.

Isay, R. A. (1986). The development of sexual identity in homosexual men. *Psychoanalytic Study of the Child, 41,* 467–489.

Isay, R. A. (1987). Fathers and their homosexually inclined sons in childhood. *Psychoanalytic Study of the Child, 42,* 275–294.

Isay, R. A. (1988). Homosexuality in heterosexual and homosexual men. *Psychiatric Annals, 18*(1), 43–46.

Isay, R. A. (1989). *Being homosexual: Gay men and their development.* New York: Avon.

Isay, R. A. (1991). The homosexual analyst: Clinical considerations. *Psychoanalytic Study of the Child, 46,* 199–216.

Isay, R. A. (1996). Psychoanalytic therapy with gay men. In R. P. Cabaj & T. S. Stein (Eds.), *Textbook of homosexuality and mental health* (pp. 451–469). Washington, DC: American Psychiatric Press.

Isensee, R. (1996). *Love between men: Enhancing intimacy and keeping your relationship alive.* Boston: Alyson.

Isensee, R. (1997). *Reclaiming your life. The gay man's guide to love, self-acceptance, and trust.* Boston: Alyson.

Island, D., & Letellier, P. (1991). *Men who beat the men who love them: Battered gay men and domestic violence.* New York: Harrington Park Press.

Israelstam, S. (1986). Alcohol and drug problems of gay males and lesbians: Therapy, counseling, and prevention issues. *Journal of Drug Issues, 16*(3), 443–461.

Israelstam, S., & Lambert, S. (1986). Homosexuality and alcohol: Observations and research after the psychoanalytic era. *International Journal of the Addictions, 21*(4 & 5), 509–537.

Israelstam, S., & Lambert, S. (1989). Homosexuals who indulge in excessive use of alcohol and drugs: Psychosocial factors to be taken into account by community and intervention workers. *Journal of Alcohol and Drug Education, 34*(3), 54–69.

Issroff, R. (1988). The difficulty of understanding a borderline patient. *Psychoanalytic Psychotherapy, 3*(3), 259–269.

Jacobs, S. E. (1968). Berdache: A brief review of the literature. *Colorado Anthropologist, 1,* 25–40.

Jacobs, S. E. (Ed.). (1997). *Two-spirit people: Native American gender identity, sexuality, and spirituality.* Urbana: University of Illinois Press.

Jacobson, S., & Grossman, A. H. (1996). Older lesbians and gay men: Old myths, new images, and future directions. In R. C. Savin-Williams & K. M. Cohen (Eds.), *The lives of lesbians, gays, and bisexuals: Children to adults* (pp. 345–373). Fort Worth, TX: Harcourt Brace.

Jafri, A. B., & Greenberg, W. M. (1991). Fluoxetine side effects. *Journal of the American Academy of Child and Adolescent Psychiatry, 30*(5), 852.

James, S. E., & Murphy, B. C. (1998). Gay and lesbian relationships in a changing social context. In C. J. Patterson & A. R. D'Augelli (Eds.), *Lesbian, gay, and bisexual identities in families: Psychological perspectives* (pp. 99–121). New York: Oxford University Press.

James, W. (1928). *The varieties of religious experience: A study of human nature.* New York: Longmans, Green.

Jay, K., & Young, A. (1977). *The gay report: Lesbians and gay men speak out about sexual experiences and lifestyles.* New York: Summit Books.

Jenks, R. J. (1988). Nongays' perceptions of gays. *Annals of Sex Research, 1*(1), 139–150.

Jensen, K. L. (1999). *Lesbian epiphanies: Women coming out in later life.* Binghamton, NY: Haworth Press.

Johnson, K. G. (1998). *Dance with the stars: A personal journey to spirituality.* Tarpon Springs, FL: Spiritual Awareness Productions.

Johnson, E. C., & Johnson, T. (2000). *Gay spirituality: The role of gay identity in the transformation of religious thought.* Boston: Alyson.

Johnson, S. R., Smith, E. M., & Guenther, S. M. (1987). Comparison of gynecologic health care problems between lesbians and bisexual women: A survey of 2,345 women. *Journal of Reproductive Medicine, 32*(11), 805–811.

Johnson, T. W., & Keren, M. S. (1996). Creating and maintaining boundaries in male couples. In J. Laird & R. J. Green (Eds.), *Lesbians and gays in couples and families: A handbook for therapists* (pp. 231–250). San Francisco: Jossey-Bass.

Johnston, D., Stall, R., & Smith, K. (1995). Reliance by gay men and intravenous drug users of friends and family for AIDS-related care. *AIDS Care, 7*(3), 307–319.

Jones, B. E., & Hill, M. J. (1996). African American lesbians, gay men, and bisexuals. In R. P. Cabaj & T. S. Stein (Eds.), *Textbook of homosexuality and mental health* (pp. 549–561). Washington, DC: American Psychiatric Press.

Jones, D. A. (1996). Discrimination against same-sex couples in hotel reservation policies. *Journal of Homosexuality, 31*(1–2), 153–159.

Jones, E. E., & Thorne, A. (1987). Rediscovery of the subject: Intercultural approaches to clinical assessment. *Journal of Consulting and Clinical Psychology, 55,* 488–495.

Jones, M. A., & Gabriel, M. A. (1999). Utilization of psychotherapy by lesbians, gay men, and bisexuals: Findings from a nationwide survey. *American Journal of Orthopsychiatry, 69*(2), 209–219.

Jordan, J. V., Kaplan, A. G., Miller, J. B., Stiver, I. P., & Surrey, J. L. (Eds.). (1991). *Women's growth in connection: Writings from the Stone Center.* New York: Guilford Press.

Jordan, K. M. (2000). Substance abuse among gay, lesbian, bisexual, transgender, and questioning adolescents. *School Psychology Review, 29*(2), 201–206.

Julien, D., Arellano, C., & Turgeon, L. (1997). In W. K. Halford & H. J. Markman (Eds.), *Clinical handbook of marriage and couples interventions* (pp. 107–127). Chichester, UK: Wiley.

Julien, D., Chartrand, E., & Begin, J. (1996). Males couples' dyadic adjustment and the use of safer sex within and outside of primary relationships. *Journal of Family Psychology, 10*(1), 89–96.

Jurek, M. R. (1999). Psychosocial factors predicting high risk sexual behavior in HIV-negative gay men. *Dissertation Abstracts International, 60*(6-B), 2947. (University Microfilms No. AAI99–36655)

Jussim, L., Nelson, T. E., Manis, M., & Soffin, S. (1995). Prejudice, stereotypes, and labeling effects: Sources of bias in person perception. *Journal of Personality and Social Psychology, 68*(2), 228–246.

Kadushin, G. (2000). Family secrets: Disclosure of HIV status among gay men with HIV/AIDS to the family of origin. *Social Work in Health Care, 30*(3), 11–17.

Kahn, M. J. (1991). Factors affecting the coming out process for lesbians. *Journal of Homosexuality, 21*(3), 47–70.

Kahn, M. J., & Nutt, R. L. (1991, August). *Factors affecting the coming out process for lesbians.* Paper presented at the 99th annual meeting of the American Psychological Association, San Francisco.

Kahn, Y. H. (1989). Judaism and homosexuality: The traditionalist/progressive debate. *Journal of Homosexuality, 18*(3–4), 47–82.

Kain, C. D. (1996). *Positive: HIV affirmation counseling.* Alexandria, VA: American Counseling Association.

Kalichman, S. C., Tannenbaum, L., & Nachimson, D. (1998). Personality and cognitive factors influencing substance use and sexual risk for HIV infection among gay and bisexual men. *Psychology of Addictive Behaviors, 12*(4), 262–271.

Kaplan, H. S. (1977). Hypoactive sexual desire. *Journal of Sex and Marital Therapy, 3,* 3–9.

Kaplan, H. S. (1979). *Disorders of sexual desire.* New York: Brunner/Mazel.

Kaplan, H. S. (1983). *The evaluation of sexual disorders.* New York: Brunner/Mazel.

Kassoff, B. (1995). Lesbian couples in therapy: Expanding the frame of gender and of couples therapy. In J. M. Glassgold & S. Iasenza (Eds.), *Lesbians and psychoanalysis: Revolutions in theory and practice* (pp. 254–261). New York: Free Press.

Kassoff, E. (1988). Nonmonogamy in the lesbian community. *Women and Therapy, 8*(1–2), 167–182.

Katz, J. N. (1983). *Gay/lesbian almanac: A new documentary.* New York: Harper & Row.

Kauth, M. R., Hartwig, M. J., & Kalichman, S. C. (2000). Health behavior relevant to psychotherapy with lesbian, gay, and bisexual clients. In R. M. Perez, K. A. DeBord, & K. J. Bieschke (Eds.), *Handbook of counseling and psychotherapy with lesbian, gay, and bisexual clients* (pp. 435–456). Washington, DC: American Psychological Association.

Kear, L. (1999). *We're here: An investigation into gay reincarnation.* Atlanta, GA: Brookhaven.

Kehoe, M. (1986a). A portrait of the older lesbian. *Journal of Homosexuality, 12*(3–4), 157–161.

Kehoe, M. (1986b). Lesbians over 65: A triply invisible minority. *Journal of Homosexuality, 12*(3–4), 139–152.

Kehoe, M. (1989). *Lesbians over sixty speak for themselves.* Binghamton, NY: Haworth Press. [Also published in *Journal of Homosexuality,* 1988, *16*(3–4)]

Kellock, D., & O'Mahony, C. P. (1996). Sexually acquired metronidazole-resistant trichomoniasis in a lesbian couple. *Genitourinary Medicine, 72*(1), 60–61.

Kelly, J. A., & Kalichman, S. C. (1998). Reinforcement value of unsafe sex as a predictor of condom use and continued HIV/AIDS risk behavior among gay and bisexual men. *Health Psychology, 17*(4), 328–335.

Kelly, J. J. (1977). The aging male homosexual: Myth and reality. *The Gerontologist, 17*(4), 328–332.

Kenney, J. W., & Tash, D. T. (1992). Lesbian childbearing couples' dilemmas and decisions. Lesbian health: What are the issues? [Special issue]. *Health Care for Women International, 13*(2), 209–219.

Kerns, J. G., & Fine, M. A. (1994). The relation between gender and negative attitudes toward gay men and lesbians: Do gender role attitudes mediate this relation? *Sex Roles, 31*(5–6), 297–307.

Kertzner, R. (1999). Self-appraisal of life experience and psychological adjustment in midlife gay men. *Journal of Psychology and Human Sexuality, 11*(2), 43–64.

Kertzner, R. M., & Sved, M. (1996). Midlife gay men and lesbians: Adult development and mental health. In R. P. Cabaj & T. S. Stein (Eds.), *Textbook of homosexuality and mental health* (pp. 289–303). Washington, DC: American Psychiatric Press.

Kettelhack, G. (1999). *Vastly more than that: Stories of lesbians and gay men in recovery.* City Center, MN: Hazelden.

Kilbourn, S. (1999, Winter). Cause for alarm: HIV/AIDS statistics point to need for comprehensive prevention plan. *HRC Quarterly*, p. 18.

Kilhefner, D. (1988). Gay people at a critical crossroad: Assimilation or affirmation? In M. Thompson (Ed.), *Gay spirit: Myth and meaning*. New York: St. Martin's Press.

Kimberly, J. A., & Serovich, J. M. (1999). The role of family and friend social support in reducing risk behaviors among HIV-positive gay men. *AIDS Education and Prevention*, 11(6), 465–475.

Kimmel, D. C. (1977). Psychotherapy and the older gay male. *Psychotherapy: Theory, Research and Practice*, 14(4), 386–393.

Kimmel, D. C. (1978). Adult development and aging: A gay perspective. *Journal of Social Issues*, 34(3), 113–130.

Kimmel, D. C. (1992). The families of older gay men and lesbians. *Generations*, 16(3), 37–38.

Kimmel, D. C., & Sang, B. E. (1995). Lesbians and gay men in midlife. In A. R. D'Augelli & C. J. Patterson (Eds.), *Lesbian, gay, and bisexual identities over the lifespan* (pp. 190–214). New York: Oxford University Press.

King, M., & Mc Donald, E. (1992). Homosexuals who are twins: A study of 46 probands. *British Journal of Psychiatry*, 160, 407–409.

Kinsey, A. C., Pomeroy, W. B., & Martin, C. E. (1948). *Sexual behavior in the human male*. Philadelphia: Saunders.

Kinsey, A. C., Pomeroy, W. B., Martin, C. E., & Gebhard, P. H. (1953). *Sexual behavior in the human female*. Philadelphia: Saunders.

Kippax, S., Noble, J., Prestage, G., & Crawford, J. M. (1997). Sexual negotiation in the AIDS era: Negotiated safety revisited. *AIDS*, 11(2), 191–197.

Kirby, D. (1999a, April 13). Risky business. *The Advocate*, pp. 41–45.

Kirby, D. (1999b, June 22). The next generation. *The Advocate*, pp. 68–71.

Kirby, D. (2000a, April 11). Teaching schools a lesson. *The Advocate*, pp. 29, 31–33.

Kirby, D. (2000b, May 23). Taking a break. *The Advocate*, pp. 37–38.

Kirkpatrick, M. (1989). Lesbians: A different middle age? In J. Oldham & R. Liebert (Eds.), *New psychoanalytic perspectives: The middle years* (pp. 135–148). New Haven, CT: Yale University Press.

Kirkpatrick, M. (1991). Lesbian couples in therapy. *Psychiatric Annals*, 21(8), 491–496.

Kirkpatrick, M. (1996). Lesbians as parents. In R. P. Cabaj & T. S. Stein (Eds.), *Textbook of homosexuality and mental health* (pp. 353–370). Washington, DC; American Psychiatric Press.

Kirschner, R. (1988). Judaism and homosexuality: A reappraisal. *Judaism*, 37(4), 450–458.

Kitano, H. H. L. (1989). A model for counseling Asian Americans. In P. B. Pedersen, J. G. Draguns, W. J. Lonner & J. E. Trimble (Eds.), *Counseling across cultures* (pp. 139–152). Honolulu: University of Hawaii Press.

Kite, M. E. (1992). Individual differences in males' reactions to gay males and lesbians. *Journal of Applied Social Psychology*, 22(15), 1222–1239.

Kite, M. E., & Deaux, K. (1986). Attitudes toward homosexuality: Assessment and behavioral consequences. *Basic and Applied Social Psychology*, 7(2), 137–162.

Kite, M. E., & Deaux, K. (1987). Gender belief systems: Homosexuality and the implicit inversion theory. *Psychology of Women Quarterly*, 11(1), 83–96.

Kite, M. E., & Whitley, B. E., Jr. (1996). Sex differences in attitudes toward homosexual persons, behaviors, and civil rights: A meta-analysis. *Personal and Social Psychology Bulletin*, 22(4), 336–353.

Kitzinger, C. (1991). Lesbians and gay men in the workplace: Psychosocial issues. In M. J. Davidson & J. Earnshaw (Eds.), *Vulnerable workers: Psychosocial and legal issues* (pp. 223–240). Chichester, UK: Wiley.

Klein, F. (1990). The need to view sexual orientation as a multivariable dynamic process: A theoretical perspective. In D. P. McWhirter, S. A. Sanders, & J. M. Reinisch (Eds.), *Homosexuality/heterosexuality: Concepts of sexual orientation* (pp. 277–282). New York: Oxford University Press.

Klein, F. (1993). *The bisexual option* (2nd ed.). New York: Harrington Park Press.

Klein, F., Sepekoff, B., & Wolf, T. (1985). Sexual orientation: A multi-variate dynamic process. *Journal of Homosexuality*, 11(1–2), 35–49.

Kleinberg, S., & Zorn, P. (1995). Rekindling the flame: A therapeutic approach to strengthening lesbian relationships. In J. M. Glassgold & S. Iasenza (Eds.), *Lesbians and psychoanalysis: Revolutions in theory and practice* (pp. 125–143). New York: Free Press.

Klinger, R. L. (1995). Gay violence. *Journal of Gay and Lesbian Psychotherapy*, 2(3), 119–134.

Klinger, R. L. (1996). Lesbian couples. In R. P. Cabaj & T. S. Stein (Eds.), *Textbook of homosexuality and mental health* (pp. 339–352). Washington, DC: American Psychiatric Press.

Klinger, R. L., & Stein, T. S. (1996). Impact of violence, childhood sexual abuse, and domestic violence and abuse on lesbians, bisexuals, and gay men. In R. P. Cabaj & T. S. Stein (Eds.), *Textbook of homosexuality and mental health* (pp. 801–818). Washington, DC: American Psychiatric Press.

Klitzman, R. L., Pope, H. G. Jr., & Hudson, J. I. (2000). MDMA ("Ecstasy") abuse and high-risk sexual behaviors among 169 gay and bisexual men. *American Journal of Psychiatry*, 157(7), 1162–1164.

Knopp, L. M. (1990). Social consequences of homosexuality. *Geographical Magazine*, 62, 20–25.

Knox, S., Kippax, S., Crawford, J., Prestage, G., & Van de Ven, P. (1999). Non-prescription drug use by gay men in Sydney, Melbourne and Brisbane. *Drug and Alcohol Review*, 18(4), 425–433.

Koh, A. S. (2000). Use of preventive health behaviors by lesbian, bisexual, and heterosexual women: Questionnaire survey. *Western Journal of Medicine*, 172(6), 379–384.

Kolodny, D. R. (Ed.). (2000). *Blessed bi spirit: Bisexual people of faith*. New York: Continuum.

Kominars, S. B. (1989). *Accepting ourselves: The twelve-step journey of recovery from addiction for gay men and lesbians*. San Francisco: Harper & Row.

Kourany, R. F. (1987). Suicide among homosexual adolescents. *Journal of Homosexuality*, 13(4), 111–117.

Krafft-Ebing, R. von (1965). *Psychopathia sexualis* (F. S. Klaf, Trans.). New York: Bell. (Original work published 1884)

Krajeski, J. P. (1986). Psychotherapy with gay men and lesbians: A history of controversy. In T. S. Stein & C. J. Cohen (Eds.), *Contemporary perspectives on psychotherapy with lesbians and gay men* (pp. 9–25). New York: Plenum Medical.

Krajeski, J. (1996). Homosexuality and the mental health professions: A contemporary history. In R. P. Cabaj & T. S. Stein (Eds.). *Textbook of homosexuality and mental health* (pp. 17–31). Washington DC: American Psychiatric Press.

Kreider, R. S. (Ed.). (1998). *From wounded hearts: Faith stories of lesbian, gay, bisexual, and transgendered people and those who love them*. Gaithersburg, MD: Chi Rho Press.

Krestan, J. (1987). Lesbian daughters and lesbian mothers: The crisis of disclosure from a family systems perspective. *Journal of Psychotherapy and the Family*, 3(4), 113–130.

Krestan, J., & Bepko, C. S. (1980). The problem of fusion in the lesbian relationship. *Family Process*, 19(3), 277–289.

Kruks, G. (1991). Gay and lesbian homeless/street youth: Special issues and concerns. *Journal of Adolescent Health*, 12(7), 515–518.

Krumboltz, J. D. (1979). A social learning theory of career decision making. In A. M. Mitchell, G. B. Jones, & J. D. Krumboltz (Eds.), *Social learning and career decision making* (pp. 19–49) Cranston, RI: Carroll Press.

Krumboltz, J. D. (1996). A learning theory of career counseling. In M. L. Savickas & W. B. Walsh (Eds.), *Handbook of career counseling theory and practice* (pp. 55–80). Palo Alto, CA: Davies-Black.

Kübler-Ross, E. (1969). *On death and dying*. New York: Macmillan.

Kurdek, L. A. (1987). Sex role self schema and psychological adjustment in coupled homosexual and heterosexual men and women. *Sex Roles*, 17(9–10), 549–562.

Kurdek, L. A. (1988a). Correlates of negative attitudes toward homosexuals in heterosexual college students. *Sex Roles*, 18(11–12), 727–738.

Kurdek, L. A. (1988b). Perceived social support in gays and lesbians in cohabiting relationships. *Journal of Personality and Social Psychology*, 54(3), 504–509.

Kurdek, L. A. (1988c). Relationship quality of gay and lesbian cohabiting couples. *Journal of Homosexuality*, 15(3–4), 93–118.

Kurdek, L. A. (1989). Relationship quality in gay and lesbian cohabiting couples: A 1–year follow-up study. *Journal of Social and Personal Relationships*, 6(1), 39–59.

Kurdek, L. A. (1991). Correlates of relationship satisfaction in cohabiting gay and lesbian couples: Integration of contextual, investment, and problem-solving model. *Journal of Personality and Social Psychology, 61*(6), 910–922.

Kurdek, L. A. (1992). Relationship stability and relationship satisfaction in cohabiting gay and lesbian couples: A prospective longitudinal test of the contextual and interdependence models. *Journal of Social and Personal Relationships, 9*(1), 125–142.

Kurdek, L. A. (1994). The nature and correlates of relationship quality in gay, lesbian, and heterosexual cohabiting couples: A test of the individual difference, interdependence, and discrepancy models. In B. Greene & G. M. Herek (Eds.), *Lesbian and gay psychology: Theory, research, and clinical applications* (pp. 133–155). Thousand Oaks, CA: Sage.

Kurdek, L. A. (1995a). Developmental changes in relationship quality in gay and lesbian cohabiting couples. *Developmental Psychology, 31*(1), 86–94.

Kurdek, L. A. (1995b). Lesbian and gay couples. In A. R. D'Augelli & C. J. Patterson (Eds.), *Lesbian, gay, and bisexual identities over the lifespan* (pp. 243–261). New York: Oxford University Press.

Kurdek, L. A. (1996). The deterioration of relationship quality for gay and lesbian cohabiting couples: A five-year prospective longitudinal study. *Personal Relationships, 3*(4), 417–442.

Kurdek, L. A. (1997a). Adjustment to relationship dissolution in gay, lesbian, and heterosexual partners. *Personal Relationships, 4*(2), 145–161.

Kurdek, L. A. (1997b). Relation between neuroticism and dimensions of relationship commitment: Evidence from gay, lesbian, and heterosexual couples. *Journal of Family Psychology, 11*(1), 109–124.

Kurdek, L. A. (1997c). The link between facets of neuroticism and dimensions of relationship commitment: Evidence from gay, lesbian, and heterosexual couples. *Journal of Family Psychology, 11*(4), 503–514.

Kurdek, L. A., & Schmitt, J. P. (1986a). Relationship quality of gay men in closed or open relationships. *Journal of Homosexuality, 12*(2), 85–99.

Kurdek, L. A., & Schmitt, J. P. (1986b). Relationship quality of partners in heterosexual married, heterosexual cohabitating, gay, and lesbian relationships. *Journal of Personality and Social Psychology, 51*, 711–720.

Kurdek, L. A., & Schmitt, J. P. (1987a). Partner homogamy in married, heterosexual cohabiting, gay, and lesbian couples. *Journal of Sex Research, 23*(2), 212–232.

Kurdek, L. A., & Schmitt, J. P. (1987b). Perceived emotional support from family and friends in members of homosexual, married, and heterosexual cohabiting couples. *Journal of Homosexuality, 14*(3–4), 57–68.

Kurtz, S. P. (1999). Without women: Masculinities, gay male sexual culture and sexual behaviors in Miami, Florida. *Dissertation Abstracts International, 60*(6-A), 2242. (University Microfilms No. AAM99-36877)

Kus, R. J. (1987). Alcoholics Anonymous and gay American men. In E. Coleman (Ed.), *Integrated identity for gay men and lesbians: Psychotherapeutic approaches for emotional well-being* (pp. 253–276). New York: Harrington Park Press.

Kus, R. J. (1988). Alcoholism and non-acceptance of gay self: The critical link. *Journal of Homosexuality, 15*(1–2), 25–41.

Kus, R. J. (1989). Bibliotherapy and gay American men of Alcoholics Anonymous. *Journal of Gay and Lesbian Psychotherapy, 1*(2), 73–86.

Kus, R. J. (1990). Alcoholism in the gay and lesbian communities. In R. J. Kus (Ed.), *Keys to caring: Assisting your gay and lesbian clients* (pp. 66–81). Boston: Alyson.

Kus, R. J. (1991). Sobriety, friends, and gay men. *Archives of Psychiatric Nursing, 5*(3), 171–177.

Kus, R. J. (Ed.). (1995). *Addiction and recovery in gay and lesbian persons.* Binghamton, NY: Haworth Press.

LaFromboise, T. D. (1988). American Indian mental health policy. *American Psychologist, 43*(5), 388–397.

LaFromboise, T. D., Trimble, J. E., & Mohatt, G. V. (1993). Counseling intervention and American Indian tradition: An integrative approach. *Counseling Psychologist, 18*(4), 628–654.

Lai, D. S. (1999). Self-esteem and unsafe sex in Chinese-American and Japanese-American gay men. *Dissertation Abstracts International, 59*(9-B), 5093. (University Microfilms No. AAM99-07530)

Laird, J. (1998). Invisible ties: Lesbians and their families of origin. In C. J. Patterson & A. R. D'Augelli (Eds.), *Lesbian, gay, and bisexual identities in families: Psychological perspectives* (pp. 197–228). New York: Oxford University Press.

Laird, J., & Green, R. J. (Eds.). (1996). *Lesbians and gays in couples and families: A handbook for therapists.* San Francisco: Jossey-Bass.

Lambert, C. (1954). Homosexuals. *Medical Press, 2,* 523–526.

Lance, L. M. (1987). The effects of interaction with gay persons on attitudes toward homosexuality. *Human Relations, 40*(6), 329–336.

Landolt, M. A., & Dutton, D. G. (1997). Power and personality: An analysis of gay male intimate abuse. *Sex Roles, 37*(5–6), 335–359.

Laner, M. R. (1979). Growing older female: Heterosexual and homosexual. *Journal of Homosexuality, 4*(3), 267–275.

Lang, N. G. (1991). Stigma, self-esteem, and depression: Psycho-social responses to risk of AIDS. *Human Organization, 50*(1), 66–72.

LaSala, M. C. (2000). Lesbians, gay men, and their parents: Family therapy for the coming-out crisis. *Family Process, 39*(1), 67–81.

Lauver, D. R., Karon, S. L., Egan, J., Jacobson, M., Nugent, J. Settersten, L., & Shaw, V. (1999). Understanding lesbians' mammography utilization. *Womens Health Issues, 9*(5), 264–274.

Leaity, S., Sherr, L., Wells, H., Evans, A., Miller, R., Johnson, M., & Elford, J. (2000). Repeat HIV testing: High-risk behavior or risk reduction? *AIDS, 14*(5), 547–552.

Leavy, S. A. (1985/1986). Male homosexuality reconsidered. *International Journal of Psychoanalytic Psychotherapy, 11,* 155–174.

Lee, J. A. (1977). Going public: A study in the sociology of homosexual liberation. *Journal of Homosexuality, 3*(1), 49–78.

Lee, J. A. (1987). What can homosexual aging studies contribute to theories of aging? *Journal of Homosexuality, 13*(4), 43–71.

Lee, J. A. (1991). Foreword. In J. A. Lee (Ed.), *Gay midlife and maturity* (pp. xiii–xix). New York: Harrington Park Press.

Lee, K. G., & Busto, R. (1991, Fall). When the spirit moves us. *OUT/LOOK, 14,* 83–85.

Lehmann, J. B., Lehmann, C. U., & Kelly, P. J. (1998). Development and health care needs of lesbians. *Journal of Womens Health, 7*(3), 379–387.

Leiblum, S. R., Palmer, M. G., & Spector, I. P. (1995). Non-traditional mothers: Single heterosexual/lesbian women and lesbian couples electing motherhood via donor insemination. *Journal of Psychosomatic Obstetrics and Gynaecology, 16*(1), 11–20.

Leland, J. (2000, March 20). Shades of gay. *Newsweek,* pp. 46–49.

Leland, J., & Miller, M. (1998, August 17). Can gays convert? *Newsweek,* pp. 47–50.

Lemle, R., & Mishkind, M. E. (1989). Alcohol and masculinity. *Journal of Substance Abuse Treatment, 6*(4), 213–222.

Lenderking, W. R., Wold, C., Mayer, K. H., Goldstein, R., Losina, E., & Seage, G. R. III (1997). Childhood sexual abuse among homosexual men: Prevalence and association with unsafe sex. *Journal of General Internal Medicine, 12*(4), 250–253.

Lesbian health: Experts outline recommendations at scientific meeting. (2000, Summer). *HRC Quarterly,* p. 24.

Letellier, P. (1994). Gay and bisexual domestic violence victimization: Challenges to feminist theory and responses to violence. In L. K. Hamberger & C. Renzetti (Eds.), *Domestic partner abuse* (pp. 1–21). New York: Springer.

LeVay, S. (1991, August). A difference in hypothalamic structure between heterosexual and homosexual men. *Science,* pp. 1034–1037.

LeVay, S., & Hamer, D. H. (1994, May). Evidence for a biological influence in male homosexuality. *Scientific American,* pp. 44–49.

Lever, J. (1994, August 23). Sexual revelations: The 1994 Advocate survey of sexuality and relationships: The men. *The Advocate,* pp. 17–24.

Lever, J., Kanouse, D. E., Rogers, W. H., & Carson, S. (1992). Behavior patterns and sexual identity of bisexual males. *Journal of Sex Research*, 29(2), 141–167.

Levine, M. P. (1989). The status of gay men in the workplace. In M. S. Kimmel & M. A. Messner (Eds.). *Men's lives* (pp. 261–276). New York: Macmillan.

Levinson, D. J. (with C. N. Darrow, E. B. Klein, M. H. Levinson, & B. McKee). (1978). *The seasons of a man's life*. New York: Knopf.

Levitt, E. E., & Klasser, A. D. (1974). Public attitudes toward homosexuality: Part of the 1970 survey of the Institute for Sex Research. *Journal of Homosexuality*, 1(1), 131–134.

Lewin, E. (1993). *Lesbian mothers: Accounts of gender in American culture*. Ithaca, NY: Cornell University Press.

Lewis, C. E., Saghir, M. T., & Robins, E. (1982). Drinking patterns in homosexual and heterosexual women. *Journal of Clinical Psychiatry*, 43, 277–279.

Lewis, L. A. (1984). The coming-out process for lesbians: Integrating a stable identity. *Social Work*, 29(5), 464–469.

Lhomond, B. (1993). Between man and woman: The character of the lesbian. [Special Issue: Gay studies from the French cultures: Voices from France, Belgium, Brazil, Canada, and the Netherlands: I). *Journal of Homosexuality*, 25(1–2), 63–73.

Liddle, B. J. (1995). Sexual orientation bias among advanced graduate students of counseling and counseling psychology. *Counselor Education and Supervision*, 34(4), 321–331.

Liddle, B. J. (1996). Therapist sexual orientation, gender, and counseling practices as they relate to ratings of helpfulness by gay and lesbian clients. *Journal of Counseling Psychology*, 43, 394–401.

Liddle, B. J. (1999a). Gay and lesbian clients' ratings of psychiatrists, psychologists, social workers, and counselors. *Journal of Gay and Lesbian Psychotherapy*, 3(1), 81–93.

Liddle, B. J. (1999b). Recent improvement in mental health services to lesbian and gay clients. *Journal of Homosexuality*, 37(4), 127–137.

Lie, G., & Gentlewarrier, S. (1991). Intimate violence in lesbian relationships: Discussion of survey findings and practice implications. *Journal of Social Service Research*, 15(1–2), 41–59.

Lie, G., Schlitt, R., Bush, J., Montagne, M., & Reyes, L. (1991). Lesbians in currently aggressive relationships: How frequently do they report aggressive past relationships? *Violence and Victims*, 6(2), 121–135.

Lilling, A. H., & Friedman, R. C. (1995). Bias toward gay patients by psychoanalytic clinicians: An empirical investigation. *Archives of Sexual Behavior*, 24(5), 562–570.

Lima, G., Lo Presto, C. T., Sherman, M. F., & Sobelman, S. A. (1993). The relationship between homophobia and self-esteem in gay males with AIDS. *Journal of Homosexuality*, 25(4), 69–76.

Linde, R. (1998). Discussion: Eros in a gay dyad. *Gender and Psychoanalysis*, 3(3), 347–353.

Lindenbaum, J. (1985). The shattering of an illusion: The problem of competition in lesbian relationships. *Feminist Studies*, 11(1), 85–103.

Lipman, A. (1986). Homosexual relationships. *Generations*, 10(4), 51–54.

Liu, P. L., & Chan, C. S. (1996). Lesbian, gay, and bisexual Asian Americans and their families. In J. Lard & R. Green (Eds.), *Lesbians and gays in couples and families* (pp. 137–153). New York: Jossey-Bass.

Lock, J., & Steiner, H. (1999). Gay, lesbian, and bisexual youth risks for emotional, physical, and social problems: Results from a community-based survey. *Journal of the American Academy of Child and Adolescent Psychiatry*, 38(3), 297–304.

Lockhart, L., White, B., Causby, V, & Isaac, A. (1994). Letting out the secret: Violence in lesbian relationships. *Journal of Interpersonal Violence*, 9(4), 469–492.

Loiacano, D. K. (1989). Gay identity issues among Black Americans: Racism, homophobia, and the need for validation. *Journal of Counseling and Development*, 68(1), 21–25.

Logue, P. M. (2000, Winter). Family matters: Lambda's family work explained. *The Lambda Update*, pp. 6–7.

Lone Dog, L. (1991). Coming out as a Native American. In B. Sang, J. Warshow, & A. J. Smith (Eds.), *Lesbians at midlife: The creative transition* (pp. 49–53). San Francisco: Spinsters.

Lott-Whitehead, L.,& Tully, C. T. (1993). The family lives of lesbian mothers. [Special Issue: Lesbians and lesbian families: Multiple reflections]. *Smith College Studies in Social Work, 63*(3), 265–280.

Lottes, I. L., & Kuriloff, P. J. (1992). The effects of gender, race, religion, and political orientation on the sex role attitudes of college freshmen. *Adolescence, 27*(107), 675–688.

Loulan, J. (1984). *Lesbian sex.* San Francisco: Spinsters.

Loulan, J. 1986). Psychotherapy with lesbian mothers. In T. S. Stein & C. J. Cohen (Eds.), *Contemporary perspectives on psychotherapy with lesbians and gay men* (pp. 181–208). New York: Plenum.

Loulan, J. (1987). *Lesbian passion: Loving ourselves and each other.* San Francisco: Spinsters/Aunt Lute.

Loulan, J. (1988). Research on the sex practices of 1566 lesbians and the clinical applications. *Women and Therapy, 7*(2–3), 221–234.

Love, S. M. (2000). *Dr. Susan Love's breast book* (3rd ed.). New York: Perseus.

Lucco, A. J. (1987). Planned retirement housing preferences of older homosexuals. *Journal of Homosexuality, 14*(3–4), 35–56.

Lukes, C. A., & Land, H. (1990). Biculturality and homosexuality. *Social Work, 35*(2), 155–161.

Lundy, S. E., & Leventhal, B. (1999). *Same-sex domestic violence: Strategies for change.* Thousand Oaks, CA: Sage.

Lutgendorf, S. K., Antoni, M. H., Ironson, G., & Klimas, N. (1997). Cognitive-behavioral stress management decreases dysphoric mood and herpes simplex virus-Type 2 antibody titers in symptomatic HIV-seropositive gay men. *Journal of Consulting and Clinical Psychology, 65*(1), 31–43.

Lynch, F. R. (1987). Non-ghetto gays: A sociological study of suburban homosexuals. *Journal of Homosexuality, 13*(4), 13–42.

Lynch, J. M., & Murray, K. (2000). For the love of the children: The coming out process for lesbian and gay parents and stepparents. *Journal of Homosexuality, 39*(1), 1–24.

Lynch, J. M., & Reilly, M. E. (1986). Role relationships: Lesbian perspectives. *Journal of Homosexuality, 12*(2), 53–69.

MacEwan, I. (1994). Differences in assessment and treatment approaches for homosexual clients. *Drug and Alcohol Review, 13*(1), 57–62.

Mackey, R. A., O'Brien, B. A., & Mackey, E. F. (1997). *Gay and lesbian couples: Voices from lasting relationships.* Westport, CT: Praeger/Greenwood.

Magee, M., & Miller, D. C. (1996). Psychoanalytic views of female homosexuality. In R. P. Cabaj & T. S. Stein (Eds.), *Textbook of homosexuality and mental health* (pp. 191–206). Washington, DC: American Psychiatric Press.

Maguen, S., Armistead, L. P., & Kalichman, S. (2000). Predictors of HIV antibody testing among gay, lesbian, and bisexual youth. *Journal of Adolescent Health, 26*(4), 252–257.

Maguire, D. C. (1984). The morality of homosexual marriage. In R. Nugent (Ed.), *A challenge to love: Gay and lesbian Catholics in the church* (pp. 118–134). New York: Crossroad.

Malcolm, T. (1999a, July 30). Pair dealt a lifetime ban on ministry to homosexuals. *National Catholic Reporter,* pp. 3–4.

Malcolm, T. (1999b, July 30). Vatican ban ends years of investigation. *National Catholic Reporter,* p. 5.

Mallet, P., Apostolidis, T., & Paty, B. (1997). The development of gender schemata about heterosexual and homosexual others during adolescence. *Journal of General Psychology, 124*(1), 91–104.

Malyon, A. K. (1982). Psychotherapeutic implications of internalized homophobia in gay men. In J. C. Gonsiorek (Ed.), *Homosexuality and psychotherapy: A practitioner's handbook of affirmative models* (pp. 59–69). Binghamton, NY: Haworth Press.

Manalansan, M. F., IV. (1993). (Re)locating the gay Filipino: Resistance, postcolonialism, and identity. *Journal of Homosexuality, 26*(2–3), 53–72.

Manalansan, M. F., IV. (1996). Double minorities: Latino, Black, and Asian men who have sex with men. In R. C. Savin-Williams, & K. M. Cohen (Eds.), *The lives of lesbians, gays, and bisexuals: Children to adults* (pp. 393–415). Ft. Worth, TX: Harcourt Brace.

Marc Morrison v. State Board of Education, 74 Cal. Rptr. 116; 1 Cal. 3d 214; 461 P.2d 365; 82 Cal. Rptr. 175 (1969).

Marcus, E. (1992). *The male couple's guide: Finding a man, making a home, building a life* (rev. ed.). New York: HarperCollins.

Marcus, E. (1999). *Together forever: Gay and lesbian couples share their secrets for lasting happiness.* New York: Anchor/Doubleday.

Marder, J. R. (1985). Getting to know the gay and lesbian shul. *Reconstructionist, 51*(2), 20–25.

Maret, S. M. (1984). Attitudes of fundamentalists toward homosexuality. *Psychological Reports, 55,* 205–206.

Marion, M. (1996). Living in an era of multiple loss and trauma: Understanding global loss in the gay community. In C. J. Alexander (Ed.), *Gay and lesbian mental health: A sourcebook for practitioners* (pp. 61–93). New York: Harrington Park Press.

Markovic, N., & Aaron, D. J. (2000). *Sexual orientation identification and self-reported history of mental health concerns.* Paper presented at the 108th annual meeting of the American Psychological Association, Washington, DC.

Marmor, J. (1980). *Homosexual behavior: A modern reappraisal.* New York: Basic Books.

Marmor, J. (1996). Nongay therapists working with gay men and lesbians: A personal reflection. In R. P. Cabaj & T. S. Stein (Eds.), *Textbook of homosexuality and mental health* (pp. 539–545). Washington, DC: American Psychiatric Press.

Marrazzo, J. M., Koutsky, L. A., Stine, K., L., Kuypers, J. M., Grubert, T. A., Galloway, D. A., Kiviat, N. B., & Handsfield, H. H. (1998). Genital human papillomavirus infection in women who have sex with women. *Journal of Infectious Diseases, 178*(6), 1604–1609.

Marrazzo, J. M., Stine, K., & Koutsky, L. A. (2000). Genital human papillomavirus infection in women who have sex with women: A review. *American Journal of Obstetrics and Gynecology, 183*(3), 770–774.

Martin, A. (1993). *The lesbian and gay parenting handbook: Creating and raising our families.* New York: HarperCollins.

Martin, A. D. (1982). Learning to hide: The socialization of the gay adolescent. *Adolescent Psychiatry, 10,* 52–65.

Martin, A. D., & Hetrick, E. S. (1988). The stigmatization of the gay and lesbian adolescent. *Journal of Homosexuality, 15*(1–2), 163–183.

Mason, H. R. C., Marks, G., Simoni, J. M., & Ruiz, M. S. (1995). Culturally sanctioned secrets? Latino men's nondisclosure of HIV infection to family, friends, and lovers. *Health Psychology, 14*(1), 6–12.

Mass, L. (1983). The new narcissism and homosexuality. In M. Denneny, C. Ortleb, & T. Steele (Eds.), *The Christopher Street reader* (pp. 340–347). New York: Coward-McCann.

Masters, W. H., & Johnson, V. E. (1970). *Human sexual inadequacy.* Boston: Little, Brown.

Mathieson, C. M. (1998). Lesbian and bisexual health care. *Canadian Family Physician, 44,* 1634–1640.

Matt, H. J. (1978). Sin, crime, sickness or alternative life style? A Jewish approach to homosexuality. *Judaism, 27*(1), 13–24.

Matt, H. J. (1987). Homosexual rabbis? *Conservative Judaism, 39*(3), 29–33.

Matteson, D. R. (1996). Psychotherapy with bisexual individuals. In R. P. Cabaj & T. S. Stein (Eds.), *Textbook of homosexuality and mental health* (pp. 433–450). Washington, DC: American Psychiatric Press.

Mattison, A. M., & McWhirter, D. P. (1987a). Male couples: The beginning years. *Journal of Social Work and Human Sexuality, 5*(2), 67–78.

Mattison, A. M., & McWhirter, D. P. (1987b). Stage discrepancy in male couples. *Journal of Homosexuality, 14*(1–2), 89–99.

Matthews, A. K. (1998). Lesbians and cancer support: Clinical issues for cancer patients. *Health Care for Women International, 19*(3), 193–203.

Matthews, C. (1991). *Sophia, goddess of wisdom: The divine feminine from black goddess to world-soul.* London: Mandala.

Matthews, K. A., Shumaker, S. A., Bowen, D. J., Langer, R. D., Hunt, J. R., Kaplan, R. M., Klesges, R. C., & Ritenbaugh, C. (1997). Women's health initiative: Why now? What is it? What's new? *American Psychologist, 52*(2), 101–116.

Mayne, T. J., Acree, M., Chesney, M. A., & Folkman, S. (1998). HIV sexual risk behavior following bereavement in gay men. *Health Psychology, 17*(5), 403–411.

Mays, V. M., Chatters, L. M., Cochran, S. D., & Mackness, J. (1998). African American families in diversity: Gay men and lesbians as participants in family networks. *Journal of Comparative Family Studies, 29*(1), 73–87.

Mays, V. M., & Cochran, S. D. (1988). The Black women's relationship project: A national survey of Black lesbians. In M. Shernoff & W. A. Scott (Eds.), *The sourcebook on lesbian and gay healthcare* (2nd ed., pp. 54–62). Washington, DC: National Gay and Lesbian Health Foundation.

Mays, V. M., Cochran, S. D., & Rhue, S. (1993). The impact of perceived discrimination on the intimate relationships of Black lesbians. *Journal of Homosexuality, 25*(4), 1–14.

McCaffrey, M., Varney, P., Evans, B., & Taylor-Robinson, D. (1999). Bacterial vaginosis in lesbians: Evidence for lack of sexual transmission. *International Journal of STD and AIDS, 10*(5), 305–308.

McCandlish, B. M. (1982). Therapeutic issues with lesbian couples. *Journal of Homosexuality, 7*(2–3), 71–78.

McCandlish, B. M. (1987). Against all odds: Lesbian mother family dynamics. In F. W. Bozett (Ed.), *Gay and Lesbian Parents* (pp. 23–36). New York: Praeger.

McCarthy, L. (2000). Poppies in a wheat field: Exploring the lives of rural lesbians. *Journal of Homosexuality, 39*(1), 75–94.

McConaghy, N. (1987). Heterosexuality/homosexuality: Dichotomy or continuum. *Archives of Sexual Behavior, 16,* 411–424.

McConaghy, N., & Silove, D. (1991). Opposite sex behaviours correlate with degree of homosexual feelings in the predominantly heterosexual. *Australian and New Zealand Journal of Psychiatry, 25*(1), 77–83.

McConaghy, N., & Zamir, R. (1995). Sissiness, tomboyism, sex-role, sex identity and orientation. *Australian and New Zealand Journal of Psychiatry, 29*(2), 278–283.

McDaniel, J. S., Farber, E. W., & Summerville, M. B. (1996). Mental health care providers working with HIV: Avoiding stress and burnout. In R. P. Cabaj & T. S. Stein (Eds.), *Textbook of homosexuality and mental health* (pp. 839–858). Washington, DC: American Psychiatric Press.

McDonald, G. J. (1982). Individual differences in the coming out process of gay men: Implications for theoretical models. *Journal of Homosexuality, 8*(1), 47–60.

McDonald, H. B., & Steinhorn, A. I. (1993). *Understanding homosexuality: A guide for those who know, love, or counsel gay and lesbian individuals.* New York: Crossroad.

McDonell, J. R., Abell, N., & Miller, J. (1991). Family members' willingness to care for people with AIDS: A psychosocial assessment model. *Social Work, 36*(1), 43–53.

McDougall, G. J. (1993). Therapeutic issues with gay and lesbian elders. [Special Issue: The forgotten aged: Ethnic, psychiatric, and societal minorities]. *Clinical Gerontologist, 14*(1), 45–57.

McDowell, D. M., Levin, F. R., & Nunes, E. V. (1999). Dissociative identity disorder and substance abuse: The forgotten relationship. *Journal of Psychoactive Drugs, 31*(1), 71–83.

McFarland, S. G. (1989). Religious orientations and the targets of discrimination. *Journal for the Scientific Study of Religion, 28*(3), 324–336.

McGrath, E., Keita, G. P., Strickland, B. R., & Russo, N. F. (Eds.). (1990). *Women and depression: Risk factors and treatment issues.* Washington, DC: American Psychological Association.

McGuire, M. (1996, November 4). Growing up with two moms. *Newsweek,* p. 53.

McHenry, S. S., & Johnson, J. W. (1991). *The homophobic therapist and the homophobic gay or lesbian client: Conscious and unconscious collusions in self-hate.* Paper presented at the 99th annual meeting of the American Psychological Association, San Francisco.

McKechnie, J. L. (Sup.). (1971). *Webster's New 20th century dictionary of the English language* (2nd ed.). Cleveland, OH: World.

McKenzie, M. (1993, Summer). AIDS: Reaping the whirlwind. *Christian Research Journal, 16*(1), 9–15, 39–40.

McKenzie, S. (1992). Merger in lesbian relationships. *Women and Therapy, 12*(1–2), 151–160.

McKirnan, D. J., & Peterson, P. L. (1988). Stress, expectancies, and vulnerability to substance abuse: A test of a model among homosexual men. *Journal of Abnormal Psychology, 97*(4), 461–466.

McKirnan, D. J., & Peterson, P. L. (1989a). Alcohol and drug use among homosexual men and women: Epidemiology and population characteristics. *Addictive Behaviors, 14*(5), 545–553.

McKirnan, D. J., & Peterson, P. L. (1989b). Psychosocial and cultural factors in alcohol and drug abuse: A analysis of a homosexual community. *Addictive Behaviors, 14*(5), 555–563.

McNair, L., & Neville, H. (1996). African American women survivors of sexual assault: The intersection of race and class. In M. Hill & E. Rothblum (Eds.), *Classism and feminist therapy: Counting costs* (pp. 107–118). Binghamton, NY: Haworth Press.

McNally, E. B., & Finnegan, D. G. (1992). Lesbian recovering alcoholics: A qualitative study of identity transformation. A report on research and applications to treatment. *Journal of Chemical Dependency Treatment, 5*(1), 93–103.

McNaught, A., & Spicer, J. (2000). Theoretical perspectives on suicide in gay men with AIDS. *Social Science and Medicine, 51*(1), 65–72.

McNaught, B. (1988). *On being gay: Thoughts on family, faith, and love.* New York: St. Martin's Press.

McNeal, J. L. (1997). The association of idealization and intimacy factors with condom use in gay male couples. *Journal of Clinical Psychology in Medical Settings, 4*(4), 437–451.

McNeill, J. J. (1985). *The church and the homosexual* (3rd ed.). Boston: Beacon Press.

McNeill, J. J. (1988). *Taking a chance on God: Liberating theology for gays, lesbians, and their lovers, families, and friends.* Boston: Beacon Press.

McNeill, J. J. (1995). *Freedom glorious freedom: The spiritual journey to the fullness of life for gays, lesbians, and everybody else.* Boston: Beacon Press.

McNeill, J. J. (1998). *Both feet firmly planted in midair: My spiritual journey.* Louisville, KY: Westminster John Knox Press.

McNeill, K. F., Rienzi, B. M., & Kposowa, A. (1998). Families and parenting: A comparison of lesbian and heterosexual mothers. *Psychological Reports, 82,* 59–62.

McVinney, L. D. (1998). Social work practice with gay male couples. In G. P. Mallon (Ed.), *Foundations of social work practice with lesbian and gay persons* (pp. 209–227). New York: Harrington Park Press/Haworth Press.

McWhirter, D. P., & Mattison, A. M. (1980). Treatment of sexual dysfunction in homosexual male couples. In S. R. Leiblum & L. A. Pervin (Eds.), *Principles and practice of sex therapy* (pp. 321– 345). New York: Guilford Press.

McWhirter, D. P., & Mattison, A. M. (1982). Psychotherapy for gay male couples. In J. C. Gonsiorek (Ed.), *Homosexuality and psychotherapy: A practitioner's handbook of affirmative models* (pp. 79– 91). Binghamton, NY: Haworth Press.

McWhirter, D. P., & Mattison, A. M. (1984). *The male couple.* Englewood Cliffs, NJ: Prentice-Hall.

McWhirter, D. P., & Mattison, A. M. (1996). Male couples. In R. P. Cabaj & T. S. Stein (Eds.), *Textbook of homosexuality and mental health* (pp. 319–337). Washington, DC: American Psychiatric Press.

McWhirter, D. P., Sanders, S. A., & Reinisch, J. M. (Eds.). (1990). *Homosexuality/heterosexuality: Concepts of sexual orientation.* New York: Oxford University Press.

Mencher, J. (1990). *Intimacy in lesbian relationships: A critical re-examination of fusion.* (Work in Progress, No. 42). Wellesley, MA: Wellesley College, the Stone Center.

Mercier, L. R., & Berger, R. M. (1989). Social service needs of lesbian and gay adolescents: Telling it their way. *Journal of Social Work and Human Sexuality, 8*(1), 75–95.

Merrick v. Rio Bravo–Greeley Union School District, Lambda Legal Defense and Education Fund, No. 99-03985 (1999).

Meyer, I. H. (1995). Minority stress and mental health in gay men. *Journal of Health and Social Behavior, 36*(1), 38–56.

Meyer, I. H., & Dean, L. (1998). Internalized homophobia, intimacy, and sexual behavior among gay and bisexual men. In G. M. Herek (Ed.), *Stigma and sexual orientation: Understanding prejudice against lesbians, gay men, and bisexuals* (pp. 160–186). Thousand Oaks, CA: Sage.

Meyer, J. (1989). Guess who's coming to dinner this time? A study of gay intimate relationships and the support for those relationships. *Marriage and Family Review, 14*(3–4), 59–82.

Meyer, L. (1999, April 13). The state of hate: Hostile classrooms. *The Advocate,* pp. 33–35.

Meyer-Bahlburg, H. (1984). Psychoendocrine research on sexual orientation. Current status and future options. In G. J. De Vries, J. P. C. De Bruin, H. M. B. Uylings, & M. A. Corner (Eds.), *Progress in brain research* (Vol. 61, pp. 375–398). Amsterdam: Elsevier.

Michaels, S. (1996). The prevalence of homosexuality in the United States. In R. P. Cabaj & T. S. Stein

(Eds.). *Textbook of homosexuality and mental health* (pp. 43–63). Washington DC: American Psychiatric Press.

Midanik, L. T., Hines, A. M., Barrett, D. C., Paul, J. P., Crosby, G. M., & Stall, R. D. (1998). Self-reports of alcohol use, drug use and sexual behavior: Expanding the Timeline Follow-back technique. *Journal of Studies on Alcohol, 59*(6), 681–689.

Milic, J. H., & Crowne, D. P. (1986). Recalled parent-child relations and need for approval of homosexual and heterosexual men. *Archives of Sexual Behavior, 15*(3), 239–246.

Miller, J. B. (1976). *Toward a new psychology of women.* Boston: Beacon Press.

Milliger, C., & Young, M. (1990). Perceived acceptance and social isolation among recovering homosexual alcoholics. *International Journal of the Addictions, 25*(8), 947–955.

Mills, J. K. (1990). The psychoanalytic perspective of adolescent homosexuality: A review. *Adolescence, 25*(100), 913–922.

Minnigerode, F. A. (1976). Age-status labeling in homosexual men. *Journal of Homosexuality, 1*(3), 273–276.

Minnigerode, F. A., Adelman M. R., & Fox, D. (1980). *Aging and homosexuality: Physical and psychological well-being.* Unpublished manuscript, University of San Francisco.

Miranda, J., & Storms, M. (1989). Psychological adjustment of lesbians and gay men. *Journal of Counseling and Development, 68*(1), 41–45.

Misovich, S. J., Fisher, J. D., & Fisher, W. A. (1997). Close relationships and elevated HIV risk behavior: Evidence and possible underlying psychological processes. *Review of General Psychology, 1*(1), 72–107.

Mitchell, V. (1988). Using Kohut's self psychology in work with lesbian couples. *Women and Therapy, 8*(1–2), 157–166.

Moberly, E. R. (1986). Attachment and separation: The implication for gender identity and for the structuralization of the self: A theoretical model for transsexualism, and homosexuality. *Psychiatric Journal of the University of Ottawa, 11*(4), 205–209.

Mobley, M., & Slaney, R. B. (1996). Holland's theory: Its relevance for lesbian women and gay men. *Journal of Vocational Behavior, 48*, 125–135.

Money, J. (1988). *Gay, straight, and in-between: The sexology of erotic orientation.* New York: Oxford University Press.

Money, J., & Ehrhardt, A. A. (1972). *Man & woman Boy & girl: The differentiation and dimorphism of gender identity from conception to maturity.* New York: New American Library.

Money, J., Schwartz, M., & Lewis, V. G. (1984). Adult erotosexual status and fetal hormonal masculinization and demasculinization. *Psychoneuroendocrinology, 9*, 405–414.

Mooney-Somers, J., & Golombok, S. (2000). Children of lesbian mothers: From the 1970s to the new millennium. *Sexual and Relationship Therapy, 15*(2), 121–126.

Moraga, C. (1983). *Loving in the war years: Lo que nunca paso por sus labios.* Boston: South End.

Morales, E. S. (1989). Ethnic minority families and minority gays and lesbians. *Marriage and Family Review, 14*(3–4), 217–239.

Morales, E. S. (1990). HIV infection and Hispanic gay and bisexual men. *Hispanic Journal of the Behavioral Sciences, 12*(2), 212–222.

Morales, E. S. (1992). Counseling Latino gays and Latina lesbians. In S. H. Dworkin & F. J. Gutierrez (Eds.), *Counseling gay men and lesbians: Journey to the end of the rainbow* (pp. 125–139). Alexandria, VA: American Association for Counseling and Development.

Morales, E. S. (1996). Gender roles among Latino gay and bisexual men: Implications for family and couple relationships. In J. Laird & R. J. Green (Eds.), *Lesbian and gay couples and families: A handbook for therapists* (pp. 272–297). San Francisco: Jossey-Bass.

Moran, M. R. (1992). Effects of sexual orientation similarity and counselor experience level on gay men's and lesbians' perceptions of counselors. *Journal of Counseling Psychology, 39*(2), 247–251.

Moran, N. (1996). Lesbian health care needs. *Canadian Family Physician, 42*, 879–884.

Morgan, K. S. (1992). Caucasian lesbians' use of psychotherapy: A matter of attitude? *Psychology of Women Quarterly, 16*(1), 127–130.

Morgan, K. S. (1997). Why lesbians choose therapy: Presenting problems, attitudes, and political concerns. *Journal of Gay and Lesbian Social Services, 6*(3), 57–75.

Morgan, K. S., & Brown, L. S. (1991). Lesbian career development, work behavior, and vocational counseling. *Counseling Psychologist, 19*(2), 273–291.

Morgenthaler, F. (1988). *Homosexuality, heterosexuality, perversion* (A. Aebi, Trans., P. Moor, Ed.). Hillsdale, NJ: Analytic Press. (Original work published 1984)

Morin, S. (1977). Heterosexual bias in psychological research on lesbianism and male homosexuality. *American Psychologist, 32*, 629–637.

Morin, S., & Garfinkle, E. (1978). Male homophobia. *Journal of Social Issues, 34*(1), 29–47.

Morris, J. F. (2000). *Lesbian women of color in communities: Social activities and mental health services.* Paper presented at the 108th annual meeting of the American Psychological Association, Washington, DC.

Morris, J. F., & Rothblum, E. D. (1999) Who fills out a "lesbian" questionnaire?: The interrelation of sexual orientation, years "out," disclosure of sexual orientation, sexual experience with women, and participation in the lesbian community. *Psychology of Women Quarterly, 23*, 537–557.

Morrow, D. F. (1996). Coming out issues for adult lesbians: A group intervention. *Social Work, 41*(6), 647–656.

Morrow, G. D. (1989). Bisexuality: An exploratory overview. *Annals of Sex Research, 2*(4), 283–306.

Morrow, S. L., Gore, P. A. Jr., & Campbell, B. W. (1996). The application of a sociocognitive framework to the career development of lesbian women and gay men. *Journal of Vocational Behavior, 48*(2), 136–148.

Morrow, S. L., & Hawxhurst, D. M. (1989). Lesbian partner abuse: Implications for therapists. *Journal of Counseling and Development, 68*(1), 58–62.

Morton, S. B. (1998). Lesbian divorce. *American Journal of Orthopsychiatry, 68*(3), 410–419 (discussion 420–423).

Mosbacher, D. (1988). Lesbian alcohol and substance abuse. *Psychiatric Annals, 18*(1), 47–50.

Moss, D. (1992). Introductory thoughts: Hating in the first person plural: The example of homophobia. *American Imago, 49*(3), 277–291.

Muehrer, P. (1995). Suicide and sexual orientation: A critical summary of recent research and directions for future research. *Suicide and Life-Threatening Behavior, 25*(Suppl.), 1–10.

Mulder, C. L., Antoni, M. H., Duivenvoorden, H. J., & Kauffmann, R. H. (1995). Active confrontational coping predicts decreased clinical progression over a one-year period in HIV-infected homosexual men. *Journal of Psychosomatic Research, 39*(8), 957–965.

Muller, A. (1987). *Parents matter: Parents' relationships with lesbian daughters and gay sons.* Tallahassee, FL: Naiad.

Munson, M. (1996). Eliminating the barriers to communication: Safer sex education for lesbians and bisexual women. *Women and Therapy, 19*(4), 75–84.

Murphy, B. C. (1989). Lesbian couples and their parents: The effects of perceived parental attitudes on the couple. *Journal of Counseling and Development, 68*(1), 46–51.

Murphy, T. F. (1992). Redirecting sexual orientation: Techniques and justifications. *Journal of Sex Research, 29*(4), 501–523.

Murray, S. O. (1991). "Homosexual occupations" in Mesoamerica? *Journal of Homosexuality, 21*(4), 57–65.

Myers, H. F., Satz, P., Miller, B. E., Bing, E. G., Evans, G., Richardson, M. A., Forney, D., Morgenstern, H., Saxton, E., D'Elia, L., Longshore, D., & Mena, I. (1997). The African-American Health Project (AAHP): Study overview and select findings on high risk behaviors and psychiatric disorders in African American men. *Ethnic Health, 2*(3), 183–196.

Myers, M. F. (1982). Counseling the parents of young homosexual male patients. *Journal of Homosexuality, 7*(2–3), 131–143.

Nakajima, G. A., Chan, Y. H., & Lee, K. (1996). Mental health issues for gay and lesbian Asian Americans. In R. P. Cabaj & T. S. Stein (Eds.), *Textbook of homosexuality and mental health* (pp. 563–581). Washington, DC: American Psychiatric Press.

Nardi, P. M. (1982). Alcoholism and homosexuality: A theoretical perspective. *Journal of Homosexuality*, 7(4), 9–25.

Nardi, P., & Sherrod, D. (1990, Spring). That's what friends are for: The results. *OUT/LOOK, 8,* 86.

National Coalition for the Homeless. (1990). *Fighting to live: Homeless people with AIDS.* Washington, DC: Author.

National focus for lesbian survivors. (2000, October 10). *The Advocate,* p. 20.

National Institute of Mental Health (NIMH). (1987). *National lesbian health care survey.* Washington, DC: U.S. Department of Health and Human Services.

National Opinion Research Center. (1998). GSSDIRS 98: *General Social Survey 1972–1998 Cumulative Codebook* [Online]. Available: http://www.icpsr.umich.edu/GSS/

Neisen, J. H. (1990). Heterosexism: Redefining homophobia for the 1990s. *Journal of Gay and Lesbian Psychotherapy, 1*(3), 21–35.

Neisen, J. H., & Sandall, H. (1990). Alcohol and other drug abuse in a gay/lesbian population: Related to victimization? *Journal of Psychology and Human Sexuality, 3*(1), 151–168.

Nelson, E. S. (Ed.). (1993). Preface to critical essays: Gay and lesbian writers of color [Special double issue]. *Journal of Homosexuality, 26*(2–3).

Nelson, J. A. (1997). Gay, lesbian, and bisexual adolescents: Providing esteem-enhancing care to a battered population. *Nurse Practitioner, 22*(2), 94, 99, 103.

Nelson, J. B. (1982). Religious and moral issues in working with homosexual clients. *Journal of Homosexuality, 7*(2–3), 163–175.

Nelson, J. B. (1983). *Between two gardens: Reflections on sexuality and religious experience.* New York: Pilgrim Press.

Neuringer, C. (1989). On the question of homosexuality in actors. *Archives of Sexual Behavior, 18*(6), 523–529.

Newman, B. S., & Muzzonigro, P. G. (1993). The effects of traditional family values on the coming out process of gay male adolescents. *Adolescence, 28,* 213–226.

Newman, F. (1999). *The whole lesbian sex book: A passionate guide for all of us.* Pittsburgh, PA: Cleis Press.

Newman, J. L., Fuqua, D. R., & Seaworth, T. B. (1989). The role of anxiety in career indecision: Implications for diagnosis and treatment. *Career Development Quarterly, 37,* 221–231.

Newton, D. E., & Risch, S. J. (1981). Homosexuality and education: A review of the issue. *The High School Journal, 64,* 191–202.

Nichols, M. (1982, Winter). The treatment of inhibited sexual desire (ISD) in lesbian couples. *Women and Therapy, 1,* 49–66.

Nichols, M. (1987a). Doing sex therapy with lesbians: Bending a heterosexual paradigm to fit a gay lifestyle. In Boston Lesbian Psychologies Collective (Ed.), *Lesbian psychologies: Explorations and challenges* (pp. 242–260). Urbana: University of Illinois Press.

Nichols, M. (1987b). Lesbian sexuality: Issues and developing theory. In Boston Lesbian Psychologies Collective (Ed.), *Lesbian psychologies: Explorations and challenges* (pp. 97–125). Urbana: University of Illinois Press.

Nichols, M. (1989). Sex therapy with lesbians, gay men, and bisexuals. In S. R. Leiblum & R. C. Rosen (Eds.), *Principles and practice of sex therapy: Update for the 1990s* (2nd ed., pp. 269–297). New York: Guilford Press.

Nichols, M. (1990). Lesbian relationships: Implications for the study of sexuality and gender. In D. P. McWhirter, S. A. Sanders, & J. M. Reinisch (Eds.). *Homosexuality/heterosexuality: Concepts of sexual orientation* (pp. 350–364). New York: Oxford University Press.

Nicholson, W. D., & Long, B. C. (1990). Self-esteem, social support, internalized homophobia, and coping strategies of HIV+ gay men. *Journal of Consulting and Clinical Psychology, 58,* 873–876.

Nicoloff, L. K., & Stiglitz, E. A. (1987). Lesbian alcoholism: Etiology, treatment, and recovery. In Boston Lesbian Psychologies Collective (Ed.), *Lesbian psychologies: Explorations and challenges* (pp. 283–293). Urbana: University of Illinois Press.

Nicolosi, J., Byrd, A. D., & Potts, R. W. (2000). Beliefs and practices of therapists who practice sexual reorientation psychotherapy. *Psychological Reports, 86,* 689–702.

Nugent, R. (Ed.). (1984a). *A challenge to love: Gay and lesbian Catholics in the church.* New York: Crossroad.

Nugent, R. (1984b). Priest, celibate and gay: You are not alone. In R. Nugent (Ed.), *A challenge to love: Gay and lesbian Catholics in the church* (pp. 257–277). New York: Crossroad.

Nugent, R., & Gramick, J. (1992). *Building bridges: Gay and lesbian reality and the Catholic church.* Mystic, CT: Twenty-Third Publications.

O'Brien, K. (1992). Primary relationships affect the psychological health of homosexual men at risk for AIDS. *Psychological Reports, 71*(1), 147–153.

O'Connor, M. F. (1992). Psychotherapy with gay and lesbian adolescents. In S. H. Dworkin & F. J. Gutierrez (Eds.). *Counseling gay men and lesbians: Journey to the end of the rainbow* (pp. 3–21). Alexandria VA: American Association for Counseling and Development.

O'Connor, N., & Ryan, J. (1993). *Wild desires & mistaken identities: Lesbianism & psychoanalysis.* New York: Columbia University Press.

O'Hanlan, K. A. (1995, March 7). Homophobia in lesbian health care. *The Advocate,* pp. 47–49.

O'Hanlan, K. (2000). Health concerns of lesbians. In R. M. Eisler & H. Hersen (Eds.), *Handbook of gender, culture, and health* (pp. 377–404). Mahwah, NJ: Erlbaum.

O'Hanlan, K. A., & Crum C. P. (1996). Human papillomavirus-associated cervical intraepithelial neoplasia following lesbian sex. *Obstetrics and Gynecology, 88*(4, Pt. 2), 702–703.

O'Neill, C., & Ritter, K. (1992). *Coming out within: Stages of spiritual awakening for lesbians and gay men.* San Francisco: Harper.

Oordt, M. S. (1990). Ethics of practice among Christian psychologists: A pilot study. *Journal of Psychology and Theology, 18*(3), 255–260.

Orzek, A. M. (1992). Career counseling for the gay and lesbian community. In S. H. Dworkin & F. J. Gutierrez (Eds.), *Counseling gay men and lesbians: Journey to the end of the rainbow* (pp. 23–33). Alexandria VA: American Association for Counseling and Development.

Ostrow, D. G. (1996). Mental health issues across the HIV-1 spectrum for gay and bisexual men. In R. P. Cabaj & T. S. Stein (Eds.), *Textbook of homosexuality and mental health* (pp. 859–879). Washington, DC: American Psychiatric Press.

Outland, O. (1998). *The principles: The gay man's guide to getting (and keeping) Mr. Right.* New York: Kensington.

Page, S., & Yee, M. (1985). Conception of male and female homosexual stereotypes among university undergraduates. *Journal of Homosexuality, 12*(1), 109–118.

Pagtolun-An, I. G., & Clair, J. M. (1986). An experimental study of attitudes toward homosexuals. *Deviant Behavior, 7*(2), 121–135.

Palerno, T. (1999). *Sex adviser: The 100 most asked questions about sex between men.* Boston: Alyson.

Paradis, B. A. (1991). Seeking intimacy and integration: Gay men in the era of AIDS. *Smith College Studies in Social Work, 61*(3), 260–274.

Paradis, B. A. (1993). A self psychological approach to the treatment of gay men with AIDS. *Clinical Social Work Journal, 21*(4), 405–416.

Paris, J., Zwieg-Frank, H., & Guzder, J. (1995). Psychological factors associated with homosexuality in males with borderline personality disorder. *Journal of Personality Disorders, 9*(1), 56–61.

Parks, C. A. (1999). Bicultural competence: A mediating factor affecting alcohol use practices and problems among lesbian social drinkers. *Journal of Drug Issues, 29*(1), 135–153.

Paroski, P. A. (1990). Gay and lesbian teens. In R. J. Kus (Ed.), *Keys to caring: Assisting your gay & lesbian clients* (pp. 160–169). Boston: Alyson.

Patel, A., DeLong, G., Voigl, B., & Medina, C. (2000). Pelvic inflammatory disease in the lesbian population—lesbian health issues: Asking the right questions. *Obstetrics and Gynecology, 95*(4, Suppl. 1), S29–S30.

Patel, S., Long, T. E., McCammon, S. L., & Wuensch, K. L. (1995). Personality and emotional correlates of self-reported antigay behaviors. *Journal of Interpersonal Violence, 10*(3), 354–366.

Patterson, C. J. (1992). Children of lesbian and gay parents. *Child Development, 63,* 1025–1042.

Patterson, C. J. (1994). Children of the lesbian baby boom: Behavioral adjustment, self-concepts, and sex role identity. In B. Greene & G. M. Herek (Eds.), *Lesbian and gay psychology: Theory, research, and clinical applications* (pp. 156–175). Thousand Oaks, CA: Sage.

Patterson, C. J. (1995a). Lesbian mothers, gay fathers, and their children. In A. R. D'Augelli & C. J. Patterson (Eds.), *Lesbian, gay, and bisexual identities over the lifespan* (pp. 262–290). New York: Oxford University Press.

Patterson, C. J. (1995b). Summary of research findings. In Committees on Women in Psychology, Lesbian and Gay Concerns, and Children, Youth, and Families, *Lesbian and gay parenting: A resource for psychologists* (pp. 1–12). Washington, DC: American Psychological Association.

Patterson, C. J. (1996). Lesbian and gay parents and their children. In R. C. Savin-Williams & K. M. Cohen (Eds.), *The lives of lesbians, gays, and bisexuals: Children to adults* (pp. 274–304). Fort Worth, TX: Harcourt Brace.

Patterson, C. J. (1997a). Children of lesbian and gay parents. *Advances in Clinical Child Psychology, 19,* 235–282.

Patterson, C. J. (1997b, October 6). *Lesbian health research* (testimony before the Committee on Lesbian Health Research Priorities, Institute of Medicine, National Academy of Sciences).

Patterson, C. J. (1998). The family lives of children born to lesbian mothers. In C. J. Patterson & A. R. D'Augelli (Eds.), *Lesbian, gay, and bisexual identities in families: Psychological perspectives* (pp. 154–176). New York: Oxford University Press.

Patterson, C. J., & Chan, R. W. (1996). Gay fathers and their children. In R. P. Cabaj & T. S. Stein (Eds.). *Textbook of homosexuality and mental health* (pp. 371–393). Washington, DC: American Psychiatric Press.

Paul, J. (1991). Ask the board: From psychology, case 1. *Journal of Gay and Lesbian Psychotherapy, 1*(4), 3–5.

Paul, J. P. (1993). Childhood cross-gender behavior and adult homosexuality: The resurgence of biological models of sexuality. *Journal of Homosexuality, 24*(3–4), 41–54.

Paul, J. P. (1996). Bisexuality: Exploring/exploding the boundaries. In R. C. Savin-Williams & K. M. Cohen (Eds.), *The lives of lesbians, gays, and bisexuals: Children to adults* (pp. 436–461). Fort Worth, TX: Harcourt Brace.

Paul, J. P., Hays, R. B., & Coates, T. J. (1995). The impact of the HIV epidemic on U. S. gay male communities. In A. R. D'Augelli & C. J. Patterson (Eds.), *Lesbian, gay, and bisexual identities over the lifespan: Psychological perspectives* (pp. 347–397). New York: Oxford University Press.

Pearlman, S. F. (1988). Distancing and connectedness: Impact on couple formation in lesbian relationships. *Women and Therapy, 8*(1–2), 77–88.

Pearlman, S. F. (1995). Making gender: New interpretations/New narratives. In J. M. Glassgold & S. Iasenza (Eds.), *Lesbians and psychoanalysis: Revolutions in theory and practice* (pp. 309–325). New York: Free Press.

Pearlman, S. F. (1996). Loving across race and class divides: Relational challenges and the interracial lesbian couple. *Women and Therapy, 19*(3), 25–35.

Penn, R. E. (1998). *The gay men's wellness guide.* New York: Henry Holt/Owl Books.

Pennington, S. (1989). *Ex-gays? There are none!* Hawthorne, CA: Lambda Christian Fellowship.

Pennington, S. B. (1987). Children of lesbian mothers. In F. W. Bozett (Ed.), *Gay and lesbian parents* (pp. 58–74). New York: Praeger.

Peplau, L. A. (1981, March). What homosexuals want. *Psychology Today,* pp. 28–38.

Peplau, L. A., & Cochran, S. D. (1980). *Sex differences in values concerning love relationships.* Paper presented at the 88th annual meeting of the American Psychological Association, Montreal, Canada.

Peplau, L. A., & Cochran, S. D. (1981). Value orientations in the intimate relationships of gay men. *Journal of Homosexuality, 6*(3), 1–19.

Peplau, L. A., & Cochran, S. D. (1990). A relationship perspective on homosexuality. In D. P. McWhirter, S. A. Sanders, & J. M. Reinisch (Eds.). *Homosexuality/heterosexuality: Concepts of sexual orientation* (pp. 321–349). New York: Oxford University Press.

Peplau, L. A., Cochran, S. D., & Mays, V. (1986). *Satisfaction in the intimate relationships of Black lesbians.* Paper presented at the 94th annual meeting of the American Psychological Association, Los Angeles, California.

Peplau, L. A., Cochran, S. D., & Mays, V. M. (1997). A national survey of the intimate relationships of African American lesbians and gay men: A look at commitment, satisfaction, sexual behavior, and HIV disease. In B. Greene (Ed.), *Ethnic and cultural diversity among lesbians and gay men* (pp. 11–38). Thousand Oaks, CA: Sage.

Peplau, L. A., Padesky, C., & Hamilton, M. (1982). Satisfaction in lesbian relationships. *Journal of Homosexuality, 8*(2), 23–35.

Peplau, L. A., Veniegas, R. C., & Campbell, S. M. (1996). Gay and lesbian relationships. In R. C. Savin-Williams & K. M. Cohen (Eds.), *The lives of lesbians, gays, and bisexuals: Children to adults* (pp. 250–273). Fort Worth, TX: Harcourt Brace.

Perkins, M. W. (1978). On birth order among lesbians. *Psychological Reports, 43*(3, Pt. 1), 814.

Perrin, E. C., & Kulkin, H. (1996). Pediatric care for children whose parents are gay or lesbian. *Pediatrics, 97*(5), 629–635.

Perry, S. T. (1995). Lesbian alcohol and marijuana use: Correlates of HIV risk behaviors and abusive relationships. *Journal of Psychoactive Drugs, 27*(4), 413–419.

Perry, S. W., Ryan, J., Fogel, K., & Fishman, B. (1990). Voluntarily informing others of positive HIV test results: Patterns of notification by infected gay men. *Hospital and Community Psychiatry, 41*(5), 549–551.

Perry, T. (1987). *The Lord is my shepherd and He knows I'm gay.* Austin, TX: Liberty Press.

Peters, D. K., & Cantrell, P. J. (1991). Factors distinguishing samples of lesbian and heterosexual women. *Journal of Homosexuality, 21*(4), 1–15.

Peterson J. L. (1992). Black men and their same-sex desires and behaviors. In G. H. Herdt (Ed.), *Gay culture in America: Essays from the field* (pp. 147–164). Boston: Beacon Press.

Peterson, J. W. (1989, April 11). In harm's way: Gay runaways are in more danger than ever, and gay adults won't help. *The Advocate,* pp. 8–10.

Phelan, S. (1993). (Be)coming out: Lesbian identity and politics. *Journal of Women in Culture and Society, 18*(4), 765–790.

Phelps, D. (2000). Why gay men should care about breast cancer [Online]. Available: http://www.advocate.com/html/washper820_washper.html.

Phillips, G., & Over, R. (1992). Adult sexual orientation in relation to memories of childhood gender conforming and gender nonconforming behaviors. *Archives of Sexual Behavior, 21*(6), 543–558.

Phillips J. C., & Fischer, A. R. (1998). Graduate students' training experiences with lesbian, gay, and bisexual issues. *The Counseling Psychologist, 26*(5), 712–734.

Pillard, R. C. (1991a). Ask the board: From psychiatry, case 1. *Journal of Gay and Lesbian Psychotherapy, 1*(4), 1–3.

Pillard, R. C. (1991b). Masculinity and femininity in homosexuality: "Inversion" revisited. In J. C. Gonsiorek & J. D. Weinrich (Eds.), *Homosexuality: Research implications for public policy* (pp. 32–43). Newbury Park, CA: Sage.

Pillard, R. C. (1996). Homosexuality from a familial and genetic perspective. In R. P. Cabaj & T. S. Stein (Eds.), *Textbook of homosexuality and mental health* (pp. 115–128). Washington, DC: American Psychiatric Press.

Pillard, R. C., Poumadere, J. I., & Carretta, R. A. (1981). Is homosexuality familial? A review, some data, and a suggestion. *Archives of Sexual Behavior, 10,* 465–475.

Pincu, L. (1989). Sexual compulsivity in gay men: Controversy and treatment. *Journal of Counseling and Development, 68*(1), 63–68.

Platzer, H. (1998). The concerns of lesbians seeking counseling: A review of the literature. *Patient Education and Counseling, 33*(3), 225–232.

Pleak, R. R. (1999). Ethical issues in diagnosing and treating gender-dysphoric children and adolescents. In M. Rottnek (Ed.), *Sissies and tomboys: Gender nonconformity and homosexual childhood* (pp. 34–51). New York: New York University Press.

Pleck, J. H., Sonenstein, F. L., & Ku, L. C. (1994). Attitudes toward male roles among adolescent males: A discriminant validity analysis. *Sex Roles, 30*(7–8), 481–501.

Plummer, K. (1975). *Sexual stigma: An interactionist account.* London: Routledge & Kegan Paul.

Ponse, B. (1978). *Identities in the lesbian world: The social construction of self.* Westport, CT: Greenwood Press.

Ponticelli, C. M. (1998). *Gateways to improving lesbian health and health care: Opening doors.* Binghamton, NY: Haworth Press.

Pope John Paul II. (1995). *Catechism of the Catholic Church.* New York: Image, Doubleday.

Pope, M. (1995). Career interventions for gay and lesbian clients: A synopsis of practice knowledge and research needs. *Career Development Quarterly, 44,* 191–203.

Pope, M. (1996). Gay and lesbian career counseling: Special career counseling issues. In A. L. Ellis & E. D. B. Riggle (Eds.), *Sexual identity on the job: Issues and services* (pp. 91–105). New York: Haworth Press.

Potgieter, C. (1997). From apartheid to Mandela's constitution: Black South African lesbians in the nineties. In B. Greene (Ed.), *Ethnic and cultural diversity among lesbians and gay men* (pp. 88–116). Thousand Oaks, CA: Sage.

Powell-Cope, G. M. (1995). The experiences of gay couples affected by HIV infection. *Qualitative Health Research, 5*(1), 36–62.

Prairielands. (2000). *Centers of excellence for substance abuse among lesbian, gay, bisexual and transgendered persons: Substance abuse treatment provider survey results.* Iowa City, IA: Prairielands Addiction Technology Transfer Centee [Online]. Available: http://www.uiowa.edu/~attc/attc_cofe_lgbt_survey.html.

Price, J. H., & Telljohann, S. K. (1991). School counselors' perceptions of adolescent homosexuals. *Journal of School Health, 61,* 433–438.

Prichard, J. G., Dial, L. K., Holloway, R. L., & Mosley, M. (1988). Attitudes of family medicine residents toward homosexuality. *Journal of Family Practice, 27*(6), 637–639.

Prime Timers Worldwide. (1997). *Original prime timers worldwide: Who are prime timers?* [Online]. Available: http://www.teleport.com/~pt.

Prince, J. P. (1997). Career assessment with lesbian, gay, and bisexual individuals. *Journal of Career Assessment, 5*(2), 225–238.

PsycINFO [Electronic data tape]. (1997). Washington, DC: American Psychological Association [Producer and Distributor].

Quam, J. K., & Whitford, G. S. (1992) Adaptation and age-related expectations of older gay and lesbian adults. *Gerontologist, 32*(3), 367–374.

Questions for couples: The results. (1989, Summer). *OUT/LOOK, 5,* 86.

Quick facts: Hate crimes. (2001). *Human Rights Campaign.* [Online]. Available: http://www.hrc.org/issues/hate_crimes/quickfacts.asp.

Quinodoz, J. M. (1989). Female homosexual patients in pyschoanalysis. *International Journal of Psycho-Analysis, 70,* 55–63.

Raab, B. (2000, June 20). A very open house. *The Advocate,* pp. 105–106.

Radkowsky, M., & Siegel, L. J. (1997). The gay adolescent: Stressors, adaptations, and psychosocial interventions. *Clinical Psychology Review, 17*(2), 191–216.

Radonsky, V. E., & Borders, L. D. (1995). Factors influencing lesbians' direct disclosure of their sexual orientation. *Journal of Gay and Lesbian Psychotherapy, 2*(3), 17–37.

Ramos, J. (Ed.) (1994). *Compañeras: Latina lesbians.* New York: Routledge.

Rankow, E. J. (1995). Lesbian health issues for the primary care provider. *Journal of Family Practice, 40*(5), 486–496.

Ratner, E. (1988). Model for the treatment of lesbian and gay alcohol abusers. *Alcohol Treatment Quarterly, 5*(1–2), 25–46.

Ratti, R. (Ed.). (1993). *A lotus of another color: An unfolding of the South Asian gay and lesbian experience.* New York: Alyson.

Razzano, L. A., Hamilton, M. M., & Hughes, T. L. (2000). *Mental health services utilization patterns among lesbians and heterosexual women.* Paper presented at the 108th annual meeting of the American Psychological Association, Washington, DC.

Reece, R. (1982). Group treatment of sexual dysfunction in gay men. In J. C. Gonsiorek (Ed.), *Homosexuality and psychotherapy: A practitioner's handbook of affirmative models* (pp. 113–129). Binghamton, NY: Haworth Press.

Reece, R. (1987). Causes and treatments of sexual desire discrepancies in male couples. *Journal of Homosexuality, 14*(1–2), 157–172.

Reece, R., & Segrist, A. E. (1981). The association of selected "masculine" sex-role variables with length of relationship in gay male couples. *Journal of Homosexuality, 7*(1), 33–47.

Reid, J. D. (1995). Development in late life: Older lesbian and gay lives. In A. R. D'Augelli & C. J. Patterson (Eds.), *Lesbian, gay, and bisexual identities over the lifespan* (pp. 215–240). New York: Oxford University Press.

Reilly, M. E., & Lynch, J. M. (1990). Power-sharing in lesbian relationships. *Journal of Homosexuality, 19*(3), 1–30.

Reilly, P. L. (1995). *A God who looks like me: Discovering a woman-affirming spirituality.* New York: Ballantine.

Reiss, B. F. (1987). Transference and countertransference in therapy with homosexuals. *Dynamic Psychotherapy, 5*(2), 117–129.

Reiter, L. (1991). Developmental origins of antihomosexual prejudice in heterosexual men and women. *Clinical Social Work Journal, 19*(2), 163–175.

Remafedi, G. (1987a). Adolescent homosexuality: Psychosocial and medical implications. *Pediatrics, 79*(3), 331–337.

Remafedi, G. (1987b). Male homosexuality: The adolescent's perspective. *Pediatrics, 79*(3), 326–330.

Remafedi, G. (Ed.). (1994). *Death by denial: Studies of suicide in gay and lesbian teenagers.* Boston: Alyson.

Remafedi, G. (1999). Suicide and sexual orientation: Nearing the end of controversy? *Archives of General Psychiatry, 56*(10), 885–886.

Remafedi, G., Farrow, J. A., & Deisher, R. W. (1991). Risk factors for attempted suicide in gay and bisexual youth. *Pediatrics, 87*(6), 869–875.

Remafedi, G. J. (1985). Adolescent homosexuality: Issues for pediatricians. *Clinical Pediatrics, 24*(9), 481–485.

Remien, R. H., & Rabkin, J. G. (1995). Long-term survival with AIDS and the role of the community. In G. M. Herek & B. Greene (Eds.), *AIDS, identity, and community: The HIV epidemic and lesbians and gay men* (pp. 169–186). Thousand Oaks, CA: Sage.

Renzetti, C. M. (1992). *Violent betrayal: Partner abuse in lesbian relationships.* Thousand Oaks, CA: Sage.

Renzetti, C. M. (1997). Violence and abuse among same-sex couples. In A. Cascarelli (Ed.), *Violence betweeen intimate partners: Patterns, causes and effects.* Boston: Allyn & Bacon.

Renzetti, C. M., & Miley, C. H. (Eds.). (1996). *Violence in gay and lesbian domestic partnerships.* Binghamton, NY: Haworth Press.

Results of poll. (1989, June 6). *San Francisco Examiner,* p. A19.

Reynolds, A. L., & Pope, R. L. (1991). The complexities of diversity: Exploring multiple oppressions. *Journal of Counseling and Development, 70*(1), 174–180.

Rich, B. R. (2000, July 18). Ming has two mommies. *The Advocate,* p. 45.

Rich, C. L., Fowler, R. C., Young, D., & Blenkush, M. (1986). San Diego suicide study: Comparison of gay to straight males. *Suicide and Life-Threatening Behavior, 16*(4), 448–457.

Richards, D. (1990). *Lesbian lists: A look at lesbian culture, history, and personalities.* Boston: Alyson.

Richardson, D. (1987). Recent challenges to traditional assumptions about homosexuality: Some implications for practice. *Journal of Homosexuality, 13*(4), 1–12.

Richardson, J. (1996). Setting limits on gender health. *Harvard Review of Psychiatry, 4*(1), 49–53.

Ricketts, W., & Achtenberg, R. (1989). Adoption and foster parenting for lesbians and gay men: Creating new traditions in the family. *Marriage and Family Review, 14*(3–4), 83–118.

Ricks, I. (1993, December 28). Mind games. *The Advocate,* pp. 39–40.

Rimer, S. (1993, December 8). Gay rights law for schools advances in Massachusetts. *The New York Times,* p. 1.

Ristock, J. L. (1998). Community-based research: Lesbian abuse and other telling tales. In J. L. Ristock & C. G. Taylor (Eds.), *Inside the academy and out: Lesbian/gay/queer studies and social action* (pp. 137–154). Toronto: University of Toronto Press.

Ritter, K. Y., & O'Neill, C. W. (1989). Moving through loss: The spiritual journey of gay men and lesbian women. *Journal of Counseling and Development, 68,* 9–15.

Ritter, K. Y., & O'Neill, C. W. (1996). *Righteous religion: Unmasking the illusions of fundamentalism and authoritarian Catholicism.* Binghamton, NY: Haworth Pastoral Press.

Rivera, R. R. (1991). Sexual orientation and the law. In J. C. Gonsiorek & J. D. Weinrich (Eds.), *Homosexuality: Research implications for public policy* (pp. 81–100). Newbury Park, CA: Sage.

Rivers, I. (2000). Social exclusion, absenteeism and sexual minority youth. *Support for Learning, 15*(1), 13–18.

Roades, L. A., Weber, C., & Biaggio, M. (1998). *Diagnosing borderline personality: Do sexual orientation, gender, and ethnicity matter?* Paper presented at the 106th annual meeting of the American Psychological Association, San Francisco.

Roberts, S. J. (1999). *Childhood experiences with sexaul abuse among lesbians.* Paper presented at the 107th annual meeting of the American Psychological Association, Boston.

Roberts, S. J., & Sorensen, L. (1999). Health related behaviors and cancer screening of lesbians: Results from the Boston Lesbian Health Project. *Women and Health, 28*(4), 1–12.

Robins, A. G. (1998). A cross-sectional analysis of psychosocial covariates and substance use: Risky sexual practices of urban gay men. *Dissertation Abstracts International, 58*(12-B), 6522. (University Microfilms No. AAM98–20045)

Robinson, J. D., & Parks, C. W. (1999). *Daydreaming activity and its impact on relationship satisfaction among lesbian survivors of childhood sexual abuse and their partners.* Paper presented at the 107th annual meeting of the American Psychological Association, Boston.

Rocchio, G., & Merciadez, J. (1992, Spring). Race & relationships. *OUT/LOOK, 16,* 84–85.

Rochman, S. (1999a, May 25). Between women. *The Advocate,* pp. 73–74.

Rochman, S. (1999b, June 22). Taking aim at parents. *The Advocate,* pp. 78, 80.

Rochman, S. (2000, May 23). The cutting edge. *The Advocate,* pp. 29–31.

Rofes, E. E. (1983). *"I thought people like that killed themselves": Lesbians, gay men and suicide.* San Francisco: Grey Fox.

Rogow, F. (1989). Speaking the unspeakable: Gays, Jews, and historical inquiry. In C Balka & A. Rose (Eds.), *Twice blessed: On being lesbian or gay and Jewish* (pp. 71–82). Boston: Beacon Press.

Rohrbaugh, J. B. (1988). Choosing children: Psychological issues in lesbian parenting. *Women and Therapy, 8*(1–2), 51–64.

Rohrbaugh, J. B. (1992). Lesbian families: Clinical issues and theoretical implications. *Professional Psychology Research and Practice, 23*(6), 467–473.

Romer v. Evans (94-1039), 517 U.S. 620 (1996).

Rosario, M., Meyer-Bahlburg, H. F. L., Hunter, J., & Exner, T. M. (1996). The psychosexual development of urban lesbian, gay, and bisexual youths. *Journal of Sex Research, 33*(2), 113–126.

Rosario, M., Meyer-Bahlburg, H. F. L., Hunter, J., & Gwadz, M. (1999). Sexual risk behaviors of gay, lesbian, and bisexual youths in New York City: Prevalence and correlates. *AIDS Education and Prevention, 11*(6), 476–496.

Rosario, M., Rotheram-Borus, M. J., & Reid, H. (1996). Gay-related stress and its correlates among gay and bisexual male adolescents of predominantly Black and Hispanic Background. *Journal of Community Psychology, 24*(2), 136–159.

Rosario, V. A. (1996). *Science and homosexualities.* New York: Routledge.

Roscoe, W. (1987a). Bibliography of Berdache and alternative gender roles among North American Indians. *Journal of Homosexuality, 14*(3–4), 81–171.

Roscoe, W. (1987b). Living the tradition: Gay American Indians. In M. Thompson (Ed.), *Gay spirit: Myth and meaning* (pp. 69–77). New York: St. Martin's Press.

Rose, S. (1994). Sexual pride and shame in lesbians. In B. Greene, & G. M. Herek (Eds.), *Lesbian and gay psychology: Theory, research, and clinical applications* (pp. 71–83). Thousand Oaks, CA: Sage.

Rosen, W. B. (1992). *On the integration of sexuality: Lesbians and their mothers* (Work in Progress No. 56). Wellesley, MA: Wellesley College, the Stone Center.

Rosenberger, P. H., Bornstein, R. A., Nasrallah, H. A., & Para, M. F. (1993). Psychopathology in human immunodeficiency virus infection: Lifetime and current assessment. *Comprehensive Psychiatry, 34*(3), 150–158.

Rosenbluth, S. (1997). Is sexual orientation a matter of choice? *Psychology of Women Quarterly, 21*(4), 595–610.

Rosenfeld, D. (1999). Identity work among the homosexual elderly. *Dissertation Abstracts International, 60*(4-A), 1348. (University Microfilms No. AEH99–26356)

Rosenzweig, J. M., & Lebow, W. C. (1992). Femme on the streets, butch in the sheets? Lesbian sex-roles, dyadic adjustment, and sexual satisfaction. *Journal of Homosexuality, 23*(3), 1–20.

Ross, M. W. (1983). *The married homosexual man*. London: Routledge & Kegal Paul.

Ross, M. W. (1990). The relationship between life events and mental health in homosexual men. *Journal of Clinical Psychology, 46*(4), 402–411.

Ross, M. W., & Arrindell, W. A. (1988). Perceived parental rearing patterns of homosexual and heterosexual men. *Journal of Sex Research, 24*, 275–281.

Ross, M. W., & Rosser, B. R. S. (1996). Measurements and correlates of internalized homophobia: A factor analytic study. *Journal of Clinical Psychology, 52*(1), 15–21.

Rosser, B. R. S., Metz, M. E., Bockting, W. O., & Buroker, T. (1997). Sexual difficulties, concerns and satisfaction in homosexual men: An empirical study with implications for HIV prevention. *Journal of Sex and Marital Therapy, 23*(1), 61–73.

Rosser, B. R. S., Short, B. J., Thurmes, P. J., & Coleman, E. (1998). Anodyspareunia, the unacknowledged sexual dysfunction: A validation study of painful receptive anal intercourse and its psychosexual concomitants in homosexual men. *Journal of Sex and Marital Therapy, 24*(4), 281–292.

Rosser, B. S., & Ross, M. W. (1989). A gay life events scale (GALES) for homosexual men. *Journal of Gay and Lesbian Psychotherapy, 1*(2), 87–101.

Rotello, G. (2000, September 26). Denial = death. *The Advocate*, p. 88.

Roth, S. (1985). Psychotherapy with lesbian couples: Individual issues, female socialization, and the social context. *Journal of Marital and Family Therapy, 11*(3), 273–286.

Roth, S. (1989). Psychotherapy with lesbian couples: Individual issues, female socialization, and the social context. In M. McGoldrick, C. M. Anderson, & F. Walsh (Eds.), *Women in families: A framework for family therapy* (pp. 286–307). New York: Norton. (revised 1985 article by the same title)

Roth, S., & Murphy, B. C. (1986). Therapeutic work with lesbian clients: A systemic therapy view. *Family Therapy Collections, 16*, 78–89.

Rothblum E. D. (1990). Depression among lesbians: An invisible and unresearched phenomenon. *Journal of Gay and Lesbian Psychotherapy, 1*(3), 67–87.

Rothblum, E. D. (1994). "I only read about myself on bathroom walls": The need for research on the mental health of lesbians and gay men. *Journal of Consulting and Clinical Psychology, 62*(2), 213–220.

Rotheram-Borus, M. J., Hunter, J., & Rosario, M. (1994). Suicidal behavior and gay-related stress among gay and bisexual male adolescents. *Journal of Adolescent Research, 9*(4), 498–508.

Rotheram-Borus, M. J., Mann, T., & Chabon, B. (1999). Amphetamine use and its correlates among youths living with HIV. *AIDS Education and Prevention, 11*(3), 232–242.

Rotheram-Borus, M. J., Meyer-Bahlburg, H. F., Rosario, M., Koopman, C., Haignere, C. S., Exner, T. M., Matthieu, M., Henderson, R., & Gruen, R. S. (1992, Fall). Lifetime sexual behaviors among predominantly minority male runaways and gay/bisexual adolescents in New York City. *AIDS Education and Prevention*, 34–42.

Rotheram-Borus, M. J., Murphy, D. A., Reid, H. M., & Coleman, C. L. (1996). Correlates of emotional distress among HIV+ youths: Health status, stress, and personal resources. *Annals of Behavioral Medicine, 18*(1), 16–23.

Rotheram-Borus, M. J., Murphy, D. A., Swendeman, D., Chao, B., Chabon, B., Zhou, S., Birnbaum, J., & O'Hara, P. (1999). Substance use and its relationship to depression, anxiety, and isolation among youth living with HIV. *International Journal of Behavioral Medicine, 6*(4), 293–311.

Rotheram-Borus, M. J., Rosario, M., & Koopman, C. (1991). Minority youths at high risk: Gay males and runaways. In M. E. Colten & S. Gore (Eds.), *Adolescent stress: Causes and consequences* (pp. 181–200). New York: Aldyne de Gruyter.

Rotheram-Borus, M. J., Rosario, M., Van Rossem, R., & Reid, H. (1995). Prevalence, course, and predictors of multiple problem behaviors among gay and bisexual male adolescents. [Special Issue: Sexual orientation and human development]. *Developmental Psychology, 31*(1), 75–85.

Rottnek, M. (1999). Introduction. In M. Rottnek (Ed.), *Sissies and tomboys: Gender nonconformity and homosexual childhood* (pp. 1–5). New York: New York University Press.

Royse, D., & Birge, B. (1987). Homophobia and attitudes towards AIDS patients among medical, nursing, and paramedical students. *Psychological Reports, 61*(3), 867–870.

Royse, D., & Clawson, D. (1988). Sex-role egalitarianism, feminism, and sexual identity. *Psychological Reports, 63*(1), 160–162.

Rubinstein, G. (1995). The decision to remove homosexuality from the DSM: Twenty years later. *American Journal of Psychotherapy, 49*(3), 416–427.

Rudolph, J. (1988). Counselor's attitudes toward homosexuality: A selective review of the literature. *Journal of Counseling and Development, 67*(3), 165–168.

Rusbult, C. E., Zembrodt, I. M., & Iwaniszek, J. (1986). The impact of gender and sex-role orientation on responses to dissatisfaction in close relationships. *Sex Roles, 15*(1–2), 1–20.

Russell, D. (1985). Psychiatric diagnosis and the oppression of women. *International Journal of Social Psychiatry, 31*(4), 298–305.

Russell, D. (1986). Psychiatric diagnosis and the oppression of women. *Women and Therapy, 5*(4), 83–98.

Russell, P. A., & Gray, C. D. (1992). Prejudice against a progay man in an everyday situation: A scenario study. *Journal of Applied Social Psychology, 22*(21), 1676–1687.

Rust, P. C. (1993a). "Coming out" in the age of social constructionism: Sexual identity formation among lesbian and bisexual women. *Gender and Society, 7*(1), 50–77.

Rust, P. C. (1993b). Neutralizing the political threat of the marginal woman: Lesbian beliefs about bisexual women. *Journal of Sex Research, 30,* 214–228.

Rust, P. C. (1996). Monogamy and polyamory: Relationship issues for bisexuals. In B. A. Firestein (Ed.), *Bisexuality: The psychology and politics of an invisible minority* (pp. 127–148). Thousand Oaks, CA: Sage.

Rutter, V., & Schwartz, P. (1996). Same-sex couples: Courtship, commitment, context. In A. E. Auhagen & M. von Salisch (Eds.), *The diversity of human relationships* (pp. 197–226). New York: Cambridge University Press.

Ryan, C., & Futterman, D. (1998). *Lesbian and gay youth: Care and counseling.* New York: Columbia University Press.

Saad, L. (1996, December). *Americans growing more tolerant of gays* [Online]. Available: www.gallup.com/poll/news/96124.html.

Sacco, W. P., & Rickman, R. L. (1996). AIDS-relevant condom use by gay and bisexual men: The role of person variables and the interpersonal situation. *AIDS Education and Prevention, 8*(5), 430–443.

Saewyc, E. M., Bearinger, L. H., Blum, R. W., & Resnick, M. D. (1999). Sexual intercourse, abuse and pregnancy among adolescent women: Does sexual orientation make a difference? *Family Planning Perspectus, 31*(3), 127–131.

Safren, S. A. (1998). Depression, substance abuse, and suicidality in sexual minority adolescents. *Dissertation Abstracts International, 58*(8-B), 4470. (University Microfilms No. AAM98–06202)

Saghir, M. T., Robins, E., Walbran, B., & Gentry, K. A. (1970). Homosexuality, IV: Psychiatric disorders and disability in the female homosexual. *American Journal of Psychiatry, 127,* 147–154.

Saltzburg, S. (1996). Family therapy and the disclosure of adolescent homosexuality. *Journal of Family Psychotherapy, 7*(4), 1–18.

Sanders, G., & Ross-Field, L. (1986). Sexual orientation and visuo-spatial ability. *Brain and Cognition, 5*(3), 280–290.

Sanders, S. A., Reinisch, J. M., & McWhirter, D. P. (1990). Homosexuality/heterosexuality: An overview. In D. P. McWhirter, S. A. Sanders, & J. M. Reinisch (Eds.), *Homosexuality/heterosexuality: Concepts of sexual orientation.* (pp. xix-xxvii). New York: Oxford University Press.

Sang, B. E. (1991). Moving toward balance and integration. In B. Sang, J.Warshow, & A. J. Smith (Eds.), *Lesbians at midlife: The creative transition* (pp. 206–214). San Francisco: Spinsters.

Sang, B. E. (1992). Counseling and psychotherapy with midlife and older lesbians. In S. H. Dworkin, & F. J. Gutierrez (Eds.), *Counseling gay men and lesbians: Journey to the end of the rainbow* (pp. 35–48). Alexandria, VA: American Counseling Association (formerly the American Association for Counseling and Development).

Sarantokos, S. (1996). Same-sex couples: Problems and prospects. *Journal of Family Studies, 2*(2), 147–163.

Saulnier, C. F. (1999). Choosing a health care provider: A community survey of what is important to lesbians. *Families in Society, 80*(3), 254–262.

Saunders, J. M. (1999). Health problems of lesbian women. *Nursing Clinics of North America, 34*(2), 381–391.

Savin-Williams, R. C. (1988). Theoretical perspectives accounting for adolescent homosexuality. *Journal of Adolescent Health Care, 9*(2), 95–104.

Savin-Williams, R. C. (1989a). Coming out to parents and self-esteem among gay and lesbian youths. *Journal of Homosexuality, 18*(1–2), 1–35.

Savin-Williams, R. C. (1989b). Gay and lesbian adolescents. *Marriage and Family Review, 14*(3–4), 197–216.

Savin-Williams, R. C. (1989c). Parental influences on the self-esteem of gay and lesbian youths: A reflected appraisals model. *Journal of Homosexuality, 17*(1–2), 93–109.

Savin-Williams, R. C. (1990). *Gay and lesbian youth: Expressions of identity.* Washington, DC: Hemisphere.

Savin-Williams, R. C. (1994). Verbal and physical abuse as stressors in the lives of lesbian, gay male, and bisexual youths: Associations with school problems, running away, substance abuse, prostitution, and suicide. *Journal of Consulting and Clinical Psychology, 62*(2), 261–269.

Savin-Williams, R. C. (1998). *". . . And then I became gay": Young men's stories.* New York: Routledge.

Savin-Williams, R. C., & Cohen, K. M. (1996). Psychosocial outcomes of verbal and physical abuse among lesbian, gay, and bisexual youths. In R. C. Savin-Williams & K. M. Cohen (Eds.), *The lives of lesbians, gays, and bisexuals* (pp. 181–200). Fort Worth, TX: Harcourt Brace.

Savin-Williams, R. C., & Esterberg, K. G. (2000). Lesbian, gay, and bisexual families. In D. H. Demo & K. R. Allen (Eds,), *Handbook of family diversity* (pp. 197–215). New York: Oxford University Press.

Savin-Williams, R. C., & Rodriguez, R. G. (1993). A developmental, clinical perspective on lesbian, gay male, and bisexual youths. In T. P. Gullotta, G. R. Adams, R. Montemayor (Eds.), *Adolescent sexuality: Advances in adolescent development* (Vol. 5, pp. 71–101). Newbury Park, CA: Sage.

Scanzoni, L. D., & Mollenkott, V. R. (1994). *Is the homosexual my neighbor? A positive Christian response* (rev. ed.). San Francisco: Harper.

Scarce, M. (1997). *Male on male rape: The hidden toll of stigma and shame.* New York: Insight Books.

Scarce, M. (1999). *Smearing the queer: Medical bias in the health care of gay men.* Binghamton, NY: Haworth Press.

Scasta, D. (1998). Moving from coming out to intimacy. *Journal of Gay and Lesbian Psychotherapy, 2*(4), 99–111.

Schaefer, S., Evans, S., & Coleman, E. (1987). Sexual orientation concerns among chemically dependent individuals. *Journal of Chemical Dependency Treatment, 1*(1), 121–140.

Schäfer, S. (1976). Sexual and social problems among lesbians. *The Journal of Sex Research, 12,* 50–69.

Schifter, J., & Madrigal, J. (2000). *The sexual construction of Latino youth: Implications for the spread of HIV/AIDS.* Binghamton, NY: Haworth Press.

Schmitt, J. P., & Kurdek, L. A. (1987). Personality correlates of positive identity and relationship involvement in gay men. *Journal of Homosexuality, 13*(4), 101–109.

Schmitz, T. J. (1988). Career counseling implications with the gay and lesbian population. *Journal of Employment Counseling, 25*(2), 51–56.

Schneider, B. E. (1986). Coming out at work: Bridging the private/public gap. *Work and Occupations, 13,* 463–487.

Schneider, J. M. (1984). *Stress, loss, and grief*. Baltimore: University Park Press.

Schneider. J. M. (1994). *Finding my way: Healing and transformation through loss and grief*. Colfax, WI: Seasons Press.

Schneider, M. S. (1986). The relationships of cohabiting lesbian and heterosexual couples: A comparison. *Psychology of Women Quarterly, 10*(3), 234–239.

Schneider, M. (1989). Sappho was a right-on adolescent: Growing up lesbian. *Journal of Homosexuality, 17*(1–2), 111–130.

Schneider, M. (1991). Developing services for lesbian and gay adolescents. *Canadian Journal of Community Mental Health, 10*(1), 133–151.

Schneider, M., & Tremble, B. (1985/1986). Gay or straight? Working with the confused adolescent. *Journal of Social Work and Human Sexuality, 4*(1–2), 71–82.

Schneider, S. G., Farberow, N. L., & Kruks, G. N. (1989). Suicidal behavior in adolescent and young adult gay men. *Suicide and Life Threatening Behavior, 19*(4), 381–394.

Schneider, W., & Lewis, I. A. (1984). The straight story on homosexuality and gay rights. *Public Opinion, 7*(1), 16–21.

Schow, R., Schow, W., & Raynes, M. (Eds.). (1991). *Peculiar people: Mormons and same-sex orientation*. Salt Lake City, UT: Signature.

Schreurs, K. M. G., & Buunk, B. P. (1996). Closeness, autonomy, equity, and relationship satisfaction in lesbian couples. *Psychology of Women Quarterly, 20*(4), 577–592.

Schroeder, M. (1980). *Hope for relationships*. City Center, MN: Hazelden.

Schuker, E (1996). Toward further analytic understanding of lesbian patients. *Journal of the American Psychoanalytic Association, 44*(Suppl.), 485–508.

Schulenburg, J. (1985). *Gay parenting*. Garden City, NY: Anchor Press/Doubleday.

Schwartz, A. E. (1998). *Sexual subjects: Lesbians, gender, and psychoanalysis*. New York: Routledge.

Schwartz, R. D. (1989). When the therapist is gay: Personal and clinical reflections. *Journal of Gay and Lesbian Psychotherapy, 1*(1), 41–51.

Scrivner, R. (1997). Gay men and nonrelational sex. In R. F. Levant & G. R. Brooks (Eds.), *Men and sex: New psychological perspectives* (pp. 229–256). New York: Wiley.

Scrivner, R., & Benkov, L. (1995). *Ethical issues in lesbian and gay family therapy*. Paper presented at the 103rd annual meeting of the American Psychological Association, New York.

Seage, G. R. III, Mayer, K. H., Wold, C., Lenderking, W. R., Goldstein, R., Cai, B., Gross, M., Heeren, T., & Hingson, R. (1998). The social context of drinking, drug use, and unsafe sex in the Boston young men study. *Journal of Acquired Immunity Deficiency Syndromes and Human Retrovirology, 17*(4), 368–375.

Sears, J. T. (1991a). Educators, homosexuality, and homosexual students: Are personal feelings related to professional beliefs? *Journal of Homosexuality, 22*(3–4), 29–79.

Sears, J. T. (1991b). *Growing up gay in the South: Race, gender, and journeys of the spirit*. New York: Harrington Park Press.

Seltzer, R. (1992). The social location of those holding antihomosexual attitudes. *Sex Roles, 26*(9–10), 391–398.

Serovich, J. M. (2000). Helping HIV-positive persons to negotiate the disclosure process to partners, family members, and friends. *Journal of Marital and Family Therapy, 26*(3), 365–372.

Shaffer, D., Fisher, P., Hicks, R., Parides, M., & Gould, M. (1995). Sexual orientation in adolescents who commit suicide. *Suicide and Life-Threatening Behavior, 25*(Suppl.).

Shalit, P. (1998). *Living well: The gay man's essential health guide*. Boston: Alyson.

Shallenberger, D. (1998). *Reclaiming the spirit: Gay men and lesbians come to terms with religion*. New Brunswick, NJ: Rutgers University Press.

Shannon, J. W., & Woods, W. J. (1991). Affirmative psychotherapy for gay men. *Counseling Psychologist, 19*(2), 197–215.

Shapiro, J. P., Cook, G. G., & Krackow, A. (1993, July 5). Straight talk about gays. *U.S. News & World Report*, pp. 42–48.

Shenitz, B. (1999, April 27). Out of balance. *The Advocate*, pp. 30–32.

Shernoff, M. (Ed.). (1997). *Gay widowers: Life after the death of a partner.* Binghamton, NY: Haworth Press.

Shernoff, M. (Ed.). (1999). *AIDS and mental health practice: Clinical and policy issues.* Binghamton, NY: Haworth Press.

Shernoff, M., & Finnegan, D. (1991). Family treatment with chemically dependent gay men and lesbians. *Journal of Chemical Dependency Treatment, 4*(1), 121–135.

Shidlo, A. (1994a). Internalized homophobia: Conceptual and empirical issues in measurement. In B. Greene & G. M. Herek (Eds.), *Lesbian and gay psychology: Theory, research, and clinical applications* (pp. 176–205). Thousand Oaks, CA: Sage.

Shidlo, B. (1994b, June). Modern day gay dads. *Division 44 Newsletter,* pp. 22, 24.

Shidlo, A., & Schroeder, M. (1999). *Changing sexual orientation: Empirical findings on conversion therapies.* Paper presented at the 107th annual meeting of the American Psychological Association, Boston.

Shidlo, A., & Schroeder, M. (2000). *National study of sexual orientation conversion: Empirical and conceptual issues.* Paper presented at the 108th annual meeting of the American Psychological Association, Washington, DC.

Shifrin, F., & Solis, M. (1992). Chemical dependency in gay and lesbian youth. *Journal of Chemical Dependency Treatment, 5*(1), 67–76.

Shively, M. G., & DeCecco, J. P. (1977). Components of sexual identity. *Journal of Homosexuality, 3,* 31–48.

Shuster, R. (1987). Sexuality as a continuum: The bisexual identity. In Boston Lesbian Psychologies Collective (Ed.), *Lesbian psychologies: Explorations and challenges* (pp. 56–71). Urbana: University of Illinois Press.

Shuster, R. (1992). Bisexuality and the quest for principled loving. In E. R. Weise (Ed.), *Closer to home: Bisexuality and feminism* (pp. 147–154). Seattle: Seal Press.

Shuster, S. (1996). Families coping with HIV disease in gay fathers: Dimensions of treatment. In J. Laird & R. J. Green (Eds.), *Lesbian and gay couples and families: A handbook for therapists* (pp. 404–419). San Francisco: Jossey-Bass.

Siegel, K., & Epstein, J. A. (1996). Ethnic-racial differences in psychological stress related to gay lifestyle among HIV-positive men. *Psychological Reports, 79*(1), 303–312.

Siegel, S., & Lowe, E. (1994). *Uncharted lives: Understanding the life passages of gay men.* New York: Dutton.

Siegelman, M. (1972). Adjustment of homosexual and heterosexual women. *British Journal of Psychiatry, 120*(558), 477–481.

Siegelman, M. (1974). Parental background of male homosexuals and heterosexuals. *Archives of Sexual Behavior, 3,* 3–18.

Siegelman, M. (1981). Parental background of homosexual and heterosexual men: A cross-national replication. *Archives of Sexual Behavior, 10,* 504–514.

Signer, S. F. (1989). Homo-erotomania. *British Journal of Psychiatry, 154,* 729.

Silverman, M. A. (1990). The prehomosexual boy in treatment. In C. W. Socarides & V. D. Volkan (Eds.), *The homosexualities: Reality, fantasy, and the arts* (pp. 177–197). Madison, CT: International Universities Press.

Silverstein, C. (1988). The borderline personality disorder and gay people. *Journal of Homosexuality, 15,* 185–212.

Silverstein, C. (1991). Psychological and medical treatments of homosexuality. In J. C. Gonsiorek & J. D. Weinrich (Eds.). *Homosexuality: Research implications for public policy* (pp. 101–114). Newbury Park, CA: Sage.

Silverstein, C. (1993). *The new joy of gay sex* (reprint ed.). New York: HarperCollins.

Silverstein, C. (1996). History of treatment. In R. P. Cabaj & T. S. Stein (Eds.), *Textbook of homosexuality and mental health* (pp. 3–16). Washington, DC: American Psychiatric Press.

Silverstein, L. B. (1996). Fathering is a feminist issue. *Psychology of Women Quarterly, 20*(1), 3–37.

Simon, A. (1995). Some correlates of individuals' attitudes toward lesbians. *Journal of Homosexuality, 29*(1), 89–103.

Simmons, L. E. (1999). The grief experience of HIV-positive gay men who lose partners to AIDS. *Dissertation Abstracts International, 60*(3-B), 1029. (University Microfilms No. AAM99–24152)

Skinner, W. F. (1994). The prevalence and demographic predictors of illicit and licit drug use and lesbians and gay men. *American Journal of Public Health, 84*(8), 1307–1310.

Skinner, W. F., & Otis, M. D. (1996). Drug and alcohol use among lesbian and gay people in a southern U. S. sample: Epidemiological, comparative, and methodological findings from the Trilogy Project. *Journal of Homosexuality, 30*(3), 59–92.

Slater, S. (1995). *The lesbian family life cycle.* New York: Free Press.

Slome, L. R., Mitchell, T. F., Charlebois, E., Benevedes, J. M., & Abrams, D. I. (1997). Physician-assisted suicide and patients with human immunodeficiency virus disease. *New England Journal of Medicine, 336*(6), 417–421.

Slusher, M. P., Mayer, C. J., & Dunkle, R. E. (1996). Gays and lesbians older and wiser (GLOW): A support for older gay people. *Gerontologist, 36*(1), 118–123.

Smith, A. (1997). Cultural diversity and the coming-out process: Implications for clinical practice. In B. Greene (Ed.), *Ethnic and cultural diversity among lesbians and gay men* (pp. 279–300). Thousand Oaks, CA: Sage.

Smith, D. F., & Allred, G. H. (1990). Adjustment of women divorced from homosexual men: An exploratory study. *American Journal of Family Therapy, 18*(3), 273–284

Smith D. M. (1997, Winter). HRC polls America: Trail-blazing surveys help accurately describe gay community, impact of our issues. *HRC Quarterly,* pp. 8–9.

Smith, G. B. (1993). Homophobia and attitudes toward gay men and lesbians by psychiatric nurses. *Archives of Psychiatric Nursing, 7*(6), 377–384.

Smith, J. (1988). Psychopathology, homosexuality, and homophobia. *Journal of Homosexuality, 15*(1–2), 59–73.

Smith, P. P. (1992). Encounters with older lesbians in psychiatric practice. *Sexual and Marital Therapy, 7*(1), 79–86.

Smith, T. M. (1982). Specific approaches and techniques in the treatment of gay male alcohol abusers. *Journal of Homosexuality, 7*(4), 53–69.

Smith, T. M. (1987). Foreword. In D. G. Finnegan & E. B. McNally, *Dual identities: Counseling chemically dependent gay men and lesbians* (pp. 3–5). Center City, MN: Hazelden.

Smith, R. B., & Brown, R. A. (1997). The impact of social support on gay male couples. *Journal of Homosexuality, 32*(2), 39–61.

Sohier, R. (1986). Homosexual mutuality: Variation on a theme by Erik Erikson. *Journal of Homosexuality, 12*(2), 25–38.

Sohier, R. (1993). Filial reconstruction: A theory of development through adversity. *Qualitative Health Research, 3*(4), 465–492.

Solarz, A. L. (Ed.). (1999). *Lesbian health: Current assessment and directions for the future.* Washington, DC: National Academy Press. [Online]. Available: www.bob.nap.edu/html/leshealth/.

Sophie, J. (1982). Counseling lesbians. *The Personnel and Guidance Journal, 60,* 341–345.

Sophie, J. (1986). A critical examination of stage theories of lesbian identity development. *Journal of Homosexuality, 12*(2), 39–51.

Sophie, J. (1987). Internalized homophobia and lesbian identity. *Journal of Homosexuality, 14*(1–2), 53–65.

Sorensen, L., & Roberts, S. J. (1997). Lesbian uses of and satisfaction with mental health services: Results from Boston Lesbian Health Project. *Journal of Homosexuality, 33*(1), 35–49.

Spahr, J. A., Poethig, K., Berry, S., & McLain, M. V. (Eds.). (1999). *Called out: The voices and gifts of lesbian, gay, bisexual, and transgendered Presbyterians.* Gaithersburg, MD: Chi Rho Press.

Spencer, B. M. (1991). Ask the board: From social work, case 1. *Journal of Gay and Lesbian Psychotherapy, 1*(4), 5–6.

Spielman, S., & Winfield, L. (1996). Domestic partner benefits: A bottom line discussion. In A. L. Ellis & E. D. Riggle (Eds.), *Sexual identity on the job: Issues and services* (pp. 53–78). New York: Harrington Park Press/Haworth Press.

Spong, J. S. (1988) *Living in sin?* New York: Harper & Row.

Springer, C. A., & Lease, S. H. (2000). The impact of multiple AIDS-related bereavement in the gay male population. *Journal of Counseling and Development, 78*(3), 297–304.

Stack, C. (1999). Psychoanalysis meets queer theory: An encounter with the terrifying other. *Gender and Psychoanalysis, 4*(1), 71–87.

Stall, R. D., Paul, J. P., Barrett, D. C., Crosby, G. M., & Bein, E. (1999). An outcome evaluation to measure changes in sexual risk-taking among gay men undergoing substance use disorder treatment. *Journal of Studies on Alcohol, 60*(6), 837–845.

Starhawk. (1979). Witchcraft and women's culture. In C. P. Christ & J. Plaskow (Eds.), *Womanspirit rising: A feminist reader in religion.* San Francisco: Harper & Row.

Starhawk. (1982). *Dreaming the dark: Magic, sex and politics.* Boston: Beacon Press.

Steckel, A. (1985). *Separation–individuation in children of lesbian and heterosexual couples.* Unpublished doctoral dissertation, Wright Institute, Berkeley, CA.

Steckel, A. (1987). Psychosocial development of children of lesbian mothers. In F. W. Bozett (Ed.), *Gay and lesbian parents* (pp. 75–85). New York: Praeger.

Stein, T. S. (1988). Theoretical consideration with gay men and lesbians. *Journal of Homosexuality, 15*(1–2), 75–95.

Stein, T. S. (1996a). A critique of approaches to changing sexual orientation. In R. P. Cabaj & T. S. Stein (Eds.), *Textbook of homosexuality and mental health* (pp. 525–537). Washington, DC: American Psychiatric Press.

Stein, T. S. (1996b). Homosexuality and homophobia in men. *Psychiatric Annals, 26*(1), 37–40.

Stein, T. S. (1999). Commentary on "Gay and lesbian clients' ratings of psychiatrists, psychologists, social workers, and counselors." *Journal of Gay and Lesbian Psychotherapy, 3*(1), 95–100.

Stein, T. S., & Cabaj, R. P. (1996). Psychotherapy with gay men. In R. P. Cabaj & T. S. Stein (Eds.), *Textbook of homosexuality and mental health* (pp. 413–432). Washington, DC: American Psychiatric Press.

Stein, T. S., & Cohen, C. J. (1984). Psychotherapy with gay men and lesbians: An examination of homophobia, coming out, and identity. In E. S. Hetrick & T. S. Stein (Eds.), *Innovations in psychotherapy with homosexuals* (pp. 60–73). Washington, DC: American Psychiatric Press.

Steinman, R. (1990). Social exchanges between older and younger gay male partners. *Journal of Homosexuality, 20*(3–4), 179–206.

Stempel, R. R., Moulton, J. M., & Moss, A. R. (1995). Self-disclosure of HIV-1 antibody test results: The San Francisco General Hospital Cohort. *AIDS Education and Prevention, 7*(2), 116–123.

Stephan, W. G. (1973). Parental relationships and early social experiences of activist male homosexuals and male heterosexuals. *Journal of Abnormal Psychology, 82*(3), 506–513.

Stephenson, Y., & Palladino, D. (1990). Perceptions of the sexual self: Their impact on relationships between lesbian and heterosexual women. In L. S. Brown & M. P. P. Root (Eds.), *Diversity and complexity in feminist therapy* (pp. 213–254). New York: Harrington Park Press.

Sterk, C. E., & Elifson, K. (2000). *Lesbian and bisexual identity among African American female drug users.* Paper presented at the 108th annual meeting of the American Psychological Association, Washington, DC.

Stevens, P. E. (1992). Lesbian health care research: A review of the literature from 1970 to 1990. *Health Care for Women International, 13*(2), 91–120.

Stevens, P. E. (1994). Protective strategies of lesbian clients in health care environments. *Research in Nursing and Health, 17*(3), 217–229.

Stevens, P. E. (1995). Structural and interpersonal impact of heterosexual assumptions on lesbian health care clients. *Nursing Research, 44*(1), 25–30.

Stevens, P. E. (1996). Lesbians and doctors: Experiences of solidarity and domination in health care settings. *Gender and Society, 10*(1), 24–41.

Stevens, P. E., & Hall, J. M. (1990). Abusive health care interactions experienced by lesbians: A case of institutional violence in the treatment of women. *Response to the Victimization of Women and Children, 13*(3), 23–27.

Stiglitz, E. (1990). Caught between two worlds: The impact of a child on a lesbian couple's relationship. *Women and Therapy, 10*(1–2), 99–116.

Stoller, R. J. (1986). The heterogeneous homosexual. *International Journal of Psychoanalytic Psychotherapy*, *11*, 175–181.

Storms, M. D. (1980). Theories of sexual orientation. *Journal of Personality and Social Psychology*, *38*(5), 783–792.

Storms, M. D. (1981). A theory of erotic orientation development. *Psychological Review*, *88*(4), 340–353.

Strommen, E. F. (1989a). Hidden branches and growing pains: Homosexuality and the family tree. *Marriage and Family Review*, *14*(3–4), 9–34.

Strommen, E. F. (1989b). "You're a what?": Family member reactions to the disclosure of homosexuality. *Journal of Homosexuality*, *18*(1–2), 37–58.

Struzzo, J. A. (1989). Pastoral counseling and homosexuality. *Journal of Homosexuality*, *18*(3–4), 195–222.

Stuart, E. (1998). *Religion is a queer thing: A guide to the Christian faith for lesbian, gay, bisexual and transgendered people*. London, UK: Cassell Academic.

Suchet, M. (1995). "Having it both ways": Rethinking female sexuality. In J. M. Glassgold & S. Iasenza (Eds.), *Lesbians and psychoanalysis: Revolutions in theory and practice* (pp. 39–61). New York: Free Press.

Sullivan, A. (Ed.). (1995). *Issues in gay and lesbian adoption: Proceedings of the fourth annual Peirce-Warwick Adoption Symposium*. Washington, DC: Child Welfare League of America.

Sullivan, P. F., Becker, J. T., Dew, M. A., Penkower, L., Detels, R., Hoover, D. R., Kaslow, R., Palenicek, J., & Wesch, J. E. (1993). Longitudinal trends in the use of illicit drugs and alcohol in the Multicenter AIDS Cohort Study. *Addiction Research*, *1*(3), 279–290.

Sullivan, T., & Schneider, M. (1987). Development and identity issues in adolescent homosexuality. *Child and Adolescent Social Work Journal*, *4*(1), 13–24.

Sullivan, T. R. (1996). The challenge of HIV prevention among high-risk adolescents. *Health and Social Work*, *21*(1), 58–65.

Sullivan, T. R., & Dawidoff, R. (Eds.). (1999). *Queer families: Common agendas*. Binghamton, NY: Haworth Press.

Super, D. E., Savickas, M. L., & Super, C. M. (1996). The life-span, life-space approach to careers. In D. Brown & L. Brooks (Eds.), *Career choice and development* (3rd ed., pp. 121–178). San Francisco: Jossey-Bass.

Surrey, J. L. (1991). The self-in-relation: A theory of women's development. In J. V. Jordan, A. G. Kaplan, J. B. Miller, I. P. Stiver, & J. L. Surrey (Eds.), *Women's growth in connection: Writings from the Stone Center* (pp. 51–66). New York: Guilford Press.

Swaab, D. F., & Fliers, E. (1985, May). A sexually dimorphic nucleus in the human brain. *Science*, pp. 1112–1115.

Swaab, D. F., & Hofman, M. A. (1990). An enlarged suprachiasmatic nucleus in homosexual men. *Brain Research*, *537*(1–2), 141–148.

Sweasey, P. (1997). *From queer to eternity: Spirituality in the lives of lesbian, gay and bisexual people*. London: Cassell.

Szapocznik, J. (1995). Research on disclosure of HIV status: Cultural evolution finds an ally in science. *Health Psychology*, *14*(1), 4–5.

Tafoya, T. N. (1992). Native gay and lesbian issues: The two spirited. In B. Berzon (Ed.), *Positively gay* (pp. 253–260). Berkeley, CA: Celestial Press.

Tafoya, T. N. (1996). Native two-spirit people. In R. P. Cabaj & T. S. Stein (Eds.), *Textbook of homosexuality and mental health* (pp. 603–617). Washington, DC: American Psychiatric Press.

Tasker, F., & Golombok, S. (1995). Adults raised as children in lesbian families. *American Journal of Orthopsychiatry*, *65*(2), 203–215.

Tasker, F., & Golombok, S. (1997). *Growing up in a lesbian family: Effects on child development*. New York: Guilford Press.

Teague, J. B. (1992). Issues relating to the treatment of adolescent lesbians and homosexuals. *Journal of Mental Health Counseling*, *14*(4), 422–439.

Temple-Raston, D. (2000, September 7). Firms juggle stigma, needs of more workers with HIV. *USA Today*, p. A1–2.

Terndrup, A. I. (1998). *Factors that influence career choice and development for gay male school teachers: A qualitative investigation* (Doctoral dissertation, Oregon State University, 1999). *Dissertation Abstracts International*, 59(12), 4371A. (University Microfilm No. AAG99–14146)

Terry, P. (1992). Entitlement not privilege: The right of employment and advancement. In N. J. Woodman (Ed.), *Lesbian and gay lifestyles: A guide for counseling and education* (pp. 133–143). New York: Irvington.

Thomason, T. C. (1991). Counseling Native Americans: An introduction for non-Native American counselors. *Journal of Counseling and Development*, 69(4), 321–327.

Thompson, C. A. (1992). Lesbian grief and loss issues in the coming out process. *Women and Therapy*, 12(1–2), 175–185.

Thompson, M. (Ed.). (1987). *Gay spirit: Myth and meaning.* New York: St. Martin's Press.

Thompson, M. (Ed.). (1994). *Long road to freedom: The Advocate history of the gay and lesbian movement.* New York: St. Martin's Press.

Thompson, M. (Ed.). (1995). *Gay soul: Finding the heart of gay spirit and nature.* San Francisco: Harper.

Thorson-Smith, S., van Wijk-Bos, J. W. H., Pott, N., & Thompson, W. P. (Eds.). (1997). *Called out with: Stories of solidarity.* Louisville, KY: Westminister John Knox Press.

Throckmorton, W. (1998). Efforts to modify sexual orientation: A review of outcome literature and ethical issues. *Journal of Mental Health Counseling*, 20, 283–304.

Throckmorton, W. (2000). *Review of empirical findings concerning ex-gays.* Paper presented at the 108th annual meeting of the American Psychological Association, Washington, DC.

Tievsky, D. L. (1988). Homosexual clients and homophobic social workers. *Journal of Independent Social Work*, 2(3), 51–62.

Toufexis, A. (1992, August 17). Bisexuality: What is it? *Time*, pp. 49–51.

Toward a new national discussion of homosexuality. (1998, August 16). *San Francisco Examiner*, p. A-22.

Tozer, E. E., & McClanahan, M. K. (1999). Treating the purple menace: Ethical considerations of conversion therapy and affirmative alternatives. *The Counseling Psychologist*, 27(5), 722–742.

Travers, R., & Schneider, M. (1996). Barriers to accessibility for lesbian and gay youth needing addictions services. *Youth and Society*, 27(3), 356–378.

Tripp, C. (1975). *The homosexual matrix.* New York: McGraw-Hill.

Trippet, S. E., & Bain, J. (1992). Reasons American lesbians fail to seek traditional health care. *Health Care for Women International*, 13(2), 145–153.

Trippet, S. E., & Bain, J. (1993). Physical health problems and concerns of lesbians. *Women and Health*, 20(2), 59–70.

Troiden, R. R. (1979). Becoming homosexual: A model of gay identity acquisition. *Psychiatry*, 42, 362–373.

Troiden, R. R. (1984/1985). Self, self-concept, identity, and homosexual identity: Constructs in need of definition and differentiation. *Journal of Homosexuality*, 10, 97–109.

Troiden, R. R. (1988). *Gay and lesbian identity: A sociological analysis.* New York: General Hall.

Troiden, R. R. (1989). The formation of homosexual identities. *Journal of Homosexuality*, 17(1–4), 43–73.

Troiden, R. R., & Goode, E. (1980). Variables related to the acquisition of a gay identity. *Journal of Homosexuality*, 5, 383–392.

Trujillo, C. (Ed.). (1991). *Chicana lesbians: The girls our mothers warned us about.* Berkeley, CA: Third Woman Press.

Tully, C. T. (1989). What do midlife lesbians view as important? *Journal of Gay and Lesbian Psychotherapy*, 1(1), 87–103.

Tully, C. T. (1992) Research on older lesbian women: What is known, what is not known, and how to learn more. In N. J. Woodman (Ed.), *Lesbian and gay lifestyles: A guide for counseling and education* (pp. 235–264). New York: Irvington.

Turner, H. A., Catania, J. A., & Gagnon, J. (1994). The prevalence of informal caregiving to persons with AIDS in the United States: Caregiver characteristics and their implications. *Social Science and Medicine, 38*(11), 1543–1552.

Turner, H. A., Hays, R. B., & Coates, T. J. (1993). Determinants of social support among gay men: The context of AIDS. *Journal of Health and Social Behavior, 34*(1), 37–53.

Turner, P. H., Scadden, L., & Harris, M. B. (1990). Parenting in gay and lesbian families. *Journal of Gay and Lesbian Psychotherapy, 1*(3), 55–66.

Tuttle, G. E., & Pillard, R. C. (1991). Sexual orientation and cognitive abilities. *Archives of Sexual Behavior, 20*(3), 307–318.

Udis-Kessler, A. (1990). Bisexuality in an essential world: Toward an understanding of biphobia. In T. Geller (Ed.), *Bisexuality: A reader and sourcebook* (pp. 51–63). Ojai, CA: Times Change Press.

Udis-Kessler, A. (1992). Appendix: Notes on the Kinsey scale and other measures of sexuality. In E. R. Weise (Ed.), *Closer to home: Bisexuality and feminism* (pp. 311–318). Seattle: Seal Press.

Uhrig, L. J. (1986). *Sex positive: A gay contribution to sexual and spiritual union.* Boston: Alyson.

Underhill, B. L. (1991). Recovery needs of lesbian alcoholics in treatment. In N. Van Den Bergh (Ed.), *Feminist perspectives on addictions* (pp. 73–86). New York: Springer.

Unger, R. K. (1989). *Representations: Social constructions of gender.* Amityville, NY: Baywood.

Unks, G. (Ed.). (1995). *The gay teen: Educational practice and theory for lesbian, gay, and bisexual adolescents.* New York: Routledge.

Vaillant, G. (1977). *Adaptation to life.* Boston: Little, Brown.

Valanis, B. G., Bowen, D. J., Bassford, T., Whitlock, E., Charney, P., & Carter, R. A. (2000). Sexual orientation and health: Comparisons in the Women's Health Initiative sample. *Archives of Family Medicine, 9*(9), 843–853.

Vanable, P. A. (1998). Alcohol use, self-regulatory failure, and increased behavioral risk for HIV. *Dissertation Abstracts International, 58*(11-B), 6248. (University Microfilms No. AAM98–15199)

Vanable, P. A., Ostrow, D. G., McKirnan, D. J., Taywaditep, K. J., & Hope, B. A. (2000). Impact of combination therapies on HIV risk perceptions and sexual risk among HIV-positive and HIV-negative gay and bisexual men. *Health Psychology, 19*(2), 134–145.

van der Geest, H. (1993). Homosexuality and marriage. *Journal of Homosexuality, 24*(3–4), 115–123.

VanderStoep, S. W., & Green, C. W. (1988). Religiosity and homonegativity: A path-analytic study. *Basic and Applied Social Psychology, 9*(2), 135–147.

Van de Ven, P. (1995). Talking with juvenile offenders about gay males and lesbians: Implications for combating homophobia. *Adolescence, 30,* 19–42.

Van de Ven, P., Bornholt, L., & Bailey, M. (1996). Measuring cognitive, affective, and behavioral components of homophobic reaction. *Archives of Sexual Behavior, 25*(2), 155–179.

Van Wyk, P. H., & Geist, C. S. (1984). Psychosocial development of heterosexual, bisexual, and homosexual behavior. *Archives of Sexual Behavior, 13*(6), 505–544.

Vaughan, S. C. (1999). The hiding and revelation of sexual desire in lesbians: The lasting legacy of developmental traumas. *Journal of Gay and Lesbian Psychotherapy, 3*(2), 81–90.

Vincke, J., Bolton, R., & Miller, M. (1997). Younger versus older gay men: Risks, pleasures and dangers of anal sex. *AIDS Care, 9*(2), 217–225.

Vreeland, C. N., Gallagher, B. J., & McFalls, J. A. (1995). The beliefs of members of the American Psychiatric Association on the etiology of male homosexuality: A national survey. *Journal of Psychology, 129*(5), 507–517.

Wagner, G. J., Remien, R. H., & Carballo-Dieguez, A. (1998). "Extramarital" sex: Is there an increased risk of HIV transmission? A study of male couples of mixed HIV status. *AIDS Education and Prevention, 10*(3), 245–256.

Wainberg, M. L. (1999). The Hispanic, gay, lesbian, bisexual and HIV-infected experience in health care. *Mount Sinai Journal of Medicine, 66*(4), 263–266.

Waldner-Haugrud, L. K., Gratch, L. V., & Magruder, B. (1997). Victimization and perpetration rates of violence in gay and lesbian relationships: Gender issues explored. *Violence and Victims, 12*(2), 173–184.

Walters, A. S., & Curran, M. C. (1996). "Excuse me, sir? May I help you and your boyfriend?": Salespersons' differential treatment of homosexual and straight customers. *Journal of Homosexuality, 31*(1–2), 135–152.

Wassermann, E. B., & Storms, M. D. (1984). Factors influencing erotic orientation development in females and males. *Women and Therapy, 3,* 51–60.

Waterman, C. K., Dawson, L. J., & Bologna, M. J. (1989). Sexual coercion in gay male and lesbian relationships: Predictors and inplications for support services. *The Journal of Sex Research, 26*(1), 118–124.

Wechsler, D. (1955). *Manual for the Wechsler Adult Intelligence Scale.* New York: Psychological Corporation.

Weinberg, M. S., & Williams, C. J. (1974). *Male homosexuals: Their problems and adaptations.* New York: Oxford University Press.

Weinberg, M. S., & Williams, C. J. (1975). *Male homosexuals: Their problems and adaptations.* New York: Penguin.

Weinberg, M. S., Williams, C. J., & Pryor, D. W. (1994). *Dual attraction: Understanding bisexuality.* New York: Oxford University Press.

Weinberg, T. (1978). On doing and being gay: Sexual behavior and male self-identity. *Journal of Homosexuality, 4,* 143–156.

Weinberg, T. S. (1995). *Gay men, drinking, and alcoholism.* Carbondale: Southern Illinois University.

Weingourt, R. (1998). A comparison of heterosexual and homosexual long-term sexual relationships. *Archives of Psychiatric Nursing, 12*(2), 114–118.

Weinrich, J. D., Atkinson, J. H. Jr., McCutchan, J. A., & Grant, I. (1995). Is gender dysphoria dysphoric? Elevated depression and anxiety in gender dysphoric and nondysphoric homosexual and bisexual men in an HIV sample. *Archives of Sexual Behavior, 24*(1), 55–72.

Weinrich, J. D., & Williams, W. L. (1991). Strange customs, familiar lives: Homosexualities in other cultures. In J. C. Gonsiorek & J. D. Weinrich (Eds.), *Homosexuality: Research implications for public policy* (pp. 44–59). Newbury Park, CA: Sage.

Weinstein, D. L. (Ed.). (1993). *Lesbians and gay men: Chemical dependency treatment issues.* Binghamton, NY: Haworth Press.

Weinstock, J. S., & Rothblum, E. D. (Eds.). (1996). *Lesbian friendships: For ourselves and each other.* New York: New York University Press.

Weise, E. R. (Ed.). (1992). *Closer to home: Bisexuality and feminism.* Seattle: Seal Press.

Welch, S., Howden-Chapman, P., & Collings, S. C. (1998). Survey of drug and alcohol use by lesbian women in New Zealand. *Addictive Behavior, 23*(4), 543–548.

Wells, J. (Ed.). (1997). *Lesbians raising sons: An anthology.* Boston: Alyson.

Wells, J. W., & Daly, A. (1992). University students' felt alienation and their attitudes toward African-Americans, women and homosexuals. *Psychological Reports, 70*(2), 623–626.

Wells, J. W., & Kline, W. B. (1987). Self-disclosure of homosexual orientation. *Journal of Social Psychology, 127*(2), 191–197.

Wells-Lurie, L. L. (1996). Working with parents of gay and lesbian children. In C. J. Alexander (Ed.), *Gay and lesbian mental health: A sourcebook for practitioners* (pp. 159–171). New York: Harrington Park Press.

Wendland, C. L., Burn, F., & Hill, C. (1996). Donor insemination: A comparison of lesbian couples, heterosexual couples and single women. *Fertility and Sterility, 65*(4), 764–770.

Weyhing, R. S., Bartlett, W. S., & Howard, G. S. (1984). Career indecision and identity development. *Journal of Psychology and Christianity, 3*(1), 74–78.

Whitam, F. L. (1977). Childhood indicators of male homosexuality. *Archives of Sexual Behavior, 6*(2), 89–96.

Whitam, F. L. (1991). From sociology: Homophobia and heterosexism in sociology. *Journal of Gay and Lesbian Psychotherapy, 1*(4), 31–44.

Whitam, F. L., Diamond, M., & Martin, J. (1993). Homosexual orientation in twins: A report on 61 pairs and three triplet sets. *Archives of Sexual Behavior, 22*(3), 187–206.

Whitam, F. L., & Mathy, R. M. (1991). Childhood cross gender behavior of homosexual females in Brazil, Peru, the Philippines, and the United States. *Archives of Sexual Behavior, 20*(2), 151–170.

White, J. C., & Dull, V. T. (1997). Health risk factors and health-seeking behavior in lesbians. *Journal of Womens Health, 6*(1), 103–112.

White, J. C., & Levinson, W. (1995). Lesbian health care: What a primary care physician needs to know. *Western Journal of Medicine, 162*(5), 463–466.

White, M. (1995). *Stranger at the gate: To be gay and Christian in America.* New York: Plume. (Original work published 1994, New York: Simon & Schuster)

White, M. R. (1991). AIDS prevention in adolescent gays: Health locus of control and self-disclosure. *Journal of Gay and Lesbian Psychotherapy, 1*(4), 115–118.

Whitehead, E. E., & Whitehead, J. D. (1986). *Seasons of strength: New visions of adult Christian maturing.* New York: Image Doubleday.

Whitley, B. E. (1988). Sex differences in heterosexuals' attitudes toward homosexuals: It depends upon what you ask. *Journal of Sex Research, 24,* 287–291.

Whitley, B. E. (1990). The relationship of heterosexuals' attributions for the causes of homosexuality to attitudes toward lesbians and gay men. *Personality and Social Psychology Bulletin, 16*(2), 369–377.

Whitney, C. (1990). *Uncommon lives: Gay men and straight women.* New York: New American Library.

Whitney, S. (1982). The ties that bind: Strategies for counseling the gay male co-alcoholic. *Journal of Homosexuality, 7*(4), 37–41.

Wildman, S. (2000, April 25). Offensive maneuvers. *The Advocate,* pp. 28–29.

Williams, R. (1992). *Just as I am: A practical guide to being out, proud, and Christian.* New York: Crown.

Williams, R. J., & Stafford, W. B. (1991). Silent casualties: Partners, families, and spouses of persons with AIDS. *Journal of Counseling and Development, 69*(5), 423–427.

Williams, W. L. (1987). Women, men, and others: Beyond ethnocentrism in gender theory. *American Behavioral Scientist, 31*(1), 135–141.

Williams, W. L. (1996). Two-spirit persons: Gender nonconformity among Native American and Native Hawaiian youths. In R. C. Savin-Williams & K. M. Cohen (Eds.), *The lives of lesbians, gays, and bisexuals* (pp. 416–435). Fort Worth, TX: Harcourt Brace.

Willmott, M., & Brierley, H. (1984). Cognitive characteristics and homosexuality. *Archives of Sexual Behavior, 13*(4), 311–319.

Wilson, P. M. (1986). Black culture and sexuality. *Journal of Social Work and Human Sexuality, 4*(3), 29–46.

Winters, K. C., Remafedi, G., & Chan, B. Y. (1996). Assessing drug abuse among gay-bisexual young men. *Psychology of Addictive Behaviors, 10*(4), 228–236.

Wisniewski, J. J., & Toomey, B. G. (1987). Are social workers homophobic? *Social Work, 32*(5), 454–455.

Wolf, J. G. (Ed.). (1989). *Gay priests.* San Francisco: Harper & Row.

Wolfson, A. (1987). Toward the further understanding of homosexual women. *Journal of the American Psychoanalytic Association, 35*(1), 165–173.

Wolfson, E. (1996, Summer). Freedom to marry 1996: Making the transition from defensive to affirmative work. *The Lambda Update, 13*(2), 5.

Wooden, W. S., Kawasaki, H., & Mayeda, R. (1983). Lifestyles and identity maintenance among gay Japanese-American males. *Alternative Lifestyles, 5,* 236–243.

Woods, J. D. (with Lucas, J. H.). (1993). *The corporate closet: The professional lives of gay men in America.* New York: Free Press.

Woods, R. (1988). *Another kind of love: Homosexuality and spirituality* (3rd ed.). Ft. Wayne, IN: Knoll.

Woog. D. (1998, January 20). Adopting a family. *The Advocate,* pp. 69–71.

Wright, J. M. (1998). *Lesbian step families: An ethnography of love.* Binghamton, NY: Haworth Press.

Wyers, N. (1987). Homosexuality in the family: Lesbian and gay spouses. *Social Work, 32*(2), 143–148.

Yarhouse, M. A. (1998). When clients seek treatment for same-sex attraction: Ethical issues in the "right to choose: debate. *Psychotherapy, 35,* 248–259.

Yarhouse, M. A., & Burkett, L. A. 2000). *Respecting religious diversity: Possibilities and pitfalls.* Paper presented at the 108th annual meeting of the American Psychological Association, Washington, DC.

Zacks, E., Green, R. J., & Marrow, J. (1988). Comparing lesbian and heterosexual couples on the Circumplex Model: An initial investigation. *Family Process, 22*(4), 471–484.

Zanotti, B. (Ed.). (1986). *A faith of one's own: Explorations by Catholic lesbians.* Trumansburg, NY: Crossing Press.

Zeeland, S. (1993). *Barrack buddies and soldier lovers: Dialogues with gay young men in the U. S. military.* Binghamton, NY: Haworth Press.

Zeeland, S. (1995). *Sailors and sexual identity: Crossing the line between "straight" and "gay" in the U. S. Navy.* Binghamton, NY: Haworth Press.

Zeeland, S. (1996). *The masculine marine: Homoeroticism in the U. S. marine corps.* Binghamton, NY: Haworth Press.

Zeeland, S. (1999). *Military trade.* Binghamton, NY: Haworth Press.

Zera, D. (1992). Coming of age in a heterosexist world: The development of gay and lesbian adolescents. *Adolescence, 27*(108), 849–854.

Ziebold, T. O., & Mongeon, J. E. (1985). Introduction: Alcoholism and the homosexual community. In Ziebold, T. O., & Mongeon, J. E. (Eds.), *Gay and sober: Directions for counseling and therapy* (pp. 3–7). New York: Harrington Park Press.

Zigrang, T. A. (1982). Who should be doing what about the gay alcoholic? *Journal of Homosexuality, 7*(4), 27–35.

Zinik, G. (1985). Identity conflict or adaptive flexibility? Bisexuality reconsidered. In F. Klein & T. J. Wolf (Eds.), *Bisexualities: Theory and research* (pp. 7–19). Binghamton, NY: Haworth Press.

Zinkernagel, C., Ledergerber, B., Battegay, M., Cone, R. W., Vernazza, P., Hirschel, B., & Opravil, M. (1999). Quality of life in asymptomatic patients with early HIV infection initiating antiretroviral therapy. *AIDS, 13*(12), 1587–1589.

Zitter, S. (1987). Coming out to mom: Theoretical aspects of the mother-daughter process. In Boston Lesbian Psychologies Collective (Eds.), *Lesbian psychologies: Explorations and challenges* (pp. 177–194). Urbana: University of Illinois Press.

Zubenko, M. D., George, A. W., Soloff, P. H., & Schulz, P. (1987). Sexual practices among patients with borderline personality disorder. *American Journal of Psychiatry, 144*(6), 748–752.

Zucker, K. J. (1990). Psychosocial and erotic development in cross-gender identified children. *Canadian Journal of Psychiatry, 35*(6), 487–495.

Zucker, K. J. (1996). Sexism and heterosexism in the Diagnostic Interview for Borderline Patients? *American Journal of Psychiatry, 153*(7), 966.

Zucker, K. J. (1997). *Gender identity disorder in children: Science, politics, and ethics.* Invited address presented at the 105th annual meeting of the American Psychological Association, Chicago.

Zucker, K. J., & Bradley, S. J. (1995). *Gender identity disorder and psychosexual problems in children and adolescents.* New York: Guilford Press.

Zucker, K. J., Bradley, S. J., Oliver, G., Hood, J. E., Blake, J., & Fleming, S. (1992). Psychosexual assessment of women with congenital adrenal hyperplasia: Preliminary analyses. Paper presented at annual meeting of the International Academy of Sex Research, Prague, Czechoslovakia.

Zuckerman, M. J. (1999). Sexual orientation disclosure and its relationship to psychological distress, immune, and physical health status variables in HIV-infection. *Dissertation Abstracts International, 59*(12-B), 6500. (University Microfilms No. AAM99–15370)

Zuger, B. (1984). Early effeminate behavior in boys: Outcome and significance for homosexuality. *Journal of Nervous and Mental Disease, 172*, 90–97.

Zuger, B. (1988). Is early effeminate behavior in boys early homosexuality? *Comprehensive Psychiatry, 29*(5), 509–519.

Zuger, B. (1989). Homosexuality in families of boys with early effeminate behavior: An epidemiological study. *Archives of Sexual Behavior, 18*(2), 155–166.

Index